T0198230

2nd Edition

Human Development and Performance

THROUGHOUT the LIFE SPAN

Printed Number: 19   Print Year: 2024
Printed in Mexico

2nd Edition

Human Development and Performance

THROUGHOUT the LIFE SPAN

Edited by

ANNE CRONIN, PhD, OTR/L, FAOTA
Associate Professor
West Virginia University
Morgantown, West Virginia

MARYBETH MANDICH, PT, PhD
Professor and Chairperson
Division of Physical Therapy
West Virginia University
Morgantown, West Virginia

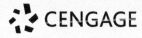

Australia • Brazil • Canada • Mexico • Singapore • United Kingdom • United States

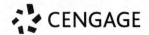

Human Development and Performance: Throughout the Life Span, Second Edition
Anne Cronin and MaryBeth Mandich

SVP, GM Skills & Global Product Management: Dawn Gerrain

Product Manager: Laura Stewart

Senior Director, Development: Marah Bellegarde

Senior Product Development Manager: Juliet Steiner

Senior Content Developer: Darcy M. Scelsi

Product Assistant: Hannah Kinisky

Vice President, Marketing Services: Jennifer Ann Baker

Marketing Manager: Michelle McTighe

Senior Production Director: Wendy Troeger

Production Director: Andrew Crouth

Senior Content Project Managers: Ken McGrath and Betty L. Dickson

Senior Art Director: Jack Pendleton

Cover image(s): © Orange Line Media/www .Shutterstock.com

© Orange Line Media/www.Shutterstock.com

© Zurijeta/www.Shutterstock.com

© bikeriderlondon/www.Shutterstock.com

© Nuzza/www.Shutterstock.com

© altanaka/www.Shutterstock.com

© Monkey Business Images/www.Shutterstock .com

© Hannamariah/www.Shutterstock.com

For product information and technology assistance, contact us at
Cengage Customer & Sales Support, 1-800-354-9706
For permission to use material from this text or product,
submit all requests online at **www.cengage.com/permissions**.

Library of Congress Control Number: 2014948327

Book ISBN: 978-1-133-95119-3

Cengage
200 Pier 4 Boulevard
Boston, MA 02210
USA

Cengage is a leading provider of customized learning solutions with office locations around the globe, including Singapore, the United Kingdom, Australia, Mexico, Brazil, and Japan. Locate your local office at: **www.cengage.com/global**

To learn more about Cengage platforms and services, register or access your online learning solution, or purchase materials for your course, visit **www.cengage.com**.

Notice to the Reader

Publisher does not warrant or guarantee any of the products described herein or perform any independent analysis in connection with any of the product information contained herein. Publisher does not assume, and expressly disclaims, any obligation to obtain and include information other than that provided to it by the manufacturer. The reader is expressly warned to consider and adopt all safety precautions that might be indicated by the activities described herein and to avoid all potential hazards. By following the instructions contained herein, the reader willingly assumes all risks in connection with such instructions. The publisher makes no representations or warranties of any kind, including but not limited to, the warranties of fitness for particular purpose or merchantability, nor are any such representations implied with respect to the material set forth herein, and the publisher takes no responsibility with respect to such material. The publisher shall not be liable for any special, consequential, or exemplary damages resulting, in whole or part, from the readers' use of, or reliance upon, this material.

Dedication

We would like to express our appreciation to West Virginia University for the time and administrative support that has supported our work on this project. We would also like to thank our faculty and staff colleagues, who helped us in so many ways, including writing case studies, editing, advising, and reviewing. As pediatric therapists, we would also like to thank all the children and their families who have so enriched our professional lives over the years and who have taught us so much. As academicians, we would like to thank all the students who have been in our classrooms, listened to our thoughts and information, and ultimately joined us as professional colleagues.

Anne Cronin: My father, Thomas Cronin, told me that he was proud of me for following a long family tradition when I chose to be a teacher. His pride continues to sustain me. My father, and my whole family, are my inspirations, teaching me much about life beyond the science that informs this text. Since the first edition of this text, I have had the opportunity to learn from occupational therapists all over the world. It is my fond hope that they will find their influences throughout the text.

MaryBeth Mandich: To my parents, Anne and Sam Mandich, children of immigrants who believed strongly in education as a path to success and who provided unfailing support in all my endeavors. To my children, Heather, Sam, Scott, and Ben, who have inspired me, helped me grow, and taught me invaluable lessons about the life span from infancy to young adulthood. Finally, I am enormously grateful for the wonderful new additions to my kinship network, Devin, Melissa, and Angie.

Contents

CHAPTER 9
The Newborn

MARYBETH MANDICH, PT, PhD

CHAPTER 10
Infancy

MARYBETH MANDICH, PT, PhD

CHAPTER 11
Family and Disability Issues through Infancy

ANNE CRONIN, PhD, OTR/L, FAOTA

CHAPTER 12
Development in the Preschool Years

ANNE CRONIN, PhD, OTR/L

CHAPTER 13
Childhood and School

ANNE CRONIN, PhD, OTR/L, FAOTA

CHAPTER 14
Adolescent Development

ANNE CRONIN, PhD, OTR/L, FAOTA

CHAPTER 20
Wellness, Prevention, and Health Promotion

*RALPH UTZMAN, PT, MPH, PhD AND
ANNE CRONIN, PhD, OTR, FAOTA*

PART 3
SPECIAL TOPICS IN HUMAN DEVELOPMENT AND PERFORMANCE

CHAPTER 21
Public Policy and Health Care

*BARBARA L. KORNBLAU, JD, OT/L, FAOTA, DMASPE,
ABDA CCM, CDMS, CPE AND
ANNE CRONIN, PhD, OTR/L*

CHAPTER 22
Assessment of Human Performance across the Life Span

*MARYBETH MANDICH, PT, PhD AND
ANNE CRONIN, PhD, OTR/L, FAOTA AND
TOBY LONG, PhD, PT*

Preface

The purpose of this text is to provide entry-level students who plan to work in health care, especially in the rehabilitation disciplines such as occupational and physical therapy, an overview of normative life tasks and roles across the life span. The Joint Commission requires that all health care providers be able to deliver age-appropriate plans of care. The unique aspect of this text is, in addition to providing information about typical human development life tasks, it discusses the impact of disease or disability on human occupations. Finally, the foregoing information is embedded in the World Health Organization's International Classification of Functioning, Disability and Health (ICF), which has now been the standard of health outcomes for over a decade, and is the foundation to the text.

Other key guiding documents and concepts include the life course model (adopted as an organizing framework by the Bureau of Maternal and Child Health), Healthy People 2020, the discipline of occupational science, and updated theoretical models from the pertinent literature of multiple disciplines. The text also serves as a resource for practicing professionals, especially those who were not educated in the conceptual framework of newer models, such as the ICF. Each chapter includes current, research-based scientific findings that offer insight into aspects of human development that may expand on earlier learning.

Since the 1960s, there has been a significant, perhaps revolutionary, change in clinical and sociologic perspectives of disability that has impacted both health services and public policy. One evidence of this impact is the passage of many pieces of legislation guaranteeing individuals with a disability the right to participate in society, including the right to education and the right to employment. In addition, as discussed in Chapter 20, the notion of health-related quality of life has become an accepted metric for judging the outcome of biomedical and psychosocial interventions. In summary, health is increasingly viewed as the ability to participate in normal and desired life roles to the maximum extent possible.

The education of health professionals, especially in the rehabilitation disciplines, must prepare professionals to deliver successful interventions in this context. Although it is often stated that there is a disconnect between academic theory and clinical practice, this text is designed to help bridge that gap with the extensive use of both clinical case studies and examples of theory applications for rehabilitation professionals. Our hope is that this compilation of science, theory, and clinical cases facilitates the learning of future generations about how to promote full participation outcomes in those individuals we serve.

NEED FOR THIS TEXT

As mentioned previously, our experience shows there is currently not an available resource that integrates information from a number of core disciplines to permit easy understanding of the newer concepts of health and participation. Professionals such as occupational and physical therapists have always studied life span human development. They have also studied medical sciences, psychology, sociology, and professional roles. However, the paradigm shifts just described will demand that rehabilitation professionals of the twenty-first century will be able to integrate knowledge of normative developmental life roles or tasks with other information to assist individuals with disabilities to participate in desired societal roles. The ICF model forms the conceptual foundation for the text, with a secondary developmental framework. Particular attention has been made to include many of the basic constructs in the field of occupational science throughout this text. The study of human occupations must be inherently grounded in the understanding of human development, and this text offers a strong adjunct to this foundation for students in this field of study.

This text meets the needs of entry-level professionals by preparing them to view both health and disability from a life tasks perspective on activity and participation. Although life span development has traditionally been considered foundational knowledge upon which to build an understanding of various health conditions, recent social and legislative trends have demanded an increased application of developmental information in setting goals and planning interventions. Increasingly, reimbursement for rehabilitation, especially occupational and physical therapy, is based on the ability to reflect and document goals directed at functional outcomes that promote individuals' health-related quality of life by participation in interpersonal, social, and environmental roles.

No prior knowledge of human development or disability models is required to use this text, commensurate with the entry-level target audience. However, exposure to basic anatomy, psychology, and physiology will help students understand the structure-function sections of each chapter. Prior courses in life span human development and sociology will allow students to apply previously learned theory to their education as health care professionals.

ORGANIZATION OF TEXT

The text is organized into three main parts: Foundations for Understanding Function, Disability, and Health; Life Stage Characteristics; and Special Topics in Human Development and Performance. The foundational section introduces readers to contemporary conceptual and theoretical models in the field of health and disability. The first three chapters in this section provide an introduction to the core frames of reference including the ICF, the life course model, and traditional developmental theories. Successful health interventions require practitioners who are culturally competent and who can apply learning and communication strategies in their therapeutic interventions. Finally, the impact of environmental contexts on health and participation are considered in this section. The second part of the book, "Life Stage Characteristics," follows a traditional developmental framework; however, basic physiologic content is presented in every chapter as an introduction, as well as the developmental characteristics of the particular life stage. Few texts combine the 360-degree approach to the study of human development across body systems, as well as dimensions of performance (motor, psychologic, and sociologic), as this text does. Interspersed in this section are chapters addressing the impact of disability at various life stages. The final section of the book, "Special Topics in Human Development and Performance," presents some contemporary topics for occupational and physical therapists, as well as others. Chapter 20, "Wellness, Prevention, and Health Promotion," prepares readers to analyze the responsibility of health care professionals to do more than treat disease and instead to participate in prevention and health promotion. The ICF contextual factor of health policy is discussed in Chapter 21, "Public Policy and Health Care." Finally, Chapter 22, "Assessment of Human Performance across the Life Span," introduces readers to the concept of accountability for evidence-based practice with documentation of outcomes at the level of activities and participation.

FEATURES OF THE TEXT

The text provides readers with a large amount of information on life span development, organized around the conceptual framework of the ICF. All chapters have case studies based on true clinical situations, which help students apply the information in the text to the practical setting. In addition, most chapters have a section called "Speaking of . . . ." These sections are informal notes from individuals—both professionals and family members of individuals with disabilities—about the application of content in the chapter. They bring to life the real challenges and experiences of individuals who have unique perspectives on the issues discussed in each chapter. These notes are intended to help readers with the "emotional intelligence" aspect of learning.

NEW TO THIS EDITION

CHAPTER 1

- Completely revised to the latest terminology and organizational frameworks in the field and the most current ICF and practice frameworks

- Reflects the evolution of ICF applications into disciplinary practice over the past decade
- Introduces the occupational model and defines human occupations in the context of the ICF and practice frameworks

CHAPTER 2

- New chapter, encompasses some content from former the Chapter 1
- Reflects the increasing demand for health to be viewed from a life span perspective
- Introduces the life course theory (LCT)
- Integrates the use of the ICF with the LCT
- Includes an increased focus on families, including the presentation of the systematic family development model (SFD) and family development theory

CHAPTER 3

- Formerly Chapter 2
- Minor revisions and updates to address new thoughts and correlate to current practices

CHAPTER 4

- Heavily revised and rewritten with a focus on understanding mainstream American cultural norms and acknowledgment and identification of cultural norms in other populations that may be encountered in practice settings
- Updated in response to the changing cultural demands and experience of competent practitioners
- Focus on occupational deprivation as illustrated in the interactions between social factors such as poverty and human occupations

CHAPTER 5

- Heavily revised chapter, with features of language structure deemphasized and an increased focus on functional communication
- Rewritten to emphasize what all health professionals should know about the development and nature of communication, emphasizing intentional communications of all types
- Cases were included to illustrate the essential role of communication for human development and human function across the life span

CHAPTER 6

- Formerly Chapter 3
- Heavily revised chapter, providing more focus on correlation to the ICF
- Incorporates discussion of contemporary neuroscience related to use-dependent brain plasticity, embodied cognition, and executive functions
- Introduces new theories and thoughts on mental functions and learning

CHAPTER 7

- Formerly Chapter 18
- Revised to reflect evolutions in understanding ICF applications
- Updates on new ideas and concepts such as universal design and virtual environments
- Expanded discussion of social and cultural environments and their potential impacts on human occupation

CHAPTER 8

- Formerly Chapter 6
- Added discussion about ethical decisions involving the embryo and fetus
- Added new information about stem cells and prenatal diagnosis and treatment
- Added/updated information about prenatal assessment and diagnosis

CHAPTER 9

- Formerly Chapter 7
- Enhanced discussion of biologic and environmental risk
- Added sections including neonatal abstinence syndrome

CHAPTER 10

- Formerly Chapter 8
- Added section about positional plagiocephaly and the Back to Sleep initiative
- Added discussions about risk and resilience, including the importance of nurturing and supportive environments in alignment with the life course theory

CHAPTER 11

- Formerly Chapter 9
- Discussed the social and economic factors related to disability and illness in children
- Introduces common disabilities and common illnesses in infancy
- Expands focus on the family and the impact of infant illness or disability of parental and sibling occupations
- Presents the best-practice standard of family-centered care

CHAPTER 12

- Formerly Chapter 10
- Reorganized around the ICF Framework
- Expands discussion of body structures and functions relevant to this life stage
- Introduces theories of sensory integration and sensory processing
- Increased focus on play and the interactions between play and development in early childhood

CHAPTER 13

- Formerly Chapter 11
- Reorganized around the ICF framework
- Expands discussion of body structures and functions relevant to this life stage
- Increased content on ADL and IADL participation during this life stage
- Updated to include changes in the social and communication demands placed on children with their increased access to digital communications and social media

CHAPTER 14

- Formerly Chapter 12
- Completely rewritten and reorganized around an ICF framework
- Increased attention to IADL activities such as driving and work
- Introduction of concepts of occupational roles including student and work roles
- Added discussions of eating disorders and enhanced discussion of other health conditions associated with adolescence

CHAPTER 15

- Formerly Chapter 13
- Expanded discussion of learning and intellectual disabilities as well as traumatic injury
- Integration of theoretical materials introduced earlier into aspects of family and child functioning
- Expanded coverage of family stress and resilience in the contexts of child illness and disability

CHAPTER 16

- Almost completely new, reflecting the changing experience of young adults, 21 to 34 years of age, including the twenty-first-century social experiences related to interpersonal, work, and family participation
- Reorganized around the ICF framework
- Introduces the construct of occupational identity
- Includes expanded content of vocational and career choices in early adulthood

CHAPTER 17

- Formerly Chapter 15 Adulthood
- Now titled Middle Adulthood and focuses on ages 40 to 65 years old
- Reorganized around the ICF framework
- Expands upon occupational science constructs introduced earlier in the text, including occupational balance and occupational deprivation
- Greatly expanded content in the areas of community, social, and civic life

CHAPTER 18

- Formerly Chapter 16 Aging
- New title, Late Adulthood, focuses on ages 65 to 80 years old
- Reorganized around the ICF framework
- Greatly expanded content in the areas of community, social, and civic life
- Expands focus on models of successful aging, integrating longitudinal research support on this topic
- Introduces construct of occupational transition and changes in occupational identity associated with aging

CHAPTER 19

- Formerly Chapter 17
- Reorganized around the ICF framework
- Expanded discussion of common disabling conditions
- Introduces readers to the disability rights movement and the constructs of self-determination and self-advocacy as they relate to individuals with disabilities
- Expands discussion of adult performance contexts including workplace contexts (sheltered workshop, supported employment, and integrated employment) and residential contexts (group home, hospice, and nursing home)

CHAPTER 20

- Formerly Chapter 19
- Completely rewritten chapter, with updates to Healthy People 2020
- Presents a broader overview of prevention, wellness, and health strategies
- Presents the view of "clients" as individuals, groups, or community
- Incorporates new theoretical paradigms about health promotion including Lifestyle Redesign and the "health belief model"

CHAPTER 21

- Formerly Chapter 20, completely revised and updated
- Presents the United Nations' *Convention on the Rights of Persons with Disabilities* and the *World Report on Disabilities* in terms of potential impact on health policy
- Updated content on U.S. legislation that impacts both individuals with disabilities and health professions
- Enhanced discussion of HIPPA
- Adds information about the Affordable Care Act and its implementation

CHAPTER 22

- Almost completely rewritten and reorganized from the former Chapter 21
- Discusses the latest assessment tools available in the fields

- Discusses challenges and opportunities in assessment of participation
- Emphasizes needs for evidence-based outcomes

SUPPLEMENTARY PACKAGE FOR INSTRUCTORS

An Instructor Companion Website is available to facilitate classroom preparation, presentation, and testing. This content can be accessed through your Instructor SSO account.

To set-up your account:

- Go to www.cengagebrain.com/login.
- Choose **Create a New Faculty Account.**
- Next you will need to select your **Institution.**
- Complete your personal **Account Information.**
- Accept the **License Agreement.**
- Choose **Register.**
- Your account creation will pend validation. You will receive an email notification when the validation process is complete.
- If you are unable to find your Institution, complete an **Account Request Form.**

Once your account is set up or if you already have an account:

- Go to www.cengagebrain.com/login.
- Enter your email address and password and select **Sign In.**
- Search for your book by author, title, or ISBN.
- Select the book and click **Continue.**
- You will receive a list of available resources for the title you selected.
- Choose the resources you would like, and click **Add to My Bookshelf.**

An instructor's manual with two main components accompanies this text. The first component is the critical-thinking guide. For each chapter, a minimum of three questions have been selected to guide the students' thinking about the content presented. The questions are suitable for in-class discussion, small-group work, or essay questions on tests. The second component of the instructor's manual is the active learning experiences designed to enhance learning of chapter content. They include such activities as web searches and analysis of current literature. Where laboratory activities are suggested, laboratory guides are presented. These components have been carefully designed to provide instructors with key tools to help facilitate student comprehension that will follow them into their professional lives.

FEEDBACK

The authors welcome comments and feedback about this text and may be contacted at the following addresses:

Anne Cronin, PhD, OTR/L, FAOTA
Division of Occupational Therapy
PO Box 1939
West Virginia University
Morgantown, West Virginia 26506-9139
acronin@hsc.wvu.edu

MaryBeth Mandich, PT, PhD
Division of Physical Therapy
PO Box 9226
West Virginia University
Morgantown, West Virginia 26506-9226
mmandich@hsc.wvu.edu

ACKNOWLEDGMENTS

We would like to acknowledge all those who provided us assistance in writing this text. First, to West Virginia University, which provided time and support for this endeavor. Second, a special thanks to our faculty colleagues who helped by taking on extra tasks so that we could be free to write.

We would like to thank all those who contributed to this book. First, to our chapter authors, who are all busy professionals and who did an outstanding job in their work on this text. Second, to all the therapists who provided case studies from their practical experience—you helped to make the text applicable and relevant. Finally, to therapists and family members of individuals with disabilities who wrote "Speaking of . . ." sections and who told us "the rest of the story"—the effort would have been much less meaningful without your contribution.

Contributing Authors

Anne Cronin, PhD, OTR/L, FAOTA
Associate Professor
Division of Occupational Therapy
West Virginia University
Morgantown, West Virginia

Garth Graebe, MOT, OTR/L
Assistant Professor
Division of Occupational Therapy
West Virginia University
Morgantown, West Virginia

Ingrid Kanics, MOT, OTR/L
Owner, Kanics Inclusive Design Services, LLC
New Castle,
Pennsylvania

Barbara L. Kornblau, JD, OT/L, FAOTA, DAAPM, CCM, CDMS
Coalition for Disability Health Equity,
  Arlington, Virginia
Florida A & M University, Tallahassee, Florida

Toby Long, PT, PhD, FAPTA
Associate Professor, Department of Pediatrics
Associate Director for Training, Center for
  Child and Human Development
Director, Division of Physical Therapy,
  Center for Child and Human Development
Georgetown University
Washington, DC

MaryBeth Mandich, PT, PhD
Professor and Chairperson
Division of Physical Therapy

Associate Dean, Professional and
  Undergraduate Programs
West Virginia University
Morgantown, West Virginia

Susannah Grimm Poe, EdD
Associate Professor
Department of Pediatrics
WVU School of Medicine
WG Klingberg Center for Child Development
Morgantown, West Virginia

Pamela Reynolds, PT, EdD
Professor
Gannon University
Erie, Pennsylvania

Winifred Schultz-Krohn, PhD, OTR, BCP, FAOTA
Professor of Occupational Therapy
San Jose State University
San Jose, California

Ralph Utzman, PT, MPH, PhD
Associate Professor
Division of Physical Therapy
West Virginia University
Morgantown, West Virginia

Elsie R. Vergara, ScD, OTR, FAOTA
Associate Professor (retired)
Occupational Therapy Program
Department of Rehabilitation Sciences
Sargent College, Boston University
Boston, Massachusetts

Contributors:
Case Studies and "Speaking of..."

Colleen Anderson
Senior Parent Network Specialist
WVU Center for Excellence in Disabilities
Robert C. Byrd Health Sciences Center
West Virginia University
Morgantown, West Virginia
"Speaking of . . ." Chapter 16

Cristina H. Bolanos, OT, PhD
Instituto de Terapia Ocupacional
General Director
Mexico City, Mexico
"Speaking of . . ." Chapter 4

Ann Chester, PhD
Vice President for Education Partnerships
Director, HSTA program
WVU Health Sciences Center
West Virginia University
Morgantown, West Virginia
"Speaking of . . ." Chapter 17

Carrie Cobun
Parent Educator, WVU Center for Excellence
  in Disabilities
Program Coordinator, WVU Department of
  Pediatrics
Klingberg Center for Child Development
West Virginia University
Morgantown, West Virginia
"Speaking of . . ." Chapter 15

Anne Cronin, PhD, OTR/L, FAOTA
Associate Professor
Division of Occupational Therapy
West Virginia University
Morgantown, West Virginia
"Speaking of . . ." Chapters 2, 3, 8, 12, 20,
  and 22
Case studies (all chapters)

Scott Davis, PT, MS, OCS
Assistant Professor
Division of Physical Therapy
West Virginia University
Case 3, Chapter 14

Garth Graebe, MOT, OTR/L
Assistant Professor
Division of Occupational Therapy
West Virginia University
Morgantown, West Virginia
"Speaking of. . ." Chapter 6

Barbara Haase, MHS, OTR, BCN
Occupational Therapist
and
Richard Haase, MA
Rehabilitation Counselor
Huron, Ohio
"Speaking of . . ." Chapter 18

Tracy Hough, MOT, OTR/L
Staff Occupational Therapist
University of Pittsburgh Medical Center
  Shadyside
Pittsburgh, Pennsylvania
"Speaking of . . ." Chapter 17

Chris Klein
BeCome AAC, blog site & AAC user
http://www.becomeaac.com, Chapter 5

Susan Lynch, MD
Associate Professor
Department of Pediatrics
Section of Neonatology
Ohio State University
Director, Comprehensive Center for
  Bronchopulmonary Dysplasia
Nationwide Children's Hospital
Columbus, Ohio
"Speaking of . . ." Chapter 10

Corrie Mancinelli, PT, PhD, GCS, CEEAA
Associate Professor
Division of Physical Therapy
West Virginia University
Morgantown, West Virginia
"Speaking of . . ." Chapter 19

MaryBeth Mandich, PT, PhD
Professor and Chairperson
Division of Physical Therapy
West Virginia University
Morgantown, West Virginia
"Speaking of . . ." Chapters 1, 7, and 9
Case 1, Chapter 8

Hannah McMonagle, RN
Parent
Morgantown, West Virginia
"Speaking of . . ." Chapter 13

Andrea Earle Mullins, MS, OTR/L
Occupational Therapist
Grafton School
Richmond, Virginia
"Speaking of . . ." Chapter 14

Hugh Murray, PT, DMDT
President, Huntington Physical Therapy
Huntington, West Virginia
"Speaking of . . ." Chapter 21

Susie Ritchie, RN, MPH, CPNP
Research Associate Professor (retired)
Department of Pediatrics
West Virginia University
Morgantown, West Virginia
"Speaking of . . ." Chapter 11

About the Editors

Anne Cronin, PhD, OTR/L, FAOTA, has been practicing pediatric occupational therapy for many years. She received her BS in occupational therapy from the University of Missouri and an MA in health services management from Webster University in St. Louis, Missouri. Her PhD was received from the University of Florida in medical sociology. Dr. Cronin has taught extensively, including content in human development, research, and clinical practice of occupational therapy, with an emphasis on practice with children and youth. Her research interests include community integration of children with disabilities, routines and time use in parenting, the establishment of healthy habit patterns in children with developmental differences, and the efficacy of occupational therapy interventions with pediatric populations. Dr. Cronin has been a leader in the exploration of assistive technology applications to support people with disabilities across the life span. In addition, Dr. Cronin has served as a member of the Board of Directors of the American Occupational Therapy Association and the Rehabilitation Engineering Society and Assistive Technology of North America. She has been a Fulbright senior specialist in Chile, Mexico, and Sri Lanka, providing occupational therapy consultation. Dr. Cronin is currently an associate professor of occupational therapy at West Virginia University.

MaryBeth Mandich, PT, PhD, has been practicing pediatric physical therapy for many years. She received BS and MS degrees in physical therapy from the Medical College of Virginia/Virginia Commonwealth University. She went on to receive a PhD in development psychology from West Virginia University, with a major area of emphasis in infancy and a minor area of emphasis in developmental neurobiology. Dr. Mandich has taught extensively, including content in neuroanatomy and neurophysiology, embryology, human development, and pediatric and adult neurologic rehabilitation and research. She teaches students from many other disciplines, such as medicine, education, occupational therapy, and nursing about neuroplasticity and the importance of early intervention and rehabilitation. Her own research interests have focused primarily on premature, high-risk infants. She has published studies on both outcome and effects of therapeutic intervention for this population. She maintains an active clinical practice in high-risk infant follow-up. Dr. Mandich is currently associate dean for professional and undergraduate programs in the School of Medicine at West Virginia University. She holds an appointment as professor and chairperson of the Division of Physical Therapy.

PART 1

Foundations for Understanding Function, Disability, and Health

CHAPTER 1

Human Performance: Function as an Organizing Framework

Mary Beth Mandich, PT, PhD,
Professor and Chairperson,
Division of Physical Therapy,
West Virginia University, Morgantown,
West Virginia
and
Anne Cronin, PhD, OTR/L, FAOTA,
Associate Professor, Division of
Occupational Therapy, West Virginia
University, Morgantown, West Virginia

Objectives

Upon completion of this chapter, readers should be able to:

- Define *quality of life,* and relate the definition to health outcomes;

- Define the concept of disablement and apply the concept to practical situations;

- Describe the medical and the social models of function, activity limitation, and disability;

- Define and give examples of the framework dimensions of ICF: "Body Structure and Function," "Activity and Participation," "Personal Factors," and "Environmental Factors";

- Differentiate contextual factors in the process of human activity; and

- Discuss how the ICF impacts the rehabilitation professional frame of reference.

Key Terms

activity	environmental factor	nonnormative
activity limitation	facilitator	nonnormative influences
activity of daily living (ADL)	frame of reference	normative
affective domain	function	occupations
age-normative influence	health	occupational model
barrier	history-normative influence	participation
body functions	instrumental activity of daily	personal factors
body structure	living (IADL)	psychomotor domain
capacity	International Classification of	quality of life
cognitive domain	Functioning, Disability and	risk factor
contextual factor	Health (ICF)	social model
disability	interprofessional education (IPE)	
disablement	medical model	

INTRODUCTION

Human beings are complex creatures capable of a myriad of accomplishments. As students of human performance and health, it is essential to understand the complex interplay of biological, behavioral, psychological, social, and environmental factors that influence individual humans over the course of their life. Like all living things, human beings have a life cycle: birth, infancy, puberty, adulthood, and old age, eventually leading to death. It is now possible for the human lifespan to encompass a century or more. During that century of life expectancy, humans have the unique capacity to study, learn about, and analyze mental processes within the self. No other creature displays the curiosity, the cognition, and the drive to attempt to explain its own behavior and actions.

Throughout the human life course there unfolds an array of challenges or tasks that must be accomplished. Some of these tasks are normative, consistent with general patterns and experiences seen within a population, such as the usual timing and sequence associated with learning to walk or to read. Some of the tasks are nonnormative. These are not consistent with general patterns seen within a population. An example of a nonnormative challenge would be adapting to a disease or disability. Throughout this text, the authors will emphasize normative patterns in human development and performance as well as the potential impact of the nonnormative experiences on future life course experiences. Another term for nonnormative is atypical. In some cases the two descriptors may be used interchangeably. The next chapter will present and explain recent theoretical models that tie the life span experience to human health.

Quality and quantity of life are separate issues. Quality of life may be defined as a perception of life satisfaction through fulfillment of both basic and complex needs. Maslow defines human needs as a hierarchy, from the most basic need for sustenance to the need for self-actualization and love (Maslow, 1954). A good quality of life implies that all the individual's needs are being adequately met.

DEFINING HEALTH, FUNCTION, AND DISABLEMENT

The most widely accepted definition of health is that of the World Health Organization (WHO) found in the 1946 preamble to its constitution, where *health* is defined as a state of complete physical, mental, and social well-being, not merely the absence of disease and infirmity (WHO, 1948). It includes the motivation to become engaged in life, a sense of control over one's actions, and a desire to interact and connect with others, and perhaps most importantly, engages the individual's self-esteem. Health is a potential for all humans that can be supported through societal efforts including social policies, community support systems, and environments that enhance health, optimal development, and quality of life. For those professions seeking to promote a high quality of life for all individuals, it is important to understand these complex factors, both those intrinsic to individuals, and social and environmental factors extrinsic to individuals.

The WHO definition of health is operationally present when an individual is *functioning* at a level appropriate to achieve desirable outcomes. Function has been defined generally as the purpose for which a person or thing exists, including synonyms such as *purpose* and *occupation* (Merriam-Webster,

Incorporated, 2014). In 1965, a sociologist named Nagi, in a landmark paper, proposed that *function* was not inherent in a given *disease* or *health condition*. For example, two people might have the health condition known as chronic low back pain. One of these people may have been accommodated to the workplace and life activities, and may continue to participate in the accommodated environment. Another person may become quite sedentary, removed from normal roles such as vocation, and hence may be very depressed. Therefore, the functional status of these individuals is not defined by the medical condition, that is, chronic low back pain.

This premise that disease or health condition is a factor, but not a determinant, of function is a sociologic concept known as **disablement**. Disablement is a *sociomedical* concept describing **disability** as the product of the impact of a health condition on function, taking into account personal and environmental factors that serve as risk factors, interventions, or exacerbators (Verbrugge & Jette, 1994). A **risk factor** is a personal or environmental factor that diminishes health, leaving an individual less likely to realize their full developmental potential (UHHS, 2010). *Disability* is a term used to encompass problems with various dimensions of human function, activity, and participation (WHO, 2001b).

CONCEPTUAL FRAMEWORKS OF DISABLEMENT

The concept of disablement merges two core conceptual frameworks traditionally used to discuss health. The first is the **medical model**, which emphasizes the person, and that person's impairments, as a cause of disease, trauma, or some other health condition (World Health Organization, 2001b). Within the medical model, disability is a feature of the person that requires medical care provided in the form of individual treatment by professionals to "correct"

the problem. The focus of intervention is medical care, and the principal feature of intervention is to change health care policy. Therapy clinicians working within the medical model will identify impairments such as weakness, and develop strategies to improve the individual's abilities or to help him learn to compensate for the impairments. For example, in the case of a person with a spinal cord injury, a therapist offers activities to strengthen muscles at the same time she is training the person in new ways to complete activities of daily living. **Activities of daily living (ADL)** are the daily self-care activities within any of an individual's routine environments (home, leisure, work, and so on). Special equipment such as wheelchairs and adapted vehicles are examples of additional compensations. This is the traditional approach presented in the rehabilitation literature.

The **social model** views the loss of function associated with a disease, trauma, or health condition, as an attribute of the social environment, which is managed by change in social policy. For example, using the person with the spinal cord injury example again, this model would argue that the individual becomes disabled, not by the spinal cord injury itself, but because he cannot access local stores, public transportation, and theaters. The focus on the problem is change in social policy. An example of such policy in the United States is the 1990 Americans with Disabilities Act (ADA), which assures accessibility and civil rights to individuals with potentially disabling health conditions. In another illustration, perhaps the person with a spinal cord injury needs an adapted motor vehicle to be able to drive to work or school but is unable to obtain the financial resources necessary to purchase such a vehicle. Access to adequate financial resources is a social condition, not a medical condition. **Figure 1-1** offers two images of a young man with a spinal cord injury. The picture on the left illustrates a caring but contextually limited *medical model*. The picture on the right shows the young man as an active participant in a valued activity within a community setting. This second picture illustrates the *social model*.

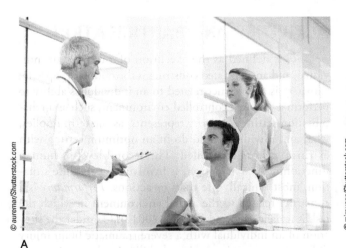
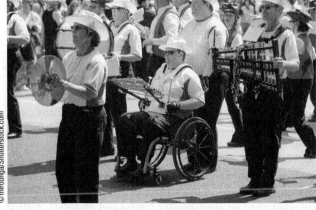

A

B

Figure 1-1   A. The Medical Model **B.** The Social Model

In a subtler example, the condition of attention deficit disorder has received a lot of attention in the last 20 years. This disorder has a rising incidence in the United States and western Europe. At the same time, the incidence is relatively low in eastern Europe, South America, and Africa. The difference in frequency of identifying this as a health condition seems to lie in societal expectations for a child's behavior. Impulsivity, distractibility, and high activity levels are disruptive in large elementary school classrooms. Cultures that offer alternative educational and social options for children may not identify such behavior as a disability.

THE INTERNATIONAL CLASSIFICATION OF FUNCTIONING, DISABILITY AND HEALTH (ICF)

The World Health Organization has long been the recognized source for universal classification of disease, with the International Classification of Disease (ICD) serving as the basis for reimbursement coding in the United States health care system. The ICD is a health care classification system that provides codes to classify diseases and a wide variety of signs and symptoms, as well as social circumstances and external causes of injury or disease. This ICD was the first in the WHO Family of International Classifications (WHO-FIC) and was designed to promote international comparability in the classification and presentation of international health statistics (World Health Organization, 2014).

In 2001, WHO member nations endorsed a new classification system, representing the culmination of several decades of attempts to classify disablement for purposes of research, reporting, and establishment of benchmarks. WHO (1993) had developed its own precursor model in 1980, known as the International Classification of Impairments, Disability, and Handicap (ICIDH); however, by the end of the century, it had rejected that model in favor of a newer model, entitled the **International Classification of Functioning, Disability and Health**, known by the acronym **ICF**. Unlike previous classifications, the ICF has the stated purpose of emphasizing health and de-emphasizing the concept of disability, hence the acronym ICF does not include the term *disability* as part of the title. The WHO (2001a) states, on its ICF home page, that any human can have a decrement in function at any time, thereby "mainstreaming" the notion of disability. Therefore, a continuum of function is the underlying construct, which avoids previous negative connotations associated with the term *disability*. In addition, the ICF acknowledges the impact of factors on function that can be attributed to an individual (person) or to an environment (social and physical). A final note is that the ICF helps to operationally define components of health and related quality of life.

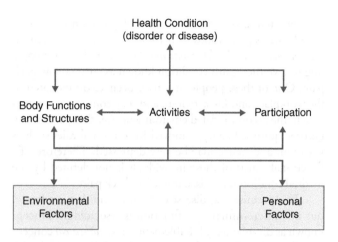

Figure 1-2   This model reflects the ICF view of the interactive relationship between health conditions and contextual factors.
Source: Towards a Common Language for Functioning, Disability, and Health (ICF), World Health Organization (2002).

The current ICF model can be imagined as a matrix with major two components: (1) health condition and (2) contextual factors (environmental and personal). These are illustrated as the top and the bottom of **Figure 1-2**. As illustrated, disability and functioning are viewed as outcomes of interactions between health condition and contextual factors. At the center of the diagram is the activity that the individual wishes to engage in.

BODY STRUCTURE AND FUNCTION

Body structures are anatomically categorized by body part, such as the nervous system or structures related to movement. **Body functions**, as the name implies, are physiological in nature and organized by functional system, such as mental functions, cardiovascular functions, or movement-related functions (WHO, 2001b). **Table 1-1** is a summary of Body Structures and Functions as presented in the current ICF model (WHO, 2001b).

ACTIVITIES AND PARTICIPATION

Activity is defined as the execution of a task by an individual, and an associated construct is the notion of capacity. **Capacity** is a construct related to an individual's ability to perform a task in a controlled environment, such as a rehabilitation setting. *Capacity* represents, as the term implies, what an individual could do in an optimum setting with extrinsic factors controlled. The second level of human functioning, **participation**, is involvement in a life situation, most typically life tasks or actions. *Performance* is a construct related to the actual environment in which the task is usually executed (WHO, 2001b). Consider the situation of an individual with a severe traumatic brain injury (TBI). At some point in the rehabilitation hospital experience, professionals will work to assure the individual can

TABLE 1-1 Body Structures and Functions	
Body Structures	**Body Functions**
Structures of the nervous system	Mental functions
The eye, ear, and related structures	Sensory functions and pain
Structures involved in voice and speech	Voice and speech functions
Structures of the cardiovascular, immunological, and respiratory systems	Functions of the cardiovascular, hematological, immunological, and respiratory systems
Structures related to the digestive, metabolic, and endocrine systems	Functions of the digestive, metabolic, and endocrine systems
Structures related to the genitourinary and reproductive systems	Genitourinary and reproductive functions
Structures related to movement	Neuromusculoskeletal and movement-related functions
Skin and related structures	Functions of the skin and related structures
Source: Towards a Common Language for Functioning, Disability, and Health (ICF), World Health Organization (2002).	

walk, talk, and perform self-care activities. However, the fact that the individual can dress herself under the supervision of an occupational therapist in the rehab setting does not guarantee that, once at home, the individual will get up every day and perform self-care routines independently. Therefore, the individual has the capacity for independence in some functional tasks, but performance will only be assured once the individual is doing the activity within a typical environmental context, without the support of the professionals and routines encountered in rehabilitation. **Table 1-2** summarizes the Activities and Participation dimensions of the ICF (WHO, 2001b).

TABLE 1-2 Activities and Participation
Learning and Applying Knowledge
General Tasks and Demands
Communication
Mobility
Self-Care
Domestic Life
Interpersonal Interactions and Relationships
Major Life Areas
Community, Social, and Civic Life
Source: Towards a Common Language for Functioning, Disability, and Health (ICF), World Health Organization (2002).

CONTEXTUAL FACTORS

One of the most notable aspects of the ICF is the incorporation from the social model of the notion of *Contextual Factors* as the second part of the classification. **Contextual factors** are shown in relationship to activity and the ICF model in **Figure 1-2**. Contextual factors may be either *personal (intrinsic)* or *environmental (extrinsic)*. **Personal factors** include attributes of the individual that impact health, including such things as motivation, cultural perspectives such as fatalism, or personality. **Environmental factors** include the physical, social, and attitudinal environmental context in which an individual lives. **Table 1-3** lists some examples of environmental factors as they are described in the ICF. Personal factors may include individual characteristics such as age, gender, education, profession, coping style, faith, social background, past, and current experiences.

ICF QUALIFIERS AND CODING

Because the ICF is a coding system, qualifiers are applied to each component along the continuum of functioning and disability.

Body structures and functions are qualified by a general scale indicating extent or nature of impairment ranging from none to complete, with the negative qualifier termed *impairment.* Body structures also have a qualifier for nature of the change in the body structure, such as whether there are deviations in structure such as a malformation (for example, a club foot) versus absence of the part in question (for example, amputation). There is also a location qualifier for body structure, indicating limbs or sides of the body affected.

TABLE 1-3	ICF Environmental Factors
Domain	**Sample Components**
Products and Technology	Products and technology for consumption, ADLs, mobility, communication, employment, recreation, and building design for public and private use
Natural and Human-Made Changes to Environment	Physical geography, population, climate, light, sound, air quality
Support and Relationships	Immediate and extended family and friends, professionals
Attitudes	Individual attitudes and societal norms
Services, Systems, and Policies	Architecture policies, policies for production of consumer goods, housing services, public places, communication and media services, civil and legal services, economic policies, health services

Adapted from—Source: Towards a Common Language for Functioning, Disability, and Health (ICF), World Health Organization (2002).

Activities and participation are represented on a continuum of function, which is biased towards "*functioning*" when the qualifiers are positive and towards "*disability*" when the qualifiers are negative. Activity is qualified by the general magnitude scoring scale, with the positive qualifier being *function* and the negative qualifier termed *activity limitation*. In the ICF, activity limitation is a descriptor which moves the continuum of function into the range of disability.

Likewise, Participation is qualified by magnitude, with the positive qualifier being *Performance* and the negative qualifier termed a *participation restriction*. Like its counterpart of activity limitation, the negative qualifier of participation restriction implies the individual is functioning in the range of disability. By employing ICF codes and qualifiers, it is possible to avoid focus on disability per say, but rather to objectively describe the individual's activities and participation as a snapshot on a continuum of function.

Contextual factors are qualified in a dichotomous system as either *barriers* or *facilitators* (WHO, 2001b). A barrier is a factor, such as low socioeconomic status, which limits the individual's access to factors that support health. Conversely, a facilitator is a factor that supports healthy participation. A high socioeconomic status, for example, may permit an individual who has lower extremity paralysis to live quite independently in his own home because he can afford to modify the home for his needs.

PUTTING THE ICF INTO PRACTICE

A simple application of ICF principles that has appeared recently in the physical therapy literature is in reference to the function of walking or gait. Fritz and Lusardi (2009) suggest that gait velocity, that is, how fast someone walks, should be considered a "vital sign." The authors base this premise upon research demonstrating correlations between how fast someone walks and other aspects of independence. To be considered able to walk in the community, which underlies participation, a person must walk about 3.1 miles per hour. Physical therapists often time a 10-meter walk in the clinical setting. To be ambulatory in a community, a person should be able to walk 10 meters in about 7 seconds. The time taken to do a 10-meter walk in the clinical (or standard) setting represents the capacity of the person for ambulation activity. If the person has the capacity to be a community ambulatory, participation would be determined by other factors, such as motivation, opportunity, or terrain. These are also contextual factors. Performance is the actual ambulation in the community setting, which reflects both capacity and contextual factors. Furthermore, Fritz and Lusardi (2009) make a convincing argument that not only does gait velocity relate to ability to move about and participate in community functions, it also relates to other aspects of activity and participation such as ADL independence. These interrelationships are summarized in **Figure 1-3**.

Activities and participation as defined in the ICF focus on normative behaviors of adulthood. In 2007, the World Health Organization introduced a version of the ICF especially focusing on children and youth, which is known as ICF-CY (WHO, 2007). The framework of the ICF-CY mirrors that of the ICF, but it addresses children in the context of their developmental continuum. It attempts to capture impacts of physical and social environment, such as malnutrition, and permits the inclusion of children with developmental delay in the classification system (Lollar & Simeonsson, 2005).

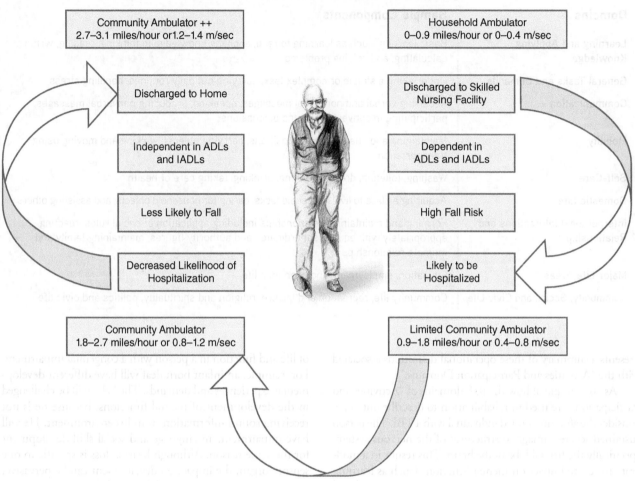

Figure 1-3 Relationship of Gait Velocity to Other Dimensions of Activity

DOMAINS OF PERFORMANCE AND FUNCTION

Traditionally, in the psychological study of human development, three domains have been addressed: cognitive, affective, and psychomotor. The **cognitive domain** involves thought, the **affective domain** involves feelings, and the **psychomotor domain** involves movement. The ICF has a much more specific and detailed analysis of behaviors that can be tested and used to infer capabilities. ICF combines the categories cognitive, affective, and psychomotor into the single category of "Mental Functions." Mental functions will be described in detail in Chapter 6 of this text (WHO, 2001a). These broad domains of human behavior, or body structure/function in ICF terminology, provide the matrix upon which function occurs.

The ICF operationally defined the list of functional domains categorized as "Activities and Participation," summarized in **Table 1-2**. These functional domains incorporate long-existent terminology associated with function. For example, in the ICF domain of "Self-Care" are behaviors traditionally referred to as activities of daily living (ADLs). Examples of ADLs are personal hygiene (toileting, bathing, feeding, dressing, and grooming). The ICF domain of "Domestic Life" incorporates a more complex set of functional behaviors traditionally known as **instrumental activities of daily living (IADLs)**. These are the activities of daily living that typically involve cognitive sequencing as well as chains of behaviors. Examples are grocery shopping, managing money, planning and preparing meals, and using transportation. The ICF domain of "Mobility" incorporates physical function, including the ability to maneuver in the environment through some means of locomotion. Physical function abilities underlie the execution of work, productive activities, and leisure. **Table 1-4**

TABLE 1-4	ICF Activities and Participation Domains

Domains	Sample Components
Learning and Applying Knowledge	Basic learning such as learning to read, applying knowledge in thinking, reading, writing, calculating, and solving problems
General Tasks and Demands	Undertaking a simple or complex task, carrying out daily routines, handling stress
Communication	Receiving verbal and nonverbal messages, speaking, producing nonverbal messages, participating in conversations and discussions
Mobility	Maintaining and changing body positions, carrying objects, walking and moving using transportation
Self-Care	Washing, toileting, dressing, eating, drinking, taking care of health
Domestic Life	Acquiring a place to live, household tasks, caring for household objects, and assisting others
Interpersonal Interactions and Relationship	Forming and maintaining relationships including application of social rules, reacting appropriately with equals, subordinates and authority figures, maintaining family and intimate relationships
Major Life Areas	Education, employment, and economic life
Community, Social, and Civic Life	Community life, recreation and leisure, religion and spirituality, politics and civic life

presents a summary of these operational definitions associated with the "Activities and Participation Domains."

As an example of how the ICF domains of "Activities and Participation" are used in rehabilitation to describe outcome, consider the aforementioned individual with a TBI. The person sustained severe damage to structures of the nervous system, specifically the frontal lobe of the brain. This results in a moderate to severe impact on mental functions (such as learning and memory), speech functions, and movement-related functions. As a result of these impairments in body structure and function, the individual has activity limitations. She may not be able to participate in self-care or feed herself. She may not be able to walk or propel a wheelchair. She is not able to behave appropriately in environmental contexts. Therefore, for the time being, she has severe participation restrictions. She cannot function in her home environment, much less return to work or school. Her intimate relationships are altered because of her dependence. Leisure is not available. If the resources permit and she enters a period of appropriate activity-focused rehabilitation, the goal is that she will ultimately return to work, school, leisure, and family life in age-appropriate roles. Thus, her participation restrictions will be lifted, and her place on the continuum of function moves away from the negative aspect of disability and toward functioning.

This example illustrates the use of the ICF for an individual with an acquired impairment. In the example given, the individual was following a normative developmental and functional performance path until she had an accident resulting in a TBI. From that point on, her life course was altered. The ICF can also be useful in understanding quality of life and function in a person with a congenital impairment. For example, an infant born deaf will have different developmental experiences and demands. The baby will be challenged in the development of mental functions, because he is not receiving sound information from his environment. He will have impairments in language and social skill development for the same reason. Although hearing loss is specific to one sensory organ, the impact on development can be pervasive, and without identification of the problem, or intervention, the boy may develop very differently from his peers.

In the case of a congenital problem, like deafness, intervention would focus on strategies that will help the boy have a more normative developmental experience, with typical developmental opportunities. In this example, a technological intervention, a cochlear implant, can offer sound input and help restore his developmental trajectory. Other interventions might include speech therapy, developmental therapy, and special education.

CLINICAL FRAMES OF REFERENCE

Rehabilitation professionals have embraced the disablement concept as a *frame of reference* for practice. A **frame of reference** is the theoretical perspective or viewpoint that organizes the approach to client management. Two professional groups, occupational therapy and physical therapy, have slightly different historical frames of reference in the management of disability. Frames of reference guide clinical reasoning in the health professions. They support the identification of assessment strategies, intervention goals, discharge planning, and offer support for advocacy and community engagement activities.

Occupational therapy has historically had strong ties to social models of disability, as well as medical models. In the practice guidelines for occupational therapy, a careful differentiation is made between the medical model, with its focus on the absence of disease, and the occupational model, with its more societal focuses on competence in performance in desired human occupations. Throughout this text, the term *occupation* is used as a descriptor for "all that people need, want, or are obliged to do; what it means to them" (Wilcock, 2006, p. 9). The interdisciplinary study of occupation, called occupational science, focuses on daily human occupation and how they are invested with meaning, value, and power.

Throughout this text we explore occupation in terms of how people typically occupy their time at differing developmental periods, what factors influence people's choice of occupations, and how occupation impacts heath and participation in society.

The *Occupational Therapy Practice Framework (OTPF)* closely parallels the ICF model and reflects an occupational perspective, especially in its unique emphasis on contextual factors. The OTPF describes occupations as "engagements in which people participate in their daily life and throughout their lifetime. Occupations occur in context and are products of the interplay among client factors, performance skills, and performance patterns. Occupations occur over time; have purpose, meaning, and perceived utility to the client; and can be observed by others (e.g., preparing a meal) or be known only to the person involved (e.g., learning while reading a textbook)" (AOTA, 2014, p. 9). The OTPF cites as the domain of occupational therapy "supporting health and participation in life through engagement in occupation" and terminology closely parallels the ICF model, as illustrated in **Figure 1-4**.

The *Occupational Therapy Practice Framework* (2014) also emphasizes that the target of intervention, that is, the client, may be people, groups, or populations. Physical therapy has

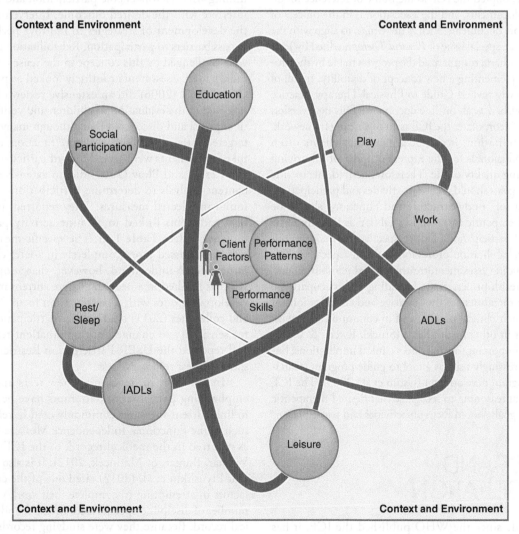

Figure 1-4   Occupational Therapy's Domain

Source: American Occupational Therapy Association. (2014). Occupational Therapy Practice Framework: Domain and process (3rd ed.) Bethesda, MD: AOTA Press.

a deeper history in the medical model, but has more recently adopted the disablement perspective as a key frame of reference. In a landmark paper published in *Physical Therapy*, the profession's flagship journal, Alan Jette proposed a disablement model adaptation based on a Nagi revision and closely aligned with the WHO's ICIDH model (Jette, 1994). The proposed model includes terms such as *pathology, impairment, functional limitation,* and *disability.* Jette related disablement to *quality of life*, which he defined as emotional well-being, behavioral competence, sleep and rest, energy, vitality, and general life satisfaction. Jette further posited that quality of life is impacted at the level of functional limitation and handicap or disability (Jette, 1994). Jette's paper and associated terminology was incorporated into the *Guide to Physical Therapy Practice*, published in 1997 and revised in 2001 by the American Physical Therapy Association (APTA). Jette (2006) summarized the history of incorporation of the disablement concept into models by the World Health Organization and others, and recommended the adoption of the ICF as the path toward a "common language" for function, disability, and health. In 2008, the APTA House of Delegates adopted the ICF as the frame of reference for all subsequent documents, and the association is in the process of revising its core documents, such as the *Guide*, to align with the ICF. In 2011, a special issue of *Physical Therapy*, edited by Jette and Nancy Latham, summarized the progress made by the profession in implementing a new concept of disability. In fall of 2014, the newly revised Guide to Physical Therapy Practice 3.0 was published as an on-line document. This new version of the Guide incorporates the ICF as an organizing framework.

In rehabilitation, it can be argued that clients often seek out professionals for the express purpose of improving or maintaining quality of life. Therefore, desired therapeutic outcomes or goals should focus on activities and participation. The domains of "Body Structure and Function" should be a focus of therapeutic intervention ONLY as they underlie activities and participation. This perspective has major implications for rehabilitation professionals, in all aspects of their practice including assessment, treatment, and reimbursement.

Many health professionals, including both occupational and physical therapists use the language and classifications of the ICF in their clinical practice and in communicating with professionals in other health fields (Stucki, Ewert, & Cieza, 2003). This important tool has direct clinical implications, but has been increasingly used as a tool to guide program evaluation and program development (Üstün et al., 2003). The ICF guides clinical reasoning to recognize that desired therapeutic outcomes or goals should focus on activities and participation.

THE ICF AND REHABILITATION

In the decade since the WHO published the ICF, it has increasingly become the standard for terminology applied to rehabilitation outcomes in key publications (Frontera,

Grimby, Basford, Muller, & Ring, 2008). Therefore, it is imperative all professionals understand and use the terms correctly. The standardization brought to the field by the ICF and ICF-CY has been interdisciplinary in nature, with benefits that are widely referenced (Cramm, Aiken, & Stewart, 2012). Over the decade, an increasing number of disciplines have adopted or recommended use of ICF terminology. For example, Linden (2012) proposed ICF terminology as the solution to the need for operational definitions in the mental health professions.

Steiner and colleagues (2002) discussed using the ICF as a clinical problem-solving tool for rehabilitation practice. One issue related to using the ICF for clinical purposes is incorporating the terminology and concepts into assessment. Goldstein, Cohn, and Coster (2004) suggested the ICF implies a top-down approach to assessment. As will be discussed in Chapter 22 of this text, a top-down assessment is one that initiates the assessment process by asking what the outcome should be in terms of participation. The remainder of the assessment process then focuses on determining what factors enable participation and what factors interfere with the desired outcome. Intervention involves the development of strategies to improve performance or bypass barriers to participation. Rehabilitation professionals were challenged by this concept in the sense that few commonly used assessments routinely looked at participation. O'Neil et al. (2006) did an extensive review of assessment involved in the evaluation of children and youth with spastic diplegia and discovered that although many assessments targeted activity and body structure/function, only a handful of assessments were geared toward participation.

Resnik and Plow (2009) did an extensive review and content analysis to determine participation-related items found in selected measures. They reported five measures that had items linked to all nine activity-participation dimensions (see **Table 1-2**). The specific measures found will be discussed more completely in a later chapter. It is important to understand, however, that adoption of the ICF has resulted in a need to analyze current measures and develop new ones with a participation focus. Van der Zee and colleagues (2011) studied four participation measures for sensitivity to change during outpatient rehabilitation and reported the USER-Participation Restriction scale to show the best responsiveness.

In addition to developing new tests and measures emphasizing participation, attempts have been reported to link current measures commonly used in rehabilitation, such as the Functional Independence Measure (FIM) score as reported in the medical record, to the ICF (Ptyushkin, Vidmar, Burger, & Marincek, 2012). It is also noteworthy that Ptyushkin et al. (2012) cited one of the complicating factors in attempting to complete their work was the large number of discipline-specific assessments found in the medical record. Because they were studying records of patients with traumatic brain injury (TBI), which traditionally involves a large multidisciplinary team, the authors were particularly enthusiastic about the potential for ICF terminology to provide standardization of outcome measures.

There is growing literature about how the ICF and ICF-CY influence clinical practice. Sullivan and Cen (2011) used a technique known as knowledge translation (KT) involving a variety of statistical analysis techniques to assess individuals with post-stroke walking disability. The authors reported the direct effect of impairment on participation was not statistically significant; however, the indirect effect through activity was significant. Therefore, the notion that rehabilitation outcomes should focus on activity and participation domains was validated. Darrah, Wiart, and Magill-Evans (2008) surveyed pediatric physical therapists to determine their use of participation as a concept in establishing therapy goals. The authors found 78 percent of therapists established at least some goals at the level of activity or participation; however, they also found therapists *assumed* spontaneous translation to participation from achievement of goals at lower levels. The ICF has also forced a more long-term community-based outcomes focus to the rehabilitation process, as exemplified by a study identifying long-term needs of survivors of stroke (Sumathipala, Radcliffe, Sadler, Wolfe, & McKevitt, 2012). These authors concluded that the ICF framework was particularly useful to investigate the influence of contextual factors on long-term needs of post-stroke survivors.

It is important to note one of the key potentials cited in ICF literature is the improvement in interprofessional communication in team-based health care. As the United States health care system undergoes changes in the twenty-first century, the health care team is considered an important founding principle to high-quality, cost-efficient care (Sheldon et al., 2012). In a paper discussing implementation of the ICF in a neurorehabilitation setting, the "team" is considered the working unit, rather than the individual treatment discipline (Rentsch et al., 2003). These authors stated that adoption of the ICF in daily practice of neurorehabilitation improved team communication and documentation, the quality of interdisciplinary work, and ultimately resulted in a more systematic approach to rehabilitation (Rentsch et al., 2003). In fact, to address emerging trends in health care, professional education programs in the health professions have begun to adopt **interprofessional education (IPE)** into professional curricula. IPE is defined by the Centre for the Advancement of Interprofessional Education (CAIPE) as: "… when two or more professions learn with, from and about each other to improve collaboration and quality of care" (2002). In a 2008 survey, Mueller, Klingler, Paterson, and Chapway asked physical and occupational therapists their perception of IPE. Of the responses, 97 percent reported a favorable perception, with 65 percent believing IPE should occur in the clinical setting, and 26 percent in the classroom setting.

Predictably, the enthusiasm with which the ICF and ICF-CY have been greeted is tempered with some concerns. Stucki, Ewert, and Cieza (2002) discussed the application of the ICF to rehabilitation and commented that, although the ICF classification system is comprehensive, it is also unwieldy and impractical in its original form. Haglund and Henriksson (2003) assessed the utility of ICF concepts in classification as applied to the profession of occupational therapy. They compared ICIDH-2 classifications with two discipline-specific classifications of 33 clients with learning disabilities, as rated by a panel of occupational therapy experts, and concluded that the ICF in isolation was insufficiently inclusive of occupational therapy concepts to replace discipline-based assessment and classification systems. One key complaint appearing in the literature is the difficulty in differentiating between the concepts of activity and participation. It has been noted that, although they are conceptually separate, by putting them in a single category for classification, the WHO made it difficult to clearly code problems identified in clinical practice (Cramm et al., 2012; Jette, 2006). In a published commentary, Ring (2010) stated the ICF was not a useful research tool, because the categories and frameworks were too imprecise to be useful. Wiegand and colleagues (2012) reviewed global diffusion and clinical implementation of the ICF and found that, although the terminology and concepts had successfully permeated rehabilitation, the effect on rehabilitation practice was idiosyncratic.

Despite problems and, in some cases, calls for modification, the ICF and ICF-CY have had an enormous impact on how disability is viewed and categorized. Many of the concepts embedded in the ICF framework, such as focus on long-term participation as the outcome and consideration of the impact of contextual factors on outcome, complement other emerging trends in health care such as life course theory (LCT), the occupational therapy practice framework, IPE, and team-based health care. All health professionals should be able to apply the ICF to their niche in the health care system and work to ensure integration at all levels of engagement.

DIMENSIONS OF HUMAN FUNCTION OVER THE LIFE SPAN

To study human function over the life span, it will be important to keep in mind that both development and aging are continuous processes. There is not a point in the life span where development ceases, and although we tend to prefer the word *maturation* when considering the very young, aging begins with conception. The focus of this text is normal aging. Normal aging is a developmental process that involves changes in function that are the result of maturation or the passage of time. Three types of influences on aging will be considered as you progress through this text:

(1) age-normative influences, (2) history-normative influences, and (3) nonnormative influences.

AGE-NORMATIVE INFLUENCE

Age-normative influences are the aspects of development that are chronological (Hayslip, Patrick, & Panek, 2011). Many age-normative changes are physiological and reflect the maturation of an organism. As you learn about development in the prenatal period and in infancy, many age-normative patterns of development will be presented. The developmental milestones used to screen young children for developmental delay are an example of age-normative developmental expectations. In Chapter 2, developmental models will be discussed as they impact health across the life span.

HISTORY-NORMATIVE INFLUENCE

A cohort is a generational group as defined in demographics. One of the most famous cohorts in recent American experience is the cohort of the "baby boomers." The baby boomers are a generation of Americans who were born in a "baby boom" following World War II, roughly between 1944 and 1964. **History-normative influences** are the aspects of development that affect a cohort in time (Hayslip et al., 2011). For example, the baby boomers were born in a prosperous time, with a strong belief that they will achieve more than their parents before them. American history influenced the worldview of the baby boomers to such a degree, that the cohort has been described as having characteristics that are unique, and not common to all Americans. The baby boomer generation is identified as confident, independent, and self-reliant. Because members of this generation grew up in an era of reform, they entered adulthood believing they could change the world. Baby boomers have also been described as "work-centric," motivated by position, perks, and prestige.

Chapter 4 of this text introduces the idea of *subcultures*. In some ways, history-normative influences, such as those baby boomers experienced, result in a subculture that is distinctive. Students of development will find few history-normative influences in the study of young children, but from adolescence all history becomes an important factor influencing development. For example, young adults entering college today are described as being part of the "net generation" (or *Internet* generation). The historical influences on this generation include the perception that computers are a natural part of their environment, and the virtual world is an extension of their real world. This perception is unique in human history, and we are only now beginning to see how it influences adult function and decision making. Chapter 16 addresses how the experience of today's young adults has been greatly influenced by the global economic recession. Chapter 17 describes the generation split, with older people in this age span as members of the baby boomers, and the younger half of this age cohort described as generation X. As we consider human performance and function in middle adulthood, it will be vital to also consider the history-normative influences in order to understand developmental trends.

NONNORMATIVE INFLUENCE

The final type of influence on development that we will consider is the nonnormative influence. **Nonnormative influences** are factors that influence development that are not related to either age or personal history. Nonnormative influences will be mentioned in many chapters as we give examples of types and impacts of disabilities. Other nonnormative influences we will consider are the impact of family violence, illness, and poverty.

SUMMARY

The study of human performance and function is vital to understanding the contexts within which people seek rehabilitation or other interventions to restore quality of life. Participation in daily life occupations is central to positive developmental and health outcomes and will be addressed throughout the text. Normative and nonnormative influences on behavior and development will be considered as they relate to each age cohort described in Part 2 of this text. Rehabilitation professionals must understand the complex relationships that allow individuals to be healthy, in the fullest use of the term. This chapter has introduced basic terminology and constructs that will serve as a guide to the study of human performance across the life span. In Case 1, you will meet Jayden, a young man with a developmental delay that is congenital and that potentially limits his participation in activities and major life areas. Linda, in Case 2, was well established in her community and was able to assist her daughter in providing child care prior to acquiring a health condition. In her case, she has life roles she hopes to return to. These two cases illustrate applications of the ICF with congenital and acquired health impairments.

As you move through Part 1 of this text, you will see the WHO ICF terminology used, often in parallel with more commonly used clinical terms for the same concept.

Part 1 of the text covers the large overarching frameworks that influence human performance and function at all levels of development. This section of the book focuses on contexts and influences on occupations that may impact individuals at any developmental period. In Part 2 of the text, readers will be moved sequentially through life span development. In all of Part 2 of this book, readers will see the ICF framework used to structure the chapter. After the chapter introduction, each chapter will begin with significant issues in body functions and structures, and then move on to areas of activities and participation. Examples of occupations that are typical within the developmental period on which the chapter focuses will be offered. Human occupations become more varied and complex throughout the life span, and this is reflected in the text as well.

Engagement in activities in the preschool period expands with a child's growing skills, and from this point on become a central focus of the book. Readers will note that the bulk of the chapters on adulthood focus on activities and participation. Because this change in focus reflects changes in the developmental life course, the focus returns to body functions and structures in the chapter on late adulthood.

The final part of this text focuses on specific societal and professional trends that impact functional performance and our ability as health professionals to support people to achieve a high quality of life. Throughout the text, case studies and clinical examples have been introduced to help readers understand the impact of developmental issues on everyday function.

CASE 1

Jayden

Jayden is 2 years and 6 months old. He has typical mental and sensory functions for his age, but has impairments in neuromusculoskeletal and movement-related functions. With secondary to poor muscular control, Jayden also has unclear speech production, known as dysarthria. He has incoordination of all large muscles limiting postural control, mobility, communication, and fine motor control. Jayden communicates through gestures and facial expression with some vocalizations. He currently attends a special needs preschool. He has attended occupational therapy (OT), physical therapy (PT), and speech therapy (ST) since birth and has been making steady gains in motor control over the past 2 years.

Jayden is very social but does not communicate well verbally because of his dysarthric speech patterns. He is intellectually able to keep up with classroom activities, and he especially loves story time. His parents want him to be able to go to the neighborhood school and attend regular classes when he is 5 years old. They are interested in learning how to best support him so that he can achieve this. Communication, mobility, and self-care are the three biggest participation areas that need additional support if Jayden is to achieve this goal. His physical therapist has been exploring mobility options for Jayden. He is working on walking with a walking frame in the clinic, but in the community his parents use a baby stroller to take him around. The focus of physical therapy intervention will be to maximize the movement and mobility abilities that he has while offering assistive technology (leg braces, wheelchairs, or power scooters) to be sure that he can keep up with his age peers and access the school environment independently.

Because of his limited physical mobility and poor muscle coordination, Jayden has had difficulty learning to dress himself, to bath himself, and to use the toilet. His family helps him with tasks that are difficult for him, and Jayden relies on them to organize and direct his play as well as his self-care activities. Jayden does not have much interaction with other children his age. Occupational therapy will work to adapt clothing and tasks so that Jayden can learn to take care of himself in dressing and personal hygiene tasks. The therapist will work with the family to arrange his clothing and other task-specific items in a way that he can reach them without adult help. In addition, the occupational therapist will help Jayden develop some play

Continues

Case 1   *Continued*

activities that he can do by himself and with other children. This may include using electronic games, board games, or imaginative play.

The focus of speech therapy will be on helping Jayden communicate verbally with both adults and age peers. The speech therapist may choose to use an alternative communication system, such as a picture board, to serve as a tool to aid communication while Jayden works on articulation skills. Because communication is integral to all aspects of school performance, the OT, PT, and ST will need to work together so that Jayden is able to communicate in all settings and across all tasks. Jayden is unlikely to gain typical age-normative skills in mobility, self-care, play, or communication without the use of assistive devices. The goal of therapy is to maximize his skills and to offer alternative methods of participating in tasks when he lacks the performance abilities to participate in a typical manner.

Guiding Questions

Some questions to consider:

1. What do you think normal *activity and participation* roles for a 2½-year-old child should be?
2. How would Jayden's case be viewed from a frame of reference that arises from the medical model, the social model, and a disablement model?
3. What environmental (contextual) factors need to be considered in Jayden's case?
4. How is an interprofessional model of care used in this case?

CASE 2

Linda

Linda is a 60-year-old woman who had a right cerebrovascular accident (CVA) with left weakness. Linda spent five weeks in the hospital and then in rehabilitation to aid in her recovery. Linda has now returned home. She lives in a single-family home with her 30-year-old daughter and her two grandchildren. She is able to walk independently with "toe drag" on the left, and is walking throughout the ground floor of the house using a standard walker.

Linda is able to feed and groom herself, given setup. She needs minimum assists in transfers to and from chairs and needs assistance to get out of bed. She uses her right hand for most tasks, and will use the left arm as a gross assist in some activities. Her left shoulder and elbow are weak, with muscles scoring in the "fair" grade of strength. She has only gross movement and control of her distal arm.

Linda had been helping her daughter with child care before her CVA and is concerned that the extra burden of caring for her will be too much for her daughter. A physical therapist and occupational therapist have been visiting her home to assist Linda in returning to daily life tasks. Areas of emphasis have been an analysis of the home environment to reduce Linda's risk for falls and to modify the home with safety grab bars and easy-access handles so that Linda can manage independently. PT will focus on Linda's mobility in

Continues

Case 2 *Continued*

the home, helping her gain strength and control in walking. Both the OT and PT will work together to help Linda regain her independence in activities of daily living. Linda wants to regain her previous life roles and participate more in cooking and child care tasks. The occupational therapist will work with Linda to both regain physical control, and also to help organize tasks so that they are easier for Linda to complete. Linda may need home modifications and assistive devices as well as therapy to regain these skills.

Even with these supports, Linda is likely to continue to need assistance in some areas of domestic life, such as acquisition of necessities, household tasks, and assisting others. With Linda and her daughter, the OT and PT may be involved in helping renegotiate roles and expectations within the home. For example, Linda may be able to do more child care and less housework with her current physical condition. Linda may also need support as she returns to old leisure pursuits or explores new leisure options. To fully return to adult roles and participation, Linda will need therapy supports to extend beyond the rehabilitation hospital and as she reenters community life.

Guiding Questions

Some questions to consider:

1. How do the participation roles in Linda's case differ from those in Jayden's case? Discuss this from a view of age-related participation expectations.
2. What contextual factors might affect Linda's ability to participate in her normal life tasks?
3. Can you apply the domains of activity and participation presented in Table 1-4 to Linda's current level of performance? Are all domains equally affected by the CVA? If not, which ones are most affected?

Speaking of
The ICF in Practice

MARYBETH MANDICH, PT, PHD
PEDIATRIC PHYSICAL THERAPIST

Many years ago, when I was a young therapist, I was working with a young man, probably 12 or 13 years old, who had spina bifida. In the fairly recent past, before I started working with him, he had given up attempts at walking. Because he was paralyzed from the waist down, he was confined to a wheelchair, and he was pretty good at getting around that way. The reason he had given up walking, it turns out, had nothing to do with energy expenditure or laziness or weight gain. The reason he had stopped walking was very simple—every time he stood up, he had a reflexive bowel movement. Now, I don't remember if this was a recently developed problem or one that he had previously, but with the onset of adolescence, he was unwilling to "pay the price" of walking.

As a brand new therapist, armed with lots of knowledge and very little wisdom, I determined that it would be an important treatment goal for this young man to regain the ability to ambulate. I had pretty good rapport with him, probably because I was so young myself, so he agreed to give it a try. Every day, he and I would leave his classroom, lock his braces up, and begin gait training. Every day, to avoid anyone else knowing his problem, I would perform the required hygiene after the inevitable bowel accident occurred. We kept this up for weeks. Eventually, however, I was

Continues

Speaking of Continued

forced to admit what this young man had feared—this reflexive reaction simply wasn't going to become accommodated, and, at the young man's request, we stopped the gait training.

Now, there are good reasons for encouraging walking in individuals with spinal cord injury, including congenital problems like spina bifida. Walking helps keep the bones strong. The energy used to walk helps control weight gain. Many individuals like the idea of being upright with their peers who are able-bodied.

However, I was approaching the issue with what I am now able to see in hindsight was a blatant disregard for this young man's functional abilities. I was focusing at the body structure and function level, and to some extent, at the activity level (the activity of walking). What I missed entirely was the focus on participation. In fact, by having this young man put such an emphasis on walking, I was in fact limiting his activities and severely restricting his participation. However, in the end, it was the ability to participate with his peers that mattered most.

What the ICF and its predecessor, the ICIDH model, have taught us is to expand our worldview in defining outcomes and setting goals for individuals with disabilities. As discussed in this chapter, it is entirely possible to have restrictions in body structure and function but not be limited in activities and participation. Conversely, it is possible to have no restriction on activity but be unable to attend a social function because of environmental or societal barriers. In order to work effectively with individuals who have disabilities, it is important to remember that activity and participation are part of normal functioning, and restoration of these abilities is part of every intervention program. This provides a mandate to the rehabilitation professional. No longer can we view our clients and patients within a single treatment area or department or gym. We have to look out to the world. We need to understand what their developmental and functional needs are in the context of their physical, social, and cultural environment. Where society puts up barriers, we need to become advocates for barrier removal.

The ICF helps us categorize and gives us a classification system to reference. But to apply the ICF correctly, we need to understand normative developmental and functional tasks across the life span. Our hope is that this text and others like it will help rehabilitation professionals learn to incorporate this frame of reference into their interventions.

REFERENCES

American Occupational Therapy Association. (2014). *Occupational therapy practice framework: Domain and process* (3rd ed.). Bethesda, MD: AOTA Press.

American Physical Therapy Association. (2001). *Guide to physical therapist practice* (2nd ed.). Alexandria, VA: American Physical Therapy Association.

American Physical Therapy Association. (2014). Guide to physical therapist practice 3.0 (3rd ed.). Alexandria, VA: American Physical Therapy Association. Retrieved from: http://guidetoptpractice.apta.org/. Accessed 10/30/2014. American Physical Therapy Association. (1997). *Guide to physical therapist practice* (1st ed.). Alexandria, VA: American Physical Therapy Association.

Centre for the Advancement of Interprofessional Education (CAIPE). *The definition and princples of inter professional education.* (2002). Retrieved from www.caipe.org.uk

Cramm, H., Aiken, A., & Stewart, D. (2012). Perspectives on the International Classification of Functioning, Disability and Health: Child and Youth Version (ICF-CY) and occupational therapy practice. *Physical & Occupational Therapy in Pediatrics.* Retrieved from http://informahealthcare.com/potp

Darrah, J., Wiart, L., & Magill-Evans, J. (2008). Do therapists' goals and interventions for children with cerebral palsy reflect principles in contemporary literature? *Pediatric Physical Therapy, 20*(4), 334–339.

Fritz, S., & Lusardi, M. (2009). Walking speed: The 6th vital sign. *Journal of Geriatric Physical Therapy, 32*(2), 2–5.

Frontera, W. R., Grimby, G., Basford, J., Muller, D., & Ring, H. (2008). Publishing in physical & rehabilitation medicine. *American Journal of Physical Medicine and Rehabilitation, 87*(3), 215–220.

Goldstein, D., Cohn, E., & Coster, W. (2004). Enhancing participation for children with disabilities: Application of the ICF enablement framework to pediatric physical therapist practice. *Pediatric Physical Therapy, 16*, 114–120.

Haglund, L., & Henriksson, C. (2003). Concepts in occupational therapy in relation to the ICF. *Occupational Therapy International, 10*(4), 253–268.

Hayslip, B., Patrick, J., & Panek, P. (2011). *Adult development and aging* (5th ed.). Malabar, FL: Krieger Publishing Company.

Jette, A. M. (1994). Physical disablement concepts for physical therapy research and practice. *Physical Therapy, 74,* 380–386.

Jette, A. M. (2006). Toward a common language for function, disability, and health. *Physical Therapy, 86*(5), 726–734.

Jette, A. M., & Latham, N. K. (2011). Disability research: Progress made, opportunities for even greater gains. *Physical Therapy, 91*(12), 1708–1710.

Linden, M. (2012). What is health and what is positive? The ICF solution. *World Psychiatry, 11*(2), 104–105.

Lollar, D. J., & Simeonsson, R. J. (2005). Diagnosis to function: Classification for children and youths. *Developmental and Behavioral Pediatrics, 26*(4), 323–330.

Maslow, A. (1954). *Motivation and personality.* New York: Harper & Row.

Merriam-Webster, Incorporated (2014). Function. *Merriam-Webster Dictionary.* Retrieved from www.merriam-webster.com /dictionary/function

Mueller, D., Klingler, R., Paterson, M., & Chapman, C. (2008). Entry-level interprofessional education: Perception of physical and occupational therapists currently practicing in Ontario. *Journal of Allied Health, 37*(4), 189–195.

Nagi, S. (1965). Some conceptual issues in activity limitation and rehabilitation. In M. Sussman (Ed.), *Sociology and rehabilitation* (pp. 100–113). Washington, DC: American Sociological Association.

O'Neil, M., Fragala-Pinkham, M., Westcott, S. L., Martin, K. Chiarell, L., Valvano, J., & Rose, R. (2006). Physical therapy clinical management recommendations for children with cerebral palsy-spastic diplegia: Achieving functional mobility outcomes. *Pediatric Physical Therapy, 18,* 49–72.

Ptyushkin, P., Vidmar, G., Burger, H., & Marincek, C. (2012). Use of the International Classification of Functioning, Disability and Health in traumatic brain injury rehabilitation: Linking issues and general perspectives. *American Journal of Physical Medicine and Rehabilitation, 91*(13), 548–554.

Rentsch, H., Bucher, P., Dommen Nyfeler, I., Wolf, C., Hefti, H., Fluri, E., Wenger, U., Walti, C., & Boyer, I. (2003). The implementation of the "International Classification of Functioning, Disability and Health" (ICF) in daily practice of neurorehabilitation: An interdisciplinary project at the Kantonsspital of Lucerne, Switzerland. *Disability and Rehabilitation, 25*(8), 411–421.

Resnik, L., & Plow, M. A. (2009). Measuring participation as defined by the International Classification of Functioning, Disability and Health: An evaluation of existing measures. *Archives of Physical Medicine and Rehabilitation, 90,* 856–866.

Ring, D. (2010). Commentary: The World Health Organization's International Classification of Functioning, Disability and Health: Invaluable framework, questionable research tool. *Journal of Hand Surgery of America 35*(11), 1806.

Sheldon, M., Cavanaugh, J., Croninger, W., Osgood, W., Robnett, R., Seigle, J., & Simonson, L. (2012). Preparing rehabilitation healthcare providers in the 21st century. *Work, 41*(3), 269–275.

Steiner, W., Ryser, L., Huber, E., Uebelhart, D., Aeschlimann, A., & Stucki, G. (2002). Use of the ICF model as a clinical problem-solving tool in physical therapy and rehabilitation medicine. *Physical Therapy, 82,* 1098–1107.

Stucki, G., Ewert, T., & Cieza, A. (2003). Value and application of the ICF in rehabilitation medicine. *Disability and Medicine, 25*(11–12), 628–634.

Sullivan, K. J., & Cen, S. Y. (2011). Model of disablement and recovery: Knowledge translation in rehabilitation research and practice. *Physical Therapy, 91*(12), 1892–1904.

Sumathipala, K., Radcliffe, E., Sadler, E., Wolfe, C. D., & McKevitt, C. (2012). Identifying the long-term needs of stroke survivors using the International Classification of Functioning, Disability and Health. *Chronic Illness, 8*(1), 31–44.

U.S. Department of Health and Human Services Health Resources and Services Administration Maternal and Child Health Bureau (USHHS). (2010). *Rethinking MCH: The life course model as an organizing framework.* Bureau of Maternal and Child Health. Retrieved from http://mchb.hrsa.gov/lifecourse/rethinkingmchlifecourse.pdf

Üstün, T. B., Chatterji, S., Bickenbach, J., Kostanjsek, N., & Schneider, M. (2003). The International Classification of Functioning, Disability and Health: A new tool for understanding disability and health. *Disability and Rehabilitation, 25,* 565–571.

van der Zee, C. H., Kap, A., Rambaran, M., Schouten, E., & Post, M. (2011). Responsiveness of four participation measures to changes during and after outpatient rehabilitation. *Journal of Rehabilitation Medicine, 43*(11), 1003–1009.

Verbrugge, L., & Jette, A. (1994). The disablement process. *Social Science and Medicine, 38,* 1–14.

Wiegand, N. M., Belting, J., Fekete, C., Gutenbrunner, C., & Reinhardt, J. (2012). All talk, no action?: The global diffusion and clinical implementation of the International Classification of Functioning, Disability and Health. *American Journal of Physical Medicine and Rehabilitation 91*(7), 550–560.

Wilcock, A. (2006). *An occupational perspective of health* (2nd ed.). Thorofare, NJ: SLACK Incorporated.

World Health Organization (WHO). (1948). *Definition of health.* World Health Organization. Retrieved from www.who.int /about/definition/en/print.html

World Health Organization. (1993). *International Classification of Impairments, Disabilities and Handicaps.* World Health Organization. Retrieved from http://whqlibdoc.who.int/publications /1980/9241541261_eng.pdf

World Health Organization. (2001a). *ICF: International classification of functioning, disability and health.* World Health Organization. Retrieved from http://www.who.int/classifications/icf/en/

World Health Organization. (2001b). *ICF: International classification of functioning, disability and health.* Geneva, Switzerland: World Health Organization.

World Health Organization (2014). Risk Factor. Retrieved from http://www.who.int/topics/risk_factors/en/

World Health Organization. (2007). *International classification of functioning, disability and health—children and youth version.* Geneva, Switzerland: World Health Organization.

World Health Organization. (2014). *The WHO Family of International Classifications.* Retrieved from www.who.int/classifications/en/

CHAPTER 2

Human Performance: The Life Course Perspective

MaryBeth Mandich, PT, PhD,
Professor and Chairperson,
Division of Physical Therapy,
West Virginia University,
Morgantown, West Virginia
and

Anne Cronin, PhD, OTR/L, FAOTA,
Associate Professor, Division of
Occupational Therapy, West
Virginia University, Morgantown,
West Virginia

Objectives

Upon completion of this chapter, readers should be able to:

- Define and describe key terms associated with development, including functional differentiation of the terms *development, maturation,* and *growth;*

- Discuss life course theory (LCT) and associated implications;

- Reflect on the implications of the Human Genome Project and the increased influence of behavioral genetics in the study of human participation;

- Discuss the concept of early programming as it impacts both health and educational policy and best practices;

- Discuss a systems theory of human development and motor control, including correct application of key terms; and

- Define key terms in genetics and apply them to behavior development and health.

Key Terms

agonist
allele
antagonist
anticipatory control
autonomic nervous system (ANS)
behavioral genetics
cardiopulmonary system
central nervous system (CNS)
competence promotion
control parameter
cumulative impact
degrees of freedom
determinant
development
developmental milestone
developmental systems theory (DST)
dynamical systems theory
early programming
effector system of motor control

emergent control
environmental constraint
epigenesis
epigenetics
evolutionary psychology
family development theory
genomics
genotype
health disparity
health trajectory
heritability
hierarchical model
Individuals with Disabilities
    Education Act (IDEA)
learning
life course health development
    model
life course theory (LCT)
maturation

motor control
mutation
neuroplasticity
occupational engagement
peripheral nervous
    system (PNS)
phenotype
prevention science
proprioceptor
protective factor
resilience
risk factor
risk reduction
sensitive period
skill
somatosensory
special senses
systemic family development
    model (SFD)

INTRODUCTION

If you look at paintings of children from the nineteenth century or earlier, most twenty-first-century viewers would find the portraits somewhat grotesque in proportional scale (see **Figure 2-1**). This is because the artistic expression of the pre-twentieth-century era reflects the commonly held societal belief that children are merely quantitatively different from adults. Taking the fact that children are obviously smaller, the artists projected adult proportions in smaller dimensions, making the paintings appear as unrealistic representations.

From the second decade of the twentieth century, at the close of the First World War, there began to be a scientific interest in discovering the nature of human development. A key factor in this field of study was predicated on federal funding, which was made available to study human development based on interest in prediction of factors such as intelligence and motor aptitude. The nineteenth-century work of Charles Darwin suggested that humans could adapt to environments and that positive traits enhance survival. Throughout the twentieth century until today, human development has been an area of study with an emphasis on qualitative changes. Most of the key theories of human development, discussed in the next chapter, were part of this surge of interest in understanding how humans change over the life span, with emphasis on the early years.

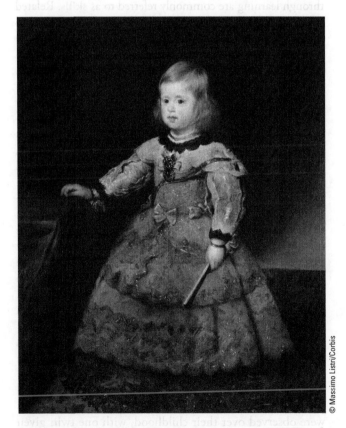

Figure 2-1   In this portrait of "The Infant Margarita at the Age of Three" by Diego Velazquez, the "infant" looks very much like an adult.

© Massimo Listri/Corbis

LIFE SPAN BEHAVIORAL CHANGE

An individual acquires an increasing number of behaviors across the life span, particularly in early life. Qualitative changes related to organizational and process change may be considered maturation. Maturation, in this context, refers to the process of an individual growing biologically, socially, and emotionally over time, changing gradually from a simple to a more complex level of function. The quantitative changes that occur over time in humans (changes in height, weight, and physical characteristics) are categorized as growth. The process of development refers to those changes in performance that are heavily influenced by maturational processes and growth, such as learning to walk (Payne & Isaacs, 2012). For example, maturation of the brain plays a key role in support of early behavioral acquisition, particularly in early childhood. Despite wide varieties of environmental influences, when all body systems are sufficiently mature, most infants will begin walking. Behaviors acquired largely through maturation, such as rolling over or crawling, are referred to as developmental milestones. Another fundamental process, learning, is the acquisition of new behavior through interaction with the environment. Learning is dependent not only on environmental exposure, but also on such factors as feedback and practice. Behaviors acquired through learning are commonly referred to as skills. Related to this is the concept of occupational engagement, used to describe "people doing occupations in a manner that fully involves their effort, drive, and attention" (Christiansen & Townsend, 2010, p. 8). As individuals learn and gain skills, they also gain in ways in which they can engage in occupations in their everyday life.

The question of the role of maturation versus learning, with the former based primarily on biologic processes and the latter based primarily on environmental interaction, led to one of the biggest debates of the early developmental theorists, known as the *nature-nurture controversy*. The theorists who believed developmental change over time was inevitable due to the nature of humans were in direct opposition to those individuals who believed human behaviors arose solely from environmental exposure. Although essentially resolved by the understanding that *all* behaviors have differing contributions from nature and nurture, advances in the study of neuroscience and genetics in the late twentieth century have resurrected a new iteration of the debate, which will be discussed later in this chapter.

An example of the theoretical dispute of the 1930s to the 1950s was between the motor theories of Myrtle McGraw and Arnold Gesell (Payne & Isaacs, 2012). McGraw is remembered today for her classic 1930 studies of the identical twins, Johnny and Jimmy. The twins were observed over their childhood, with one twin given more toys and overall greater opportunities for stimulation

(McGraw, 1935). Several key findings of these classic studies are still accepted today. For example, some skills, such as roller-skating, appear to be learned and retained better when introduced at an early age. Children will not learn to roller-skate or without exposure and practice. The young girl in **Figure 2-2** is gaining skill with skating. However, skills such as walking, creeping, and so on are less affected by environmental exposure. Arnold Gesell, on the other hand, believed firmly in the unfolding of developmental acquisitions irrespective of environmental experience.

Of course, as we look back on these controversies from our twenty-first-century perspective, we know there are no dichotomies. Contemporary scientific findings in genetics and neuroscience show it is a question of extent rather than absolutes. For example, acquisition of behaviors such as rolling over, while heavily maturational, can be influenced if the environment is extremely deprived. Cross-cultural studies have revealed infant caregiving practices, if relatively supportive, result in children being able to walk at around 1 year of age. However, in extremely deprived environments, even

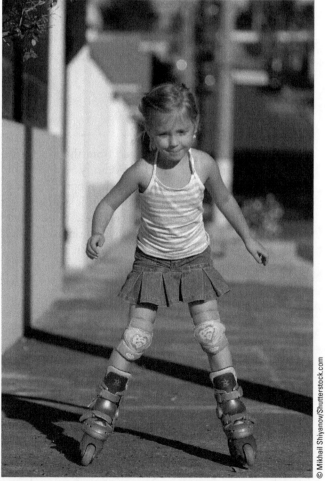

Figure 2-2 Learning to skate using in-line skates requires practice and exposure; based on McGraw's studies, this is a skill best introduced early in life.

© Mikhail Shiyanov/Shutterstock.com

such a maturational milestone can be delayed. Likewise, although skills such as playing the violin certainly depend on environmental exposure and practice, there is no question that a certain amount of growth and maturation have to occur prior to even the youngest children learning how to play the violin.

NEUROSCIENCE AND LIFE COURSE DEVELOPMENT

One of the key factors that placed the nature-nurture controversy in perspective is the explosion of information arising from *neuroscience,* or the study of the nervous system. Functional imaging studies of the human brain in the latter part of the twentieth century tell us the young brain is very responsive to environmental influences, and this responsiveness persists in diminishing quantity throughout the human life span.

While all body systems undergo life span change, there is no question the **central nervous system (CNS)** is a key factor underlying developmental changes in behavior. The central nervous system, for the purposes of this text, is the brain and spinal cord, that is, the parts of the nervous system that are protected by the bony covering of skull and vertebral column. The **peripheral nervous system (PNS)** consists primarily of nerves and nerve roots that connect the control centers of the CNS to external sites, such as muscles, glands, or skin. The **autonomic nervous system (ANS)** is the part of the peripheral nervous system that acts as a control system functioning largely below the level of consciousness, and controls visceral functions. The ANS is directed by special parts of the brain and peripheral nervous system. The parts of the ANS that communicate with the periphery are subdivided into the sympathetic and parasympathetic systems. The sympathetic nervous system controls "fight or flight" behaviors and is associated with a high level of arousal. Conversely, the parasympathetic nervous system mediates basic physiologic behaviors such as digestion, elimination, and sexual function.

As mentioned earlier, our understanding of the role of the CNS in human behavior has changed considerably over the years. As early as 1945, Myrtle McGraw attempted to specifically tie the acquisition of developmental milestones such as rolling to the level of brain maturation. Her work was an example of a hierarchical model of development. A **hierarchical model** of development suggests that as the CNS matures, the behavior displayed represents the function of that level. A hierarchical model was supported by motor maturational theorists, like McGraw, who hoped to show specific motor behaviors and reflexes tied to functions of certain levels of the CNS hierarchy.

Several areas of developmental study in the 1960s were responsible for the merging of neuroscience and child development studies. First, studies of language development supported a biological predisposition for language in human infants, and second, Nobel prize–winning studies of development of the visual part of the brain were influential in support of McGraw's earlier efforts to link brain maturation with behavioral development (Segalowitz & Schmidt, 2003). The latter studies by Hubel and Wiesel (1962) were also instrumental in the evolution of the science of *neuroplasticity.* **Neuroplasticity** refers to the ability of the human brain to change as a result of one's experience, that the brain is "plastic" and "malleable," and structural and functional changes in the brain are driven by environmental experience. It was once believed the direction of influence was that genes direct brain growth, which directs brain function, thereby ultimately directing behavior (the hierarchical model). However, it is now clear the model is not unidirectional in a top-down flow. In other words, as a child spontaneously engages in a challenging activity because of maturation of the brain, the CNS functions associated with the activity are then modified by virtue of engaging in such activity (Segalowitz & Schmidt, 2003). The role of genetic influences on the cellular and metabolic functions as well as the connectivity of the central nervous system has given rise to a field of study known as **behavioral genetics.** Behavioral genetics is the field of study that examines the role of genetics of behavior in all animals, including humans. Behavioral geneticists study the inheritance of behavioral traits. In humans this is most often seen in twin studies or studies of people who have been adopted. The goal of developmental behavioral genetics is to determine how genetic and environmental influences direct the development of behavior, as mediated by the nervous system (Saudino, 2009).

GENETICS AND LIFE COURSE DEVELOPMENT: NATURE-NURTURE REVISITED

In 2001, the rough draft of the human genome was published, with the completion of the sequence filled in a few years later. The genome is the entire set of genetic instructions in the cell nucleus, and **genomics** is the study of the genetic code in the context of the genome. The goal of genomics and related fields is to create a full picture of how living things are assembled and operate (Watson, 2003). The **genotype** is the genetic makeup of a cell, an organism, or an individual (that is, the specific allele makeup of an individual). The genotype of an organism is the inherited instructions it carries within its genetic code. Not all organisms with the same genotype look or act the same way because appearance and behavior are modified by environmental and developmental conditions. Likewise, not all organisms that look alike necessarily have the same genotype.

A **phenotype** is the composite of an organism's observable characteristics or traits, behavior, and products of behavior. Phenotypes result from the expression of an organism's genes as well as the influence of environmental factors and the interactions between the two. Thus, to the extent the genotype and phenotype are identical, the characteristic can be attributed to the genotype; however, to the extent they vary, some other factor must explain variance in the phenotype. The term **heritability** is used to describe the amount of variability in the phenotype that is attributable to the genotype (Saudino, 2009).

Over recent decades, a field known as **evolutionary psychology** has received increasing attention. Evolutionary psychology is defined as the application of evolutionary biology to psychology, including the notion that the human brain, as the source of behavior, has specialized mechanisms that evolve to solve recurrent problems encountered by the organism in the environment (Bjorklund, Ellis, & Rosenberg, 2007). Core assumptions of evolutionary psychology include the notion that behaviors reflect mechanisms that are designed by nature to be responsive to a particular range of stimuli. Evolutionary psychology has been criticized by some as simply a contemporary form of genetic determinism. Evolutionary psychology has also been criticized as incapable of explaining the enormous variation in phenotype seen among individuals (Bjorklund et al., 2007). In fact, there has been little success in the prediction of phenotype from simple knowledge of genotype (Wermter et al., 2010). Some of this difficulty may arise from the nature of the genome itself.

The Human Genome Project produced the first complete sequences of individual human genomes. At this time thousands of human genomes have been completely sequenced, and many more have been mapped at lower levels of resolution. The resulting data are being used in medicine and many branches of science. There is a widely held expectation that genomic studies will lead to advances in the diagnosis and treatment of diseases. The human genome contains approximately 20,000 protein-coding genes, and protein-coding sequences account for only a very small fraction of the genome (approximately 1.5 percent), and the rest is associated with noncoding ribonucleic acid

(RNA) molecules, regulatory DNA sequences, and other sequences. The code is represented by pairs of nucleotide bases that, in triplet sequence, code for amino acids. Amino acids are the building blocks of protein. One important factor of note is that the gene does not directly encode functions or behaviors (Bjorklund et al., 2007). Another important factor is that genes do not constantly exert their influence, but are switched on and off by triggers, which may be other genes sensitive to environmental effects. Finally, genes can be changed or mutated. A **mutation** is a change of the DNA sequence within a gene or chromosome of an organism resulting in the creation of a new character or trait not found in the parental type. One common type of mutation that has been extensively studied in medical genetics is the *single nucleotide polymorphism* (SNP). As implied, an SNP mutation involves only one base pair; however, it may have enormous effects in phenotypic expression of disease, such as mental health disorders or cancer (Wermter et al., 2010). An **allele** is one member of a pair or series of genes that occupy a specific position on a specific chromosome. Alleles can be preexisting or the result of mutation.

Wahlsten (2003) summarized the possibilities inherent in the study of the effect of genes on behavior. "Either genes or environment" was once considered obsolete, but has been resurrected by some claims that long-term changes in the brain and underlying behavior are results of genes that are adaptable over time. The premise "genes plus environment" was the compromise of the late twentieth century and underlies the concept of heritability, that is, given any trait or behavior, the contribution of genetic variability to the overall variability can be quantified, with the remainder of the variability due to environmental influence. A third approach emphasizing "interdependence of heredity and environment," is notable for asserting bidirectional influences between genes and environment. In this school of thought, the notion of determinism is eliminated. Rather, the context in which development occurs is a critical feature. The context may be broadly interpreted to include not only factors acting on the organism, but also the time in the organism's life when the extrinsic factors exert their influence (Wahlsten, 2003). For example, as shown in **Figure 2-3**,

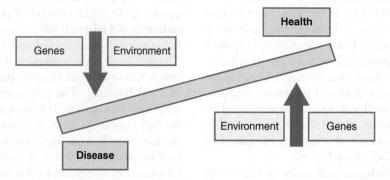

Figure 2-3   Environment-Genetic Interactions on Health

genetic influences and environmental influences can interact in the same direction to promote health or produce disease. On the other hand, healthy lifestyle behaviors can offset genetic influences and tip the scale away from the disease condition.

Wermter and colleagues (2010) reviewed some key examples of gene-environment bidirectional influences. These authors theorize that phenotypic variance may be explained in one of two ways. First, environmental factors may lead to a change in the phenotype, but only in the presence of a certain genotype. Alternatively, a certain genotype may lead to a disorder, only in the presence of certain environmental conditions. For example, in the study of depression, the neurotransmitter serotonin is a key element, and there is a polymorphism associated with the transporter gene for serotonin. The effect of early environmental exposure to maltreatment affected only individuals who carried a certain allele affecting the transport system.

Wermter and colleagues (2010) also presents an interesting review of gene/environment interactions in the problem of obesity, currently a huge public health concern in industrialized countries. The authors report the surge in obesity in recent years suggests environmental factors, including lifestyle, clearly have had an impact. More than 10 genes have been reported as having a role in regulating appetite and body size, with different mutations involved in producing obesity and associated conditions, such as diabetes. Although the two conditions overlap, the effect of restriction of calories and nutritional supplementation has differing effects on the phenotype of obesity and diabetes, depending on the allele form of certain genes carried by the individual (Wahlsten, 2003). Likewise, the effect of genotypes associated with obesity are expressed only when the environment (diet and lifestyle) support the genotype. Researchers in health fields, including those studying development of new drugs, cite the importance of **epigenetics** toward developing an understanding of how to treat health conditions, including such serious conditions as cancer. Epigenetics involves the study of how an individual's genotype may change in response to the prevailing environment, as opposed to how the genotype directs the environmental response. Many of these changes are thought to occur in noncoding parts of an individual's DNA and RNA. If these environmental alterations that direct genes to switch on or off could be thoroughly understood, then behaviors or drugs could help control these "switches" and therefore decrease an individual's likelihood of developing obesity and diabetes, for example (Duarte, 2013).

With respect to behavior, Saudino (2009) reported that, in summarizing across many study designs and methods, there is little doubt temperament has a genetic component. This means that shared environments, such as those siblings experience, do not explain differences in temperament, which must then be attributed to genetic influences. In a recent review article on the nature of temperament,

Shiner et al. (2012) introduce the concept of "differential susceptibility" as a paradigm for interpretation of life span influences on temperament. These authors define differential susceptibility as an extension of the "goodness of fit" concept, meaning some traits (such as fearlessness) will result in positive adaptations in certain environmental circumstances and negative adaptations in others. These authors conclude that future studies of genetic and environmental influences on behavior will need to include the notion of differential susceptibility in assessment of risk and resiliency. Guerra & Leidy (2008) summarized recent advances in the study of childhood aggression, stating there have been a large number of studies documenting moderate genetic and nonshared environmental influences, with small shared environment contributions. This means individuals who have temperament characteristics such as low agreeability and low conscientiousness, when placed in an adverse environment, are more likely to develop violent behaviors. There is a wealth of literature on many aspects of behavior that reflect these interaction effects between genetics and environment in a bidirectional manner.

Like the studies mentioned previously with respect to obesity, the clear take-home message in study of human development and behavior is that outcomes must take into account bidirectionality of multiple environmental and genetic interactions in an attempt to understand, and predict outcomes, in hopes of leading to implementation of health and social policies that optimize human potential.

DEVELOPMENTAL SYSTEMS THEORY

Developmental theory has traditionally been regarded as an attempt to explain, predict, and influence change in behavior over time. As evident from the preceding discussion, a simple hierarchical attempt to explain human development is considered to be obsolete. Instead, the concept of systems has been introduced in many contexts to attempt to address the complexity of interactions that influence human behavior and health. **Developmental systems theory (DST)** is a term often applied to a collection of models of biological development and evolution that attempt to incorporate the multiple scientific advances discussed previously. Developmental systems theory embraces a range of positions, from the view that biological explanations need to include more elements than genes and natural selection, to the view that modern evolutionary theory profoundly misconceives the nature of living processes (Oyama, Griffiths, & Gray, 2001). This theory emphasizes the co-occurring contributions of genes, environment, and epigenetic factors on developmental processes. Developmental systems theory has been described as an attempt to resolve the nature-nurture controversy by relational interactions

(Lerner, 2002). In other words, interactions between an individual at multiple levels (genetic, neural, and behavioral) and the environment at multiple levels (physical, social) occur over time and result in the emergence of a more mature individual. **Epigenesis** describes the development of an organism as it moves from a relatively unstructured state to a more ordered and differentiated state over the course of developmental time. During epigenesis the action of the organism influences its own development. For example, as a child attends to a favorite story being read, the process of attending improves the neural mechanisms that underlie attention (Bjorklund, et al., 2007). A general overview of developmental system theory is presented here. There are many more specialized approaches that use developmental systems approaches.

SYSTEMS THEORY OF MOTOR CONTROL

The psychomotor domain of human function has been viewed from a systems perspective for over two decades. In fact, developmental systems theory was pre-dated and developed in tandem with dynamical systems theory. **Dynamical systems theory** developed from the fields of physics and mathematics that refers to self-organization of complex particles. This theory deals with the long-term qualitative behavior of complex dynamical systems. The original theory addressed the motion of systems that are primarily mechanical in nature such as planetary orbits and the behavior of electronic circuits. Dynamical systems theory has been assimilated into many other fields relevant to the study of human development and performance. In particular, dynamical systems theory has recently been used to explain aspects of human development (Miller, 2009). Within this framework, human development is viewed as constant, fluid, emergent or nonlinear, and multidetermined (Spencer et al., 2006).

Dynamical systems theory has been extensively discussed in the literature by Esther Thelen and colleagues (Thelen & Bates, 2003). In the context of human development, dynamical systems theory emphasizes the notion that behaviors are self-organizing and will emerge according to the context or environment in which they are active. Thelen's work on infant movement and motor learning has greatly influenced the practice of occupational and physical therapy. Her work will be referred to in the context of development in later chapters in this text. Important to this discussion of development and theory, dynamical systems theory has been frequently applied to the neuroscientific study of how movements are produced, the field of study known as **motor control**. The dynamical systems view of development and motor control has three critical features that separate it from older models. First is the idea that

behavior at any given point in time is the result of variable interaction of a number of complex systems. This interaction occurs in accordance with control parameters and environmental constraints (Kamm, et al., 1991). **Control parameters** are the conditions in existence at the time the task is executed. A control parameter could be a function of change in any one of the subsystems within dynamical systems theory. An **environmental constraint** is any factor in the environment that slows, limits, or restricts a behavior or process within dynamical systems theory.

Second, a dynamic system is dependent on time. In this case time might be considered the age of the person, or where the person is within the trajectory of human development. The current motor performance skills of an individual provide insight into both past experience and potential future experiences.

The third feature of dynamical systems theory that readers should understand is that dynamical systems are relatively stable and include *control parameters* that support the systems' stability.

The generation of a motor program, which represents a pattern of CNS commands about the movement, is not prescriptively generated, but must be flexible, according to what is going on in the environment. For example, consider the task of ringing a doorbell. One option for the CNS to program is a simple elevation and advancement of the arm so the tip of the index finger hits the button. But, consider the situation where a person is holding a heavy box. In that case, the task of hitting the button may be done by moving the body in space so the individual can hit the doorbell with an elbow. In this example, a *control parameter* would be holding the heavy box. The motor program is flexible and emerges based on what is happening in a number of systems. Using the definition common to the field of physics, any of the minimum number of coordinates required to completely specify a motion are called **degrees of freedom**. In the context of this book, the flexibility in the motor program is referred to as its degree of freedom.

Environmental constraints are the prevailing environmental conditions that help shape the movement and typically limit the degrees of freedom. In our example, not having hands free to hit a doorbell would be a constraint, because options for moving would be restricted. As is implied by the preceding discussion, in systems theory, the CNS is no longer the prime determinant of human motor function but is rather one of the key subsystems mediating the motor behavior. Likewise, the outcome of systems processing is probabilistic, not deterministic (Shumway-Cook & Woollacott, 2012).

A second key element of dynamical systems theory is the idea of **emergent control** of behavior, meaning that an individual will alter a task in myriad ways to meet the current conditions. Emergent control goes along with the idea of **anticipatory control**, meaning that the motor program is adjusted even before any interaction with the environment.

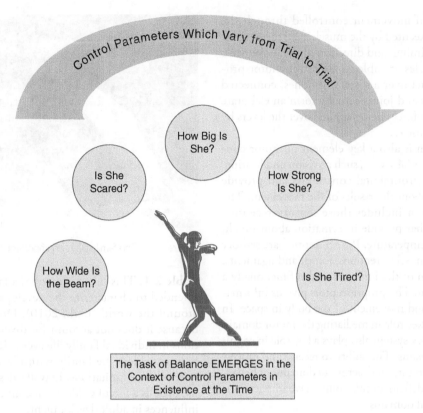

Control Parameters Which Vary from Trial to Trial

How Big Is She?

Is She Scared?

How Strong Is She?

How Wide Is the Beam?

Is She Tired?

The Task of Balance EMERGES in the Context of Control Parameters in Existence at the Time

Figure 2-4 Systems theory represented as number of interacting systems, indicated by circles, producing the emergent task of balancing on the beam.

For example, if someone said to you: "Be careful in picking up that box … it is very heavy!" the motor program generated would dictate more stiffness in the limbs and more muscle tension than if you expected the box to be empty. Moreover, behavior from a systems perspective is believed to be self-organizing. This concept implies that there is an extremely complex interaction between systems, which act together in an infinite number of ways to produce a behavioral result (Kamm et al., 1991). **Figure 2-4** shows a common representation of systems theory as a series of interlocking circles or control parameters acting within a given system, in this case for a motor task.

Dynamical systems theory addresses the importance of systems and subsystems other than the CNS in determining psychomotor behavior. One of the key systems in executing motor behavior is the *musculoskeletal system,* considered to be the **effector system of motor control**. The specific parameters of how the musculoskeletal system is to act are coded in a message called the motor program, sent from the CNS to the spinal cord and out to the muscles. The muscles act in accordance with this program. For example, the motor program may specify the amount of reciprocal versus co-contraction of agonist and antagonist muscles. An **agonist** muscle is the prime mover, as the biceps muscle is in the flexion of the elbow, as shown in **Figure 2-5**. The **antagonist** muscle to elbow flexion would be the triceps muscle.

When there is a lot of reciprocal inhibition specified by the motor program, the elbow flexor (biceps) would be

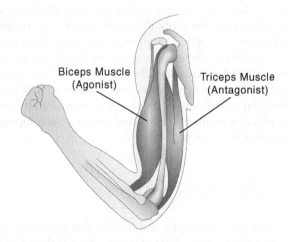

Biceps Muscle (Agonist)

Triceps Muscle (Antagonist)

Figure 2-5 The active muscle in this picture is the elbow flexor, the biceps. During elbow flexion, the antagonist triceps muscle is reciprocally inhibited.

relatively inactive during elbow extension, permitting a very pliable elbow joint as it moves into extension. An example of a task requiring a relatively pliable elbow joint is playing the violin. However, when the CNS specifies a large amount of co-contraction of antagonist muscles, the joint is relatively stiff. An example of a task requiring a relatively stiff elbow would be stabilizing the elbows to pick up a pot of boiling water. Therefore, the motor program specifies the amount and pattern of muscle contraction to control joint stiffness.

Other aspects of movement controlled through the motor program, as executed by the muscles, are the amount of force or tension, timing, and direction of the movement. Of course, the muscles are able to affect the motor program because they act over a system of bones, connected by joints. The bones and joints actually form an elaborate system of levers, with forces being applied over the levers by the contraction of muscles.

Sensory function is also a key element of motor control. The organs of special senses, such as vision and hearing, inform us about environmental constraints and provide important feedback about the results of the movement. The somatosensory system includes those sensory receptors located in the skin that provide information about touch, pressure, pain, and temperature. Proprioceptors are sensory receptors located in muscles, tendons, joints, and ligaments. The vestibular system of the inner ear is also functionally a proprioceptive system. The proprioceptors give us information about position and movement of the body in space. In addition to playing a key role in mediating the motor domain of function, the sensory system also plays a key role in cognitive and affective domains. The ability to receive and process sensory input is important, then, across all domains of behavior, and, conversely, deficits in this ability have implications for all three behavioral domains.

Another key physiologic system in mediating behavior, particularly motor behavior is the *cardiopulmonary system*. The cardiopulmonary system is made up of the heart and lungs. It is from the cardiopulmonary system that oxygenated blood is supplied to all organs, permitting normal function. When cardiopulmonary function is normal, the motor control systems have the oxygen needed to perform. Cardiopulmonary deficits can lead to motor control problems, even though muscle physiology is normal. In the context of motor control the cardiopulmonary system supports endurance in motor performance.

FAMILY SYSTEMS

Returning to the cognitive and affective domain of function, an integral contextual factor for individuals is their family. Families are a central feature of human development in all life stages. An understanding of families and family development is essential to creating a vision of the whole individual and to providing a contextually relevant understanding of life course pressures and supports (see **Figure 2-6**). **Family development theory** emphasizes the evolution of families over time. Early family development theorists assumed that all families develop in the same way and designated stages through which families are alleged to develop (Laszloffy, 2002). A central defining attribute of family development theory is that its focus is on families rather than individuals.

Duvall's model (1957) identified eight stages of family development. These eight stages are presented in

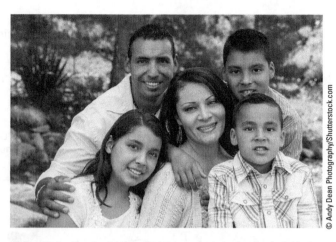
© Andy Dean Photography/Shutterstock.com

Figure 2-6   The family plays an important role in shaping individuals.

Table 2-1. This theory describes a family life cycle that is intended to characterize the development of most families around the world (Berk, 2010). Duvall's model is dated because it does not account for diversity or possible variations in individual family life cycles. In addition, this model only considers the family within a single generation. In spite of these limitations, Duvall's description of the family life cycle is a useful guide when considering the stresses and influences in adult development.

The systemic family development model (SFD) is a process-oriented model grounded in systems theory. This model recognizes that all families share a common process of development; however, within individual families, there is variation in how this process manifests. Laszloffy (2002) asserts that within the SFD model, the common process that all families experience is "the emergence of a stressor (a phenomenon that exerts force on a family system thereby pressuring it to change and adapt)" (p. 207). The end result of the process of changing and adapting is a developmental transition. When a family makes a transition, shifts in family roles and relationships inevitably occur. A strength of the SFD model is that the model assumes that families are complex, multigenerational systems that cannot be reduced to a single generational level.

SYSTEMS AND HEALTH: LIFE COURSE THEORY AND HEALTH DEVELOPMENT MODEL

Systems theories and their various applications, such as developmental, dynamical, and family systems, currently enjoy widespread support. Many new theories have arisen with their foundations directly tied to systems theories. One such theory is known as life course theory (LCT). LCT is a multidisciplinary paradigm for the study of people's lives, structural contexts, and social change. The authors will use

TABLE 2-1   Stages of the Family Life Cycle

Stage	Developmental Tasks
Stage 1: Family of origin experiences	Maintaining relationships with parents, siblings, and peers Completing secondary education
Stage 2: Leaving home	Differentiation of self from family of origin and parents Developing adult-to-adult relationships with parents Developing intimate peer relationships Beginning work, developing work identity Financial independence
Stage 3: Premarriage stage	Selecting partners Developing a romantic relationship Deciding to establish own home with someone
Stage 4: Childless couple stage	Developing a way to live together both practically and emotionally Adjusting relationships with families of origin and peers to include partner
Stage 5: Family with young children	Realigning family system to make space for children Adopting and developing parenting roles Realigning relationships with families of origin to include parenting and grandparenting roles Facilitating children to develop peer relationships
Stage 6. Family with adolescents	Adjusting parent-child relationships to allow adolescents more autonomy Adjusting family relationships to focus on midlife relationship and career issues Taking on responsibility of caring for families of origin
Stage 7: Launching children	Negotiating adult-to-adult relationships with children Adjusting to living as a couple again Adjusting to including in-laws and grandchildren within the family circle Dealing with disabilities and death in the family of origin
Stage 8: Later family life	Coping with physiological decline in self and others Adjusting to children taking a more central role in family maintenance Valuing the wisdom and experience of the elderly Dealing with loss of spouse and peers Preparation for death, life review, reminiscence, and integration

the life course theoretical (LCT) paradigm described by Lu and Halfon (2003) to consider both human development, quality of life, and current health trends such as childhood obesity, asthma, diabetes, and developmental and behavioral issues, all of which are influenced by the social, economic, and physical context of an individual. Life course theory has received major contributions from Glen H. Elder, Jr., who summarized four central principles to the theory. First, human development occurs over changing times and places. Second, a human life occurs within a specific point in time.

For example, overall intelligence quotients have increased 9 to 20 points over the last 100 years in industrialized nations, the so-called Flynn effect. This means someone born in 2012 would likely have a higher measured intelligence than someone born in 1912. It is not likely this change can be attributed to wholesale genetic change; therefore, changes in education, health, and nutrition over the last century must play the most significant role (Watson, 2003, p. 381). Third, there is interplay between human development and social phenomena. For example, spending early years in a postrevolutionary society may influence the course of a person's life. Finally, Elder views choice as a parameter that affects lifelong development. For example, an individual may be placed into an education system, such as a magnet school for the arts, which could have a lifelong impact on the person (Elder, 1998; Lerner, 2002). As a member of the family of developmental systems theories, the LCT has recently enjoyed a significant influence on health policy in the United States.

In 2010, the U.S. Department of Health and Human Services Maternal and Child Health Bureau published a paper entitled, *Rethinking MCH: The Life Course Model as an Organizing Framework*. The proposed outcome arising from adoption of the life course model is to guide policy development that maximizes health of individuals and populations (USHHS, 2010a).

The theoretical underpinning of this position paper is an updated understanding of how biology and environment interact, in conjunction with a discussion of issues such as health equity and disparity. The **life course health development model** (Halfon & Hochstein, 2002) holds that health is more than the absence of disease and is affected by multiple determinants over the life course, a fundamental premise underlying this text.

Life course theory (LCT) and the associated life course health development model were adopted by the Bureau of Maternal and Child Health as a way to examine and explain health and disease patterns across populations of people over time. LCT is a tool to help researchers identify factors that influence the capacity of individuals and/or populations to reach their full potential. It also serves as a tool to understand the persistence of health disparity across population groups. **Health disparity** refers to the differences in the quality of health and health care across different populations that includes differences in the incidence of disease, health outcomes, or access to health care across racial, ethnic, and socioeconomic groups. The nation's most recent public health agenda, known as Healthy People 2020, defines health disparity as "a particular type of health difference that is closely linked with social, economic, and/or environmental disadvantage. Health disparities adversely affect groups of people who have systematically experienced greater obstacles to health based on racial or ethnic group; religion; socioeconomic status; gender; age; mental health; cognitive, sensory, or physical disability; sexual orientation or gender identity; geographic location; or other characteristics historically linked to discrimination and exclusion" (UHHS, 2010b). Like the ICF presented in Chapter 1, Healthy People 2020 acknowledges health is more than simply the absence of disease. A **determinant** is an influencing or determining element or factor. In health, determinants include biology, genetics, and also factors such as socioeconomic status and access to health care (UHHS, 2010b). Healthy People 2020 is discussed extensively in Chapter 20 of this text. LCT incorporates an in-depth understanding of human development, and also considers personal and social factors

that may lead to health disparities in groups of people within a society. In keeping with the emerging agenda of public health, LCT considers broad social, economic, and environmental factors as possible causes of persistent inequalities in health across population groups (Halfon & Hochstein, 2002). The LCT offers a population-focused scope to the ICF, with its foundational focus on the individual as part of a community.

The LCT offers several important concepts that will be addressed throughout this text. The first of these is attention to **health trajectories**. In physics, a trajectory is the path made by an object moving forward under the influence of external forces like gravity or a physical thrust. In health, a trajectory is a predicted pattern of health or disablement that is likely given the internal and external influences on individuals as they develop and mature. Health trajectories may be started and change over an individual's life course. The LCT considers health trajectories not just for individuals, but also trajectories for groups such as populations and communities.

Early programming is another conceptual focus of the LCT. The literature in human development shows that early experiences can "program" an individual's future health and development (USHHS, 2010a). This early programming can have either a positive or a negative effect on the health of an individual. The recognition that there are critical or **sensitive periods** is not new, but this recognition is taken beyond its original scope in the realization that although adverse events and exposures can have an impact at any point in a person's life course, the impact will be greatest if the adverse event occurs during a sensitive period of development. An example of this would be an individual's loss of hearing. If this loss occurs in infancy, the impact on language learning and communication is profound. The sensitive period for human language learning is between birth and age 6. Hearing loss can derail this intense language learning period. The same hearing loss acquired in adulthood will certainly impact an individual, but will not limit the individual's understanding of language, as an adult who has already learned to communicate will be able to compensate effectively for the loss.

In addition to recognizing sensitive periods in terms of a health trajectory, the LCT model also considers the **cumulative impact**, the impact resulting from increasing or frequent influences during the developmental period being considered. Cumulative experiences, both positive and negative, can result in programming that impacts an individual's future patterns of health and development. This concept is similar to the early programming concept, but differs in that it accepts that even a small stressor, repeated often over time, may have a profound impact on the individual's health and development. Similar in effect to cumulative impact, the LCT emphasizes the importance of risk and protective factors. **Risk factors** are characteristics of family and community environments that are known to predict increased likelihood of a negative health outcome. For example, parents with sedentary lifestyles that frequently serve fast food at family meals provide a risk factor for childhood obesity. **Protective** factors exert a positive influence or buffer against the negative influence of risk, thus a family that shares healthy meals may reduce the negative influence of more unhealthy peer and community eating habits. Through the influence of risk and protective factors, health trajectories are changeable.

The USHHS concept paper titled *Rethinking MCH: The Life Course Model as an Organizing Framework* (2010a) summarized the key life course concepts described earlier into four key ideas:

- Today's experiences and exposures influence tomorrow's health. (Timeline)

- Health trajectories are particularly affected during critical or sensitive periods. (Timing)

- The broader community environment—biological, physical, and social—strongly affects the capacity to be healthy. (Environment)

- While genetic makeup offers both protective and risk factors for disease conditions, inequality in health reflects more than genetics and personal choice. (Equity) (USHHS, 2010a, p. 4)

As is made clear by these features, systems theories in general, and the LCT in particular, has given rise to **prevention science** as a field of study. Gest and Davidson (2011) define prevention science as an interdisciplinary field with roots in disciplines such as developmental, community, and clinical psychology; psychiatry; public health; epidemiology; and psychopathology. In the area of mental health, these authors give examples of government initiatives that focus on risk reduction and competence promotion. **Risk reduction**, as the name implies, involves reducing risk factors. **Competence promotion** involves education and public health initiatives designed to increase resilience. **Resilience** is a concept that describes the emergence of a desired outcome despite periods of stress and change. The ability to weather each period of disruption and reintegration leaves people better able to deal with the next change. As prevention science addresses the complexity of gene-environment interactions, some authors have called for the ICF to be modified to reflect health-facilitating natural environmental factors (Day, Theurer, Dykstra, & Doyle 2012). Prevention science is discussed more thoroughly in Chapter 20.

HEALTH PROFESSIONALS AND THE KNOWLEDGE OF HUMAN DEVELOPMENT

The Joint Commission is the national accrediting body for hospitals and hospital-affiliated clinics. In 1991, The Joint Commission published standards requiring all practitioners responsible for the assessment, treatment, and care of patients be competent in the delivery of "age-appropriate

care." This resulted in the necessity of training programs being developed for all health professionals in order to demonstrate compliance (Haxton & Van Dyke, 1992). Merging the concepts of the ICF with those of LCT, and in keeping with the Healthy People guidelines for setting public health policy, the new health care system evolving in the United States places a great emphasis on the participation of individuals in every meaningful aspect of life. That participation is variable across the life course: For example, for a 6-year-old with cerebral palsy, participation means being able to attend school, as well as play with friends on the playground and in community recreation activities. However, for a 40-year-old with low back pain, participation means being able to earn a living, attend the activities of children, maintain a household, engage in intimate relations with a spouse, and participate in meaningful leisure activities. Although it is important to individualize goals of intervention, it is important that all rehabilitation professionals have a general frame of reference about age-appropriate assessments, interventions, and goals. This text attempts to give an overview for developing that perspective.

LIFE COURSE THEORY, THE ICF, AND SYSTEMS

From the discussion in this chapter of various systems theories that apply to human life span development, there are important relationships that can be drawn to the ICF presented in Chapter 1. It is important for rehabilitation professionals to understand these relationships. First, all systems theories, like the ICF, avoid simple determinants of outcome. Rather, the notion of dynamic interaction of multiple systems or factors is foundational. In other words, issues such as a disease diagnosis or place of birth do not predict what is going to happen. It is understood that there is a dynamic interplay involved in predicting outcome. This is critical for rehabilitation professionals to understand. For example, children with Down syndrome have an extra 21st chromosome as part of their genotype. Even at the level of the genotype, this is not deterministic. Individuals with Down syndrome can have wide-ranging profiles of activity and participation. Some of that relates to other genetic factors, as the 21st chromosome does not represent the entire genetic code. We know it is very important that children with Down syndrome receive early intervention services to maximize available neuroplasticity for learning. For example, critical or sensitive periods for acquiring language certainly are in the first 5 years of life. If a child, such as the one in **Figure 2-7**, receives appropriate services from developmental specialists who teach the parents how to create an enriched and supportive environment, the cumulative negative impact of the extra chromosome is minimized. Today, the IQ of a child with Down syndrome is typically higher than a child 40 to 50 years ago (Lerner, 2002).

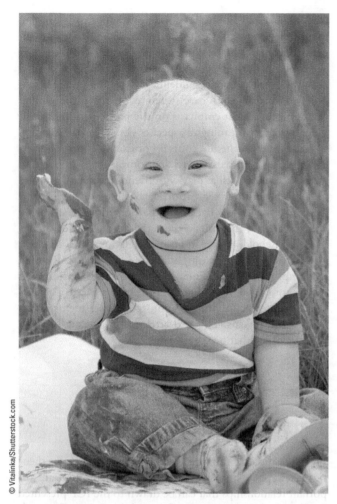

© Vitalinka/Shutterstock.com

Figure 2-7   With an early enriched and supported environment, this young boy with Down syndrome has a bright future.

In accordance with LCT, this favorable outcome implies that a child with Down syndrome is born in a place where early intervention services are available.

The United States has early intervention services of some form in every state as part of the **Individuals with Disabilities Education Act (IDEA)**, which will be discussed in Chapter 21 of the text. The Individuals with Disabilities Education Act (IDEA) is a United States federal law that governs how states and public agencies provide early intervention, special education, and related services to children with disabilities. It addresses the educational needs of children with disabilities from birth to age 21. Although the term *early intervention* was used in IDEA to describe early programming to minimize disability, many countries have similar initiatives that are given different names. Many countries, particularly poorer or developing countries do not have such programs. In this case the policy might continue to segregate or even institutionalize children with Down syndrome. In addition to national policies and early programming models, parents who have sufficient resources all over the world can support their children with special needs through programs such as swimming, horseback riding, gymnastics, or dance. In the LCT, optimizing a child's environment would be viewed as a *protective factor* to reduce the known *risk factors* associated with Down syndrome. In the ICF, these factors would be viewed as contextual factors, which are either facilitatory or inhibitory. In all theoretical frameworks, the systems and the ways they interact predict the outcomes for children with Down syndrome. It is important that both health and education professionals involved with such children over their life course understand the systems and theoretical frameworks of the ICF and LCT because they are both part of the systems as well as potential organizers of the systems' impact.

SUMMARY

Throughout this text, readers will see an emphasis on cohorts of people with shared experiences in both developmental and social aspects of daily life. Occupational engagement will be a central focus as patterns of engagement reflect the skills and abilities of individuals as they progress developmentally. Patterns of occupational engagement and social participation have a strong and persistent influence on health.

Trajectories in development require health care practitioners to take a longer view and to consider patterns of stability and change. Transitions between developmental stages will be discussed in future chapters. The case reports at the end of each chapter are intended to help students in the health professions apply the chapter's information in a clinical context and to help promote the consideration of developmental trajectories. The cases offered in this chapter will help illustrate this pattern. In both cases, the individual has type 1 diabetes, a serious medical condition

requiring medical attention and lifestyle adaptations. The adolescent in Case 1 views her condition by how it makes her different from her peers, reflecting the developmental focus of her age cohort on peers. In the second case, an older woman who has been living with the condition for 60 years is not focused on either her diabetes or her peers, but on maintaining important life roles.

The developmental life course model also considers more individualized influences such as life events or turning points. In this text the life event focus has been on patterns of impairment and disability. Although examples of impairments and disabling conditions are offered in each of the life stage chapters, specific information on family function and the impact of disability within family and social contexts is offered in separate chapters (Chapters 11, 15, and 19), pulling together the information from preceding chapters with examples and further exploration of the interaction of development and lived experience.

CASE 1

Meredith (at 16 years of age)

Meredith is a 16-year-old girl who has just been diagnosed with type 1 diabetes. She lives at home with her parents. She is a middle child. Her older brother is a senior this year and plays football. Her parents are very involved with going to his games and supporting him. Meredith's younger sister is 8 years old and is very good at gymnastics. Meredith herself plays the flute and has been in the school band the past 2 years. Although she loves the band, somehow she always felt her parents were disappointed she wasn't good at sports like her siblings.

Meredith began to have "spells" of feeling dizzy and weak. That is what caused her to go to the doctor and ultimately to get diagnosed. Meredith has been taught to do blood glucose monitoring. She has also had to learn to give herself insulin injections.

Meredith has always been shy and has had one best friend, unlike her siblings, who are very popular. Meredith is worried about being able to continue to participate in the band, especially band camp. She is also worried that she will be made fun of and kept out of any groups. She really would like to have a boyfriend, but thinks no one will want to go out with someone who has diabetes because of the "hassle." She has become increasingly sad and moody. However, because she is by nature very compliant, she is almost obsessive about monitoring blood glucose and insulin.

Guiding Questions

Some questions to consider:

1. How do you think Meredith's age is a factor in her response to the diagnosis?
2. Using the material in the text, apply the term *epigenetics* to the condition of diabetes.
3. Diabetes places individuals at risk for a number of associated health conditions. Apply the terms *risk reduction, competence promotion,* and *resilience* to this early-stage postdiagnosis for Meredith. How could you, as a health professional, implement these concepts?
4. Apply Elder's four tenets of life course theory to Meredith's case.
5. How are family systems both potential barriers and facilitators to Meredith's coping with this new diagnosis?

CASE 2

Meredith (at 76 years of age)

Meredith is a 76-year-old woman who lives in her own home with her husband. She has a diagnosis of type 1 diabetes, for which she has been taking insulin since she was a teenager. As a teen, she was very focused on managing her diabetes and on how that condition impacted her ability to engage in social and recreational activities. She has managed her diabetes successfully for many years and has been successful in her chosen adult roles of spouse, mother, homemaker, and church leader. Now, after her children have left home, Meredith has been spending more time with her church group. At this time, she also has some long-term complications of this condition, including severe visual impairment due to diabetic retinopathy and coronary artery disease.

Meredith is an elder in her church, and she and Darrel (her husband) are active participants in their church's senior activity program. Meredith typically spends 10 to 12 hours a week in church-related activities. At home Darrell is "sometimes confused" and relies on her to manage and direct their daily activities.

Because of increasing "dizzy spells," Meredith sought medical attention. At this time, she was admitted to the hospital where tests revealed an infarction of the right middle cerebral artery and evidence of several past small strokes (partially reversible ischemic neurological deficits). Within 24 hours, the transient ischemic attack (TIA) symptoms had stabilized and Meredith was referred to a skilled nursing facility (SNF) for rehabilitation and further assessment. In the SNF, Meredith walks independently but has poor endurance and is unable to sustain physical activity during self-care routines, needing frequent rests. She uses her right hand for most tasks, and will use the left arm as a gross assist in some activities. Her left shoulder and elbow are weak, with muscles scoring in the "fair" grade of strength. She has only gross movement and control of her distal arm.

Meredith wants to return home. She says that she is able to function far better at home, where she knows where things are and how they work. Things such as eating and personal hygiene, which she manages independently at home, require assistance now, because of her poor vision. She also needs moderate physical assistance with showering/bathing, lower extremity dressing, and hair care. She would prefer to get rehabilitation and support at home. Meredith has made many accommodations for her poor vision at home, and feels that in that environment she is fully functional. Also, Meredith sees herself as Darrell's caregiver and has been worried about leaving him at home alone. Darrell has been receiving meals-on-wheels since Meredith has been in the hospital. He has never done housework before, and, according to his pastor (who has visited him at home), he is just letting things pile up.

Meredith's diabetes greatly impacts her ability to perform activities of daily living in the rehabilitation setting. Because this condition has developed gradually, Meredith had been able to plan for and accommodate this condition in her home environment. Until her recent TIA events, Meredith has been able to participate fully in her home and community activities, in spite of serious chronic health conditions. Meredith's focus is not on her condition, but on her valued life roles, including her roles of caregiver, homemaker, and church leader.

Guiding Questions

Some questions to consider:

1. How can you apply the concepts of the life course health development model to Meredith's case from adolescence to late adulthood?
2. Meredith has problems with walking due to weakness and fatigue. Can you apply the terms of systems theory to her motor skills, using any selected task, such as climbing stairs or doing laundry?
3. How does the concept of cumulative impact discussed in the chapter apply to Meredith?
4. Using the ICF model presented in Chapter 1, work through Meredith's health status before and after her stroke.
5. Discuss with your peers how you, as a health professional, can apply the life span theories and perspectives presented in this chapter to Meredith's case.

Speaking of
Turning Points

ANNE CRONIN, PHD, OCCUPATIONAL
THERAPIST AND TEACHER

The process of becoming a health professional requires an immersion in anatomy, physiology, neurobiology, and many other highly complex and technical areas of study. When we first begin to interact as professionals in clinical settings, it is the mechanics of practice, the assessment and documentation procedures, and the utilization of specialized intervention strategies that new therapists focus on as we try to understand how to help our clients return to valued life roles and to remain functional in their lifestyles. This is an important focus for all clinicians.

After several years of clinical practice, I began to encounter people who I had seen as clients years before. What surprised me was that what they remembered about their rehabilitation experience was far less focused on the treatments than on the relationships they built, the information they learned, and the attitude of the people around them about what they should focus their energy on. They would laugh at the hours spent doing some task, such as putting on socks, when they did not use this task in their everyday life. They also talked about places where we therapists missed the mark. One older woman told me of her physical therapist who worked with her to walk with the use of a walking frame, and the occupational therapist reviewed safety features of the car, made sure that she could still operate all of the car's devices. When she got home she found that she had difficulty maneuvering her walking frame down the stairs to her garage, she could not lift the walking frame into her car, and without the walking frame, could drive only to places with drive-through services because her walking frame was waiting for her in her garage.

For this woman, who lived alone in a suburban area with no public transportation, her inability to use both her walker and her car in the same trip was significantly disabling. With a greater attention to the person's context and life stage, the therapy goals might have focused a little less on the return of physical skills and more on the application of the skills to maintain her community mobility. Within the life course model, a hip fracture may serve as a turning point leading to an increasingly isolated way of life due to decreased mobility. Similarly, the loss of the ability to drive a car may be a turning point with similar results. Taking a life course view should help health care practitioners to understand the turning points facing their clients and try to minimize the negative impact to the greatest degree possible.

I have been teaching students of health professions for about 20 years now. I have always tried to use many clinical cases and clinical examples in my teaching. Because of this I find myself writing many case studies for my students' use. A few years ago, in the throes of writer's block, I realized that I could use the same basic case, in terms of background medical and functional performance features, and change the age, the family context, the community, and the personal goals, and have a whole different clinical reasoning problem. The influences of the culture and of life events can completely change the focus of both personal interests and quality of life experiences. It is important to keep individuals, their developmental experiences, as well as their dreams, desires, and values always at the forefront of any assessment, treatment, or discharge planning.

REFERENCES

Berk, L. (2010). *Exploring lifespan development* (2nd ed.). Prentice Hall.

Bjorklund, D. F., Ellis, B. J., & Rosenberg, J. S. (2007). Evolved probabilistic cognitive mechanisms: An evolutionary approach to gene X environment X development interactions. In R. V. Kail (Ed.), *Advances in child development and behavior* (vol. 35; pp. 1–36). New York: Elsevier.

Christiansen, C., & Townsend, E. (2010). *Introduction to occupation: The art and science of living* (2nd ed.). New Jersey: Pearson.

Day, A. M., Theurer, J. A., Dykstra, A. D., & Doyle, P. C. (2012). Nature and the natural environment as health facilitators: The need to reconceptualize the ICF environmental factors. *Disability and Rehabilitation, 34*(26), 2281–2290.

Duarte, J. (2013). Epigenetics primer: Why the clinician should care about epigenetics. *Pharmacotherapy, 33*(12), 1362–1368.

Duvall, E. M. (1957). *Family development, 1st edition*. Philadelphia: J. B. Lippincott.

Elder, G. H., Jr. (1998). The life course and human development. In W. Damon (Series Ed.) & R. M. Lerner (Vol. Ed.), *Handbook of child psychology: Vol. 1. Theoretical models of human development* (5th edition, pp. 939–991). New York: Wiley.

Gest, S. D., & Davidson, A. J. (2011). A developmental perspective on risk, resilience, and prevention. In M. K. Underwood & L. H. Rosen (Eds.), *Social development: Relationships in infancy, childhood, and adolescence* (pp. 427–454). New York: The Guilford Press.

Guerra, N. G., & Leidy, M. (2008). Lessons learned: Recent advances in understanding and preventing childhood aggression. In R. V. Kail (Ed.), *Advances in child development and behavior* (vol. 35; pp. 287–330). New York: Elsevier.

Halfon, N., & Hochstein, M. (2002). Life-course health development: An integrated framework for developing health, policy, and research. *Milbank Quarterly, 80,* 433–479.

Haxton, R. K., & Van Dyke, P. (1992). Age-appropriate care: A system designed to make it happen. *Journal for Healthcare Quality, 14*(4), 20–23.

Hubel, D. H., & Wiesel, T. N. (1962). Receptive fields, binocular interaction and functional cat's visual cortex. *Journal of Physiology (London), 160*(1), 106–154.

Kamm, K., Thelen, E., & Jensen, J. (1991). A dynamical systems approach to motor development. In J. Rothstein (Ed.), *Movement science* (pp. 11–23). Alexandria, VA: American Physical Therapy Association.

Laszloffy, T. (2002). Rethinking family development theory: Teaching with the systemic family development (SFD) model. *Family Relations, 51,* 206–214.

Lerner, R. M. (2002). *Concepts and theories of human development* (3rd edition) New Jersey: L. Erlbaum & Associates.

Lu, M., & Halfon, N. (2003). Racial and ethnic disparities in birth outcomes: A life-course perspective. *Maternal & Child Health Journal. 7*(1), 13–30.

McGraw, M. (1935). *Growth: A study of Johnny and Jimmy*. New York: Appleton-Century-Crofts.

McGraw, M. (1945). *Neuromuscular maturation of the human infant* (1962 reprint of 1945 edition). New York: Hafner Press, 1962.

Miller, P. (2009). *Theories of developmental psychology* (5th ed.). New York: Worth Publishers.

Oyama, S., Griffiths, P. E., & Gray, R. D. (2001). *Cycles of contingency: Developmental systems and evolution*. Cambridge: MIT Press.

Payne, V. G., & Isaacs, L. D. (2012). *Human motor development: A lifespan approach*. New York: McGraw-Hill.

Saudino, K. J. (2009). The development of temperament from a behavioral genetics perspective. In Patricia Bauer (Ed.), *Advances in child development and behavior* (vol. 37). Burlington, MA: Academic Press, Elsevier.

Segalowitz, S. J., & Schmidt, L. A. (2003). Developmental psychology and the neurosciences. In J. Valsiner & K. Connolly (Eds.), *Handbook of developmental psychology* (pp. 48–71). London, England: Sage Publications.

Shiner, R. L., Buss, R. A., McClowry, S. G., Putnam, S. P., Saudino, K. J., & Zentner, M. (2012). What is temperament now? Assessing progress in temperament research on the twenty-fifth anniversary of Goldsmith, et al. (1987). Child *Development Perspectives, 6*(4), 436–444.

Shumway-Cook, A., & Woollacott, M. (2012). Motor control issues and theories. In *Motor control: Translating research into clinical practice* (4th ed., pp. 1–20). Baltimore: Lippincott, Williams and Wilkins.

Spencer, J. P., Clearfield, M., Corbetta, D., Ulrich, B., Buchanan, P., & Schöner, G. (2006). Moving toward a grand theory of development: In memory of Esther Thelen. *Child Development, 77,* 1521–1538.

Thelen, E., & Bates, E. (2003). Connectionism and dynamic systems: Are they really different? *Developmental Science, 6,* 378–391.

Wahlsten, D. (2003). Genetics and the development of brain and behavior. In J. Valsiner & K. Connolly (Eds.), *Handbook of developmental psychology* (pp. 18–47). London, England: Sage Publications.

Watson, J. D. (2003). *DNA: The secret of life*. New York: Alfred A. Knopf, Random House.

Wermter, A., Laucht, M., Schlmmelmann, B., Banaschweski, T., Sonuga-Barke, E., Rietschel, M., & Becker, K. (2010). From nature versus nurture, via nature and nurture, to gene x environment interactions in mental disorders. *Early Childhood and Adolescent Psychiatry, 19,* 199–210.

U.S. Department of Health and Human Services Health Resources and Services Administration Maternal and Child Health Bureau (USHHS). (2010a). Rethinking MCH: The life course model as an organizing framework. Bureau of Maternal & Child Health. Retrieved from http://mchb.hrsa.gov/lifecourse/rethinkingmchlifecourse.pdf

U.S. Department of Health and Human Services (USHHS). (2010b). *Healthy People 2020*. Retrieved from http://healthypeople.gov/2020/

CHAPTER 3

Classic Theories of Human Development

MaryBeth Mandich, PT, PhD,
Professor and Chairperson,
Division of Physical Therapy,
West Virginia University, Morgantown,
West Virginia

Objectives

Upon completion of this chapter, readers should be able to:

- Define and describe the applications of theory;

- Define and correctly apply classifications of theory;

- Recognize and describe the contributions of key classic developmental theorists according to domain of function;

- Apply theoretical constructs to various domains of human performance; and

- Reflect on the role of theory in understanding human development.

Key Terms

accommodation	Dewey, John	open-loop theory
Ainsworth, Mary	empiricist school	operant conditioning
applied behavior analysis (ABA)	Erikson, Erik	Pavlov, Ivan
assimilation	Freud, Sigmund	Piaget, Jean
Bandura, Albert	Gesell, Arnold	reinforcement
behaviorism	Gestalt school	Sears, Robert
Bowlby, John	Gibson, Eleanor	self-actualization
Case, Robbie	Kohlberg, Lawrence	sensitive period
Chess, Stella	Maslow, Abraham H.	Skinner, B. F.
classical conditioning	McGraw, Myrtle	temperament
closed-loop theory	modeling	Thomas, Alexander
constructivist theories	motor behavior	Vygotsky, Lev
critical period	motor learning	Watson, John
developmental theory	nativist school	zone of proximal development

INTRODUCTION

The word *theory* is widely used, and most people would agree that they have a general idea of the meaning of the term. Perhaps in its broadest sense, a theory is understood to mean an explanation of a phenomenon. For example, an individual might have a theory about why a certain type of behavior occurs. Theory is typically defined as an attempt to explain human behavior through a series of propositions or hypotheses about how a phenomenon works. The purpose of a theory is to attempt to explain, predict, or control the phenomenon. As seen in **Figure 3-1**, a theory often attempts to address complex interactions between multiple variables. Thomas (2001), in the introduction to his book summarizing theories of human development, defines a theory as a proposal identifying critical variables and how these variables interact. Miller (1983) observes that a theory should meet certain criteria: It should be logically and empirically sound, meaning that it should be internally consistent as well as observationally validated. Furthermore, it should be testable, cover a broad scope of observed phenomena, and contain a manageable number of constructs and propositions. Typically, a **developmental theory** addresses changes that are attributed proportionately more to maturation than

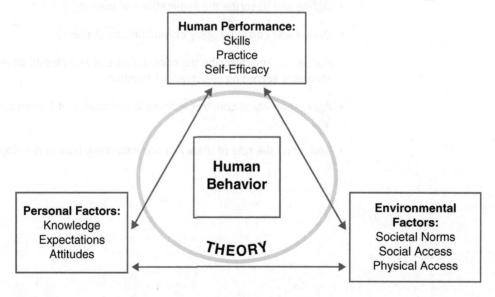

Figure 3-1 Theory attempts to explain human behavior as an interaction of various factors.

to environmental experience. For this reason, developmental change tends to be less sensitive than other types of change to such influences as the practice of the skill, past experiences, and cultural variation in sequence and type of skills expected. The complex interplay of nature and nurture, although strongly debated in early years of developmental study, is now accepted as an assumption.

A theory is typically formed to explain a series of observations that are considered fact. However, because the theory itself is not fact, it can be disproved. Some of the theories discussed in this chapter have indeed been disproved, although they are important to know about because of their impact on the field. Others, such as that of Piaget, have been significantly altered by growth in knowledge and further study. The theories discussed here are considered "classic" because of their impact. Those that have not been rejected remain under constant evaluation, with potential for rejection, revision, or strengthening.

Therapists and others who work with individuals to help them recognize their full human potential often use theory to guide their interventions. As mentioned in Chapter 1, when theoretical material is organized and functionally translated into practice, it becomes a *frame of reference*. For example, one person might approach a given clinical scenario from a developmental frame of reference while another approaches the same problem from a learning frame of reference.

CLASSIFICATION OF THEORY

Theories may be classified in a number of ways. Understanding where a theory falls under a given classification paradigm helps to get a perspective of relationships among theories. Traditionally, developmental theories have been classified along a continuum according to the classification systems discussed as follows.

NATURE VERSUS NURTURE

As discussed extensively in Chapter 2, the classification of nature versus nurture reflects a historical perspective regarding the amount of influence that genetics has in determining a behavior versus the role of environmental experience. In the past, the nature-nurture argument was a focal point of developmental psychology and even philosophy. In the twenty-first century, it is accepted that behavior is inevitably a product of both nature and nurture; however, theorists continue to debate the relative contribution of each. The nature-nurture debate is also described as innate-acquired, maturation learning, biology-culture, and nativism-empiricism (Miller, 1983). The role of contemporary scientific methods, including study of the human genome, has provided new dimensions to the nature-nurture debate, as discussed in Chapter 2.

QUALITATIVE VERSUS QUANTITATIVE

A *qualitative* theory says that individuals are distinct and may differ from one another based on some quality or characteristic rather than on some quantity or developmental milestone. For example, a theory that emphasizes the qualitative nature of behavior acquisition would state that behaviors at a point in time reflect maturational qualities in the individual. Until those qualities develop, the behavior cannot be observed. Qualitative theories often present behavior as developing in sequential stages. A *quantitative* theory sees development as primarily the acquisition of a number of skills; therefore, the appearance of an ability or the lack thereof is related merely to the presence or absence of a sufficient number of prerequisite exposures or skills.

STABILITY VERSUS INSTABILITY

A theory that emphasizes *stability* implies that the rules for anticipating behavior are consistent across the life span; hence, future behavior is predictable from current behavior. A theory that classifies behavior as *unstable* holds that different rules apply at different points in an individual's life; therefore, one must know the applicable set of rules before prediction can occur. Another classification that is sometimes used in a similar fashion is continuity versus discontinuity. *Continuity* in theory states that the same developmental laws apply across the life span; *discontinuity* states that there are different laws at different points in the life span.

REDUCTIONIST VERSUS NONREDUCTIONIST

A *reductionist* theory states that behavior is the sum of a number of smaller behavior links; a *nonreductionist* theory is one that sees behavior as a total that cannot be broken into component parts with any degree of meaning.

ORGANISMIC VERSUS MECHANISTIC

In a theory classified as organismic, human beings act on the environment and can change environmental circumstance by virtue of that action. In the *mechanistic* model, human beings react to the environment, so the environment rather than the person initiates a behavior. A machine does not start itself or act in the absence of an outside influence, hence the name mechanistic or "*like a machine*" (Miller, 1983; Reese & Overton, 1970).

As mentioned previously, classifying theories helps to provide some quick reference to the overall perspective taken by the theorist as well as allowing for comparison among theories. Classifications are not mutually exclusive.

For example, a mechanistic theory is also likely to be reductionist, stable, and quantitative. An organismic theory is likely to be unstable, nonreductionist, and qualitative.

A final way to classify theories, which will be used here for purposes of discussion, is by the area of behavior the theory purports to address. The domains of human performance addressed in Chapter 1 are affective, cognitive, and psychomotor. The following theories ultimately seek to explain, describe, and predict human function in a variety of contexts by domain of performance.

AFFECTIVE DOMAIN

The affective domain includes those characteristics that underlie feeling. It includes some aspects of intelligence, which will be discussed in the cognitive domain, as well as personality and temperament. This section will include theories that emphasize an understanding of the affective domain.

FREUDIAN THEORY

One of the most significant theorists detailing the development of personality was **Sigmund Freud**. Born in 1856 in Moravia (in the modern Czech Republic), Freud spent most of his life in Austria, where his theory of development became the foundation of the school of psychoanalysis. Key aspects of the theory include the dynamic conflict between destructive and loving instincts. The latter came to be known as *libido*. Freud defined human mental processes according to the *id, ego,* and *superego*. The id represents the most basic instincts and drives. The ego represents intellectual activities and logical thought. The superego represents the conscience and awareness of right and wrong. Freud viewed dreams as a reflection of unconscious mental processes and used dream interpretation in psychoanalysis.

Freud saw development as qualitative and in stages. He proposed a theory of child development based on his observations and clinical work with women suffering from hysteria. In the development of young children, before 5 years of age, Freud identified three stages: oral, anal, and phallic. The oral stage roughly was that of infancy, concerned with feeding and oral exploration. The anal phase roughly coincided with toilet training and was concerned with gratification and the development of control. The phallic stage was the early exploration of the genitals and awareness of sexual differences. These stages were followed by a lengthy period of latency, terminating in the genital stage of adolescence and the awakening of sexuality (Puner, 1947). The resolution of these stages determines not only characteristics of sexual functioning, but also how children relate to self and others (Miller, 1983).

Two early members of Freud's school, Alfred Adler and Carl Jung, eventually split from Freud and established their own schools of psychologic thought. Both Adler and Jung downplayed the role of sexual factors in personality. Jung's approach tended to emphasize ethics and religion, but remained true to some classic Freudian concepts such as the importance of dreams, whereas Adler eventually opposed most classic Freudian tenets (Puner, 1947). Adler emphasized social rather than biologic factors in explaining human motivations. He never practiced psychoanalysis, but rather employed a philosophy in which therapist and client are on equal footing. His approach became known as *individual psychology* (Chaplin & Krawiec, 1960).

Although many of his ideas have been disproved, Freud's impact on the study of psychology was significant in several ways. Although it seems intuitive today, Freud was one of the first to realize that development was a worthwhile pursuit of study—that is, that the antecedents of adult behavior could be found in the past. Moreover, Freud was one of the first to devote attention to the psychology of motivation and played a role in the evolution of clinical psychology as a discipline. Prior to Freud, the role of mental health professionals such as psychiatrists was primarily to diagnose and describe. Through psychoanalysis, Freud laid the groundwork for the notion of psychological intervention (Chaplin & Krawiec, 1960). Freudian theory also impacted a number of other psychologists, including Erik Erikson, Rene Spitz, Robert Sears, and Margaret Mahler (Thompson & Goodman, 2011). Freud's daughter, Anna Freud, spent most of her career developing techniques for analysis of children and adolescents. She spent more time in direct observation than her father, and she developed a diagnostic profile, which emphasized developmental lines to personality function, especially the action of the ego (Austrian, 2002).

ERIKSON'S THEORY

Among the key theorists in developmental psychology, **Erik Erikson** plays a unique role. His theory, which addresses primarily psychosocial development, was one of the few stage theories to cover the life span; hence, it is frequently found useful in studying human development. Like many others who had a major impact on the field of development in the twentieth century, Erikson's roots were in the Freudian tradition and, as such, are sometimes classified as "neo-Freudian." Like Freud, Erikson believed in the dynamic influences of psychological structures; however, he rejected Freud's strict biologic approach, addressing instead the sociocultural influences on development (Miller, 1983). After Erikson fled Europe to escape the Nazis, he worked with two prominent anthropologists, Margaret Mead and Ruth Benedict, which explains his attention to the role of culture and society in the development of personality (Austrian, 2002). **Table 3-1** compares the basic stages described by these two important theorists.

Erikson viewed development as a series of conflicts or crises that must be resolved. These crises can be resolved in either a positive or a negative mode, which determines future function. The Erikson stages are summarized in **Table 3-2**. Erikson's contributions to the field of

TABLE 3-1 Comparison of Freud's and Erikson's Theories on Dynamic Influences of Psychological Structures

Positive Outcomes of Erikson's Stages of Personality Development

1	2	3	4	5	6	7	8
Trust vs. Mistrust	*Autonomy vs. Shame/Doubt*	*Initiative vs. Guilt*	*Industry vs. Inferiority*	*Intimacy vs. Isolation*	*Identity vs. Role Confusion*	*Generativity vs. Stagnation*	*Ego Integrity vs. Despair*
The infant must form a loving, trusting relationship.	The child is motivated toward the development of functional movement.	The child is motivated by social challenges, becoming more confident.	The child is faced with peer comparisons and demands for new skills.	There is pressure to develop intimate relationships in friendships and romances.	The individual is motivated to achieve a sense of identity in adult occupational roles.	The individual is motivated toward the development of satisfaction in chosen occupational roles.	The individual is motivated to seek a sense of fulfillment and life satisfaction.

Freud's Biologic Stages

Oral	Anal	Phallic	Latency	Genital			

Adapted from Erikson, 1963; Feldman, 1999; Miller, 1983; Thomas, 2001.

TABLE 3-2 Summary of Erikson's Stages

Stage	Age (approx.)	Task or Purpose	Adverse Resolution
I. Trust vs. Mistrust	Birth to 1 year	Infants learn that needs will be met; parents will return after absence; contingencies.	Fearful toward others.
II. Autonomy vs. Shame/Doubt	1 to 2 years	Differentiation of "self" wishes from others; learns control over basic physiologic functions and social exchange (saying NO!).	Insecurity, dependency.
III. Initiative vs. Guilt	3 to 5 years	Begins to make or construct things in play; accepts parents as role models; "busy."	Belief that thoughts and actions are wrong, inferior, or bad.
IV. Industry vs. Inferiority	Childhood, 6 to 12 years	Entering school; child is very proud of accomplishments.	Consistent failure may lead to a sense of inferiority.
V. Identity vs. Identity diffusion	Adolescence	Importance of peer relationships; separation from parents; tries out new roles; integration of previous resolutions.	Inability to identify roles, establish a self-identity and awareness.
VI. Intimacy vs. Isolation	Young adult	Uses identity established in previous stages; forms intimate relationships with friends, family, spouse.	Inability to form meaningful relationships; fear of commitment.
VII. Generativity vs. Stagnation	Adult	Becomes part of larger picture; wants to leave lasting mark on society through family and/or work.	Believes that life is meaningless; extreme self-absorption.
VIII. Ego Integrity vs. Despair	Older adult	Belief that life was worth living; made a lasting contribution; life is what it was—minimal regrets.	Regret for what one has done or not done.

Adapted from Erikson, 1963; Feldman, 1999; Miller, 1983.

developmental psychology were significant. As mentioned previously, the idea that developmental change occurs across the life span was new. Some tenets of Erikson's theory have been confirmed by research (Feldman, 1999), and his view of culture and society as important factors in shaping an individual's personality fits well with contemporary views of culture. But Erikson's theory is limited in predictive ability as well as in specific mechanisms of development (Feldman, 1999; Miller, 1983).

Freud and the neo-Freudians were essentially pursuing a psychology of motivation to answer several questions, the primary one being what drives people to act as they do. In particular, Freud's dynamic exchange among personality structures of id, ego, and superego revealed the unconscious nature of motivation.

MASLOW'S THEORY

Another individual who specifically attempted to address human motivations was **Abraham H. Maslow**. Maslow's theory is organismic and is summarized by the concept of a *hierarchy of needs,* usually represented by a pyramid as shown in **Figure 3-2**. At the base of the pyramid are the physiologic needs, followed by safety. Then, progressing up the pyramid are love and belonging, esteem, and self-actualization. According to Maslow, a person acts according to the priority of needs at any given point in time. If a basic need, such as food, is denied, the individual will be obsessed with satisfying that need; however, as the basic needs become satisfied, the individual is free to seek higher-level needs. Love and belonging reflect the need for intimacy and close interpersonal relationships; esteem is the need to be thought well of by self and others and relates to mastery and competence. **Self-actualization** is the need to become all that one can be (Chaplin & Krawiec, 1960). The issue of disability is an interesting one to discuss under the Maslow paradigm. According to the ICF model, there may be intrinsic and extrinsic barriers to individuals with disabilities realizing self-actualization.

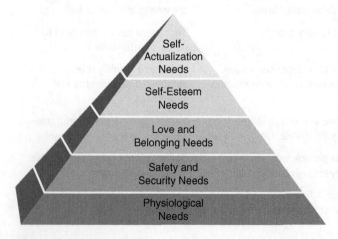

Figure 3-2 Maslow's Hierarchy of Needs

KOHLBERG'S THEORY

Related to the study of motivation is the study of moral behavior and altruism. Psychologists wish to understand not only what developmental processes underlie the development of morality, but also what factors produce antisocial and violent behaviors. **Lawrence Kohlberg** was specifically concerned with the development of higher-level behaviors of morality and social consciousness. He identified three levels of moral thinking: preconventional, conventional, and postconventional, or autonomous (Kohlberg, 1974).

In the *preconventional level,* typically represented in children aged 4 to 10, rules are obeyed primarily based on an understanding of rewards and punishment. As with all three levels, two stages are further characterized. In the first stage, rules are obeyed to avoid punishment, and in the second, rules are followed primarily to gain personal benefit—the concept of *pragmatic reciprocity.*

In the *conventional level,* typically represented by pre-adolescents, rules are obeyed to preserve status in society as good and responsible people. In Stage 3, individuals obey rules to maintain the respect of others; in Stage 4 they do so to conform to society's rules, expressing an understanding of the importance of maintaining order in the society.

The final level is *postconventional morality.* In this level, the moral principles to which individuals subscribe are seen as transcending the dictates of a particular societal structure. In Stage 5 individuals operate on the concept of a *social contract,* an understanding of generally agreed-upon rights. In this stage, individuals understand that personal values may dictate individual understanding of right and wrong but that there must be procedural rules founded on principles that protect all. The American Constitution reflects this stage of morality. Finally, Stage 6 consists of adherence to rules of conscience and self-chosen ethical principles (Feldman, 1999; Kohlberg, 1974). Of course, these stages of moral thinking are inextricably linked to the development of cognitive processes that underlie these judgments, and Kohlberg states that the highest stage is unobtainable before the age of approximately 13, due to lack of development in cognitive structures. Furthermore, according to Kohlberg, not all individuals develop to the highest stage.

Kohlberg's theory is a stage theory, based on the concept that there is a linear path of development in the individual's moral growth. Stage theories such as this have come under heavy criticism because they are culturally influenced and not representative of an individual with unusual or atypical life experiences. Although some studies have findings that can be viewed as supportive of Kohlberg's theory, it has been criticized on several points. First, Kohlberg's theory is more applicable to moral judgments than to moral behavior, meaning that individuals may make judgments reflecting the highest stage, but their judgments do not necessarily coincide with behavior. It is also argued that Kohlberg's theory emphasizes justice to the exclusion of other moral values, such as caring (Gilligan, 1982). Finally, Kohlberg's theory has been criticized as being descriptive of morality as conceived in postindustrial Western cultures and constrained to the time frame within which he worked (Harkness, Edwards, & Super, 1981).

TEMPERAMENT THEORIES

Whereas personality represents the enduring emotional and behavioral characteristics of an individual, **temperament** is conventionally used to refer to a predisposition of response (Feldman, 1999). Temperament is described in the ICF as a global mental function and will be discussed in some detail in Chapter 6. Theories of temperament evolved from the work of **Alexander Thomas** and **Stella Chess**. These scientists were dissatisfied with the explanatory and predictive ability of either the psychoanalytic or behavioral schools. The classifications they determined, have led to extensive research on the stability and predictive utility of these different temperament classifications (Kagan, 2005). A reason for the current significance of temperament work is based in neuropharmacology. The notion that the relative amounts of chemical neurotransmitters present in the brain in any individual at any point in time play a large role in determining an individual's pattern of behavior and response is the foundation of a great deal of research in today's laboratories. **Table 3-3** summarizes the concepts presented by Thomas and Chess.

Contemporary thought regarding temperament suggests it is an ordered but changing reflection of the brain's basic chemical organization, which is both genetically and environmentally influenced (Kagan, 2005). Human genetic science has also significantly contributed to the study of temperament across the life span. It is estimated that genetic influences on temperament range from 20 to 60 percent, with remaining influences attributed to the environment (Saudino, 2009). This explains how temperament tends to be relatively stable across the life span. However, it is important to apply the discussion from Chapter 2 of the dynamic interactions between genes and environment in reaching any conclusion about the stability of temperament. Furthermore, how temperament is measured is an important factor in interpreting current studies on the subject (Saudino, 2009).

BOWLBY'S THEORY

A discussion of the affective domain would be incomplete without some discussion of the affective elements of a human being's interactions with others in social relationships. Once again, an individual exposed early in his career to the Freudian school of thought developed a theory that had widespread significance. **John Bowlby** was a psychiatrist who had observed that family experience was related to emotional well-being. After World War II, Bowlby was invited to become the director of a mental health clinic. In this pursuit, he established a research division focused on the study of mother-child separation. Bowlby formulated a belief that an intimate and continuous relationship with the mother was necessary for an infant and young child to develop normal emotional attachments. He incorporated

TABLE 3-3	Chess and Thomas's Dimensions of Temperament
Activity Level	Motor activity and the proposition of active and inactive periods
Rhythmicity	The predictability or unpredictability of biologic functions
Approach/Withdrawal	The individual's response to new or altered situations
Adaptability	Overall (not immediate) response to new or altered situations
Sensory Threshold	Level of sensory stimulation needed to evoke a response
Quality of Mood	Relative proportions of positive and negative mood behavior
Intensity of Reactions	The energy level of the person's responses
Distractibility	The degree to which outside stimuli interfere in ongoing behavior
Persistence	The continuation of an activity in the face of obstacles
Attention	The length of time an activity is pursued without interruption

Adapted from Chess & Thomas, 1987.

ethological work into his theory, becoming fascinated with data on imprinting and critical periods in animal development. He also presented work detailing the phenomenon of separation anxiety.

In 1950, Bowlby formed a relationship with **Mary Ainsworth** that was to further immortalize his work. Ainsworth brought her talents in methodology to the research. She worked with Bowlby in England for a while, then traveled to Uganda, where she studied the quality of mother-infant interaction. Ainsworth developed the classic *Strange Situation* experimental paradigm consisting of sequential scenarios of mother-infant play, separation, rejoining, and introduction of a stranger (Bretherton, 1994).

Ainsworth and Bowlby described three categories of attachment: secure, avoidant, and ambivalent. Infants are classified in these categories in accordance with the child's response to being reunited with the mother after separation. Securely attached children use the mother as a "home base," referencing to her when she is present. They are upset when the mother leaves and happy to see her when she returns. Avoidant children do not seek initial proximity to the mother and avoid her when she returns. Ambivalent children may have decreased exploratory behavior in the mother's presence, are distressed when she leaves, and, when she returns, alternate between a desire to be comforted and aggression toward the mother (Feldman, 1999). Ainsworth also identified the importance of the mother's sensitivity to the child's cues as one determinant of quality of attachment.

These theories of development in the affective domain have an impact on all domains of human function: physical, cognitive, and social. The domains of human function represent competence in the environment, whatever it may be. As these theories become increasingly removed from current scientific literature, it is important to respect the contributions made by the theorists. Current study of social development, especially in the light of high-profile violent behavior in children and youth, is particularly attuned to understanding risks and vulnerabilities of early development with associated practice implications for intervention in high-risk children and youth (Thompson & Goodman, 2011).

COGNITIVE DOMAIN

The cognitive domain, according to the ICF, includes both global and specific mental functions. These functions provide the foundation of all aspects of human cognition, and will be described in detail in Chapter 6. An understanding of how cognitive functions develop, how they are impacted by the environment, and how they are sustained is important in designing learning, prevention, and remediation paradigms. Historical cognitive theories will be presented here. The field of cognitive neuroscience is growing rapidly, and cognitive theory has been changing to reflect the growing scientific understanding of cognition.

PIAGET'S THEORY

By far, the "classic" stage or qualitative theory of cognitive development is **Jean Piaget**'s theory of cognitive development, which has charted the path toward understanding how human beings come to know what they know. Born in 1896 in Switzerland, Piaget displayed an early interest in biology, publishing his first paper at the age of 10. After receiving his doctorate in 1918 at age 21 (with a thesis on mollusks), Piaget went to study at the Sorbonne in Paris, where he met Theodore Simon. Simon worked with Alfred Binet in Paris and suggested that Piaget assist in the standardization of intelligence tests by interviewing Parisian children. This experience stimulated Piaget to attempt to ascertain the nature of intelligence through meticulous empirical observation (Miller, 1983). Piaget returned to Switzerland as a director of studies at the J. J. Rousseau Institute, where he began the series of experiments that formed the basis for his theory of cognitive development.

Piaget's theory is complex and still evolving even after his death. From his background in biology, Piaget postulated two functional invariants: organization and adaptation. Organization is the tendency for integration of parts to a higher order (Austrian, 2002; Miller, 1983). Adaptation is a basic biologic need to permit functioning in a given environment. From adaptation, Piaget further identified the processes of *assimilation* and *accommodation,* which are integral to his theory. **Assimilation** is the process of changing elements of the environment so they can be incorporated into the organism's structure. The function of adaptation, illustrated in **Figure 3-3**, is to modify observations and experiences to fit the child's cognitive structures (Flavell, 1963). For example, when a young child labels all animals with four legs as dogs, assimilation has occurred. The child has modified the existing observation (cow, dog, horse) into the existing structure (dogs have four legs). **Accommodation** is changing of function in accordance with the environment (Flavell, 1963). For example, as a child learns, she might call a cow a "big dog." This shows modification of the concept of dog learned previously.

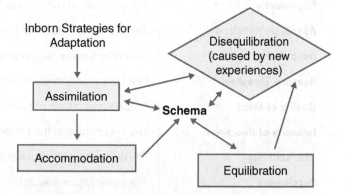

Figure 3-3   Adaptation and Formation of Schema as Described by Piaget adapted from Beilin, 1994. Reference Crediting : Beilin, H. (1994). Jean Piaget's enduring contribution to developmental psychology. In R. D. Parke, P. A. Ornstein, J. J. Rieser, & C. Zahn-Waxler (Eds.), A century of developmental psychology (pp. 257–290). Washington, DC: American Psychological Association.

In time, the child will learn to differentiate the salient features of "cow" by the process of accommodation.

The cognitive structures of Piaget's theory are known as *schema*. A schema refers to a class of similar sequences of action or mental representations that are related (Flavell, 1963; Miller, 1983). The process by which assimilation and accommodation are balanced is known as *equilibration*. Equilibration is achieved when neither assimilation nor accommodation is dominant. Conversely, *disequilibration* is when either the organism or the environment is changing and out of balance (Miller, 1983).

Piaget is a classic example of a hierarchical, or stage, theorist. He named four stages of cognitive development in which thought processes are qualitatively different from previous stages. There is some quantitative element to Piaget's theory, however, in that the number of schema and number of facts change over time (Miller, 1983). Despite the small quantitative aspect to his theory, the stages are some of the most classic elements.

Sensorimotor Stage

The first stage is the sensorimotor stage, which can be divided into six substages. Although the stages are not equivalent to chronologic change, the sensorimotor stage is generally considered to run from birth to 2 years of age. The first substage is *reflexive*, lasting from approximately birth to one month. During this stage, the infant performs little volitional activity; most of the activity is reactive to stimuli. For example, the infant displays sucking and kicking patterns. Substage 2 is *primary circular reactions*, from approximately 1 to 4 months. Neonatal reflexes begin to be altered, so that the infant can repeat interesting actions volitionally. For example, the infant will begin to swipe or bat at objects repetitively. In the third substage, *secondary circular reactions*, the infant begins to act more upon objects, with the goal of making events that are interesting last longer. Secondary circular reactions roughly coincide with 4 to 8 months of age. An example that is often given in this stage is picking up a rattle and shaking it. The fourth substage is *coordination of secondary circular reactions*. During this period, from approximately 8 to 12 months, the infant begins to use objects instrumentally, in order to accomplish a goal. Intention is a hallmark of this stage.

Another key acquisition is first evident in Substage 4 of the sensorimotor stage: the development of the concept of *object permanence*, in which the infant knows that something continues to exist even when it is out of sight. One of the exercises infants will do to "test" this hypothesis is to drop things off the high-chair tray, visually following the object to the floor. When the parent obligingly returns the object to the tray, the infant drops it again. Through this and a number of such exercises, the infant "learns" that objects exist even when out of sight.

The second year of life is composed of two Piagetian substages, 5 and 6, lasting from 12 to 18 and 18 to 24 months, respectively. In Substage 5, *tertiary circular reactions* occur, in which means and ends are combined in order to experiment with actions to determine consequences. In this stage, children can solve problems with new means, by trial and error. A classic example would be to use a rod or stick to draw a toy that is out of reach closer. Substage 6 is *invention of new means through mental combinations*. In this stage, children are able to mentally, without overt experimentation, devise means of manipulating the environment (Flavell, 1963; Feldman, 1999; Miller, 1983).

Preoperational Stage

The preoperational stage follows the sensorimotor stage and generally occurs between 2 and 7 years of age. In the preoperational stage, several key aspects of cognitive development occur. The first is *symbolic function*, where children are able to use signs and symbols to stand for something else. Piaget uses the concept of signs to refer to universally accepted signifiers that bear little or no concrete relationship to what they represent. Words are the most common signs. Symbols, on the other hand, are internal signifiers that usually have some resemblance to what they stand for. Piaget is very clear that language develops as a result of the development of symbolic function, not vice versa (Flavell, 1963).

Other characteristics of the preoperational stage include the notion of *egocentrism*, which is the inability to take another person's viewpoint. For example, when young children play hide-and-seek, they might hide in plain view, believing that because others cannot be seen, others cannot see them (Feldman, 1999). Another classic example of egocentrism is the Swiss mountain experiment in which toy mountain climbers are placed at various places along a mountain model. Children in this stage cannot understand how a person viewing the mountain from the other side of the table will see something different.

Still another characteristic of preoperational thought is *centration*. In centration, children focus on one salient aspect of a stimulus to the exclusion of others. For example, when a child looks at containers of different widths, she focuses on the width only, such that when a given amount of liquid is poured before her eyes into another container, she still does not see the volume as equal, because of an inability to decenter from focus on container width (Flavell, 1963). Children in preoperational thought cannot see the reversibility of actions. In the later preoperational stage, a transition from the more centered, rigid, and irreversible thought occurs in preparation for the transition to concrete operations.

Concrete Operations

The next period in Piaget's theory is concrete operations and generally occurs between 7 and 12 years of age. In the period of concrete operations, children are able to decenter, using an organized cognitive structure to organize and manipulate the environment. At this point they are capable of understanding the reversibility of actions and hence can grasp mathematical concepts of addition, subtraction, multiplication, and division. Now they grasp the concept of *identity,* that things are the same despite differences in shape or size. This permits the concept of *conservation* to evolve fully. Children in concrete operations are also able to understand relationships, such as those between distance, time, and speed (Feldman, 1999).

Formal Operations

The final stage of Piaget's theory is formal operations and generally occurs between 12 years of age and up. It is important to note that, according to Piaget, not every individual reaches the stage of formal operations. Typically, formal operations are characterized by highly symbolic thought and representation and appear when individuals have been exposed to more complexity in cognitive challenges. Individuals who reach this stage are able to perform mental operations on abstract representations. Formal operations also permit hypothetico-deductive reasoning (Feldman, 1999). **Table 3-4** presents the basic stages described by Piaget next to those described by Erikson and Freud. This table gives some perspective on the differences between these three important theorists.

The preceding is a very brief overview of Piagetian theory, on which volumes have been written. Piaget's significance to the field of developmental psychology is enormous. It is agreed that one of his most important contributions was to make observable the study of the mind,

involving cognition and learning. Previously it was believed that such topics could be approached only philosophically. Piaget's stages of cognitive development influenced educators to reevaluate their practices. His conceptualization of the child as a dynamic force caused his theory to be labeled as constructivist, indicating that children actively construct knowledge through interaction with the environment (Thompson & Goodman, 2011). **Constructivist theories** emphasize learning and an approach to education that lays emphasis on the ways that people create meaning of the world through a series of individual constructs. Constructivist theories reflect a learning process that allows students to experience an environment firsthand and the students are required to act upon the environment to both acquire and test new knowledge.

Although Piaget's theory was rooted in biology, it incorporated the social and physical environments as key aspects of cognitive development (Beilin, 1994). In the more than half a century since his theory was first made known, it has been criticized and modified by many. One of the main criticisms of the theory was leveled at a process Piaget called *decalage* (meaning displacement), which was the idea that children do not enter a different stage of cognitive development uniformly across all dimensions. In other words, each child will show lags in some areas while moving forward in others. A developmental psychologist named **Robbie Case** has attempted to address this problem by reclassifying the stages after the sensorimotor stage and identifying substages for the latter three stages, much as Piaget did with the sensorimotor stage. Case also proposed that there is a feedback loop connecting specific contextual knowledge and general knowledge. He concluded that early cognitive

TABLE 3-4 Comparison of Basic Stages Described by Erikson, Freud, and Piaget

Erikson's Stages of Personality Development							
1	2	3	4	5	6	7	8
Trust vs. Mistrust	Autonomy vs. Shame/Doubt	Initiative vs. Guilt	Industry vs. Inferiority	Intimacy vs. Isolation	Identity vs. Role Confusion	Generativity vs. Stagnation	Ego Integrity vs. Despair
Freud's Biologic Stages							
Oral	Anal	Phallic	Latency	Genital			
Piaget's Stages of Cognitive Development							
Sensorimotor	Preoperational	Concrete Operation	Formal Operations				

Adapted from Beilin, 1994; Erikson, 1963; Feldman, 1999; Miller, 1983; Thomas, 2001.

function is primarily a reflection of biologic factors, but as children age, cultural and social influences tend to take over (Thomas, 2001).

Like all the theories discussed in this chapter, there is a diminishing influence of Piaget's work on contemporary practice. Partly, this is because his study was limited to a small racial and cultural sample, which does not transpose well to a diverse society. In addition, the strict stagelike acquisition of cognitive processes has been disproven (Thompson & Goodman, 2011). Finally, the ability to study acquisition of knowledge through study of brain electrical activity and functional imaging has dramatically changed the landscape in cognitive psychology.

VYGOTSKY'S THEORY

Another developmental theorist who studied cognitive development was the Russian **Lev Vygotsky** (1896–1934). Vygotsky's initial impact was not as noticeable as that of Piaget, in part because of his relatively short life; however, his work continues to stimulate investigation in the latter half of the twentieth century. Vygotsky differed from Piaget in his emphasis on sociocultural influences on cognitive development. This theory somewhat reflected the communist thought of the early postrevolution period, that is, the importance of communal support for children. Vygotsky argued that to understand cognitive development, we need to evaluate what is significant in the cultural milieu in which the child is living. Vygotsky used the term **zone of proximal development (ZPD)** to refer to a child's being nearly prepared to comprehend a fact or perform a task such that a minimal support from others will allow her to successfully complete the task. **Figure 3-4** illustrates the four stages of this process.

The support from others is known as *scaffolding.* Vygotsky also cited the importance to cognitive development of *private speech,* the talking to oneself that children do as they solve a puzzle, for example. He theorized this private speech was integral to learning, but that children began to internalize this speech into mental processes by approximately 9 years of age (Feldman, 1999). Psychologists have used Vygotsky's work to continue to study, among other things, the impact of culture on a child's learning and development. A psychologist named Valsiner has expanded Vygotsky's concepts, including the addition of two zones: the zone of free movement and the zone of promoted action. The *zone of free movement* refers to all the resources available to children in an environment at a given point in time. The *zone of promoted action* refers to those actions or impulses that are promoted by the caregivers within the zone of free movement (Thomas, 2001). It is easy to see how this work is deemed invaluable in today's social and intellectual environment, which seeks to support cultural identity and diversity.

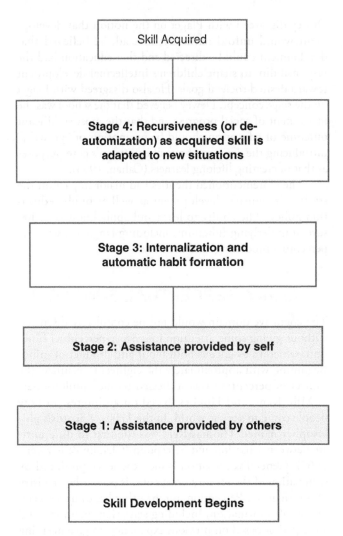

Figure 3-4   Vgotsky's Zone of Proximal Development adapted from Feldman, 1999, & Thomas, 2001. Reference Crediting: Feldman, R. S. (Ed). (1999). Child development: A topical approach. Upper Saddle River, NJ: Prentice Hall.; Thomas, R. M. (Ed). (2001). Recent theories of human development. Thousand Oaks, CA: Sage.

DEWEY'S THEORY

Piaget's work influenced educators in many ways, including the concepts of *active learning* and *readiness.* Vygotsky's work spawned educational innovations such as group learning and peer teaching. However, no one has had greater impact on the American educational system than **John Dewey** (1859–1952). Dewey was less of a developmental psychologist than a social psychologist and educational philosopher; however, his work had such impact on the education system that a brief overview is warranted. Like Vygotsky, Dewey believed that the cultural setting was key to understanding the human mind. Like both Piaget and Vygotsky, he believed in an empirical approach to understanding. Dewey felt that there were actually two fundamental psychologies, biologic and social, both warranting investigation. He criticized, however, the psychological laboratory as lacking relevance to the world and suggested instead that the school was the perfect "laboratory" for studying how children learn.

Dewey disagreed with Piaget on the notion that development would unfold naturally; instead, he believed that development could be directed and that education had the responsibility to shape children's intellectual development toward desired societal goals. He also disagreed with Piaget on the stage concept. Dewey believed that the school was the instrument of social progress and that the most significant outcome of education should be promotion of "growth," introducing the concept of one of education's core purposes as that of creating lifelong learners (Cahan, 1994).

The aforementioned theories had major impact on the study of cognitive development as well as public education policy. The ability to learn and apply knowledge has several underlying functions, including language, sensory-perceptual processing, and memory.

SENSORY-PERCEPTUAL FUNCTION

The cognitive domain would not be completely discussed without giving some attention to sensory-perceptual function, which in essence is both input and product of mind. Beginning with approximately the eighteenth century, the subject of perception was addressed by such philosophers as Mill, Kant, and Hobbes, based on an interest in how people come to see the world. In the 1700s, a Scottish philosopher named Thomas Reid was the first to differentiate between sensation and perception (Chaplin & Kraweic, 1960). Generally, sensation is the experience produced by stimulation of the sensory organs and is primarily a registry of information. Perception, on the other hand, uses several modes of information, including sensation, memory, and anticipation based on previous experience, to give meaning to sensory information.

The early theorists on perception were of two schools: the *nativist school* and the *empiricist school.* The **nativist school** believed that genetic predisposition and innate abilities explained perception while the empiricists believed the formation of associations between various sensations was its origin (Chaplin & Kraweic, 1960). The **empiricist school** was based on belief that the formation of associations between various sensations is the foundation of perception. Hermann von Helmholtz was one key theorist of the empirical camp who wrote in the mid-nineteenth century. He developed theories of hearing and color vision and believed that spatial qualities were perceived by something called *unconscious inference,* the addition to the sensory information of other information based on memory and previous experience. The association formed by all such information was what created the perception, according to Helmholtz (Chaplin & Kraweic, 1960).

Wundt was a contemporary of Helmholtz who added other analyses to the theory of perception. Also an empiricist, Wundt believed that a group of preexisting ideas and memories, which he termed an *apperceptive mass,* was applied to pure perceptions, thereby creating *apperceptions.*

Thus, an apperception is an active, conscious product of mental processing, whereas the relatively simple *perception* is passive (Chaplin & Kraweic, 1960).

Edward Titchener (1867–1927), an American pupil of Wundt's who went on to develop his theory, utilized a methodology called *introspection,* in which a psychologist analyzes self-consciousness. Titchener's theory was called a "core context" theory and had four key points. First, sensations are clustered in accordance with attention; second, the cluster of sensations is replaced by images; and third, the images provide meaning to the sensory experience. Finally, the perception, if it is common, may pass into unconsciousness and become represented in neuronal groupings (Chaplin & Kraweic, 1960).

German psychologists, including Max Wertheimer, Wolfgang Kohler, and Kurt Koffka, founded the **Gestalt school** in the late nineteenth century. The Gestalt school argued that introspection is insufficient to explain all perceptual phenomena, based on some classic experiments in which there were repetitive sensory illusions that defied the facts of the sensory experience. Gestalt psychology simply states that perception cannot be reduced to parts, but rather, the whole is greater than the sum of the parts. **Figure 3-5** illustrates perceptual thinking within the Gestalt model.

Some key contributions of the Gestalt school that continue to have validity today include the notion that individuals will create a "best fit" perception in the face of inadequate or incomplete sensory data. This conclusion reflects the Gestalt belief that the perception is not a perfect or photographic representation of the world; hence, it is not merely a sum of sensations. Rather, the perception has a psychological form that represents the world but is not

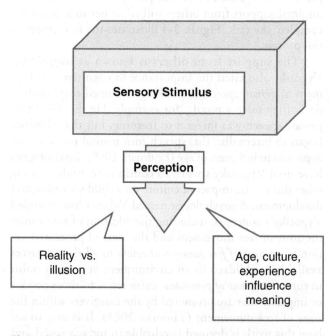

Figure 3-5 Principles of Gestalt Psychology adapted from Chaplin & Krawiec, 1960. Reference Creditng: Chaplin, J. P., & Krawiec, T. S. (Eds.) (1960). Systems and theories of psychology. New York: Holt, Rinehart and Winston.

identical to it. The Gestalt school also pioneered the study of *figure-ground perception,* that is, the ability to pick out key points of a stimulus from the background (Chaplin & Krawiec, 1960).

Moving to a more contemporary, twentieth-century study of perception, attention must be directed to the work of **Eleanor Gibson** and her husband James. The Gibsons challenged the prior notion of associationism, saying instead that the sensory stimulation itself contained numerous meaningful elements and that perceptual learning was actually learning to pay attention or differentiate more and more information from the pattern. Eleanor Gibson did a classic visual perception experiment to support this notion. She tested 7- and 9-year-olds and adults, presenting a scribble picture of a coil, followed by other pictures, asking the subjects to identify whether they were identical to or different from the initial picture. She gave no feedback and repeated the experiment. She found the expected difference in accuracy between adults and children. However, more significantly, she found that subjects' accuracy improved over trials, indicating to her that what was occurring was that subjects expanded the salient features of the pictures over trials. For example, initially the subjects might focus on the size or shape of the coil. With repetition, all the subjects, including the children, began to take note of more features, such as direction of the coil, distance between loops, and so on.

Other features of Gibson's theory included the importance of information obtained through exploratory activity and the notion of *affordance,* which is the salient property of stimuli in relationship to the explorer. Gibson supported this notion of affordance in research on infant locomotor patterns. She tested two groups of infants: a group of crawlers and a group of walkers. The infants had the choice to walk over one of two surfaces—a rigid surface or a waterbed-like surface—both with the same visual pattern. The walkers consistently chose the rigid surface, supporting the notion that for a walker, the rigidity of the surface is the salient feature.

Since the 1960s, Gibson's work has focused a great deal on the development and characteristics of perception in infancy. Perhaps she is best known for her visual cliff study with Richard Walk, in which crawling infants were allowed to crawl toward their mothers on a checkered surface that had an optical drop-off. The results showed that infants of 6 to 14 months would not crawl over the visual cliff. This pioneering work of Gibson's is anticipated to be combined with newer strategies of neurologic imaging to further our understanding of perceptual development (Pick, 1994).

PSYCHOMOTOR DOMAIN

In the first half of the twentieth century, significant gains were made in the theoretical underpinnings of child development, with a particular interest in motor behavior. For the purposes of this text, **motor behavior** is any performance of movement that can be observed or documented. Research in child development and motor behavior arose largely from a national focus, in the early part of the century, on the wars that had such an impact on the United States. The interest in child development arose around the prediction problem. When large numbers of men (and some women) entered the military, large-scale testing was carried out across a number of functions. It then became of interest to identify why individual differences in proficiency occurred and to determine if attributes could be predicted. In this climate, funding was available for large-scale studies of development, centered primarily in two places, Yale on the east coast and Berkeley on the west coast. Theories of motor development focus on the acquisition of motor behavior that is heavily maturational in origin.

GESELL'S THEORY

Arnold Gesell (1880–1961) was the director of the Yale Clinic of Child Development from 1911 to 1948, and his work continued at the Gesell Institute after his mandatory retirement from Yale in 1948. Several others, including Charles Darwin and G. E. Coghill, influenced Gesell's work. From Darwin, Gesell confirmed his commitment to the biologic framework and methodology. Coghill was an embryologist who studied the development of locomotion in salamanders, correlating the onset of motor pattern to underlying changes in neural maturation. The perspectives from Coghill's work that had a defining influence on Gesell were (1) that behavior has a characteristic pattern, (2) that the nature of that pattern reflects the underlying maturation of neural structure, and (3) that the emergence of the pattern is directly tied to the maturational process, which is genetically driven (Thelen & Adolph, 1994). Gesell's "laboratory" consisted of sophisticated cinemagraphic equipment and toys that infants and children would explore. His scientific contribution was a meticulous account of the individual child's approach to various tasks. Of course, Gesell noted individual differences in the children's performances, but he attributed these largely to innate differences.

Perhaps the most enduring contribution of Gesell's work was the publication of large-scale norms of child behavior and development. The *Gesell Schedules,* as they were called, formed the basis for numerous developmental assessments over the years. Gesell also contributed the concept of the *developmental quotient,* mirroring the intelligence quotient with a developmental age determined by a test of normative behavior in which the score was divided by the chronologic age and multiplied by 100. Because he was a pediatrician by training, in addition to being a teacher and psychologist, Gesell had a profound influence on the field of pediatrics. He was important in the establishment of the field of developmental pediatrics and in the notion that pediatricians should have some developmental training.

Gesell's theory is perhaps the most profoundly maturational of any that have been discussed here. His belief was that it was the genetically driven unfolding of the innate potential that produced acquisition of new developmental behaviors. From this belief, he formulated *laws of developmental direction.* These laws, as a group, summarized the trends of developmental milestone acquisition as follows:

1. *Development proceeds in a cephalocaudal direction.* Infants gain control progressively of the head, shoulders, down the spine, and ultimately the lower legs.

2. *Development proceeds proximal to distal.* Infants gain control of the shoulder and hip before hand and foot.

3. *Development proceeds medial to lateral.* Medial to lateral development is similar to proximal to distal; for example, in the hand, development of grasp moves from ulnar (medial) to radial (lateral).

4. *Development proceeds up against gravity.* Infants progress from completely prone to prone on elbows, then supported by hands, then supported by all four limbs, and finally standing and walking.

Other principles traced to Gesell include *functional asymmetry,* in which infants progress from initial asymmetry through symmetry and once again to asymmetry to develop handedness; *optimal realization,* in which infants are able to progress despite adverse circumstances; and finally, the important principle of *reciprocal interweaving* (Thelen & Adolph, 1994), in which there is a progressive spiral reincorporation of sequential forms of behavior. Reciprocal interweaving refers to the fact that, during development, infants will appear to show alternating dominance of antagonistic behaviors: for example, flexion extension and approach avoidance. However, the nondominant behavior has not disappeared but will reappear at a higher functional level (the progressive spiral). A simplistic example of this is seen in locomotor development. An infant first displays reflexive supporting and stepping responses when supported upright. These responses disappear, and the infant will enjoy a "bouncing game," withdrawing legs when placed in standing (astasia) at the age of around 5 to 6 months. Shortly thereafter, the infant will resume standing again, but this time it is more mature in terms of postural control.

Gesell's influence on the study of child development had some unexpected negative consequences. First, his work on motor development was so persuasive in attributing development to biologic mechanisms that for several decades the processes of motor development were not considered of interest for further study (Thelen & Adolph, 1994). A second, more pervasive influence was brought about by Gesell's maturational focus. Because he believed that development was relatively unaffected by external forces, he was responsible for the "wait and see" attitude many pediatricians and child care professionals adopted

toward developmental problems. In other words, if a parent had a concern that a child had not yet walked, the first approach was to give the child more time, as it was believed that there was little that could be done to change the course of development. The last 20 years of study and experience have challenged these notions.

McGRAW'S THEORY

A contemporary of Gesell's who also had a lasting influence on the field of motor development, first mentioned in Chapter 2, was **Myrtle McGraw**. McGraw is classified as a maturationist, because, like Gesell, she was interested in correlation of change in underlying structure with change in function. McGraw differed from Gesell in that she saw the environment as having a greater influence than he did, and she believed that environment could potentially change the influences of developing structures.

McGraw disputed a strict biologic explanation for development. She introduced the notion of *critical periods.* A **critical period** is a limited time in which a developmental event can occur, the time when an organism is most receptive to learning a certain kind of behavior. She was explicit, however, in saying that critical periods were not exclusive, they just referred to a time when children are most receptive and learning is most efficient. McGraw's critical periods have been widely accepted in both education and neuroscience. One example of a contemporary application is the research table presented in **Figure 3-6**. The more contemporary term, used in the life course model, is sensitive periods. A **sensitive period** is a more extended period of time during development when individuals are especially receptive to specific types of environmental stimuli, and therefore are more predisposed to learning.

McGraw disagreed with the notion that environment had little influence on development. She believed that many of the emerging behaviors she observed had the qualities of learned components. McGraw also identified a period of disorganization and deterioration of function in times of transition to higher levels. Her theory differs from Gesell's theory of reciprocal interweaving in that Gesell never proposed an actual deterioration of function. McGraw believed such a period occurred as the underlying structures were reorganizing to support new behaviors (Bergenn, Dalton, & Lipsitt, 1994). For example, very young infants were observed to display holding of breath and more rhythmic motions when placed in water than did slightly older infants, who seemed to flail and struggle. McGraw viewed the seeming deterioration as a period of reorganization prior to development of true swimming behavior (McGraw, 1945). Studies of neural development and plasticity support the notion that the developing nervous system is shaping a synaptic pattern, which includes both activation and development of synapses as well as synapses becoming dormant or disappearing.

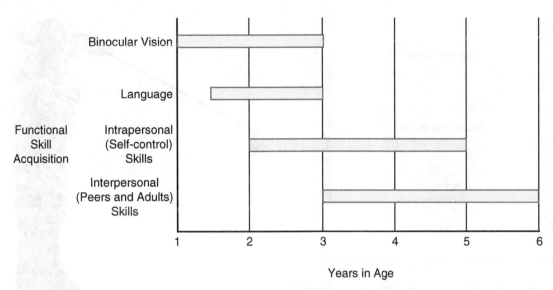

Figure 3-6   Examples of McGraw's Critical Periods adapted from Bergenn, V. W., Dalton, T., & Lipsitt, L. P., 1994. Reference crediting: Bergenn, V. W., Dalton, T., & Lipsitt, L. P. (1994). Myrtle B. McGraw: A growth scientist. In R. D. Parke, P. A. Ornstein, J. J. Rieser, & C. Zahn-Waxler (Eds.), A century of developmental psychology (pp. 389–423). Washington, DC: American Psychological Association.

THEORIES OF MOTOR LEARNING

We have differentiated motor development from motor learning along a continuum of relative influence of the environment. **Motor learning** theories incorporate both a specific type of learning and an approach to therapeutic intervention following injury that is directed toward searching for a motor solution that emerges from an interaction of the individual with the task and the environment. *Motor control* was first presented in Chapter 2, and involves the study of the control of posture and movement, usually emphasizing the role of the central nervous system. Motor learning itself cannot be measured but only inferred from motor performance. There are several classic theories of motor learning.

Closed-Loop Theory

One is the **closed-loop theory**. Another way to think about closed-loop theory is feedback-dependent (hence, the stimulus-response-stimulus loop is closed). In the closed-loop theory, proposed by Jack A. Adams, sensory feedback is believed to guide the successive improvement of performance of a motor skill in the following paradigm: The individual has a *memory trace* of a movement or a movement approximation, if the movement is totally novel. When the goal is established, the person generates a *perceptual trace,* which is a sensorimotor plan based on the memory trace, modified by sensory experience or feedback. At the end of each session of practice, the new memory trace is stored. An analogy for this model is to think of word processing using a computer. You use a word processing program (the neural network) to generate a written document, which you save (the memory trace). Later, you want to edit that document, so you pull it into active memory (perceptual trace), edit it, and store it once again.

The closed-loop theory of motor learning has been criticized on two main points. First, some movements, such

as throwing, occur too rapidly to be modified by feedback during the movement itself. Second, studies on animals and humans who lack input over sensory nerves have shown that capabilities to produce movement continue to exist, even though learning of new skills is severely impaired.

Open-Loop Theory

One of Adams's contemporaries, Richard Schmidt, proposed an **open-loop theory** of motor learning that addressed some of the limitations of closed-loop theory. In the open-loop theory, a motor response *schema* exists, consisting of a set of rules for directing movement. These rules are known as *response specifications* and, as a whole, create the motor program that directs the movement through neural pathways acting on the motor neurons. During and after the movement has occurred, a number of sensory channels provide intrinsic and extrinsic feedback to the system, as described earlier. The actual sensory consequences, obtained through feedback, are compared to the expected sensory consequences, generated as part of the schema and response specifications. If an error is detected, the schema is adjusted. This theory of motor learning assigns a *comparator* with the job of comparing actual and expected sensory consequences (Shumway-Cook & Woollacott, 2012). The open-loop theory of motor learning implies that practice is best done as variable practice—that is, under a variety of conditions. Research has supported this best in young children and to a lesser extent in adults (Shumway-Cook & Woollacott, 2012).

Stage Theories

In addition to open- and closed-loop theories of motor learning, there are theories that describe the overt aspects of motor learning in terms of characteristic stages. Paul Fitts and Michael Posner identified three stages of motor learning:

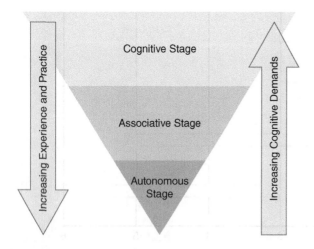

Figure 3-7   Fitts and Posner's Three Stages of Motor Learning

cognitive, associative, and autonomous (Shumway-Cook & Woollacott, 2012). These stages are illustrated in **Figure 3-7**. The *cognitive stage* is characterized by verbal rehearsal, where individuals recite, often audibly, the steps to a task. Anyone who has ever taken a dance class has participated in an example of verbal rehearsal. The early cognitive stage of learning requires that learners initiate the movement; too much feedback or coaching in this stage can be disruptive. On the other hand, in the *associative stage*, feedback and coaching are very helpful in correcting and improving the motor skill. In the final, *autonomous stage,* the movement proceeds automatically. In fact, once a skill has been well learned, excessive attention to the skill can result in the phenomenon known as *"paralysis by analysis."* The term *paralysis by analysis* has been used in the study of sports performance and refers to the disruption of a familiar and well-learned motor pattern when an athlete thinks about the movement excessively. In this instance, the skill worsens the more attention is paid to it. A baseball player in the middle of a hitting slump suffers from this condition. Another example would be the need to pause instructions when teaching a familiar task, because in describing the task to a novice, the instructor must bring the skill back into conscious processing because it has been relegated to an automatic mode. The cumulative result of the stages of motor learning is acquisition of a new motor skill as seen in **Figure 3-8**.

Hierarchical models of motor control had widespread acceptance from the mid- to late twentieth century, paralleling the work of Coghill, Gesell, and McGraw in describing the neural mechanisms that mediate movement. Whereas the aforementioned authors emphasized the developmental hierarchy, this model of motor control emphasized the increased role of higher centers in regulating movement as maturation progressed. The motor patterns, primarily reflexes, which were elicited solely at the spinal level, were most primitive. As a baby matured, the mid-level of control, represented by first the postural reflex patterns and then the mature postural reactions (righting, protective extension, and equilibrium), developed. The behavioral manifestation of movement was believed to directly reflect

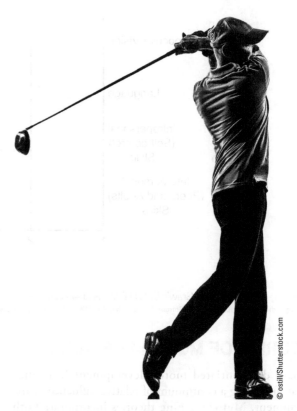

© ostill/Shutterstock.com

Figure 3-8   Golfer Who Has Passed through Stages of Motor Learning

the level of central nervous system maturation. If damage to the nervous system occurred, it was believed that lower centers of control once again exerted dominance in motor systems, and it was the task of the rehabilitation process to attempt to activate the higher levels of control.

The hierarchical model of control is no longer accepted as the definitive theory of motor control. Some reasons for its rejection include the fact that development does not perfectly reflect CNS maturation, and top-down control has been disproven. The accepted model of motor control today views a number of systems acting in parallel with elaborate multidirectional communication between neural centers (Horak, 1991). Most of today's literature emphasizes the dynamical systems theory of motor control discussed in Chapter 2. The attractiveness of the systems theory as applied to motor control is that it explains several phenomena, such as the aforementioned fact that different responses can be elicited from stimulation of the same neural pathways. In systems theory, the organization and interaction of the participating systems would change in accordance with the new environmental task constraints.

CONTINUOUS MULTI-DOMAIN: BEHAVIORISM

A final set of theories of performance exists that cannot be placed under a single domain. This theoretical perspective, known as **behaviorism**, covers all domains of behavior. The origins of behaviorism are in the **classical conditioning** experiments by the Russian scientist **Ivan Pavlov.** Pavlov documented how hungry dogs could be conditioned to salivate to the sound of a bell by pairing the sound of the bell with the presentation of meat (Feldman, 1999). Salivation was the conditioned response (CR), the sound of the bell the conditioned stimulus (CS), and the presentation of the meat the unconditioned stimulus (UCS). Pavlov's contributions to the field of psychology

are founded in systematic experimentation and objective recording of results (Chaplin & Krawiec, 1960). **Figure 3-9** illustrates classical conditioning. Note that the previously neutral stimulus elicits a "conditioned" response. This type of learning occurs below the level of consciousness and can be difficult to counteract.

An important feature of classical conditioning is that the subject is passive, and an outside person or event reinforces desired behavior. This has proved to be a productive model

Stage 1 Sight of bottle causes no response, but being fed from bottle elicits pleasurable responses such as sighs and coos

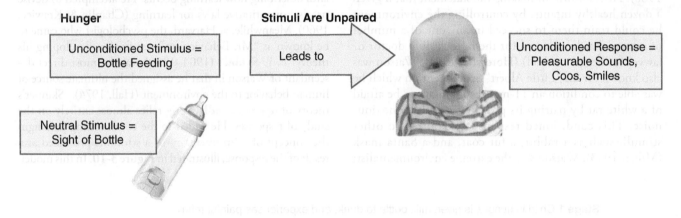

Stage 2 Sight of bottle is paired with administration of bottle

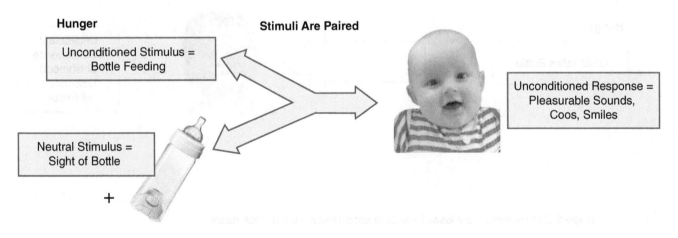

Stage 3 Now sight of bottle alone elicits pleasurable response

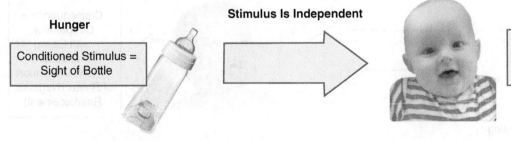

Figure 3-9 Classical Conditioning Process adapted from Kaplan & Sadock, 1998

for psychological research but is less applicable in natural human environments. For therapists hoping to assist clients in positive behavior change, the strategies discussed in subsequent paragraphs utilizing an active subject are more often appropriate.

The first American to adopt the theory of behaviorism was **John Watson** (1878–1958). In 1913 Watson proposed that behavioral psychology is objective and seeks to predict and control behavior (Horowitz, 1994). Watson saw the stimulus-response relationship as the essential one between organism and environment (Chaplin & Krawiec, 1960). He is known for making the statement that if given a dozen healthy infants, by controlling the environment he could train them to succeed in any one of a number of careers that he selected for them, including doctor or lawyer (or beggar or thief) (Horowitz, 1994). Watson was also known for his "Little Albert" experiment, in which he was able to condition an 11-month-old infant to be afraid of a white rat by pairing its presentation with a noxious noise. This conditioned response generalized to other stimuli, such as a rabbit, a fur coat, and a Santa mask (Miller, 1983). Watson was the extreme environmentalist;

although he acknowledged some role for heredity, he saw it primarily in terms of dictating structure rather than function.

In the next cohort of behaviorists, Clark Hull, known for his deductive methodology, led a group at Yale. He introduced to the stimulus-response paradigm the "O" variables, which are unobservable factors. One example of such a factor is the sensory processing that occurs within the organism in response to a stimulus. Hull's learning paradigm looked something like S-O-R, in which S is the stimulus, O is the organism's processing, and R is the emitted response. Hull derived postulates describing how learning occurs. He attempted to devise precise, quantitative laws for learning (Chaplin & Krawiec, 1960). Meanwhile, at Harvard, the psychologist who came to be known as "Mr. Behaviorism" was further developing his theory. **B. F. Skinner** (1904–1990) was the most direct descendant of Watson in that he assigned the ultimate source of human behavior to the environment (Hall, 1974). Skinner's theory of **operant conditioning** relies almost entirely on the study of responses. He added to the conditioning paradigm the concept of **reinforcement**, or a stimulus produced as a result of the response, illustrated in **Figure 3-10**. In this model,

Stage 1 Child is hungry, is given milk bottle to drink, and experiences painful reflux.

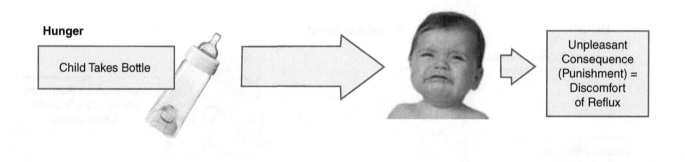

Stage 2 Child is hungry but loses interest in eating because it is unpleasant.

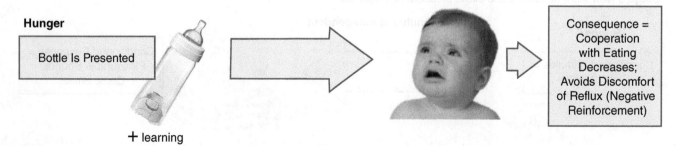

Figure 3-10   Operant Conditioning Process adapted from Kaplan & Sadock, 1998

learning is conscious, and the type and rate of responses are directly related to the outcome the individual desires. Skinner classified behaviors that were elicited in response to a determined stimulus, such as the food or the bell in Pavlov's experiments, as *respondents*. However, Skinner argued that the majority of behavior could not be studied from the perspective of a specific eliciting stimulus. Rather, he posited, most behaviors are emitted, meaning that specific stimuli are not identifiable. These behaviors are the *operants* (such as an infant exhibiting the behavior of taking a bottle). Reinforcers are the result of the operant behavior. Positive reinforcers (for example, the pleasant feelings of satiety associated with bottle feeding) are desired outcomes that lead to an increase in the behavior. However, negative reinforcers are outcomes leading to a decrease in the behavior. **Figure 3-10** illustrates a common clinical scenario. In that scenario, infants who have gastroesophageal reflux experience a negative reinforcer from taking the bottle. This tends to result in feeding avoidance behaviors. Occupational therapists often work with infants who have developed feeding avoidance behaviors due to aversive consequences associated with feeding.

Punishment is a potential consequence of a response, but Skinner describes punishment as an ineffective method of behavior control because it only temporarily eliminates the response, but not permanently. In other words, the organism learns to avoid punishment, but when the punishment is removed, the behavior is likely to recur, because the strength of the behavior, or operant, has not been affected (Chaplin & Krawiec, 1960). Reinforcement schedules could focus on intervals (elapsed time) or ratios (number of responses required for response) and could be continuous, fixed, or variable. Using the notorious "Skinner box," which was a box with a bar that the animal pressed to receive a pellet of food, Skinner studied the effect of various reinforcement schedules on operant behavior. He also studied the contingencies under which response rate decreases as a result of withdrawal of reinforcement. Generally, it was found that continuously reinforced behaviors were quicker to undergo extinction than those that had been variably reinforced. Extinction occurred more rapidly than forgetting, which is a time decay of the operant (Chaplin & Krawiec, 1960).

The contributions of the behaviorists, and Skinner in particular, to the study of human behavior are immense. First, they popularized the idea that empirical methods could be used to answer every question of importance in understanding human performance. Second, they had a major impact on society, especially child-rearing practices and the notion of reward and punishment. Finally, they provided scientists with a means to shape animal behavior to perform numerous studies on effects of manipulations on behavior. Skinner's operant conditioning principles have given rise to a form of behavior management known as **applied behavior analysis (ABA)**.

ABA uses the principles of antecedent, consequence, and reinforcement to manage desirable and undesirable behaviors, in order to shape appropriate behavioral responses. Although ABA, like operant conditioning, is often criticized for ignoring innate characteristics, it is one of the best documented and widely used therapeutic approaches in the management of autism (Rosenwasser & Axelrod, 2001).

SOCIAL LEARNING THEORY

A natural legacy of the behaviorist perspective is social learning theory, which turns its attention to how children learn the rules and behavior of social functioning. Two names inextricably linked to social learning theory are **Robert Sears** and **Albert Bandura**, who were colleagues at Stanford University, although they never collaborated on any major work. Each made significant contributions independently. The social learning theory developed by Sears had its foundation in the work of Hull; however, in the organism's functions, Sears applied the concepts of psychoanalytic theory. For example, Sears explained how a child becomes dependent on the mother. He postulated that the mother is consistently paired with the reduction of drive states, such as hunger, discomfort, and so forth, such that she ultimately becomes a reinforcer for the child. He further stated that, because the young child cannot distinguish between self and mother, the child begins to reproduce the mother's actions through imitation, which in itself becomes reinforcing (Grusec, 1994). Eventually, social learning theorists began to decrease the emphasis on drive and look more closely at the chain of behaviors evident in a dyad or triad of interactions (Miller, 1983). Sears did not view social development as occurring in stages; rather, he offered three mechanisms of explanation: learning, physical maturation, and social standards of expectation (Grusec, 1994).

Bandura's work never incorporated psychoanalytic theory; from its inception, operant principles were emphasized. However, his theory evolved over time to incorporate cognitive information processing as a key element. Bandura's legacy is perhaps most tied to the concept of **modeling**, which was how he attempted to resolve the issue of learning novel responses. Basically, Bandura and his colleague Walters speculated that children need not be directly reinforced or punished for a behavior. Instead, a process known as *vicarious reinforcement* could occur in which the child observed the reinforcement of others' behavior and thus learned rules of reinforcement by observation. Bandura named four essential components in the process of modeling: (1) attention to the model, (2) retention of past experiences, (3) ability to reproduce the response physically, and (4) motivation to produce the response.

Bandura elaborated on the interactional dynamics of social exchange, coining the term *reciprocal determinism* for the concept that the person's actions themselves help to create or determine the environment in which social exchange occurs (Miller, 1983). Although once again maintaining its origin in the behaviorist tradition, in its final form Bandura's social learning theory is best classified as an information-processing theory, involving memory, imagery, and problem solving (Grusec, 1994).

SUMMARY

All of the theories discussed in this chapter have had a major impact on the field of psychology and the understanding of human behavior. In this chapter a number of different theories have been presented regarding the nature and development of human behavior. As illustrated in **Figure 3-1**, theory attempts to explain human behavior, taking into account performance and contextual factors. Theory, as mentioned at the beginning of this chapter, is not fact. Therefore, theory can change, be proved, or disproved. The important contribution of theory to the analysis of human function is that it leads to a set of rules that are subject to investigation. These rules also guide practice, as we've seen in the child-rearing impact of Skinner's theory and the educational impact of Vygotsky's, Piaget's, and Dewey's theories. Theories help us propose plans for interventions that will maximize human functioning; however, it is only through ongoing analysis and investigation that we will refine our ability to create interventions that optimize human potential under a number of internal and external conditions.

CASE 1

Missy

Missy is a former preterm infant born with neonatal abstinence syndrome (NAS) due to substance abuse by her mother. She was briefly placed with her mother, but she was removed from the home by Child Protective Services. She has been in several foster homes. Missy is now 15 months old (adjusted) and has been with the current foster family for 12 months. They would like to adopt her. The mother has been in a drug rehabilitation program and hopes to bring Missy home with her in the future. During supervised visits, Missy tends to cling to her foster mother and be unwilling to separate. When the early intervention team comes to the house to work with her, she cries when her foster mother puts her down. In addition to being shy and clingy, Missy is delayed in motor development as well as in her cognitive and language development. She is not yet walking, but pulls to stand and cruises. She does not have any words except for babbling ma-ma and da-da, generically and not as names.

Guiding Questions

Some questions to consider:

1. Analyze Missy's temperament along the dimensions discussed by Chess and Thomas. What genetic and environmental influences may be factors in her temperament?
2. As a development specialist, how would you get Missy to interact in treatment?
   a. Using principles of operant conditioning
   b. Using interactive learning, such as Piagetian principles
3. Discuss Missy's attachment issues according to the Ainsworth frame of reference.
4. What Erikson stage is Missy in? How does she demonstrate her resolution of the developmental tasks associated with that stage?

CASE 2

Bryan

Bryan is a 4-year-old boy who has been diagnosed with autism spectrum disorder (ASD). His gross motor behavior is characterized by the ability to walk and run, but activities requiring balance and coordination are difficult for him. He would like to learn to ride a tricycle without training wheels. He does not have much spoken language, but uses gestures and utterances to indicate his wants and needs. When he gets upset, he displays problem behaviors such as pinching himself or others. He is in a public school program, and has an ABA therapist to coach the teachers and aides about how to work with him.

Guiding Questions

Some questions to consider:

1. Applied behavior analysis (ABA) is largely based on the principles of operant conditioning. Take a positive behavior (uttering a word) or an undesirable behavior (pinching) and describe how to apply the principles of operant conditioning to either increase a desirable behavior or decrease an undesirable behavior.
2. Apply motor learning theory and stages to the process of teaching Bryan how to ride a tricycle.
3. Analyze social learning theory (Sears and Bandura) in the context of Bryan's behavior. Does the theory apply to children with autism? Defend your answer.

Speaking of
Who Really Cares about Theory?

ANNE CRONIN, PHD, OTR/L,
PEDIATRIC OCCUPATIONAL THERAPIST

I, like many of you, first learned about many of the theorists discussed in this chapter in my first "General Psychology" course. It was not exciting, but Pavlov and the dogs were kind of interesting. In all, it meant very little to me. Later, as a graduate student, I saw that every class seemed to have its own take on theory, and sociology theories were applied to management, and economic theories were applied to human behavior, and I plodded through them all—sometimes with interest, other times just to get through.

My first job as an occupational therapist was in an intermediate care facility for developmentally delayed adults. Part of my job was to help people transition from the institution to the community. Ricky, in his middle 30s, had been institutionalized at birth. He had severe spastic cerebral palsy, had no ability to speak, and was dependent on others in all aspects of self-care. In spite of this, Ricky was social and playful, had a wonderful sense of humor, and although untestable by traditional means, appeared to have excellent reasoning abilities. Ricky was recognized as exceptional

Continues

Speaking of   Continued

and given special status in the institution. He had his own room and his choice of caregivers, and was allowed to share meals with the staff rather than with the other residents. Our ambitious team of young therapists and social workers worked for about 2 years to get Ricky equipment and build community connections. It wasn't until we started taking Ricky out to look at apartments that Ricky really understood our goal. All of us were dumbfounded as Ricky systematically "lost" the ability to use his communication device and began having bouts of aggression. We were confused and hurt by Ricky's sudden rejection of all that we had worked on.

It wasn't until I began working on my doctorate in medical sociology that the importance of theory and an understanding of Ricky came together for me. I had been keeping up with the developments in occupational therapy theory and had begun teaching occupational therapy. I was a good therapist, and strongly believed in the premises of my profession. Then, as I came face to face with the theories of Karl Marx, Emile Durkheim, and Karl Mannheim, I was forced to take on a societal rather than a clinical perspective. Tackling those giants in theory development, I learned how their theories had shaped beliefs and understanding, and influenced all of science for generations to come.

As I reflected on Durkheim's ideas about isolation and alienation, I understood that the challenge of a clinician is not just to collect information about people's lives and their personal expectations, but also to problem-solve in a complex way that supports the individual while integrating the best your profession has to offer. I then understood that for Ricky, the institution was home. He was truly loved there and was always singled out for a lot of special attention. The community was a fearsome jungle to him. He was viewed as a freak and was avoided by others. In Ricky's view, we were replacing his home, his family, and his security with alienation and isolation. How stupid I felt. While focusing on our professional goals and values, we had lost awareness of the human being and the occupations he most valued. Ricky taught me that knowledge without perspective may result in "progress" without influencing participation in meaningful everyday contexts. Theory is a dynamic tool to help us integrate knowledge and research to address the very real human factors influencing functional performance across the life span.

REFERENCES

Austrian, S. G. (2002). *Developmental theories through the life cycle.* New York: Columbia University Press.

Beilin, H. (1994). Jean Piaget's enduring contribution to developmental psychology. In R. D. Parke, P. A. Ornstein, J. J. Rieser, & C. Zahn-Waxler (Eds.), *A century of developmental psychology* (pp. 257–290). Washington, DC: American Psychological Association.

Bergenn, V. W., Dalton, T., & Lipsitt, L. P. (1994). Myrtle B. McGraw: A growth scientist. In R. D. Parke, P. A. Ornstein, J. J. Rieser, & C. Zahn-Waxler (Eds.), *A century of developmental psychology* (pp. 389–423). Washington, DC: American Psychological Association.

Bretherton, I. (1994). Origins of attachment theory. In R. D. Parke, P. A. Ornstein, J. J. Rieser, & C. Zahn-Waxler (Eds.), *A century of developmental psychology* (pp. 431–471). Washington, DC: American Psychological Association.

Cahan, E. D. (1994). John Dewey and human development. In R. D. Parke, P. A. Ornstein, J. J. Rieser, & C. Zahn-Waxler (Eds.), *A century of developmental psychology* (pp. 145–167). Washington, DC: American Psychological Association.

Chaplin, J. P., & Krawiec, T. S. (Eds.) (1960). *Systems and theories of psychology.* New York: Holt, Rinehart and Winston.

Chess, S., & Thomas, A. (1987). *Know your child: An authoritative guide for today's parents.* New York: Basic Books.

Erikson, E. H. (1963). *Childhood and society.* New York: Norton.

Feldman, R. S. (Ed). (1999). *Child development: A topical approach.* Upper Saddle River, NJ: Prentice Hall.

Flavell, J. H. (1963). *The developmental psychology of Jean Piaget.* Princeton, NJ: D Van Nostrand.

Gilligan, C. (1982). In a different voice: Women's conceptions of self and morality. *Harvard Educational Review, 47*(4).

Grusec, J. E. (1994). Social learning theory and developmental psychology: The legacies of Robert Sears and Albert Bandura. In R. D. Parke, P. A. Ornstein, J. J. Rieser, & C. Zahn-Waxler (Eds.), *A century of developmental psychology* (pp. 473–497). Washington, DC: American Psychological Association.

Hall, M. H. (1974). An interview with "Mr. Behaviorist," B. F. Skinner. In *Readings in Psychology Today* (pp. 114–119). Del Mar, CA: Ziff-Davis.

Harkness, S., Edwards, C. P., & Super, C. M. (1981). The claim to moral adequacy of a highest stage of moral judgment. *Developmental Psychology, 17*(5), 595–603.

Horak, F. (1991). Assumptions underlying motor control for neurologic rehabilitation. In M. J. Lister (Ed.), *Contemporary management of motor control problems: Proceedings of the II step conference* (pp. 11–27). Alexandria, VA: Foundation for Physical Therapy.

Horowitz, F. D. (1994). John B. Watson's legacy: Learning and environment. In R. D. Parke, P. A. Ornstein, J. J. Rieser, and C. Zahn-Waxler (Eds.), *A century of developmental psychology* (pp. 233–256). Washington, DC: American Psychological Association.

Kagan, J. (2005). Temperament. *Encyclopedia on Early Childhood Development.* Retrieved from http://www.child-encyclopedia .com/en-ca/home.html

Kohlberg, L. (1974). The child as moral philosopher. In *Readings in Psychology Today* (pp.186–191). Del Mar, CA: Ziff-Davis.

McGraw, M. (1945). *Neuromuscular maturation of the human infant.* New York: Columbia University Press.

Miller, P. H. (Ed). (1983). *Theories of developmental psychology.* San Francisco: W. H. Freeman.

Pick, H. L. (1994). Eleanor J. Gibson: Learning to perceive and perceiving to learn. In R. D. Parke, P. A. Ornstein, J. J. Rieser, & C. Zahn-Waxler (Eds.), *A century of developmental psychology* (pp. 527–544). Washington, DC: American Psychological Association.

Puner, H. W. (Ed.) (1947). *Freud: His life and his mind.* New York: Grosset and Dunlap.

Reese, H. S., & Overton, W. F. (1970). Models of development and theories of development. In L. R. Goulet & P. B. Baltes (Eds.), *Life-span developmental psychology.* New York: Academic Press.

Rosenwasser, B., & Axelrod, S. (2001). The contribution of applied behavior analysis to the education of people with autism. *Behavior Modification, 25*(5), 671–677.

Saudino, K. J. (2009). The development of temperament from a behavioral genetics perspective. In P. Bauer (Ed.), *Advances in child development and behavior* (pp. 201–231). New York: Elsevier.

Shumway-Cook, A., & Woollacott, M. (2012). *Motor control: Translating research into clinical practice* (4th ed.). Philadelphia: Lippincott, Williams and Wilkins.

Thelen, E., & Adolph, K. (1994). Arnold L. Gesell: The paradox of nature and nurture. In R. D. Parke, P. A. Ornstein, J. J. Rieser, & C. Zahn-Waxler (Eds.), *A century of developmental psychology* (pp. 357–387). Washington, DC: American Psychological Association.

Thomas, R. M. (Ed.). (2001). *Recent theories of human development.* Thousand Oaks, CA: Sage.

Thompson, R. A., & Goodman, M. (2011). *The architecture of social developmental science: Theoretical and historical perspectives.* In M. K. Underwood & L. H. Rosen (Eds.), *Social development: Relationships in infancy, childhood, and adolescence* (pp. 3–28). New York: The Guilford Press.

CHAPTER 4

Culture and Development

Anne Cronin, PhD, OTR/L, FAOTA,
Associate Professor,
Division of Occupational Therapy,
West Virginia University, Morgantown,
West Virginia
With contributions by
**Winifred Schultz-Krohn, PhD,
OTR, BCP, FAOTA,**
Professor of Occupational Therapy,
San Jose State University,
San Jose, California

Objectives

Upon completion of this chapter, readers should be able to:

- Discuss the impact of norms and values in making everyday decisions;

- Describe the essential components of cultural awareness and cultural competence;

- Recognize how culture shapes individual perceptions, beliefs, and values;

- Discuss the complex interaction and differences between the terms *culture, ethnicity,* and *race;*

- Describe cultural differences in communication, control, and definition of self;

- Understand how developmental expectations and developmental progression are culturally influenced;

- Describe how poverty and socioeconomic factors influence development; and

- Define paralanguage and offer examples of how it relates to culture and life span development.

Key Terms

acculturation

acute poverty

causal attribution

chronic poverty

collectivistic cultural
characteristics

cultural awareness

cultural broker

cultural competence

cultural fluidity

culture

developmental niche

egalitarianism

ethnicity

ethnocentric

expressive/overt communication

habit

health literacy

individualistic cultural
characteristics

interdependence

linguistic competence

occupational deprivation

paralanguage

poverty

proxemics

racism

religion

restrained formal communication

routine

self-representation

subculture

values

CASE 1

Nangane

Nangane is a 76-year-old widow from Sri Lanka. When Nangane's husband died last year, her son brought her to stay with his family in Chicago. In Sri Lanka, children, especially sons, are expected to assume responsibility for their aging parents. Asoka, Nangane's son, is 51 years old and has lived in the Chicago area for 20 years. Asoka, his wife, and two teenaged daughters are naturalized U.S. citizens. Asoka and his wife are both research scientists who work full time at a local university.

Nangane fell and broke her hip. She was sent to a skilled nursing facility (SNF) for therapy. To return home, Nangane needed to be ambulatory with a walker, she needed to be independent in toileting and to have stabilized her blood pressure, and she needed to improve her overall strength and endurance. She had been independent in dressing and involved in cooking for the family before her fall, and hoped to return to those tasks as well.

Nangane expressed anger at her daughter-in-law for "locking her up" rather than caring for her at home. In the SNF, Nangane was noncompliant in most areas of care. Nangane was refusing all "American" medications, even though persistent pain limited her ability to participate in therapy. She refused to participate in PT at all. She was willing to participate in some self-care activities with the OT, but her noncompliance was enough that she was about to be discharged rather than treated.

To address Nangane's needs, the therapy team met with the family. With her teenaged granddaughter serving as a cultural broker, it became clear that Nangane did not understand the temporary nature of the SNF, and the opportunity for specialized care that it offered. A devout Buddhist, Nangane had performed morning meditations all of her life. This routine was disrupted in the SNF, where she lacked the privacy and quiet needed in the early morning, and she felt the loss of this support profoundly.

As you explore this chapter, we will come back to the challenges facing Nangane and her family in the context of optimizing her health care and her quality of life.

Continues on page 76

INTRODUCTION

In Chapter 2 of this text, the life course theory (LCT) was introduced. As presented earlier, the four key concepts of this theory are: (1) Today's experiences and exposures influence tomorrow's health, (2) health trajectories are particularly affected during critical or sensitive periods, (3) the broader community environment—biologic, physical, and social—strongly affects the capacity to be healthy, and (4) although genetic makeup offers both protective and risk factors for disease conditions, inequality in health reflects more than genetics and personal choice (USHHS MCH, 2010, p. 4). This life course perspective has been widely accepted and endorsed because of advances in science and an increasing understanding of social contexts.

As few as two generations ago, many Americans never met a person from another country or needed to learn another language to interact with people in their own community. Increasingly, through immigration, social media, and travel, the average person is much more aware of the great ethnic diversity that exists in the world (Balcazar, Suarez-Balcazar, Taylor-Ritzler, & Keys, 2011). People today are often exposed to new healthy and unhealthy lifestyles through personal contacts, television, social media, and the Internet. Socioeconomic disparity, cultural values, and cultural barriers are all significant factors to today's health care workplaces.

Norms are the agreed-upon expectations and rules that guide individual function within a group. Norms can vary based on many factors, including age, gender, place, and culture. In this chapter, our emphasis will be on cultural norms. Cultural norms support the development of conformity and consistency of behavior that is appropriate to the group or society that individuals must function within (Scott & Marshall, 2009). For individuals living within a culture, norms may not be explicitly stated, but are understood as rules by members of the group. **Values** are broad preferences concerning appropriate courses of action or outcomes. Values often reflect a person's sense of right and wrong such as "Equal rights for all." Values function as a justification for the norms, as well as the concepts of good and bad, desire and disgust. *Cultural norms* provide rules, while *values* provide the guidance for judging and evaluating actions.

With globalization, increasingly diverse racial and ethnic populations are in much of the world. One of the greatest challenges for health professionals now is the need to respect, address, and bridge differences between people while supporting health and quality of life. This includes recognizing our own cultural norms and values as well as learning about the cultures of others and learning to serve as support and mediator for our clients as they face challenges of all types. This need to be sensitive to cultural differences and to gain skills to interact positively and productively with people whose culture differs from our own is essential for all health care professionals (Royeen & Crabtree, 2006). In this chapter, we will consider culture as an influence on the developmental life course. For example, one cultural group may view a baby's first steps as a significant event, whereas another cultural group places far greater emphasis on a child's ability to help with household chores or care for the family's animals. Similarly, in the case of Nangane, elders within the family were revered and the cultural expectation was that they would be cared for in the home of their adult children. Although Nangane's son may have held the same values as his mother, the American health care system offers rehabilitation services in residential skilled nursing facilities. He had to choose between getting excellent state of the science care or keeping her at home with the limited home therapy services that he could arrange. His choice of the skilled nursing facility was best from an American point of view, but was offensive to Nangane and her own traditional values.

An additional emphasis in this chapter will be an understanding of the interconnectedness between race, culture, and disparity. The LCT idea of *early programming* described in Chapter 2 posits that early experiences can "program" an individual's future health and development (USHHS MCH, 2010). This early programming can have either a positive or a negative effect on the health of an individual. Working within the medical model, there is an assumption that an ideal outcome is a cure or to regain full functional abilities. In Western medicine and rehabilitation, there is an expectation that individuals (the clients) will actively work toward their own recovery, a recovery leading to a life of independent participation in daily life activities (Royeen & Crabtree, 2006). Although this is an ideal in the United States, in neighboring Mexico, the ideal is to return to the loving and supportive care of an extended family. Bolanos (2003) reports that it is often difficult to motivate elderly Mexicans to work toward independence in rehabilitation, because the need for independence in old age is considered necessary only when your family will not support you.

The purpose of this chapter is to provide an understanding of influence of culture on human development and performance across the life course. Several terms will first be defined to aid readers.

DEFINITION OF TERMS

Some of the concepts in this chapter are multidimensional and may be defined differently in different contexts. The definitions that follow for the terminology related to culture will be used consistently in this text.

CULTURE

Culture refers to "the sum of experiences, values, beliefs, ideals, judgments, and attitudes that shape and give continuous form to each individual" (Royeen & Crabtree, 2006). Spector (2012) adds that culture is an interlinked web of symbols, and serves as a device for creating and limiting human choices. Culture is learned as people experience the complexity of social life, and although much of culture is conscious, over time culture becomes deeply embedded in personality and becomes

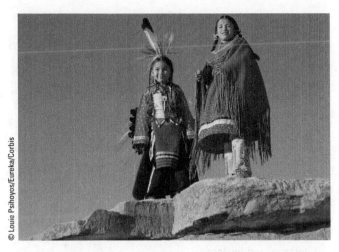

Figure 4-1 These young girls reflect pride in their heritage through wearing traditional tribal costumes.

unconscious. Culture is typically taught to the young by the adults in their community. **Figure 4-1** shows young Native American children in tribal dress. Competitions and gatherings like the North American "Gathering of Nations" are one way in which cultural heritage is preserved.

Because cultures are so varied and multidimensional, individuals are unlikely to ever gain the specific skills needed to be socially competent in all cultural contexts. Although many authors discuss cultural competence on an individual level, a more accurate ideal is the development of cultural fluidity. **Cultural fluidity** is an understanding of cultural differences

and how they manifest in everyday occupations that allows individuals to consider their own primary culture as a reference point from which new values and beliefs are considered and understood. The development of cultural fluidity requires active self-examination of one's own cultural beliefs and the ability to weigh those influences with cultural sensitivity to others to support positive interpersonal exchanges. All individuals working in health care are expected to demonstrate cultural fluidity in client care and workplace interactions.

The term *cultural competence* is used widely and often interchangeably with the construct of cultural fluidity. The term cultural competence is an older term, widely used in health care settings. In this text, the term **cultural competence** will be considered as defined by Cross, Bazron, Dennis, and Isaacs (1989) as "a set of congruent behaviors, attitudes, and policies that come together in a system, agency, or among professionals and enable that system, agency, or those professions to work effectively in cross-cultural situations" with a focus on group and institutional considerations. There is some controversy about the use of the word "competence" in this context because it implies that there is a finite skill set, rather than the ongoing dynamic process that is needed for interacting effectively with persons of other backgrounds. Alfred Irving ("Pete") Hallowell was an anthropologist whose main field of study was Native Americans, proposed the term cultural proficiency. He reported that cultural responses to social diversity can be seen on a continuum reflecting overt cultural destructiveness at the negative end with institutionalized cultural proficiency as the optimal response. **Figure 4-2** presents the continuum of

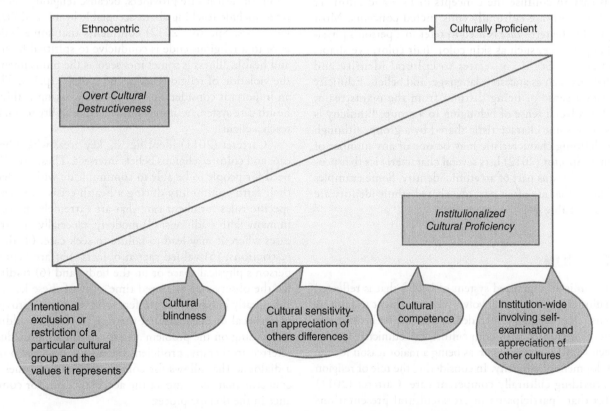

Figure 4-2 This diagram illustrates a cultural behavioral continuum that leads to cultural proficiency on an institutional level.

cultural behaviors described by Cross et al. (1989). This figure illustrates a continuum of cultural behaviors leading to the ideal of cultural proficiency on an institutional level.

RACE

There is consensus in the scientific community that the racial categories that are commonly used to describe population groups (Caucasoid, Mongoloid, Negroid, Australoid) are socially constructed, and that racial groups cannot be biologically defined (Williams & Templeton, 2003). Social conceptions and groupings of races have varied throughout human history and are grounded in the beliefs and social experience of regional groups. Most typically the popular use of the word *race* refers instead to a particular social group. For example, the terms *Hispanic* and *Latino* refer not to a race but to a cultural group, although it has been listed as a racial category on some reporting forms.

Racism is a pattern of actions, practices, or beliefs that are based in the view that there are indeed human races, and that some of these races are inherently superior or inferior to others. Definitive genomic data show there are no true human races in the scientific sense. As an action, racism is the act of discriminating against people of difference races or ethnic origins.

ETHNICITY

It is easy to confuse the concepts of race and ethnicity because both are culturally constructed concepts. Most typically, the term *race* is used to refer to a person's physical appearance, such as skin color, hair color, eye shape, and so on. **Ethnicity** relates to cultural identity and behaviors such as ancestry, language, and beliefs. Ethnicity carries a sense of being distinct from the mainstream, and involves a sense of belonging to a group. Ethnicity is based on some characteristic shared by a group, although the defining characteristic may be one of any number of things. Spector (2012) lists several characteristics that people may share as part of an ethnic identity. Some examples of things that are often part of a shared ethnic identity are listed in **Table 4-1**.

RELIGION

Religion is an organized system of beliefs that is reflected in cultural systems, and involves a commitment to faith. A discussion of religion is included in this chapter because it is closely interrelated with both culture and ethnicity. In fact, Spector (2012) cites religion as being a major reason for the development of ethnicity. In considering the role of religion in providing culturally competent care, Carteret (2011) notes that "participants in cross-cultural presentations

TABLE 4-1 Characteristics that may be Shared by People as Part of an Ethnic Identity

Common geographic origin
Migratory status
Race
Language and dialect
Religious faith or faiths
Shared traditions, values, symbols
Literature and folklore
Food preferences
Music and musical instruments
Dance
Discipline and child-rearing practices

often ask how to separate an individual's cultural beliefs and behaviors from those that are based on the person's religion. The best answer to this very complex question is to think of culture and religion as being two sides of the same coin" (p. 1). Religion is a particularly important consideration for health care providers, because religious teachings often include teaching about acceptable health and lifestyle behaviors. Spector (2012) comments that some "adherence to a religious code is conducive to spiritual harmony and health. Illness is sometimes seen as the punishment for the violation of religious codes and morals" (p.12). This is an important consideration for people working within the health care system, as it may influence the ability to guide or teach a client.

Carteret (2011) identifies six key areas where health care and culture/religious beliefs intersect. These are (1) the need for people to be able to communicate with leaders of their faith community during a health crisis; (2) gender-specific rules for client care that are extremely important in many faith traditions; (3) modesty, especially in extreme cases where it may lead to failure to seek care; (4) dietary restrictions; (5) valued sacred objects that are kept in a person's physical space or on the body; and (6) traditions for the observance of sacred time. Any of these key areas can greatly enhance or interfere with successful provision of physical or occupational therapy services. In addition to focusing on the problem area for which an individual is referred to therapy, proficient therapists should also open a dialogue that allows for communication of values and concerns that may impact the acceptance and/or compliance in the therapy process.

In the case of Nangane, she had a faith tradition of morning meditation and prayer. The early morning routine in the SNF interfered with her faith practices at a time when she was struggling to deal with significant personal and health challenges. Although chaplain services were available to residents of the SNF, Nangane's Buddhism was not a faith that either the nursing home staff or the chaplain services understood well. By failing to offer her spiritual support, Nangane's rehabilitation was profoundly impacted.

SUBCULTURE

A subculture is a cultural subgroup differentiated in some way from the dominant cultural group. For example, a person may be American culturally, then female as a subculture, then work in rehabilitation as another subculture, and be an occupational therapist in an even smaller subculture. Most individuals are a part of many cultures and subcultures, and the influence of these cultures varies by the social and emotional context of the individual at any given point in time. Subcultures can be based on many features; some of the most common are status, ethnic background, religion, education, and place of residence (Royeen & Crabtree, 2006).

Culture is not a single organized influence on an individual, but is an amalgam of an individual's experiences of the social world. People may describe themselves as bicultural, perceiving themselves as influenced by two dominant cultures. An example of this might be an Asian child adopted by parents in the United States or a person with one African American parent and one Anglo-American parent. A culture can be specific to career or professional issues; for example, there is a subculture of providers in the American health care system. A single individual may have an ethnic culture, a national culture, a faith-based culture, a family culture, and a professional culture. Because no health care professional can be competent in all possible cultural affiliations, an understanding of the meaning an individual ascribes to a daily occupation is essential in providing relevant and culturally sensitive care in a clinical setting.

CULTURE AS A SYSTEM OF LEARNED VALUES

The cultural community of the individual promotes continuation of cultural traditions, as in the example of the young Native American dancer, and also builds developmental trajectories (Keller, 2007). Young children in western Europe learn to feed themselves using spoons and forks. Spoon and fork use is typically mastered around 4 years of age. Children growing up in Taiwan, however, will be expected to manage chopsticks. The use of chopsticks requires more refined hand skills, and children may be as old as 6 years before they fully master this skill. Some of these cultural trajectories lead to predictable patterns of problem solving, and people from different cultures may have differing expectations and see different problems given the same scenario. For example, if Grandmother has a stroke (cerebrovascular accident) in the United States, the ideal would be to get Grandmother into the best hospital, followed by a stay in the best rehabilitation program in the area. Grandmother would stay in rehabilitation until she was ready to return to her previous lifestyle. If she could not return to independent living, many alternatives would be considered, including moving in with a son or daughter, moving into an assisted living care home, or staying in her own home with a hired caregiver. In Mexico, the same scenario might be seen very differently. When a family member has a disability, the first resource sought is the family. Seeking support or even therapy from outsiders may be thought of as a last resort. A common Mexican cultural value is that family members take care of each other, and the elder members of the family deserve special consideration. The Mexican grandmother would still go to the best hospital, but then she would be brought to the home of one of her sons or daughters. Grandmother would be cherished and cared for, but requiring her to regain her independence might be seen as cruel and reflect a lack of caring within the family. Sending Grandmother to a residential care home or to her own home with a hired caregiver might be seen as both callous and selfish in a Mexican worldview.

CULTURAL AWARENESS

To be proficient in dealing with people with a different cultural background recognizing the influences of your own culture as well as, learning about the new cultures must occur. This learning path was illustrated in **Figure 4-2**. In this model, cultural destructiveness is characterized by an extreme lack of awareness or lack of consideration that results in attitudes or practices that are destructive to a cultural group. An example of this might be the assumption that a female client from an Arabic culture is comfortable having a male physical therapist. Many cultural groups have strongly proscribed gender roles and gender-driven patterns of interaction. Some of these general cultural beliefs and values can be found by searching the Internet. Although Internet resources will not assure competency, they can provide a starting point for consideration and assist in framing the questions that health care providers need to ask of their clients. Physical and occupational therapists may need to change their practice style or otherwise accommodate clients who have differing gender role beliefs than they do.

Cultural incapacity reflects some awareness of a problem even though there is an insufficient understanding or set of resources to respond effectively to the needs and preferences of culturally diverse people. In the example of the Arabic woman needing physical therapy, cultural incapacity would occur if a male physical therapist accepts her refusal to work with him, but then cannot find a female physical therapist who can meet her needs. Taking the example further, what if the physical therapist does not attempt to solve the problem by seeking a female through which to provide care? He may simply document that the Arabic woman refused treatment, and make no attempt to understand or resolve her concerns. When people treat all people as the same, as our physical therapist did, there is an inherent assumption that all people think and react the same. This belief is called *cultural blindness*. A culturally blind clinician is not actively discriminatory, but holds the belief that people will assimilate to the dominant culture.

Cultural awareness is recognizing that there are other ways of viewing the same scenario, and that your viewpoint is shaped by your own cultural background. Cultural awareness can help individuals recognize how culture shapes their own perceptions and values. One of the goals of this chapter is to help readers develop a basic cultural awareness with which to develop interpersonal and professional clinical communications. **Table 4-2** outlines many behaviors associated with cultural awareness.

The process of developing cultural awareness begins with self-reflection. Not surprisingly, most people tend to believe that how they see the world is correct. When people insist on their own culture as the only correct way to understand the world, they are said to be **ethnocentric**. People or social groups that consider their own group superior to others are ethnocentric. For example, learning that European-dominant mainstream normative values common in much of the United States and Canada are in fact a set of cultural values offers a useful beginning in a discussion of culture and a foundation for cultural fluidity. Royeen and Crabtree (2006) list several predominant mainstream American values for readers to consider. These include scientific orientation, progress and change, materialism, individualism, moralistic orientation, time orientation, doing rather than being, egalitarianism, role of women, and hygiene.

Scientific Orientation

In American mainstream, it is believed that there is a scientific explanation for most experiences in everyday life. This is reflected in both the proliferation of books on how to parent young children, and in the belief that all activity limitations or developmental differences should be analyzed and cured. Other cultures have an expectation that the extended family will provide all needed parenting support and that differences in development are natural, and may require accommodation rather than seeking or expecting a cure. For example, prior to attending school, the family of a 6-year-old child in rural Chile had not sought health care services of any kind for their child. On his first day of school, his mother went with him and brought some adapted school tools. Both the mother and the child had "split-hand/split-foot syndrome." The deformities associated with this syndrome are extreme, and limit both ambulation and performance of everyday tasks. When the school occupational therapist asked why they did not seek therapy earlier, the mother commented, "It runs in the family. I have brought in my things I used when I was in school so he can use them." Although medical and developmental care would have been available for this family, the family did not see the condition as either extraordinary or as needing outside help. In Chile, the therapist sought to rally the needed supports for this child in school. If the same scenario had occurred in the United States, it would have been considered child neglect and may have resulted in having the child removed from the home.

Progress and Change

Americans are described by Royeen and Crabtree (2006) as "preoccupied with the here-and-now and seek immediate results and gratification for future security and prosperity" (p. 7). Associated with this is an expectation of personal and social mobility. Americans have one of the highest rates of voluntary personal mobility in the world (Cohn & Morin, 2008). When Americans are asked why they move, the most

---

TABLE 4-2 Cultural Awareness is:

Having a firm grasp of what culture is and what it is not

Having insight into subcultures and intracultural variation

Understanding culture's important role in personal identities and life choices

Being conscious of one's own culturally shaped values, beliefs, perceptions, and biases

Reflecting on one's reactions to people whose cultures differ from one's own

Seeking and participating in meaningful interactions with people of differing cultural backgrounds

Recognizing that cultural values influence the mental and physical health of not only individuals, but also communities

common reason listed is economic opportunity. In much of the rest of the world, the idea of intentionally moving away from family is considered not only extraordinary, but rebellious.

Although most Americans consider change as an inevitable part of life, people from many other cultures tend to look upon their traditions as a guide to the future.

Materialism

Perhaps linked to the scientific orientation and the cultural value on progress, Americans often measure their success as adults through the acquisition of material goods. Royeen and Crabtree (2006) suggest that materialism is in part a way of looking for measureable results of personal efforts. People from Western cultures strive for material comforts and convenience, as seen in the assumption that devices like remote controls for televisions and automatic garage door openers are necessities.

Individualism

Western cultures, in particular the United States, encourage independence and inquisitiveness in children. Each individual is encouraged to explore personal goals, even when those goals may lead to distancing themselves from their families. For example, Korean infants and American infants were compared regarding the amount of exploration used during play (Kim, Kim, & Rue, 1997). Although both groups of infants would explore toys, "American infants used general exploration significantly more than Korean infants" (p. 190). This difference was attributed to the cultural focus of Korean mothers on interdependence instead of independence for their infants.

Moralistic Orientation

Americans have confidence in their own values, to the point of being considered *ethnocentric* by much of the rest of the world. The result of American moralism is that Americans want to win other people over to their way of thinking, assuming that their way is the best. In addition, they are likely to negatively judge other societies and other ways of approaching developmental challenges. Returning to the earlier example of the young boy with split-hand/split-foot syndrome, my first response as an American-trained therapist was a sense of outrage that this family had had no support prior to the child's start in school. It was only with reflection that I realized that the health care system in Chile had as many, or more, supports in place for children like this. The difference was that the family and community were so accepting of the disability that the family had not sought help.

Time Orientation

Time is viewed as a valued commodity in American society. Devices like dishwashers and clothes dryers that save time are common in most households. American children are

taught to organize their activities and maintain daily schedules as early as age 5, when they enter the school system. To people from cultures that focus more on the process of living, rather than the products of living, the American pace of life may seem very hectic and unrewarding.

Doing Rather than Being

Often described as a "work ethic," Americans consider activity to be a good thing. Some common expressions like "keeping busy" and "keeping out of trouble" reflect the value of using time productively in a goal-focused manner. This is not only seen in the workplace, but also in leisure pursuits. For example, rather than simply relaxing with friends, Americans frequently will plan a particular activity so that there is a focus to the leisure time. This is also seen in the health care environment. When participating in rehabilitation in the United States, there is a requirement that individuals be able to engage in at least three hours of active therapy daily. The traditional rehabilitation setting offers a strenuous schedule, with little to no time for self-reflection or contemplation of the dramatic life changes an individual is experiencing.

Egalitarianism

Egalitarianism is a belief in the equality of all people This includes people in authority and results in an expectation that rules and standards can be negotiated. Americans tend to judge individuals in terms of merit rather than based on a fixed social position. This is often one of the most challenging issues for Americans when responding to people from another cultural context. Typically Americans do not automatically show deference to people of greater wealth, greater age, or higher social status. The American tendency to call people by their first names is so deeply ingrained, that it is without thought that physical therapists address an elderly client as "Mary" rather than as Mrs. Mitchell. For older people and people from different cultures, the use of a first name by a relative stranger is perceived as a sign of disrespect. Additionally, in the United States, people are seen as having equal rights, equal social obligations, and equal opportunities to develop their own potential. The Individuals with Disabilities Education Act (IDEA) (2004) is a law ensuring school access and special education services to children with disabilities throughout the United States. This law requires that children be included in regular classrooms to the greatest extent possible, rather than segregated into special education classrooms. This approach to the education of children with special education needs is expensive in terms of resources and is not widely accepted internationally.

Role of Women

In the United States, especially the U.S. health care system, women play a public role and have more responsibility and authority than they do in many other countries. There is greater leeway in both professional and social settings in what is considered acceptable dress and behavior for women. American women who travel internationally may be distressed to find that people from other cultures make assumptions about their status and even their sexual availability based entirely on their dress and behavior. In a clinical setting, an older man of status within his own culture may object to having a young woman as a therapist. Additionally, many of the "traditional" clothing styles expected of women from different cultural backgrounds offer challenges to therapists supporting relearning of self-care skills. For example, a therapist from the United States may find it challenging to assist a client in donning the sari worn by women in India and Sri Lanka, such as the one shown in **Figure 4-3**.

Hygiene

Personal hygiene, as you will see in later chapters, is a focus of child socialization and is an expectation for adults in everyday life. Average Americans expect to bathe and change their clothes every day. Americans tend to find natural body odors unpleasant, and failure to maintain an expected level of cleanliness may have a negative effect on a person's social relationships. Although perfumes and deodorants are widely used in Western cultures, these scents may be as unsettling to people from differing cultural backgrounds as strong perspiration odors are to people in the United States.

AWARENESS OF SUBCULTURES

We hope that considering this list of "Americanisms" will help students gain a deeper understanding of the dynamic nature of culture. Having reviewed the generalities of United States culture, it is time to consider some subculture. Within mainstream American culture, there are many subcultures. "Digital natives" is a term commonly used to describe today's college undergraduates. This is the generation of individuals who have spent their entire lives with access to, and influenced of, the World Wide Web. Digital natives, such as the young man pictured in **Figure 4-4**, use communication technology and social media extensively, changing how information is distributed and used all over the world. As we move into our discussion of developmental life stages, the cultural influence of the Internet will be considered.

Other American subcultures include cohorts defined by their place in historical time, such as the "baby boomers" or the "millennials"; these cohorts are subcultures that have shared social and historical experiences that set them apart from the American mainstream. Subcultures can be historical, but they can also be defined based on other characteristics. They can be regional, as is reflected in terms such as *Southerner, hillbilly,* and *Yankee.* Labels such as *Joe Six-pack, soccer mom,*

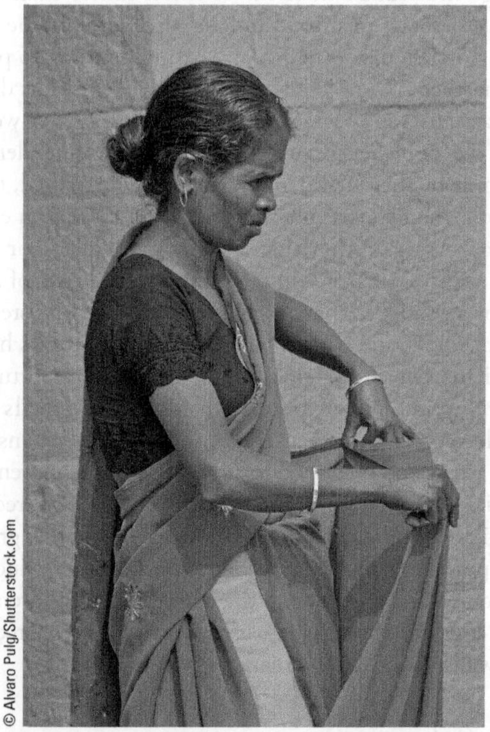

Figure 4-3   The family of a traditional woman of Indian background may have to teach therapists raised in the United States to manage a sari if the therapists are to help her learn to dress again.

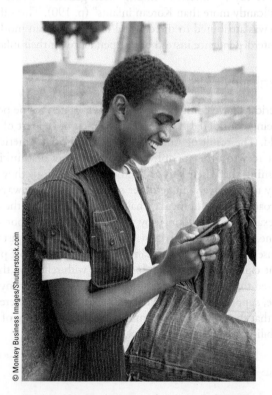

Figure 4-4   Smartphones encourage not only texting, but a continuous link to the Internet and social media that is unprecedented in human history.

and *upper crust* reflect subcultures based on social class rather than age, geography, or ethnicity. There are Internet-based subcultures as well; these can be based around specific topics like gaming, around blog sites like Tumblr or Internet fan sites for various aspects of popular media.

This discussion of cultural norms in the United States provides a foundation for developing cultural awareness, and illustrates the need for reflection in interactions with people from different cultural backgrounds. The influence of culture is pervasive and shapes the occupations that any individual engages in. Associated with this are habits and routines, patterns of behavior that are culturally expected or prescribed. These patterns of behavior are so interrelated with culture that the term *culture* is often part of the definition of the term. For example, *habit* is defined as a "customary practice or use" (Dictionary.com, 2014). In a broader sense, a **habit** is a learned behavior pattern regularly followed until it has become automatic. A routine is more complex than a habit. A **routine** is a predictable and constantly repeated pattern of actions. Routines offer structure to everyday activities. Routines can be explicit, such as the daily schedule of activities for a preschool classroom, or implicit, such as the pattern and timing of task performance that fills your time in the period between waking up and leaving for work in the morning. A routine, such as a morning routine, may include one or more habits. Much of the average person's day is shaped by routines and habits. Culture influences how, why, when, and where people engage in habits and routines.

ACCULTURATION

Acculturation is the process of outsiders getting used to the way people are within a particular community, while retaining core cultural values from their ethnic cultural upbringing. Acculturation is typically seen in immigrants to a new culture. Humans learn culture, consciously and unconsciously, throughout our lives. As we pick up and incorporate parts and pieces of a culture different from our own, we become acculturated. An example of acculturation is an American residing in Australia who embraces the "un-American" ritual of afternoon tea.

In the United States, the use of designations such as Mexican Americans, Polish Americans, and African Americans acknowledge both the original ethnic culture and a shared national culture. These designations also reflect that most people are members of more than one cultural group. In the case of immigrant groups, it is common that the children of immigrants identify themselves as bicultural or multicultural. Bicultural individuals are able to interact effectively and easily in two cultures and may speak more than one language fluently. Individuals who self-identify as multicultural can be particularly effective in health care settings because they can function as **cultural brokers** serving as a communication bridge between people of differing

cultural background. Jezewski and Sotnik (2001) defined cultural brokers as communicators who work to bridge or mediate between groups or people of differing cultural backgrounds in order to reduce conflict or produce change. The role of cultural broker typically covers more than being an interpreter, although this is an important attribute in cross-cultural situations where language is part of the role.

CULTURAL CHARACTERISTICS

This use of broad categories to characterize groups of people is not useful in the overall trajectory toward developing cultural proficiency. **Table 4-3** offers some examples of commonly noted cultural characteristics. Some of these cultural characteristics reflecting differing cultural worldviews will be presented to offer readers insight into "non-Western" points of view.

Each of the four contrasting cultural characteristics presented in **Table 4-3** will be further discussed briefly. It is important for readers to understand both these general trends and that these generalities oversimplify cultural behaviors when you are considering individuals acting in a social context. For example, in Nangane's case, her son has the same basic cultural background and cultural belief systems as she does. In spite of this, he and she are in conflict because he has weighed the options for her health care within the context of the American health care system and made a decision that she was not comfortable with.

Culture influences the occupations people choose to fill their time. Culture may influence diverse daily activities such as self-care routines, social relationships, health behaviors, and achievement orientation. Although culture has a pervasive influence, it is always mediated by the characteristics of the individual. A caveat is offered when discussing cultural characteristics broadly: No example provided should be viewed as an absolute descriptor of a cultural group. There is a danger of furthering cultural stereotypes when a specific characteristic is seen as representing every person within the identified cultural group.

INDEPENDENCE VERSUS INTERDEPENDENCE

This dichotomy in cultural orientation is also referred to as "individualistic versus collectivistic" when referring to cultural characteristics of independence and interdependence (Green, Deschamps, & Paez, 2005). **Collectivistic cultural characteristics** reflect principles or system of ownership and control of the means of production and distribution by the people collectively, often under the supervision of a government. In this cultural orientation, group members share responsibility for both social successes and social failures. **Individualistic cultural characteristics** reflect a value on

TABLE 4-3 Four Contrasting Cultural Characteristics

Independent/Individualistic	1	Interdependent/Collectivistic
Individuals are encouraged to pursue self-initiated interests and to be responsible for their own behavior. Their performance serves as the measure for success or failure in a task. Individual excellence is emphasized.		Group members share responsibility for behavior, and the pursuit of interests is strongly influenced by group needs. The group performance serves as the measure for success or failure. Group cohesiveness is emphasized.
Active Achievement	2	**Passive Acceptance**
Focus is on controlling circumstances and situations to benefit individuals.		Focus is on accepting circumstances and situations as part of a natural course.
Authoritarianism	3	**Egalitarianism**
Identification of a clear authority and individual freedoms are superseded by decisions made by an authority figure.		Decision making is done through negotiation between members, and individual freedoms are included in the process.
Expressive/Overt Communication	4	**Restrained Formal Communication**
Public communication style openly expresses moods and feelings in addition to content.		Public communication style is often quiet and controlled, with limited emotional tone.

assertiveness in reaching goals, with emphasis on individual over collective welfare. European Americans tend to be individualistic in their orientation and often exhibit assertive behaviors when working toward a goal (Schimmack, Oishi, & Diener, 2005). This construct has often been compared with the more collaborative orientations of many other cultural groups. The term *collectivism* has fallen out of favor, as it has been too generally and inconsistently defined in the literature (Brewer & Ya-Ru, 2007). Brewer and Ya-Ru state that "Clarification of the nature of individualism and collectivism orientations becomes important to the extent that such orientations play a role in explaining social behavior" (2007, p. 144). Rather than a focus on the four contrasting cultural characteristics presented in **Table 4-3,** these authors have considered several subtraits that can be consistently measured to use in the analysis of group social behavior. Each of these subtraits will be briefly introduced and linked to the more widely known characteristics from **Table 4-3.**

Interdependence

Interdependence is the manner of considering social exchanges. When people value interdependence, they hold the belief that closeness is the key to all relationships. Interdependence is considered social exchange in terms of perceiving there to be greater rewards in collaborating than in competing. The social exchange construct that is opposite to interdependence is independence. A cultural value of interdependence may focus on a family group or a faith community, and may not extend to broad social or governmental patterns (as described in a collectivistic cultural orientation.

A cultural orientation toward either interdependence or independence can influence the acquisition of specific developmental skills. A comparison between Asian and Western elementary schoolchildren found Asian children more willing to share with peers than Western children were. The Asian children were seen as influenced by a culture "where harmonious interactions are highly valued" and the needs of others are emphasized (Stewart & McBride-Chang, 2000, p. 333). Although Western children and Asian children displayed similar levels of empathy toward peers, the Western children's empathy "did not translate into a greater willingness to share with others" (p. 345). The cultural endorsement of community well-being over personal gain was seen as influential in the development of sharing skills in Asian elementary schoolchildren.

ACTIVE ACHIEVEMENT VERSUS PASSIVE ACCEPTANCE

Causal attributions are the explanations that people ascribe to actions and events that help them understand the world around them and/or to seek reasons for a particular event. Attributions can be explanatory, that is, "I did well on the test because I studied hard," or they can be interpersonal, that is, "I did poorly on the test because my neighbors made so much noise I could not sleep." In considering causal attributions in cultural contexts, there is a tendency for people from Western cultural groups to attribute behaviors to internal factors (self ability) and people from East Asian cultures attribute behaviors to external factors (group efforts) (Lieberman, Jarcho, & Obayashi, 2005).

Causal attribution can be influenced by many factors including religion and economic resources. The United States government and social systems were built on a tradition known as the "Protestant work ethic." The Protestant work ethic emphasizes hard work and self-denial as the path to salvation. This puts many Americans at odds with cultures that value work, but also value investments of time into the family and community.

Similarly in cultures with a more collectivistic belief system, members may look at Americans who work long hours and spend little time with their children or their parents as the source of the problems of crime and disillusionment that are common in modern America.

AUTHORITARIANISM, EGALITARIANISM, AND SELF-REPRESENTATION

Authoritarianism is the preference for obedience to a clearly identified authority, with individual freedoms viewed as unimportant. A culture that endorses an authoritarian perspective often does not provide an opportunity for dissenting views or give all members equal voice in the decision-making process. Authoritarianism may also be reflected in the structure of a family in which one member makes the decisions and input from other family members is not sought out or considered. There is an additional expectation that those who are not designated as an authority figure will be submissive (Luckman, 2000).

An egalitarian viewpoint is characterized by a belief in equal political, economic, social, and civil rights for all people and allows for negotiation in authority relationships including consideration of individual differences. In an egalitarian culture, all members are included in the decision-making process. This interactional style may be mirrored in a family in which decisions require input from several members. The term *egalitarian* is also used to reflect the equal authority of members within a specific cultural group (Downes, 1997). One investigation compared parental child-rearing practices of Chinese parents in Taiwan, first-generation Chinese parents in America, and European American parents in the United States (Jose, Huntsinger, Huntsinger, & Liaw, 2000)—all parents with either preschool or kindergarten-aged children. The parents completed several questionnaires, and the families were videotaped during playtime. Both groups of Chinese parents reported exercising more control over their children and expected greater obedience when compared with European American parents. Chinese parents also rated attributes of being calm, polite, and neat as more important than European American parents did. Of interest was that all parents exhibited warmth and concern for their children. The authoritarian Chinese parents exhibited the same degree of warmth toward their children as the egalitarian European American parents did.

Self-representation, in terms of culture, is a sort of group self-esteem. *Self-representation* is a term that reflects a group's overall evaluation or appraisal of the worth of individuals within the group and reflects the groups perceptions of their status in the power structure. In an egalitarian view point the group would expect to challenge authority to promote the groups interests. In an authoritarian view point the group would accept the role and limitations assigned to them rather than challenging the status quo. Self-representation is more complex than the other two constructs. Consider the study by Chiang, Barrett, and Nunez (2000). In this study, Taiwanese and American mothers of toddlers were compared regarding their beliefs about their children's behavior. All mothers were asked to report not only the frequency of various behaviors but also why they believed those behaviors occurred. American mothers attributed more of their children's positive behaviors to internal factors such as disposition and ability, whereas Taiwanese mothers attributed positive behaviors to external factors such as environmental support and structure. These beliefs were contrasted with beliefs about negative behaviors. Taiwanese mothers attributed negative behaviors displayed by their children—for example, hurting another child or breaking objects—to internal factors such as anger and aggressiveness. American mothers attributed these same negative behaviors displayed by their children to accidents. The results of this investigation led the authors to conclude that there is a "tendency for Americans to believe that success is a result of internal ability and failure is not one's fault" (p. 365). American mothers reported that negative behaviors occurred as a result of external forces beyond the child's control, thus removing the responsibility from the child, yet successes were considered to be due to the child's ability. Taiwanese mothers were "more ready to blame their children and themselves for misdeeds and less willing to take credit for their positive behavior than are Americans" (p. 365). This investigation reflects how cultural norms influence the mother's perception of the value of their child's behavior.

COMMUNICATION STYLE AND CULTURE

Although there are a wide variety of communication and language styles, the two extremes of potential communication styles are presented here. On one end of the continuum is the expressive/overt communication style that conveys feelings, ideas, or moods in an open rather than a hidden, or controlled, manner. On the other end of the continuum is the restrained formal communication style that requires governing one's emotions or passions and adhering to traditional standards of correctness and without emotional content. Even the quantity of verbal interaction may be limited within this form of communication style. Several Native American groups, for example, place greater importance on a child's development of observational skills than verbal skills as a method to understand the world. This cultural emphasis has led to the misdiagnosis of language delays in bilingual Native American children by professionals trained in a Western cultural orientation (Kalyanpur, 1998).

The rate of speech and frequency of pauses during speech varies across cultural groups (Canino & Spurlock,

2000; Luckman, 2000). "Navajo children usually adopt a slow, methodical speech pattern" with frequent pauses during their statements (Canino & Spurlock, 2000, p. 13). Adults from a European American culture may interpret this pause as completion of a statement and inappropriately move to another topic without allowing the child to finish the statement. Many Asian and Native American groups value the use of quiet vocal tone and emotional restraint when speaking, contrasted with individuals from a southern European background such as Italy. Italian verbal interaction tends to have wide fluctuations in tonal qualities, and speech is often rapid.

Culture is both shaped by social communication and shapes language acquisition and nonverbal communication strategies. There are many ways culture, and cultural values are communicated that do not involve words. **Paralanguage** is a term used to describe nonverbal elements of communication that are used to modify meaning and convey emotion within a cultural context. Paralanguage may be expressed consciously or unconsciously. Paralanguage helps prevent ineffective communication, by giving a cultural message that accompanies any verbal message. The most obvious form of paralanguage is body language, the language of gestures, expressions, and postures. In North America, we commonly use our arms and hands to communicate many things such as to say hello, to count, express excitement, to beckon, warn away, and to insult. While traveling in Sri Lanka, the author noted that children would seldom return a wave or a smile. When a native of the culture was asked about this, two things stood out. First, in Sinhalese, there is no word equivalent to "hello." Greetings between people were conducted differently, and waving hello was not part of the cultural experience of the children. Also, the respondent indicated that young children were kept within the home and family circle. They were not encouraged to interact with others outside the home and family context. So, the meaning of even very common gestures within your own culture may be meaningless or have a different meaning in others.

Another type of paralanguage is the sense of personal space, called proxemics. **Proxemics** is a subcategory of the study of nonverbal communication and involves "the study of the nature, degree, and effect of the spatial separation individuals naturally maintain (as in various social and interpersonal situations) and of how this separation relates to environmental and cultural factors is the study of such interaction distances and other culturally defined uses of space" (Proxemics, n.d.). North Americans (particularly North Americans of European heritage) are notorious for preferring a lot of personal space. The crowded conditions that are common in many affluent Asian cities make the average American uncomfortable. **Figure 4-5** shows the crush of shoppers in downtown Hong Kong.

Communicating with Clothes

The last area of paralanguage we will review is the message conveyed by how a person dresses. Throughout history, clothing

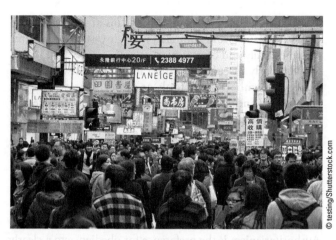

Figure 4-5 The dense crowds in many Asian cities are daunting to people from cultures where people expect more personal space between strangers.

has been both functional and a reflection of wealth and status. Clothing also reflects values, such as modesty, faith, and pride. Even within that description, what constitutes modesty is culturally determined. Clothing also is associated with group membership. People choose to dress differently in some social settings to "fit in" or to project their distinct identity. Uniforms are common in both schools and work environments because they make social relationships clear and thus simplify social interactions. Even when uniforms are not required, many students in health professions have rigid standards for dress while they are in a clinical setting. One reason for these standards is that young college students often have a very different sense of "modesty" in clothing than their elderly clients may have, and the young people may be seen as disrespectful or immature. By not adjusting to accommodate the cultural values of the people they serve in the health care area, students may actually damage a client's trust in them as clinicians. On the continuum of cultural responsiveness presented earlier in this chapter, this would be considered culturally destructive.

Tailoring the Message

In some cases, cultural backgrounds influence how individuals understand and respond to health information and the participation in preventative health behavior. For example, in the United States, the Safe to Sleep® campaign is a public health initiative that instructs parents in actions they can take to help their baby sleep safely and to reduce the baby's risk of sudden infant death syndrome (SIDS) and other sleep-related causes of infant death (Allen, Vessey, & Shapiro, 2009). American Indian/Alaska Native (AI/AN) infants have the highest rates of sudden infant death syndrome (SIDS) in the United States and are nearly three times more likely to die of SIDS than are white infants. For this reason, the National Institute of Child Health and Human Development (NICHD) worked with Native American communities to build the Healthy Native Babies Project. This project has created materials, messages, and methods for sharing safe infant sleep and other health information in native communities. These materials, messages, and methods are designed to be culturally appropriate and easily relatable to members of native communities (NICHD, 2013).

CULTURAL INFLUENCES ON DEVELOPMENT

Human learning is irreversibly intertwined with human culture. Occupational therapist Helene Polatajko notes that "how people go about understanding something depends on what it is that they want to know and how well they want to know it" (2010, p. 59). John Whiting and Beatrice Whiting were pioneers in the study of child development across cultural contexts and focused on cultural influences on development and contextual learning (Edwards & Bloch, 2010). The cultural learning environment of the Whitings was the foundation for the *early programming* consideration in the life course model (LCM) (USHHS MCH, 2010). It is widely acknowledged that experiences as varied as play, social companions, rules, and expected patterns of behavior shape children's learning and development (Worthman, 2010). Cultural influences on development extend broadly to shape who engages in what occupations. Factors such as gender, age, religion, family, and community needs all impact what children "want to know" and shape their motivation to learn.

Raghavan, Harkness, and Super (2010) described the early social learning context of the young child as a **developmental niche**. The developmental niche is seen as the interaction of children's physical and social settings, customs, child-rearing practices, and beliefs of parents about caretaking. Each of the aspects of the developmental niche is dynamic and adapts based on the age, gender, temperament, developmental level, and talents of individual children. The daily habits and routines of young children including eating, personal hygiene, social communication, and help seeking—all are culturally mediated and contribute to health and quality of life expectations. In **Figure 4-6**, you see a young child leaving for his first day of school. This is a significant life event in most Western cultures. In other cultures, education may be provided in the home, or may be considered optional, so a "first day of school" is not seen as an important event. In this way the relationship between cultural learning environments and early programming of health beliefs and behaviors is direct. Differences in the development of motor skills in various countries have been attributed to cultural experiences and expectations (Hopkins & Westra, 1990; Keller, Yovsi, & Voelker, 2002).

Children from different cultural groups have been shown to have differences in motor performance on standardized developmental instruments (Crowe, McClain, & Provost, 1999; Kerfield, Gurthrie, & Stewart, 1997). These differences have been attributed to the unique cultural expectations and the opportunity for children to engage in various activities within the cultural group. Typically developing Native Alaskan

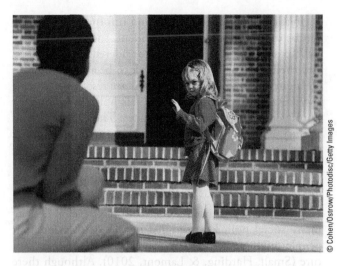

Figure 4-6   Culture determines the relative importance of daily events. In North America, a child's first day of school often includes new clothes and special attention, signifying its importance.

children were evaluated using the Denver Developmental Screening Test II (Kerfield et al., 1997). These children achieved many of the gross motor skills earlier than predicted by the Denver II. The authors postulated that cultural practices contributed to these differences. Native Alaskan children are provided with substantial freedom to engage in motor exploration, and older siblings are often responsible for the supervision of younger children. These older siblings exert few restrictions on motor behaviors, and this cultural practice creates the potential for Native Alaskan children to develop motor skills at an earlier age. Although some cultural practices may enhance motor development, other practices may restrict development.

Typically developing Native American 2-year-olds were also evaluated using the Peabody Developmental Motor Scales (Crowe et al., 1999). Children's performance was significantly poorer on the fine motor portion of this instrument, and the authors suggested that cultural expectations again played a role in this difference. The engagement in fine motor activities, particularly for this age group, is not a cultural norm or expectation. The data collected by both Crowe and colleagues (1999) and Kerfield and colleagues (1997) highlight the need for therapists to carefully select assessment tools to avoid cultural bias.

POVERTY AND DEVELOPMENT

In addition to the influence of cultural norms and expectations on development, the level of *poverty* associated with a specific ethnic group should also be considered. **Poverty** is the state of not having sufficient basic resources. No culture endorses abject poverty, but poverty is present to some degree in all human societies. *Absolute poverty* refers to the state of severe deprivation of basic human needs, which commonly includes food, water, sanitation, clothing, shelter, health care, education, and information. Poverty can be caused by a particular incident, such as the loss of a job or a major illness. This is considered **acute poverty**, and the individuals involved expect to be able to improve their circumstances as the problems are resolved. **Chronic poverty** occurs when the individuals hold little hope for improvement in their circumstances. The expectation of poverty as a way of life is what distinguishes it as a distinct subculture. The concept of a self-perpetuating subculture of poverty was first proposed by anthropologist Oscar Lewis (1998). According to Lewis, people living in the subculture of poverty reflect a strong feeling of helplessness, isolation, and dependency. Lewis's ideas led to the development of many social policies grounded in the assumption that people might cease to be poor if they changed their culture (Small, Harding, & Lamont, 2010). Although there continues to be evidence that living in chronic poverty results in changes in aspirations, coping strategies, and lifestyle choices, it is no longer viewed as a distinct culture (Copestake & Camfield, 2010).

Both the noncompletion of a high school education and incomes at or below the poverty level are statistical predictors of poor health. Limited educational achievement and poverty have been documented to reflect disparity among racial and ethnic groups. Compared with non-Hispanic whites, the disparity was greatest for Hispanics and non-Hispanic American Indians/Alaska Natives. Non-Hispanic blacks showed some disparity, but to a lesser degrees than that seen among the Hispanics and Native American groups (CDC, 2011). The Centers for Disease Control and Prevention (2011) state that "The percentage of adults with disabilities who did not complete high school was approximately double that of adults without disabilities in both 2005 and 2009 and the proportion of people with disabilities living below the poverty level was more than twice that of people without disabilities" (p. 2).

In 2009, the United Nations Economic Commission for Europe Conference of European Statisticians defined homelessness as consisting of two broad groups of people. The first of these groups, called *primary homelessness,* includes people living in the streets without a shelter that would fall within the scope of living quarters. Homeless "street people," such as the man shown in **Figure 4-7**, can be found in cities all over the world. The second and more common type, *secondary homelessness,* includes people with no place of usual residence who move frequently between various types of accommodations (including dwellings, shelters, and institutions for the homeless or other living quarters).

In the United States in 2012, the estimated odds of experiencing homelessness were 1 in 29 for people living in poverty. The group at greatest risk included poor veterans; people discharged from prisons or jails were the group with the next greatest risk (National Alliance to End Homelessness, 2012). Although we often think of the homeless as single men, as illustrated in **Figure 4-7**, children and youth in fact make up a large part of the world's homeless

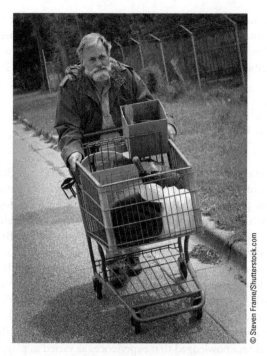

Figure 4-7 Homeless people, who carry all their belongings with them, are at risk for violence, health problems, and mental illness.

population. Children who are homeless are currently the fastest-growing segment of the homeless population and are more likely to have delayed development than other children (Nunez & Fox, 1999; Royeen & Crabtree, 2006). Children from African American, Hispanic, and Native American households are at far greater risk to experience the effects of poverty than children in European American households in the United States (Reviere & Hylton, 1999; Spector, 2012; Wright, 2002).

Homelessness has particularly adverse effects on children and youth, including poor physical and mental health, developmental delay, and missed educational opportunities. Schooling for homeless children is often interrupted and delayed, with homeless children twice as likely to have a learning disability, repeat a grade, or to be suspended from school (American Psychological Association, 2012). In addition, as of 2012, a quarter of homeless children have witnessed violence and 22 percent have been separated from their families. The result of this is that as many as half of school-age homeless children experience problems with mental health including depression, anxiety, post-traumatic stress disorder, and substance abuse problems (American Psychological Association, 2012).

The term **occupational deprivation** has been used to describe the condition when something external to an individual results in limiting his or her opportunity to participate in valued occupations. Occupational deprivation is often associated with homelessness. When the cause of the homelessness is an economic downturn or fleeing from an abusive spouse, individuals may no longer be able to pursue the occupations that they found meaningful before.

CULTURE, LANGUAGE, AND HEALTH LITERACY

Earlier in this chapter, the term *cultural competence* was defined. An important related concept is the concept of *linguistic competence*. As with cultural competence, linguistic competence is a goal set for health care providers. **Linguistic competence** is defined as "the capacity of an organization and its personnel to communicate effectively, and convey information in a manner that is easily understood by diverse audiences including persons of limited English proficiency, those who have low literacy skills or are not literate, and individuals with disabilities" (National Center for Cultural Competence, 2012a). Linguistic competency requires organizational and provider capacity to respond effectively to the health literacy needs of populations served. **Table 4-4** offers suggestions for the support of linguistic competency for organizations.

Associated with linguistic competence is the concept of *health literacy*. **Health literacy** is "the degree to which individuals have the capacity to obtain, process, and understand basic health information needed to make appropriate health decisions and services needed to prevent or treat illness" (USHHS HRSA, 2012). Health literacy includes the ability to read and understand information associated with managing yourself and your family's health. This can include diverse skills such as understanding the instructions written on prescription drug bottles, reading appointment slips, and understanding home exercise programs. Health literacy is not specifically about reading ability. A person who reads routinely at home or work may be overwhelmed or confused by the complex and unfamiliar language used in the health care environment.

The broad use of the Internet has caused challenges to health professionals trying to provide clear concise information. When people with health conditions use the Internet to search for health information, they are likely to use that knowledge to question a doctor, manage pain, or change the way they cope with a chronic condition (Fox & Purcell, 2010). Savvy Internet users who focus on their specific health concerns may be in the position of bringing new research information to their health care provider. Conversely, there is much false and unsubstantiated health information on the Internet, and discussion between and health care providers often involves clarifying facts from fiction, and explaining the importance of seeking credible health information.

In the case of Nangane, both linguistic and cultural competence were needed to meet the needs of her and her family. Through establishing a culturally sensitive dialog, Nangane was able to both understand and accept the rehabilitation process. She was able to return to her son's home and function effectively in both the community and cultural practices that she valued.

CULTURAL BELIEFS ABOUT DISABILITY

We have discussed aspects of culture and cultural influences on development and behavior, but it is also important to consider that culture influences values and

TABLE 4-4 Capabilities Needed to Support Linguistic Competency in Organizations

Bilingual/bicultural or multilingual/multicultural staff
Cultural brokers
Foreign language interpretation services including distance technologies
Sign language interpretation services
Multilingual telecommunication systems
Computer-assisted real-time translation (CART) or viable real-time transcriptions (VRT)
Print materials in easy-to-read, low-literacy, picture and symbol formats
Materials in alternative formats (e.g., audiotape, Braille, enlarged print)
Varied approaches to share information with individuals who experience cognitive disabilities
Materials developed and tested for specific cultural, ethnic, and linguistic groups
Ethnic media in languages other than English (e.g., television, radio, Internet, newspapers, periodicals)
Adapted from National Center for Cultural Competence (2012b).

CASE 1

Continuing Nangane's story . . .

Nangane believed strongly in traditional medicine (Ayurveda) and had wanted to continue her herbal medicines rather than using Western medicines to treat her arthritis and high blood pressure. Her physician had discouraged the use of her Ayurvedic medications, largely because no one in the family was able to explain what actual herbs were in the medicines. Because all the herbs had Sinhalese names, some of which had no translation, the physician and pharmacist were worried about potential drug interactions.

In this meeting, the team learned that Nangane's problem with PT was that the assigned PT was a male, and she was uncomfortable being touched and guided by a young unmarried man. Nangane understood the need for exercise and was open to reconsidering PT interventions if they were provided in private (rather than in the big therapy gym) and provided by a female therapist. Nangane said that she liked her OT, who was a middle-aged woman, but had always performed her personal hygiene tasks differently than the OT was instructing her to do. Using the granddaughter's interest in traditional Sri Lanka routines, the OT was able to open a dialog to discuss private personal habits that Nangane had not been open to before.

In this meeting, most of Nangane's concerns were addressed. It was arranged that Nangane would be the first person attended to by the nursing staff each morning, and that after her nursing and ADL activities, she would have 30 minutes in the recreation room (where it was quiet) before her breakfast. Her granddaughter agreed to learn the scientific names for the herbs in her grandmother's traditional medicines, in the hopes that they could be added to her daily regime. Nangane agreed to take the "American medicines" for the time being.

Following this meeting, Nangane was pleased with the therapy team's interest in her culture and her country. She was able to successfully complete her rehabilitation regime and return to the family home. Before her discharge, she taught all of her therapists how to wear a Kandyan sari and introduced them to Sri Lanka curries.

beliefs. Throughout this text, we will offer examples of human performance and development, reflecting typical patterns of performance and participation, as well as offering asides to give readers insight into issues related to people with disabilities. The issues related to cultural beliefs about disability will be expanded upon in many of the following chapters in this text. In Chapter 5, "Life Span Communication," we will discuss language and communication issues related to both culture and disability; in Chapter 6, "Activities and Participation: Learning and Applying Knowledge," we will discuss learning theory and social learning; and finally, in Chapter 7, "Environmental Contexts," we will look into everyday spaces and issues of accessibility and mobility.

SUMMARY

Understanding the unique contributions of culture on development affords therapists greater variety and skill in developing appropriate and effective intervention plans. Culture provides both a lens and a filter to view reality. Throughout this chapter, examples have been provided to describe the interaction of cultural expectations and development. There are cultural differences in child rearing, in activity expectations, and in the role of people with disabilities within a community, among many other things. Culturally relevant topics will be included in future chapters as they relate to the chapter topic.

No example offered in this or later chapter should be misconstrued as an absolute representation of a cultural group. Stories from clinicians and clients in differing national and cultural settings are included to offer a window to the wider world, but should simply be viewed as what they are, personal stories.

CASE 2

Juan

Juan was a 2-year, 7-month-old boy from Puerto Rico. His family had recently moved to the Northeast from Puerto Rico for the father to pursue better employment. Juan was born with a brachial plexus injury resulting in significant loss of function in his right arm. Upon arrival in the Northeast, Juan's parents enrolled him in an early intervention program. Juan had a lack of sensation and motor control in his arm. His family had "exercised" his arm for him, but he had not received any therapy support before his move.

Discussions with Juan's mother revealed that Juan did not use utensils to feed himself and he did not engage in any dressing skills. He was able to drink from a cup but preferred to use a bottle. The mother reported that Juan was healthy, and she had taken him to all his medical appointments while living in Puerto Rico, but his right arm still did not work. Although Juan was verbal, according to his mother, and primarily spoke Spanish, he spoke only a few words during the initial evaluation session and appeared shy.

A developmental assessment revealed that Juan's fine motor skills were compromised bilaterally. He had very limited use of his right arm and hand due to decreased strength and range of motion and displayed poor dexterity on his left hand. His decreased sensory awareness of his right arm posed a potential safety risk. He was referred to OT for treatment. His initial intervention plan included play activities to stretch his right arm, along with developing basic dressing and self-feeding skills. Fine motor activities were addressed through both play and use of utensils for self-feeding. Although Juan's mother agreed to the plan, she also wanted to know how she could get his "right arm to work."

The OT was able to see Juan in his home. The family lived in a small two-bedroom, one-bathroom apartment with three children, the grandmother, and both parents. The parents slept in the living room while the grandmother had one bedroom and the three children shared the other bedroom. Although Juan was the youngest child, he was also the only male child in this family. His father frequently asked the OT if she knew how strong Juan would become as he grew and if she could help him become stronger. Although both parents had verbally agreed that the suggested occupational therapy activities would be helpful, they reported that they did not have time to "exercise Juan's arm," even though the suggested activities were meant to be used during playtime.

The initial OT focus was to improve fine motor skills and motor control through the use of functional self-care tasks and play activities. The parents always agreed with the OT plan but then did not follow the suggested activities. During the third home visit, the OT noticed that both the mother and the grandmother would take great pride in dressing Juan very neatly, and his older sisters would bring him toys instead of having Juan open the small toy box to get the toys himself. The cultural orientation of interdependence was revealed in many of the actions this family performed. The OT began to understand that for the family to follow through with the recommendations would symbolize that the family did not provide adequate care for Juan. The OT intervention plan asked the family to make Juan engage in tasks that were very challenging. Although the parents agreed with the therapist's recommendations, those recommendations conflicted with the cultural stance that it would be uncaring to force Juan to use his right arm.

Then the OT changed her orientation at that point and worked with the mother and sisters to design an intervention program by which each could help Juan develop his muscles, and then explained that he should practice using his right arm to make it stronger, rather than focus on self-care skill. The practice sessions included play activities such as hammering with a toy hammer and sawing. These activities required use of both hands in activities that would be interpreted by all family members as tasks to make Juan strong.

Continues

Case 2   *Continued*

As he gained strength, the OT could progress to activities to help make Juan's fingers strong. These activities included such tasks as pulling on his socks and shoes, but the task was now framed as an exercise to help Juan strengthen his hands. Both sisters took great delight in helping Juan become strong. The cultural orientation of providing interdependent support was used as an asset in the intervention plan. During subsequent visits, Juan began to use his right hand to stabilize toys while playing and improved the dexterity of his left hand. Instead of viewing this family as noncompliant with OT intervention, the OT demonstrated cultural sensitivity and reoriented her intervention to meet the family's needs.

Guiding Questions

Some questions to consider:

1. Would a cultural worldview, such as the one Juan's family held, be best described as individualistic or collectivistic? Explain your choice?
2. The OT in this case is English speaking, but understands basic Spanish. What strategies should she have taken as she started the therapeutic relationship to be sure that the family agreed with the goals that she set for Juan?
3. Skilled nursing facilities have a structured routine, and typically these institutions do not easily accommodate individual preferences about things like the timing or frequency of showers or the protection of daily personal time for prayer. Of all the problems that Nangane had during her stay in the skilled nursing facility, which do you think the facility should have made an effort to accommodate and why?
4. What are some things the therapists might have done to better meet Nangane's needs and improve her rehabilitation experience?

Speaking of
Culture across Borders

CRISTINA H. BOLAÑOS, PHD, OT OCCUPATIONAL
THERAPIST WORKING OUTSIDE THE UNITED STATES

Although most therapists in the United States regard Mexicans as a homogenous cultural group, Mexican culture varies greatly depending on the geographical region where the person comes from, her educational background, socioeconomic level, religion, all of which influence lifestyle and occupational development. The culture in which you live influences the profession you choose and the value it is given by society.

The vast majority of occupational therapists in my country do not study occupational therapy because of the value society ascribes to our profession, which continues to be low. The main reason people study occupational therapy in Mexico is because they are genuinely interested in helping people to improve their lives. Occupational therapy offers this possibility in different stages of life and different pathologies.

Continues

Speaking of Continued

I have been working as an occupational therapist in Mexico for over 30 years. At the beginning of my studies, we were taught techniques that emphasized independence, function, and self-care. However, we lacked insight into how the culture and their socioeconomic level could support or undermine our interventions.

In Mexican culture, the family or the caregiver takes care of an ill person, rather than an external institution. Although elderly people may be able to look after themselves, their families discourage them from doing so; they are also discouraged from maintaining their own occupations. Many clients I saw who came from wealthy families were not interested in doing any household activities whatsoever. These were activities that they had not done prior to their illness or impairment, and they were not motivated to pursue them either, as part of their rehabilitation.

Later, when I moved from physical rehabilitation to work in the pediatrics area, I started working with teachers and other health professionals to facilitate the development and occupations of children in schools. Over time, I expanded my range of work to also include clinician consultant and researcher.

I have been involved as an educator since early in my career. My continuous challenge in this field has been to help students understand the importance of occupational competence and social participation while being aware of the cultural values of our country and to develop an understanding of their contribution to health through healthy occupations.

As an occupational therapist, understanding the relationship between valued occupations and culture has been critical for me to see clearly how culture influences interventions.

REFERENCES

Allen, P. J., Vessey, J. A., & Shapiro (2009). *Primary care of the child with a chronic condition* (5th ed.). St. Louis, MO: C.V. Mosby.

American Psychological Association. (2012). Effects of poverty, hunger, and homelessness on children and youth. Retrieved from http://www.apa.org/pi/families/poverty.aspx

Balcazar, F., Suarez-Balcazar, Y., Taylor-Ritzler, T., & Keys, C. (2011). *Race, culture, and disability: Rehabilitation science and practice*. Sudbury, MA: Jones and Bartlett Publishers.

Bolanos, C. (2003). Personal communication.

Brewer, M. B., & Ya-Ru, C. (2007). Where (who) are collectives in collectivism? Toward conceptual clarification of individualism and collectivism. *Psychological Review, 114*(1), 133–151.

Canino, I. A., & Spurlock, J. (2000). *Culturally diverse children and adolescents* (2nd ed.). New York: Guilford Press.

Carteret, M. (2011). The role of religion in providing culturally responsive care. *Dimensions of culture: Cross cultural communications for healthcare professionals*. Retrieved from http://www.dimensionsofculture.com/2011/09/the-role-of-religion-in-providing-culturally-responsive-care/

Centers for Disease Control and Prevention (CDC). (2011). Fact sheet—*CDC health disparities and inequalities report—U.S., 2011*. Atlanta, GA: CDC. Retrieved from http://www.cdc.gov/minorityhealth/reports/CHDIR11/FactSheet.pdf

Chiang, T., Barrett, K. C., & Nunez, N. N. (2000) Maternal attributions of Taiwanese and American toddlers' misdeeds and accomplishments. *Journal of Cross-cultural Psychology, 31,* 349–368.

Cohn, D., & Morin, R. (2008). *Who moves? Who stays put? Where's home?* Pew Social & Demographic Trends.

Copestake, J., & Camfield, L. (2010). Measuring multidimensional aspiration gaps: A means to understanding cultural aspects of poverty. *Development Policy Review, 28*(5), 617–633.

Cross, T., Bazron, B., Dennis, K., & Isaacs, M. (1989). *Towards a culturally competent system of care* (vol. I). Washington, DC: Georgetown University Child Development Center, CASSP Technical Assistance Center.

Crowe, T. K., McClain, C., & Provost, B. (1999). Motor development of Native American children on the Peabody Developmental Motor Scales. *American Journal of Occupational Therapy, 53,* 514–518.

Dictionary.com (2014). *Habit*. Retrieved from http://dictionary.reference.com/browse/habit

Downes, N. J. (1997). *Ethnic Americans: For the health professional* (2nd ed.). Dubuque, IA: Kendall/Hunt Publishing Co.

Edwards, C. P., & Bloch, M. (July, 2010). The Whitings' concepts of culture and how they have fared in contemporary psychology and anthropology. In C. P. Edwards & T. Weisner (Guest Eds.),

Journal of Cross Cultural Psychology, Special Issue, "The Legacy of Beatrice and John Whiting for Cross-Cultural Research," *41*(4).

Fox, S., & Purcell, K. (2010). *Chronic disease and the Internet, Pew Internet & American Life Project.* Washington, DC: Pew Research Center.

Green, E. G., Deschamps, J., & Paez, D. (2005). Variation of individualism and collectivism within and between 20 countries. *Journal of Cross-Cultural Psychology, 36,* 321–339.

Hopkins, B., & Westra, T. (1990). Motor development, maternal expectations, and the role of handling. *Infant Behavior and Development, 13,* 117–122.

Jezewski, M.A. & Sotnik, P. (2001). *Culture brokering: Providing culturally competent rehabilitation services to foreign-born persons.* Center for International Rehabilitation Research Information and Exchange. CIRRIE Monograph Series, John Stone, Ed. Buffalo, NY: CIRRIE.

Jose, P. E., Huntsinger, C. S., Huntsinger, P. R., & Liaw, F.(2000). Parental values and practices relevant to young children's social development in Taiwan and the United States. *Journal of Cross-Cultural Psychology, 31,* 677–702.

Kalyanpur, M. (1998). The challenge of cultural blindness: Implications for family-focused service delivery. *Journal of Child and Family Studies, 7,* 317–332.

Keller, H., Yovsi, R. D., & Voelker, S. (2002). The role of motor stimulation in parental ethnotheories. *Journal of Cross-Cultural Psychology, 33,* 398–414.

Keller, H. (2007). *Cultures of infancy.* Mahwah, NJ: Lawrence Erlbaum.

Kerfield, C. I., Gurthrie, M. R., & Stewart, K. B. (1997). Evaluation of the Denver II as applied to Alaskan Native children. *Pediatric Physical Therapy, 9,* 23–31.

Kim, W. J., Kim, L. I., & Rue, D. S. (1997). Korean American children. In G. Johnson-Powell and J. Yamamoto (Eds.), *Transcultural child development* (pp. 183–207). New York: John Wiley and Sons.

Lewis, O. (1998). The culture of poverty. *Society, 35*(2), 7.

Lieberman, M., Jarcho, J., Obayashi, J. (2005). Attributional inference across cultures: Similar automatic attributions and different controlled corrections. *Personality and Social Psychology Bulletin, 31*(7), 889–901.

Luckman, J. (2000). *Transcultural communication in health care.* Albany, NY: Delmar.

National Alliance to End Homelessness. (2012). Snapshot of homelessness. Retrieved from http://www.endhomelessness.org /section/about_homelessness/snapshot_of_homelessness

National Center for Cultural Competence. (2012a). Cultural awareness. Retrieved from http://www.nccccurricula.info /awareness/index.html

National Center for Cultural Competence. (2012b). Cultural and linguistic competence: Rationale, conceptual frameworks, and values. Retrieved from http://www.ncccurricula.info/framework/B4.html

National Institute for Child Health and Human Development (NICHD). (2013). Getting safe infant sleep messages into native communities. Retrieved from http://www.nichd.nih.gov /news/resources/spotlight/Pages/091313-HNBP.aspx

Nunez, R., & Fox, C. (1999). A snapshot of family homelessness across America. *Political Science Quarterly, 114,* 289–307.

Polatajko, H. (2010). Chapter 3: The study of occupation. In C. Christiansen & E. Townsend (Eds.), *Introduction to occupation: The art and science of living* (2nd ed., pp. 58–79). New Jersey: Pearson.

Proxemics. (n.d.). In *Merriam Webster Online.* Retrieved from http://www.merriam-webster.com/dictionary/proxemics

Raghavan, C. S., Harkness, S., & Super, C. M. (2010). Parental ethnotheories in the context of immigration: Asian Indian immigrant and Euro-American mothers and daughters in an American town. *Journal of Cross Cultural Psychology, 41*(4), 617–632.

Reviere, R., & Hylton, K. (1999). Poverty and health: An international overview. In R. L. Leavitt (Ed.), *Cross-cultural rehabilitation.* (pp. 59–69). London: W. B. Saunders.

Royeen, M., & Crabtree, J. (2006) *Culture in rehabilitation: From competency to proficiency.* Upper Saddle River, NJ: Pearson Prentice Hall.

Scott, J., & Marshall, G. (2009) *A dictionary of sociology (Oxford dictionary of sociology).* Oxford University Press, USA.

Schimmack, U., Oishi, S., & Diener, E. (2005). Individualism: A valid and important dimension of cultural differences between nations. *Personality & Social Psychology Review, 9,* 17–31.

Small, M., Harding, D. J., & Lamont, M. (2010). Reconsidering culture and poverty. *Annals of the American Academy of Political And Social Science, 629*(1), 6–27.

Spector, R. E. (2012). *Cultural diversity in health and illness* (8th ed.). Stamford, CT: Appleton and Lange.

Stewart, S. M., & McBride-Chang, C. (2000). Influences on children's sharing in a multicultural setting. *Journal of Cross-Cultural Psychology, 31,* 333–348.

United Nations. (2009). *Enumeration of homeless people, United Nations Economic and Social Council.* Economic Commission for Europe Conference of European Statisticians, Group of Experts on Population and Housing Censuses, Twelfth Meeting, Geneva, 28–30 October 2009.

U.S. Department of Health and Human Services Health Resources and Services Administration Maternal and Child Health Bureau (USHHS MCH). (2010). *Rethinking MCH: The life course model as an organizing framework concept paper,* Version 1.1.

U.S. Department of Health and Human Services, Health Resources and Services Administration (USHHS HRSA). (2012). About health literacy. Retrieved from http://www.hrsa.gov /publichealth/healthliteracy/healthlitabout.html

U.S. Public Law Individuals With Disabilities Education Act (IDEA), 20 U.S.C. § 1400 (2004).

Williams, S. M., & Templeton, A. R. (2003). Race and genomics. *New England Journal of Medicine, 348,* 2581–2582.

Worthman, C. M. (2010), The ecology of human development: Evolving models for cultural psychology. *Journal of Cross Cultural Psychology, 41*(4), 546–562.

Wright, K. (2002). *Homeless in America.* Farmington Hills, MI: Gale Group.

CHAPTER 5

Life Span Communication

Anne Cronin, PhD, OTR/L, FAOTA,
Associate Professor, Division of
Occupational Therapy, West Virginia
University, Morgantown, West Virginia

Objectives

Upon completion of this chapter, readers should be able to:

- Define communication as an aspect of human activity and participation;

- Discuss the interrelationship between culture and communication;

- Describe forms of communication commonly used in the prelinguistic period;

- Differentiate between the terms *voice, speech, expressive communication,* and *receptive communication;*

- Discuss the implications of establishing communications with people who are prelinguistic or limited to concrete symbols in communication;

- Identify possible implications or limitations that may complicate communication with individuals with language or hearing impairments;

- Articulate the developmental and social considerations associated with augmentative and alternative communication strategies; and

- Be able to paraphrase the focus and issues addressed in the communication bill of rights.

Key Terms

abstract symbols
American sign language (ASL)
assistive technology (AT)
augmentative/alternative
    communication (AAC)
communication
communication bill of rights
concrete symbols
expressive communication
hearing impairment
intelligibility
intentional behavior

language
language decoding
language disorder
language impairment
linguistic competence
literacy
meme
metalinguistic awareness
morphology
paralinguistic communication
phonology
pragmatics

prelinguistic period
pre-intentional behavior
presymbolic communication
receptive communication
semantics
speech
speech disorder
symbolic communication
syntax
voice

CASE 1

Jonathan

Jonathan is 7½ years old and attends a regular education second-grade classroom with an aide and special education support. He has normal intelligence and spastic cerebral palsy. Jonathan is very social but does not communicate verbally well because of his dysarthric speech patterns. He is intellectually able to keep up with second-grade classwork, but is unable to do the written work assigned to the class. He has been seen by OTs, PTs, and speech-language pathologists (SLPs) since birth and has made fewer gains in motor control over the past two years. At this time, Jonathan spends most of his school day in his wheelchair, and he is unable to produce any written output. Jonathan is unable to isolate a pointer finger to do computer or blackboard tasks. He has a full-time aide to assist him with writing, mobility, and other physical tasks within the school. Jonathan needs moderate assistance on individual tasks and does not function well in groups. He works well independently and communicates when assistance is needed. One of the teacher's hopes for Jonathan is that he will gain skill in negotiating and compromising, because he has mostly used his augmentative and alternative communication (AAC) device to give directions or answer direct questions to date.

Jonathan has extensive rehabilitation needs, including communication needs. As readers learn more about the nature of communication, the interrelationship between communication and other rehabilitation needs will become clear.

Continues on page 90

INTRODUCTION

Communication is a broad term that encompasses the ability of humans to interact in ways that enable them to share such functions as basic needs, wants, desires, and ideas (Owens, 2011). Developmental and rehabilitation interventions that emphasize communication are the primary domain of practice for speech-language pathologists (SLP). Although SLPs typically take the lead in the health care team in addressing communication impairments, all members of the team need communication as a foundation for building a therapeutic relationship. The focus of this chapter is on functional communication, patterns of development, and nonverbal aspects of communication, all of which are essential to effective provision of care for occupational and physical therapists.

In this chapter, we will focus on functional communication in all forms. We will also integrate cultural influences on communication and the development and maintenance of communication from birth to adulthood, differences in communication, and an introduction to communication disorders that adversely affect the communication of children and adults.

Without a "voice," Jonathan will have difficulty interacting with his peers and may be excluded socially because of this. The fact that he is in a wheelchair is far less likely to limit his participation in childhood and playground cultures than will the lack of a voice. Even with a device to help him gain a voice, Jonathan will need help using it in all of the social contexts in which he needs to function.

Specific age-related milestones for language acquisition in young children will be addressed later in the chapters devoted to those age groups.

DEFINITIONS

There are many aspects of communication, some of which were addressed earlier in the discussions of cognition and development. The National Institutes of Deafness and Other Communication Disorders differentiate between the terms *voice*, *speech*, and *language* (NIH NID, 2011b). Because they are distinct, disorders affecting any one of these three will affect an individual's ability to communicate.

VOICE

Voice is traditionally considered the sound made as air from our lungs is pushed through our larynx. It is the physiological production of sound through motor and respiratory control. Voice, in this context, is the result of the vibration of the vocal folds to create a complex tone that is composed of many frequencies. Movements and positions of the lips, teeth, and tongue, together with breath support, produce various sounds. Use your hearing skills to analyze two sounds that provide a contrast between voicing and nonvoicing. If you produce the "s" sound and place your hand on your larynx (voice box), you will not feel much in the laryngeal area. Air is taken from the lungs and forced through a narrow constriction in the mouth to produce the sound. Contrast the "s" with production of a "z," because "z" is a voiced sound. You will feel vibration of the larynx as you produce the sound. Air is taken from the lungs, and through vocal fold vibration, a complex sound is produced. A number of speech sounds are produced with voicing.

Later when we discuss alternative and augmentative forms of communication, the term *voice* will also be used to describe the digital or recorded output of electronic communication devices. In the case of Jonathan, the conception of a voice will be extended to include the sound output of a device intended to aid communication.

Voice is distinct from speech and language in that it carries meaning only in how it may be interpreted by a listener, as in a parent listening to a baby cry, or in how it is used to form speech.

SPEECH

Speech involves very skilled motor control, but also involves the expression of thoughts in spoken words. Speech therefore is learned, and reflects the culture and communication forms of the society within which the infant develops. People of all cultures and backgrounds require extensive postnatal experience to produce and decode speech sounds that are the basis of language.

LANGUAGE

Language is a system of words or signs that have understood meanings within a particular group of people. Through language, people express thoughts and feelings to each other. Language may be expressed verbally or by writing, signing, or making other gestures, such as eye blinking or mouth movements. It encompasses verbal and nonverbal communication skills and how individuals use language.

The word *language* has many meanings. Contemporary views of human language hold that:

- Language evolves within specific historical, social, and cultural contexts;

- Language, as a rule-governed behavior, is described by at least five parameters—phonologic, morphologic, syntactic, semantic, and pragmatic;

- Language learning and use are determined by the interaction of biological, cognitive, psychosocial, and environmental factors; and

- Effective use of language for communication requires a broad understanding of human interaction including such associated factors as nonverbal cues, motivation, and sociocultural roles.

(American Speech-Language-Hearing Association, 1983, p. 44)

This definition underscores the fact that language is a multifaceted behavior that is under constant change due to a number of different factors. For example, our use of advanced technologies has resulted in the introduction of new words to our vocabularies. Concepts such as tweeting, texting, or even email did not exist until the advent of the Internet and cellular telephones.

TABLE 5-1   Clarifying Speech and Language
Voice is the sound we make as air from our lungs is pushed between vocal folds in our larynx, causing them to vibrate. An individual's voice has distinctive qualities that are a combination of learning and anatomy. These qualities include pitch, resonance, and amplitude.
Speech is talking, which is one way to express language. Speech requires precisely coordinated muscle actions of the tongue, lips, jaw, and vocal tract to produce the recognizable sounds that make up language. *Articulation* is how clearly a speech sound is produced. Children or adults may have errors in speech for one specific sound, or a group of sound classes. For example, a child may say "tat" for "cat."
Language is a set of shared rules that allow people to express their ideas in a meaningful way. Language may be expressed verbally or by writing, signing, or making other gestures, such as eye blinking or mouth movements. Language may be received through listening, reading, or through the interpreting of some other coding system.
Adapted from: http://www.nidcd.nih.gov/health/voice/pages/speechandlanguage.aspx

Expressive communication is the use of language to communicate thoughts, ideas, or feelings. Expressive communication may be spoken, signed, or written language. *Expressive language* is similar in conception but focuses on the ability to express oneself through language. Expressive language includes both speech and written communication. Expressive language skills include vocabulary, semantics (word/sentence meaning), morphology, and syntax (grammar rules).

Receptive communication describes an individual's ability to receive and interpret verbal and/or nonverbal messages. In typical development, children's receptive understanding of language greatly exceeds their ability to produce speech. *Receptive language* parallels this concept; however, it is narrowed to consider communication that is language based. *Receptive language skills* include receptive vocabulary, following directions, and understanding questions.

Table 5-1 offers clear definitions of voice, speech, and language. The distinctions between voice, speech, and language will be critical for health professionals to understand as they relate to distinctly different considerations in the daily activities and participation of individuals.

COMMUNICATION IN THE ICF

Although "voice and speech functions" are described in the ICF as a subcategory under body functions and structures, the focus of this chapter will be on communication as it relates to activities and participation. The ICF definition of communication is "… general and specific features of communicating by language, signs, and symbols, including receiving and producing messages, carrying on conversations, and using communication devices and techniques" (World Health Organization, 2001, p. 12). Communication is required for functional participation and interpersonal interaction in most areas of occupation, especially education, work, and social participation. Communication is also the foundation of group occupations such as participation in home life, kinship, faith groups, and civic involvement. As the Internet has made worldwide virtual social connections possible, communication is at the forefront of many daily occupations including email correspondence, web "chats," online blogs, and online video sharing.

THE INTERRELATIONSHIP BETWEEN CULTURE AND COMMUNICATION

Thinking back to Chapter 4, when people interact over time, cultures are formed. Even in two-person relationships, a culture may develop over time. Partners will develop their own shared history, language patterns, rituals, and customs that give their relationship its unique character. So, although we tend to think of culture in terms of racial and ethnic groups, any social unit can develop a culture over time (Scott & Marshall, 2009). Although it may seem odd to start a chapter on communication with a discussion of culture, communication and culture are intimately linked. Through communication, cultures are built, and without communication and communication media, it would be impossible to preserve and pass along cultural values. In addition, cultures influence how much and what type of language we are exposed to as learners. Many cultural patterns in communication, such as gender differences in communication styles reflect this close relationship between culture and communication.

Through communication, we express ideas and values. We express these in many ways, including language, gestures, and visual images. The role of visual images as a mechanism for conveying culture is growing with the the rapid societal changes associated with increasing technology and information sharing.

The word meme was coined by the biologist Richard Dawkins to explain the spread of ideas and cultural phenomena.

A **meme** is an element of a culture or system of behavior that may be considered to be passed from one individual to another through communication. Most typically a meme is an image, video, or piece of text that becomes popular and is copied and spread across the Internet, often with slight variations. Memes, like genes, evolve and spread through communication between individuals. Memes are the building blocks of functional communication and, as noted by Christiansen and Townsend, are "particularly important in the emergence of occupations that express culture through creative thought" (2010, p. 185).

COMMUNICATION DEVELOPMENT

Communication is central to all human cultures and in all stages of development. Typically, we think of language as the focus of communication, and often this is true. We express our ideas through written or spoken words. However, communication often occurs without verbal exchange. Rowland (2011) has developed and published an online assessment tool, the *Communication Matrix*. This assessment tool is designed to clearly describe communication skills in individuals who are in one of the earliest stages of communication development, regardless of age. This instrument was used in this chapter to describe early, nonverbal, and prelinguistic communication development.

The **prelinguistic period** is the period from birth to approximately 12 months of age and is characterized by children's exploration of the environment with their caregivers. This period is characterized by unintentional and intentional nonspeech communication. When this period ends, the children begin to use words as referents, which is the hallmark of linguistic development. **Table 5-2** offers details of specific communication milestones in the prelinguistic period. This is a particularly important period of communication development to understand, because many developmental disabilities that include delays in language development are best treated when they are identified early. This is especially true of the autism spectrum disorders.

UNINTENTIONAL COMMUNICATION

When the newborn infant cries, and flails her arms, her father comes and picks her up. She did not intend to call him over, but the father recognized her distress, interpreted it, and responded. **Pre-intentional behavior** communicates even though the behavior is not under an individual's own control, but rather reflects his or her general state (hungry) and the caregiver interprets the meaning from the infant's

TABLE 5-2 Communication Milestones in the Prelinguistic Period				
Expected Age of Development	**Play and Cognitive Skills**	**Receptive Language**	**Expressive Communication**	**Sound Production**
0 to 3 months	Children make eye contact Are alert to sounds Watch a speaker's mouth Engage in vocal play	Discriminate between angry and friendly voices	Have distinct cries for hunger, discomfort, and boredom Vocalize to show pleasure	Make cooing sounds: "ah, ah, ah, ah"
3 to 6 months	Maintain eye contact with speakers Imitate facial expressions Are attracted to objects and people in the immediate environment	Begin to recognize their own name Respond to "no"	Take turns vocalizing Will show you toys	Make razzing sounds and consonant/vowel combinations: "bah, bah, bah"
6 to 9 months	Imitate gestures in play Search for hidden objects Looks to see if you are watching when playing with toys Do things to make you laugh	Move toward or look for familiar people or pets when they are named	Shout or squeal to gain attention Smile or laugh when looking at parents	Variegated babbling: "bah, bah, tah, tah, dah" Vocal inflection patterns resemble adult patterns
9 to 12 months	Play gesture games like "peekaboo" Hold out toy to show others Are interested in playing with a variety of objects	Respond to some verbal requests such as "Give me..." or "Want up?"	Wave "hi" and "bye" Look at the toy when you point to it across a room Will point to show you things	

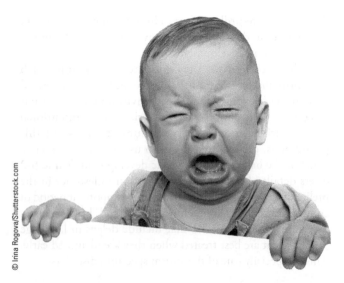

Figure 5-1 Crying to express distress is an example of pre-intentional communication. Note that, in addition to the use of voice, the use of paralanguage is also prominent.

body movements, facial expressions, and sounds. The unhappy baby shown in **Figure 5-1** would cause most adults in his immediate vicinity to stop and talk to him. The attention he gets helps him understand the value of communication. Pre-intentional behavior is a normal form of communication in typically developing children between 0 and 3 months of age (Rowland, 2011). With experience, infants learn that they can initiate actions that cause results.

The pre-intentional interactions of infants typically become paired with verbal communication, as in the previous example, the father speaks to his daughter to comfort her and engage her attention. Through this interaction, the infant learns that her vocalizations lead to positive social interactions and often result in increased personal comfort. The infant quickly learns that the behavior (crying) results in something good (her father's attention) and learns to use the behavior to get other things.

This learning leads to a second level of behavioral communication called intentional behavior. In the **intentional behavior** stage, the behavior is intentional but what it communicates is not always clear. This state is still considered unintentional communication because, although the child intentionally engages in a behavior, what that behavior communicates must be determined through interpretation of the caregiver. In typically developing children, this stage occurs between 3 and 8 months of age, and there is a gradual transition between stages one and two as infants learn through interactions with others (Rowland, 2011).

When children are delayed in the acquisition and development of communication skills, they may continue to rely on behavioral communication, and caregivers must learn to interpret the meaning of the child's behaviors to meet the child's needs. In the first three months of life, when unintentional communication is predominant, infants do have a voice. Through different types of cries, infants are capable of clearly communicating—among other things—anger, hunger, fatigue, discomfort, and boredom.

INTENTIONAL COMMUNICATION

The earliest form of intentional communication is called unconventional communication. At this level, behaviors are used intentionally to communicate. For example, when the infant girl wants to drink from her father's cup, she will look at the cup, stretch her arm toward it, and grunt or squeal to get her father's attention. This communicative behavior is unique to the infant and the situation. This communication is considered unconventional because it may not be interpreted correctly by people not familiar with the infant initiating the communication. Unconventional communications are not considered socially acceptable for us to use as we grow older. In typically developing children, this stage occurs between 6 and 12 months of age. This type of unconventional communication reflects early paralinguistic communication. Paralanguage was defined in Chapter 4 as the nonverbal elements of communication that are used to modify meaning and convey emotion within a cultural context. **Paralinguistic communication** is the use of manner of speaking, including tone, rhythm, pacing, and inflection to communicate particular meanings.

Infants' unconventional and paralinguistic communications will result in social interactions, and from these the children begin to imitate the behaviors of the people around them. Camaioni, Aureli, Bellagamba, and Fogel (2003) note that with the onset of intentional communication, infants also begin to use word-like sounds for communicative purposes. For example, a baby may point and vocalize "da" to direct her father's attention to an interesting toy. Through this process, gestures and verbalizations rapidly become productively combined.

Conventional communicative behaviors include pointing, nodding or shaking the head, waving, hugging, and looking from a person to a desired object. The meanings of some gestures may be unique to the culture in which they are used. Conventional communication behaviors emerge in typically developing children between 12 and 18 months of age, often concurrent with the child's first use of spoken words. Conventional communicative behaviors are socially acceptable, and we continue to use them to accompany our language as we mature (Rowland, 2011). **Figure 5-2** shows early conventional communication as a baby reaches out to be picked up.

SYMBOLIC COMMUNICATION

All of the early communication behaviors described so far are considered presymbolic forms of communication. **Presymbolic communication** refers to communication that does not use symbols such as words or signs. This kind of communication therefore does not have a shared meaning for others. Presymbolic communications can only be interpreted by looking at the context. When an infant imitates behaviors, such as waving her hand while she says "bye-bye," there is a cultural meaning to the gesture that does not change with context. This use of a gesture in a uniform, culturally consistent manner that

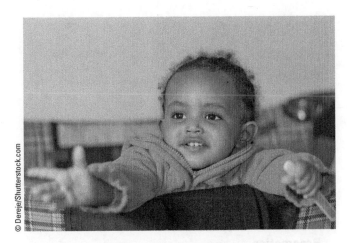

Figure 5-2 This little girl is communicating that she wants to be picked up using paralanguage to express her intention.

can be interpreted by others is the beginning of **symbolic communication**. Symbolic communication refers to communication that involves a shared message between a sender and a receiver. Symbolic gestural communication often emerges approximately at the same developmental period during which children produce their first words to label objects (for example, *toy, bottle, cookie*) or to regulate social interaction (for example, *hello, bye-bye, no*) (Camaioni et al.,

2003). This early symbolic communication uses concrete symbols that physically resemble what they represent.

Concrete symbols include the use of actual objects, gestures (such as raising arms to say "pick me up"), and sounds (such as making a barking sound to mean dog) (Rowland, 2011). Most typically developing children will quickly assimilate concrete words for common things, for example, the sight of an approaching dog triggers the referent "doggie" from a child, thus providing evidence that the child has developed the concept of a dog and can produce a word that represents the internal concept. Most early words of young children consist of object names and actions. A child may be hungry and express a need for food with the action word *eat*. Similarly, labels for others in the environment may be produced, such as "muh-muh" for "mommie." The word shapes children use are simple types consisting of consonant-vowel (bye), vowel-consonant (eat), or repetitions of the simple types (muh-muh).

Abstract symbols in communication may include pictograms and alphabets, and are used to indicate a concept, quality, or abstract idea in a way that is not physically similar to what they represent. **Figure 5-3** presents some common international signs. These signs are accepted abstract symbols that are consistently used to convey information in public places around the world, especially in public places like airports and bus stations that frequently include people

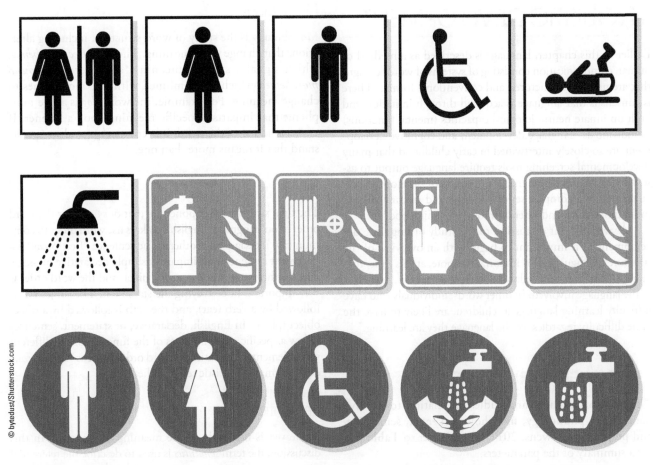

Figure 5-3 These symbols are widely used internationally to help people find resources without needing to know the local language.

with differing language and cultural backgrounds. As with concrete symbols, children start using abstractions in both their verbal and nonverbal communications at about the same time. In typically developing children, this stage occurs between 12 and 24 months of age (Rowland, 2011).

The first three years of life are recognized as a *sensitive period* for language development (NIH NID, 2011b). During this early period, a maturing brain is most open to acquiring speech and language skills. Most babies begin producing sounds at about 7 months (babbling), but congenitally deaf infants show obvious deficits in their early vocalizations. If early differences are identified and addressed through supportive interventions or the provision with an alternative form of symbolic expression the infant is likely to develop a communication impairment. Physical and occupational therapists often work with newborn and very young infants with delays in development. This group of children is at high risk for developing communication impairments. With an understanding of prelinguistic communication, early intervention therapy providers will be better able to identify children with possible communication delays and refer the children to a speech-language pathologist (SLP) for assessment. Because of the sensitive period for language development, delays in referring children for communication support may have a lasting negative impact on the children.

LINGUISTIC DEVELOPMENT

Earlier in this chapter, language is described as a method of human communication consisting of systems of words or signs that are used in a structured and conventional format. There is consensus that language is acquired through imitation and built on innate neurobiological capacities (mental functions) in individuals. Language development and cognitive development are so closely intertwined in early childhood that many developmental screening tools require language output to assess cognitive development. The process of developing language within a complex set of linguistic and cultural rules is multidimensional and extends throughout childhood.

As we shift our discussion to the study of linguistic development, it is important to begin with an overview of the structure of language. It is important to note, at this time, that linguistic development follows a predictable pattern, regardless of the language involved. In other words, individuals who have difficulty learning language as children, are likely to have the same difficulty regardless of the language they are learning.

LANGUAGE STRUCTURE

The rules of language are studied in relation to the five parameters: phonology, morphology, syntax, semantics, and pragmatics (Owens, 2011). Please refer to **Table 5-3** for a summary of the parameters.

TABLE 5-3 Parameters Used to Study and Quantify Language Development
Structure
Phonology—sound system
Morphology—word structure
Syntax—word order
Meaning
Semantics—the meaning component of language
Pragmatics
Pragmatics—the rules and conventions for talking

Phonology

Phonology is the study of how sounds are organized and used in spoken languages. It includes the rules that govern combinations of phonemes producing meaningful words. Along with morphology and syntax, phonology constitutes what is referred to as the structure of language.

Morphology

Morphology is the study of word structure, including alterations that change word meaning. There are *free morphemes,* which signal a specific meaning, and there are *bound morphemes,* which are combined with free morphemes to change meaning. For example, the word *dog* is a free morpheme that imparts a specific meaning upon a listener. If an "s" is added to the word, it becomes *dogs,* and we understand that it means more than one.

Syntax

The final structural component is that of **syntax**, or the word order of our language. English speakers use word order to communicate messages with others. The sentence "I eat pizza" is a statement sentence that imparts a simple declarative message. That is, the speaker enjoys eating pizza, and the word order is very important in conveying the statement. The subject (I) is followed by a verb (eat), and the verb is followed by a direct object (pizza). In English, declarative, or statement, sentences follow a specific order in terms of the function of the different word elements. A violation of word order, such as "Eat I pizza," does not make linguistic sense to the listener.

Semantics

Semantics is the study of the meaning of language. In this discussion, the term *semantics* is used to describe the referential and relational meaning of language. *Referential meaning* is the meaning of individual words, or the word knowledge that we possess. The word *car* creates a mental image of an object that is expensive, driven by people, has doors, and so on. *Relational meaning* includes the use of words that assign or explain relationships with and between words. Many relational meaning words are verbs. So the phrase "car going" adds information about the car in relationship to the speaker and the speaker's environment. Children learn to use relational aspects of language more slowly than they gain referential information.

This example illustrates that as speakers of a language, we have an extensive vocabulary. Items in the vocabulary are organized and stored by the brain as a sequence of semantic features. This pattern continues so that by completion of high school, normal adults have a vocabulary of approximately 80,000 words (Hulit & Howard, 2005)!

Pragmatics

The final element of language structure is pragmatics. Pragmatics refers to the ways in which context of any communication contributes to the meaning of the communication. **Pragmatics** includes the social rules for talking, or the rules governing what we say and how we say it. When we engage in a conversational interchange with another speaker, we produce utterances that are classified as speech acts. A speech act must conform to the conversational context that is at hand. That is, an utterance or group of utterances must be appropriate for the context of the conversation. For example, "Pass me the milk" is a legitimate request to another for something. In the appropriate context, a speaker produces the utterance as a precursor to receiving the milk from another. The pragmatic aspects of communication are greatly influenced by culture. Basic social rules about eye contact and the use of gestures to accompany speech vary widely around the world.

MORPHOLOGIC DEVELOPMENT

The next stage of development is marked by the expansion of utterance length and modulations, or changes in meaning, through the emergence of morphology (Owens, 2011). From the acquisition of the first word (around 12 months) language structure becomes increasingly complex. Generally, children are around 27 to 30 months of age when they begin to combine words to form sentences that express their thoughts. This is when they are beginning to produce phrases ("my doggie") and clauses ("my doggie eating") when communicating with others (Hulit & Howard, 2005). The appearance of phrases and clauses signals the preparation for adult sentence structure that consists of *subject-verb-object (SVO)* relationships. For example, the utterance "Billy eats pizza" is a sentence that contains a SVO relationship. Children are working toward this goal in the formation of statement sentences, and they are developing the structural knowledge to produce questions and imperative, or command-type, sentences.

Various morphologic inflections also appear as children refine their knowledge of word meaning (Owens, 2011). *Inflections* are alterations to words that change meaning, and children begin to use inflectional morphemes. For example, changing a noun from singular to plural tense (*hat* to *hats*) involves the addition of an inflection and the internal semantic knowledge of pluralization. Similarly, a verb can be marked for tense by adding an inflection such as "I eat" versus "I eating." The subtle changes in words and the increases in utterance length are the products of both linguistic and cognitive growth.

One also needs to keep in mind that acquisition does not happen in a vacuum. Caregivers in the environment are constantly stimulating children by expanding upon a their utterances during interactions. For example, a child may say, "drinking" while drinking, and the caregiver will follow with an expansion like "Yes, you are drinking." In other cases, the caregiver may add new information to what the child says, so that there is constant stimulation and interaction.

DEVELOPMENT OF SYNTAX

The next change in language development occurs at about 31 to 34 months of age, and encompasses additional changes in language development. Some of the highlights of this period are the development of questions and imperatives. Children at this stage are forming questions with the appropriate word order, such as "Can she play now?" What and where questions are also used correctly in most utterances. Imperative or command utterances like "Give me a drink" are used to request action from others. This is an important developmental advance and one that was problematic in the case of Jonathan introduced at the beginning of this chapter.

SENTENCE EMBEDDING

The next stage in our discussion is generally observed in children between the ages of 35 and 40 months. The important linguistic feature of this period is sentence embedding. Embedding is a process wherein phrases and clauses are combined with other clauses to create more complex utterances. A prepositional phrase is added to an utterance, such as "Put it *under the table*." Another example of embedding is the combining of two clauses to create an utterance that has a main clause and a dependent clause. For example, the child might say, "I like the boy who helped." The utterance is a complex sentence with an independent/dependent clause relationship. The independent clause is "I like the boy," and the dependent clause is "who helped." Hulit and Howard (2005) emphasize that the other components of language continue to improve, including pragmatics. Turn-taking skills improve to the level that children can engage in a conversation and are capable of taking more than two turns when discussing a topic. Children are learning to

CASE 1

Jonathan . . . Continued

Jonathan has been using a specialized assistive technology device called an augmentative/alternative communication (AAC) device that allows him to touch a point on a screen to make the device speak preprogrammed words or phrases. The device he has been using is the one he was given as a 2-year-old. Now, this device cannot meet his communication needs. For Jonathan to function effectively in both the school and the community, he must be able to produce language as complex as that of his age peers. His SLP has just upgraded him to a device that allows him to compose grammatical phrases, rather than just using preprogrammed requests. A simple touch screen will not allow him the scope of control options that he needs for this new system. Jonathan is learning to scan and select using a simple switch to build his language. The SLP is involved in programming the device and assuring that he has the vocabulary he needs. However, to use this device functionally, Jonathan must have a way to access it while he is seated in his wheelchair. Placement of the switch, supportive positioning for Jonathan, the mounting of the device on the wheelchair, or the placement of the device on the class desk are all issues that both the OT and PT will need to address. This will involve the assessment of his movement patterns, his energy (and fatigue) levels, as well as an assessment of the environments he usually interacts with. For Jonathan, the new device can enhance his life in many ways, it can allow him to advance academically, it can allow him to communicate at an age-appropriate level with peers, and it can offer him options to continue to develop his language skills. Although the SLP is central to the identification of the best device for Jonathan, the ability for him to have the device when and where he needs it and have a reliable means of accessing it are the domain of both PT and OT practitioners. Without interprofessional communication and collaboration, Jonathan is unlikely to have a communication system that meets his needs.

Guiding Questions

Some questions to consider:

1. Why would the OT and PT be involved in helping Jonathan use his new device? Shouldn't this be the exclusive role of the speech therapist?
2. Because many AAC devices are expensive, some school districts do not want to let students take the devices home. How might this impact Jonathan if he is only able to use the device at school?
3. Many digital technologies, including smartphones, can read out text typed into them. Would this type of technology be useful for Jonathan? Why or why not?

perceive differences in pauses when conversing with a caregiver. A short pause means that an utterance is forthcoming, but an extended pause signals the cessation of an utterance.

COJOINING SENTENCES

The final stage is one of language mastery across the language components and is associated with children in the age range of 41 to 46 months (Owens, 2011). Although these children still have to refine some aspects of language, they are quite sophisticated in their production and com-

prehension of language. Their utterances are complete in reference to structure, and they begin to consider the perspective of listeners (Hulit & Howard, 2005). For example, a previous request for something might take the form, "Give me a pop." At this stage, a child might say, "I ate my supper. Why don't you give me some pop?" Note that the child is reminding the listener that supper was finished successfully and that a reward should be forthcoming. In the previous stage, the concept of phrase and sentence embedding was discussed, and examples of such use were provided. Children continue to refine embedding, and they begin to cojoin sentences. Before this period, cojoining of items, such as "I like cookies and milk," are noted. At this stage, sentences such as "I saw the dog and I gave him a biscuit," illustrate the combining of two sentences into a single sentence. The child's preferred connector is "and," but other connecting devices such as "if" are also noted.

REFINING LANGUAGE SKILLS

It is quite obvious that children acquire the building blocks of language in a very short period of time. The process begins at birth and continues into adulthood; however, the basic foundation is formed during the preschool years. Typically the receptive communication abilities develop first, with expressive abilities emerging later. This is seen in a toddler who can follow two- and three-step instructions while he may only be able to utter a two-word statement. As speech skills improve, so does speech intelligibility. Articulation is the ability to produce individual speech sounds clearly and combine sounds correctly for words. In early childhood, speech may be hard for people outside of the family to understand. Articulation involves very skilled control of both respiration and the oral/facial muscles.

The term **intelligibility** refers to the proportion of a speaker's output that a listener can readily understand. In typical development, as children learn to talk, they not only gain speech sounds, but those sounds also become more understandable to those around them. Family members can often understand speech intent far earlier than outsiders can. **Table 5-4** describes the pattern of increasing intelligibility with age. Most children have functionally intelligible speech (understandable even though some aspects of articulation may be imperfect) by age 5.

METALINGUISTIC AWARENESS

Metalinguistic awareness is a cognitive ability that involves thinking about language as a process as well as a communication tool. It is the ability to consciously reflect on the nature of language, including awareness that language has a structure that can be manipulated, and that language can have multiple meanings and has implicit as well as explicit

meaning (Wagner, Muse, & Tannenbaum, 2007). In older children, metalinguistic awareness is seen when a child engages in introspective tasks that reflect one's knowledge of language. Metalinguistic awareness is important in learning to read and in reading comprehension (Zipke, 2008). Typical elementary school students who enjoy riddles and word play are demonstrating emerging skills in the area of metalinguistic awareness.

WRITTEN COMMUNICATION

Concurrent with the emergence of metalinguistic awareness in young children, the use of written communication emerges in the form of reading and writing. Reading is the ability to construct linguistic meaning from written symbols that represent language. Reading is a skill that is built upon language comprehension, linguistic knowledge, and cultural knowledge. These skills are applied as individuals learn an abstract alphabetic or symbol based upon the communication system they are already fluent in. Alphabetic languages are those whose writing systems relate the written and spoken form of words systematically. Preschool children begin to understand the alphabet and the idea of representing words with written symbols through early shared reading times such as bedtime stories and formal story times in the preschool setting (Zucker, Cabell, Justice, Pentimonti, & Kaderavek, 2013).

Early shared reading is an important shared occupation that supports the development of crucial life skills in young children. Zucker and colleagues (2013) emphasized the importance of conversations during the shared reading experience that help children transition from spoken language to the use of an alphabetic language. Accomplished readers, whether they are a parent, teacher, or older sibling as illustrated in **Figure 5-4**, can support young people as they learn to use the alphabetic language as a form of communication.

TABLE 5-4	Speech Intelligibility Expectations
Ages	**Intelligibility Expectations**
1½ to 2 years	25% to 50%
2 to 3 years	50% to 75%
4 to 5 years	75% to 90%

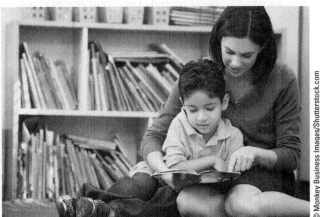

© Monkey Business Images/Shutterstock.com

Figure 5-4   Children learn to decode written language more quickly with the support of others in both traditional book and digital formats.

Language decoding is the ability to recognize written representations of words. Through decoding, learners develop an understanding of letter-sound relationships, including knowledge of letter patterns to represent words. It is only through the development of language decoding that individuals learn that alphabetic symbols can be combined in an endless variety to express language.

Literacy is the ability to read and write in the shared language of a culture (Bittman, Rutherford, Brown, & Unsworth, 2012). In considering the learning of a new generation of "digital natives," a specialized type of literacy, digital literacy, has been studied in relationship to communication and language skills. Digital literacy was defined by Bittman and colleagues as "critical thinking in the context of technology use" (2012, p. 18). Digital literacy is highly valued by young people as it supports social participation. Although motivated by social participation, digital literacy does support traditional literacy development. Studies have determined that there are higher levels of reading among Internet users, and that Internet use has been associated with higher academic performance, particularly reading performance (Bittman et al., 2012). In a finding similar to that reported by Zucker and colleagues (2013) on the importance of shared reading in the development of language decoding skills, Bittman and colleagues (2012) found that the parents' role in negotiating and discussing media use with their child was more significant than the actual digital media used in developing literacy skills.

Digital literacy includes both reading and writing. Writing is a communication tool that allows individuals to project thoughts, ideas, and to express feelings. Prior to the development of decoding skills, writing is simply the copying of abstract designs. As children decode alphabetic symbols, this skill can be translated into the formation of words through writing. People only learn to write as they learn to read, and their written communication skills do not exceed their language comprehension skills. Writing is a complex form of communication that requires not only decoding and symbolic thought, but that requires specific management of writing implements and discrete fine motor control. The motor aspects of writing will be presented later in the life span chapters.

IMPACT OF LANGUAGE SKILLS

Boroditsky (2011) argues that language not only communicates, but that it also shapes thought. Evidence from new technologies that study brain function shows that people rely on language to understand their sensory world and interpret information into perceptions. Boroditsky's studies suggest that what we consider "thinking" is actually a collection of both linguistic and nonlinguistic processes. There is also evidence, though these findings continue to be debated, that grammatical gender rules within a particular language can shape how people interpret the world in myriad ways, including color perception (Winawer, et al., 2007), space, and time (Matlock, Ramscar, & Boroditsky, 2005). Even social standards, like gender equity, are reflected in a language's gender rules for grammar (Prewitt-Freilino, Caswell, & Laakso, 2012). If language has this broad of an effect on thinking, consider the impact of fluency in more than one language. Studies consistently show that bilingual children outperform monolinguals on reasoning and analysis of word meaning (Marinova-Todd, 2012). Recent functional near-infrared spectroscopy (fNIRS) brain imaging indicates deep connections between language and thought, influencing human social skills and shaping personality (de Lange, 2012).

Finally, language is associated with identity perception (Martin, 2012). Membership in cultural and ethnic groups may be based on a shared spoken language alone. Cultural fluidity, as discussed in Chapter 4, requires that individuals must be self-reflective and demonstrate behaviors, attitudes, policies, and structures that enable them to work effectively cross-culturally. Cultural competence was described in Chapter 4 as a goal in health care settings. Similarly, **linguistic competence** is the capacity to communicate effectively and convey information in a manner that is easily understood by diverse audiences including, people of limited English proficiency, those who have low literacy skills or are not literate, and individuals with disabilities (Goode, Jones, Dunne, & Bronheim, 2007). This term is also widely supported as an ideal among persons working in health care settings. The earlier discussion about the use of a cultural broker is an example of assuring linguistic competence in communications with people from differing cultural backgrounds.

COMMUNICATION DISORDERS

Communication disorders can occur at any point in the life span. Because the understanding of language is complex and language development is integrally related to both cognitive and cultural aspects of development, the assessment and treatment of language disorders is best done by professional speech-language pathologists (SLPs). As you reflect on the material presented in this chapter about communication disorders, be aware that because different areas of the brain process receptive and expressive language, a disorder may be just receptive, meaning the person cannot understand what is said to him, but remains able to speak; it may be expressive, meaning the person may understand what is said but be unable to speak; or the disorder may be a combination of the two. Communication disorders may be caused by sensory loss, as in hearing disorder, or by motor incoordination resulting in unintelligible speech. Communication disorder may be developmental, manifesting in infancy, or acquired following an accident or illness. Most communication disorders involve the use of language, and so the terms *speech disorder, language impairment* and *communication disorder* are often used

TABLE 5-5	Classification of Communication Disorders

Speech Disorders

Speech Sound Disorders

Unknown etiology

Structural-based disorders

Sensory-based disorders

Motor speech–based disorders

Voice and Resonance Disorders

Pitch disorders

Loudness disorders

Quality disorders

Inappropriate oral-nasal coupling

Fluency Disorders

Language Impairment

Language Impairment in Children

Mental retardation/developmental disability

Autism

Hearing impairment

Specific language impairment

Neglect and abuse

Traumatic brain injury

Language Impairment in Adults

Aphasia

  Fluent aphasia

  Nonfluent aphasia

Traumatic brain injury

Dementia

interchangeably, but there are distinctions between the terms as illustrated in **Table 5-5**.

LANGUAGE IMPAIRMENT

A **language impairment** is any difference or limitation in the comprehension (understanding) or production (speaking) of the language code that results in a difference in communication but does not interfere with it. Our discussion of language impairment will deal with children and adults separately, because the origins of their impairments differ. That is, children with language impairment experience difficulty in acquiring language, whereas adults have acquired the language code but lose certain language skills due to some medical condition or disease process. The difference

in terms of delayed acquisition versus loss causes us to look at language impairment across the life span a bit differently. A **language disorder** is a type of impairment that includes a problem with the comprehension or production of the language components morphology, syntax, semantics, and pragmatics that interferes with functional communication to a significant degree. A **speech disorder** is a type of language disorder specifically related to the articulation (phonetic or phonological disorders); fluency (stuttering or cluttering); or voice (tone, pitch, volume, or rate) of spoken language.

LANGUAGE IMPAIRMENT IN CHILDREN

Paul (2001) states that most discussions of language impairment in children identify subgroups based on etiology. The different causal categories consist of mental retardation/developmental disability, autism, hearing impairment, specific language impairment, neglect and abuse, and traumatic brain injury. Accordingly, individuals from those subgroups will demonstrate language impairments that will vary as a function of the different subgroups. Keep in mind that this discussion will deal with generalities, but individual differences among children are quite evident and need to be considered (Owens, 2011). A speech-language pathologist will evaluate a child with suspected language impairment to establish a level of language function. Following assessment, a treatment program will be developed to enhance existing language skills and to incorporate caregivers and significant others in a plan to improve existing language skills. Even with treatment, children with language impairment continue to have some degree of difference in their language skills across the life span.

Autism Spectrum Disorders

Autism spectrum disorders are disorders of development characterized by impaired social interaction and communication, and by restricted and repetitive behavior (Sundberg & Partington, 2010). Children with the diagnosis of *pervasive developmental disorder, not otherwise specified* (PDD-NOS) exhibit some behaviors characteristic of people with autism, but complete criteria for a diagnosis of autism are not met. Autism is generally diagnosed when a child is very young; the onset is generally before 30 months of age. Caregivers often report that the child started to develop language, but then development stopped very abruptly. Many children with an autism spectrum disorder will have a language problem. Their ability to communicate will vary, depending upon innate intellectual abilities and social development. The majority of children with autism have difficulty using language effectively. There are some patterns of language use and behaviors that are often found in children with autism. The National Institutes of Health, National Institute on Deafness and Other Communication Disorders (NIH NID) (2009) describes these patterns as repetitive or rigid language.

Repetitive or Rigid Language

Often, children with autism who can speak will say things that have no meaning or that seem out of context in conversations with others. For example, a child may count from one to five repeatedly. Or a child may continuously repeat words he or she has heard, a condition called echolalia. *Immediate echolalia* occurs when a child repeats words someone has just said. For example, the child may respond to a question by asking the same question. A child with *delayed echolalia* will repeat words heard at an earlier time. The child may say, "Do you want something to drink?" whenever he or she asks for a drink.

Some children with autism speak in a high-pitched or singsong voice or use robot-like speech. Other children with autism may use stock phrases to start a conversation. For example, a child may say, "My name is Tom," even when he talks with friends or family. Still others may repeat what they hear on television programs or commercials.

Hearing Impairment

Hearing impairment has a significant effect on the other components of language. The severity of the language impairment will vary according to age of onset, type of loss, and degree of loss. In the case of hearing loss, an audiologist must carefully evaluate the person to quantify the type and degree of loss. Language impairment in individuals with a hearing impairment can be severe, with limited verbal output, and poor auditory comprehension. Speakers with a hearing impairment use speech and supplement expression and comprehension of language with speech reading and manual signing. If appropriate, a hearing aid is employed to amplify speech. Note that a hearing aid will assist these people, because the aid amplifies sound; however, it does not restore hearing loss.

A *cochlear implant* is a small, complex electronic device that can help to provide a sense of sound to people who are profoundly deaf or severely hard of hearing. **Figure 5-5** shows a cochlear implant on an adult. The implant consists of an external portion that sits behind the ear and a second portion that is surgically placed under the skin. The implant provides a means to receive speech and process it. A cochlear implant functions very differently from a hearing aid. Although hearing aids amplify sounds so damaged ears can detect them, the cochlear implants bypass damaged portions of the ear and directly stimulate the auditory nerve. The brain recognizes the signals from the implant as sound, but hearing through a cochlear implant is different from normal hearing and requires a period of training for users to make meaning from the transmitted sounds.

Cochlear implants are often used as early as 12 months of age so that profoundly hearing-impaired children can acquire speech, language, and social skills. Early implantation provides exposure to sounds that can be helpful during the critical period when children learn speech and language skills (NIH NID, 2011c).

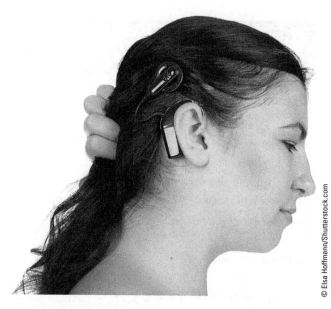

© Elsa Hoffmann/Shutterstock.com

Figure 5-5 Cochlear implants offer greater opportunities for the development of communication skills in young people with hearing loss. They are also used with adults who have lost their hearing to help them regain communication functions.

Specific Language Impairment

The subgroup of children diagnosed as having a *specific language impairment (SLI)* do not have any cognitive, social, sensory, or motor problems that would adversely affect language acquisition. However, as Bishop and Norbury (2008) point out, they show early delays in language acquisition that will continue in the event of no intervention. The lack of achievement of various linguistic milestones usually prompts caregivers to seek services when the children are young. Consequently, these children are often identified early in life and receive treatment as preschoolers, with treatment continuing into school age. Children with SLI will frequently comprehend more than they are capable of producing. They have difficulty extracting regularities from language; hence, aspects of language such as morphology are problematic. Vocabulary growth can also be a problem with these children. Finally, pragmatics, which are the rules for talking with others, are difficult for children in this subgroup to master. SLI is a strongly genetic disorder (Bishop, 2006). Only a handful of nongenetic factors have been found selectively to impact language development in children.

LANGUAGE IMPAIRMENT IN ADULTS

Most adults have acquired language without problem and are competent communicators with others in their language community. Language impairment in adults may be the result of a disruption of the blood supply to the brain, damage to neural tissue, or some degenerative pathological process (Owens, Metz, & Haas, 2000). In some cases, people may have altered or dysfluent language, but still be able to communicate and function in their daily lives. Often there are other problems that co-occur with language impairment, such as sensory or motor deficits, memory problems, poor judgment, and so on. In addition, some may also have a coexisting motor speech disorder and possibly a swallowing disorder. It is obvious that language impairment can seriously affect a person's quality of life.

Three of most the most common types of language disorders in adults—aphasia, speech apraxia, and dysarthria—occur as a result of neurological damage such as from a stroke or head injury. *Aphasia* is a type of language disorder due to brain damage or disease resulting in difficulty in formulating, expressing, or understanding language. *Speech apraxia* is a motor control disorder that impairs speech production. The speech attempts of a person with speech apraxia sound jumbled or meaningless. *Dysarthria* results from paralysis, weakness, or lack of coordination of the muscles required for speech.

ALTERNATIVE AND AUGMENTATIVE COMMUNICATION (AAC) AND ASSISTIVE TECHNOLOGY (AT)

For the remainder of this chapter, the focus will be on special issues in communication with people who do not have typical communication abilities. **Augmentative/alternative communication (AAC)** includes forms of expressive communication (other than oral speech) that are used to express thoughts, needs, wants, and ideas. AAC includes exaggerating facial expressions or gestures to make a point, the use of symbols or pictures to express words or ideas, and a wide array of specialized assistive technology devices to produce language for people who do not have a functional natural voice. **Assistive technology (AT)** is an umbrella term that includes assistive, adaptive, and rehabilitative devices for people with disabilities. AT enables people to perform tasks that they were formerly unable to accomplish by providing enhancements to, or changing methods of interacting with, the technology needed to accomplish such tasks. Some examples of assistive technology for communication impairments include voice synthesizers, text telephones, cochlear implants, and picture exchange communication systems. In all cases the AAC strategies employed by the individuals should be in collaboration with the SLP.

Augmentative communication devices run the gamut from simple picture boards or signs to speech synthesizers via computer output. Output methods that do not require equipment, such as signing or gesturing are classified as *unaided systems* of communication. *Aided systems* of communication use some form of either "low" or "high" technology. This may be a simple picture board, or may be a complex computer-based voice output system. AAC devices are matched to the level of communication development of the individual and the contexts within which the individual needs to communicate. As in the case of Jonathan presented earlier in this chapter, having an AAC device that does not match his receptive language understanding can perpetuate the language impairment it was intended to address. Research has consistently shown that the use of AAC with young children actually enhances the development of speech for children who will be able to develop speech (Branson & Demchak, 2009). Parental concerns that the use of an AAC strategy will limit the development of speech are unfounded.

THE COMMUNICATION BILL OF RIGHTS

The use of AAC devices has been slow to be accepted by the mainstream population. With the exception of Stephen Hawking, a prominent AAC user, most people have never had the experience of people using an AAC device. This lack of experience has led to a lack of enthusiasm for the use of devices by families and even by health care professionals. The negative impact of this inexperience led to the publication of a "**Communication Bill of Rights**" (The National Joint Committee for the Communicative Needs of Persons with Severe Disabilities, 1992). This document emphasizes the importance of communication to quality of life. The Communication Bill of Rights asserts that "all people with a disability of any extent or severity have a basic right to affect, through communication, the conditions of their existence" (National Joint Committee for the Communicative Needs of Persons with Severe Disabilities, 1992).

It is easy for outsiders to see an AAC device, recognize its utility, and yet not respect it as an individual's voice. It is not unheard of for children to only have their AAC devices during certain periods of the school day, or for people to have to choose between the ability to talk and the ability to drive a power wheelchair.

AAC is not simply an issue of focus for speech-language pathologists; these approaches can be used to aid both spoken and written language, and can supplement or replace speech and writing as necessary. AAC may be introduced as early as six months of age, when there is clear evidence of significant impairment that would lead to poor communication development and can support child development broadly, not simply support language development. As noted by Topia and Hocking (2012), "AAC potentially assists people with severe communication needs to meet occupational potential, engage in relationships, and participate and belong in society. Early provision can maximize the development of language skills and literacy, attaining and sharing information, experiencing accomplishment, and succeeding academically in educational settings. Mastering communicative competence can elicit feelings of self worth, dignity, and well-being" (p. 24). Although AAC prescription and training is typically managed by SLPs, both occupational and physical therapists have an important role in supporting the use of the devices through enhancing the specific skills needed to access a device, in integrating the use of a device into everyday occupations, and in collaborating with SLP to assure that the devices reflect the users' true communication needs.

SIGN LANGUAGE

The best known form of AAC is **American Sign Language (ASL)**. ASL "is a complete, complex language that employs signs made with the hands and other movements, including facial expressions and postures of the body. It is the first language of many deaf North Americans, and one of several communication options available to deaf people. ASL is said to be the fourth most commonly used language in the United States" (NIH NID, 2011a). ASL is actually a language, with syntax, semantics, pragmatics, and fluency. ASL is not a literal repetition of spoken English, but requires actual translation to communicate to its users. Sign languages vary by region and nationality, as does spoken language. Therefore, in addition to ASL, there is also a British Sign Language and an Australian Sign Language.

Often caregivers have the notion that the use of sign language and other forms of AAC will prevent future expressive language; however, studies indicate that using AAC increases an individual's verbal output (Owens, Metz, & Haas, 2000).

A popular trend has been the promotion of "baby sign language" as a tool to enhance developmental outcomes in otherwise typically developing infants. Baby sign language is the use of manual signing to communicate with infants using a limited number of "stand-alone" manual signs from ASL. The practice of introducing sign language in infancy to help a child at risk for expressive communication impairments (such as children with severe hearing loss or children with Down syndrome) is well established as a form of early intervention to support cognitive and language development. The "baby sign" trend extends this approach to infants who are not at risk for expressive communication problems. The premise is that prelinguistic infants have a desire to communicate but lack the ability to do so clearly because the production of speech lags behind receptive language in the first two years of life (Pizer, Walters, & Meier, 2007). The popularity of this trend seems grounded in the parents' desire to optimize their infants learning and language skills. This approach offers a focus for infant-parent social exchanges and can serve as a baby-enrichment resource (Pizer et al., 2007). Unfortunately, the marketing claims for baby sign extend far beyond basic enrichment and support of social interactions. In a review of 33 websites that advocate sign language for hearing children, Nelson, White, and Grewe (2012) report claims of improved language development, increased IQ, reduced tantrums, higher self-esteem, and improved parent-child bonding. Although the study found that many parents found the use of baby sign language enjoyable, the authors warn that "there is no credible research evidence to support the frequent claims on these websites that teaching sign language to young children with normal hearing will result in increased IQ, improved language development, reduced tantrums, improved self-esteem, earlier communication, and increased parent–child bonding" (Nelson et al., 2012, p. 490).

SUMMARY

Communication is a fundamental human function that we use in both social interactions with others and in our own thoughts. This chapter was designed to furnish an overview of communication that includes a consideration of both prelinguistic communication and the use of language in many contexts. Language is that aspect of communication that enables us to share our inner thoughts and feelings, influence others, and engage in introspective talking. It has been conceptualized as comprising phonology, morphology, syntax, semantics, and pragmatics. Children acquire language through the development of cognitive-linguistic rules for pairing structure with meaning in the context of rules for communicating with others. Physical and occupational therapists will often share clients and will need to understand both language impairment and aspects of presymbolic communications to communicate effectively with their clients and to support their clients' participation in daily occupations.

Communication and language are central to all human interactions, reflects culture, and allows social participation in both real life and virtual environments. Although language assessment is not typically part of the occupational or physical therapy role with clients, everything else we do relies on our ability to communicate and our ability to support the clients' ability to communicate effectively. For this reason, an understanding of communication and its close interrelationships with both culture and cognition are central to both professions. In addition to the role of physical and occupational therapy in the functional use of AAC devices mentioned earlier, in early childhood, occupational and physical therapists commonly will see children with a developmental delay earlier than the SLP and can serve an important role as referral sources so that these children can get services as early as possible.

CASE 2

Chau

Chau is 36 years old and was born with normal physical capabilities. She was involved in a motor vehicle accident at age 30, which resulted in left-sided motor incoordination and an inability to speak clearly. She was diagnosed as having hemiplegia and dysarthria. Prior to the accident, Chau was living independently and working as a computer software trainer and troubleshooter for a local university. She enjoyed spending her free time pursuing her hobby, video gaming.

Chau has complex communication problems following her injury that include problems with speech content (word finding and difficulty with abstract meanings, idioms, or proverbs). She has intact receptive language and mild dysarthria. Chau has difficulties with prosody, including flat affect, slowed initiation of speech and overall rate, and difficulty interpreting emotional intent.

Chau receives OT for ADL support and computer access, and PT for mobility. She is able to walk with a walker and is highly motivated to gain strength and endurance. In her conversations with her therapists, Chau has an inability to be concise, poor topic maintenance, and doesn't effectively seek clarification during conversations. Chau has twice overextended in her home exercise program, based on her incomplete understanding and poor communication with her PT. In OT, she is frustrated because as a computer specialist, she is frustrated with the slow rate of text entry she is able to manage. She becomes frustrated and distressed easily, and this limits her progress in therapy.

In a client-centered intervention model, Chau and all three of her therapists (SLP, PT, and OT) held a meeting to sort out her priorities and to build communication supports that extended across therapy sessions. With these in place, Chau is better able to focus on her goal of returning to work.

Guiding Questions

Some questions to consider:

1. Search the Internet for the term *visual schedules*. How might you use a visual schedule in your practice to help Chau?
2. There are many application programs (apps) for electronic devices that can serve as reminders and prompts for daily activities. Do you use any of these yourself? What would Chau need in an app to meet her needs?

CASE 1

Returning to Jonathan . . .

Both Jonathan's OT and PT have been recruited to help Jonathan understand the basic rules of social communication and social exchanges. They require that he use the device in his therapy sessions and build in negotiation about the sequence and type of therapy tasks he is to complete as part of a daily routine.

Continues

Case 1   *Continued*

Though working with the teacher and the SLP, OT, and PT can give Jonathan a safe and structured way to practice his growing communication abilities, he is making gains specific to his control of movements and the production of written work at the same time. Jonathan will not only benefit from having improved communication skills in the classroom, it is likely that his therapy progress will be greater because he will be more motivated to work for goals he has had input into.

Guiding Questions

Some questions to consider:

1. Search the Internet for videos of AAC devices using scanning. In addition to the need for understanding language, Jonathan will need several cognitive skills to perform this task. What are they?
2. Jonathan will want to access other communication devices such as a computer and a smartphone. What might be the role of OT and PT in supporting his transition to these devices?

Speaking of
Life and Relationships

CHRIS KLEIN, BeCOME: AAC

It's a Tuesday morning as I roll over in bed and notice somebody is next to me. Who is this person? What is she doing next to me? As I begin to wake up, I realize she is my wife. I was married on Monday, and I am going to spend the rest of my life with this woman, who is my best friend. What is the big deal? There is nothing special about getting married. There is nothing out of the ordinary about having a relationship. I know you are thinking to yourselves, so what?

I was born in 1973. The umbilical cord was coming out before me, so they had to do an emergency C-section. The doctors knew they were racing the clock. Forty-five minutes later, I was born. I was given CPR for another 40 minutes. The lack of oxygen caused an injury to the motor portion of my brain. I have cerebral palsy. I am classified as an athetoid, which means that my muscles never stop moving. The expectations for my life weren't high. Actually, my parents and family didn't know what to expect out of me.

I know we aren't the only family that experienced this. This is a normal thing to experience when you are faced with a disability of any kind. However, when that disability also contains a complex communication disability as well, the expectations sink even further. However, the frustration of not knowing what is bothering your child is even more frustrating and anguishing to parents.

I cannot understand what the frustration is like for a parent, but I do understand what it is like for a person who is unable to speak. For the first 6 years of my life, I couldn't express myself. I was stuck because nobody could really understand me. Everybody wondered what my mental capacity was, but these were questions nobody could answer, because I couldn't communicate.

What is communication? Why do we communicate? I feel these are two very important questions we need to answer. We need to communicate to request things. We need to communicate to tell someone our needs. We need to

Continues

Speaking of   Continued

communicate to order something or someone around. We need to communicate to share stuff. Last but not least, to communicate to share our feelings, and to build relationships.

As I grew up, I started using a picture book to communicate with my family. It solved some of the frustration, but I still couldn't communicate everything that I wanted to say. Judy, my speech therapist, wondered if I might be able to speak using a communication box, so I was given my first one when I was 6. My first sentence was "Leave me alone." I have two older brothers and two older sisters. They used to do things to me that you would cringe at. When I was able to express myself, I could finally tell them off, and our relationship grew from that point.

This technology changed the course of my life. All of a sudden, my family could see I was able to communicate. Augmentative communication gives a person like me a chance to be educated. Most importantly, it gives a person a chance to build relationships. The relationships that are built develop into a great community. That community helps a person achieve goals that nobody thought were attainable.

I believe relationships are the key to everybody's success. When I went to college, I quickly realized how important relationships were to my independence. As a freshman I did try to hire my personal attendants, and it caused me a lot of headaches. As I started developing relationships, my friends wanted to help me. The friendships developed into a great network of assistants. After graduating college, I decided I was going to stay in Holland, Michigan. I was able to achieve that goal because I had developed a great community.

Before I was married, I lived on my own and used a home care service for the morning. They would have to shower and dress me. It only took them an hour to do, and by 8:30 they were out of the door. I was by myself from 8:30 until noon. When noon came, a friend came to give me lunch. I had about 35 friends doing a lunch, dinner, or bedtime once a week. They were there for only an hour, and then the rest of the day, I was able to function on my own. My AAC device makes this possible because when I needed something, I was able to call a friend to come over. I had friends who lived right in my neighborhood, so even in an emergency, I could call a friend, and he or she could get to my house as quickly as possible.

We are living in a culture that doesn't like silence. We don't like silence when we are communicating with people. A person that is using AAC realizes it's difficult to have those deeper conversations because people don't like waiting. I believe that is causing people that use AAC to feel isolated. This is the reason why people who use AAC have a more difficult time building relationships. Many have a difficult time engaging in conversation because we are living in a fast-paced culture. It is going to be difficult to hold someone's attention.

When I think over my life, I have realized it isn't my accomplishments that I am proudest of. It is the relationships I have built. My life wouldn't be the same without my wife, or my other friendships. My AAC device gave me the ability to communicate, which give me the ability to build relationships. I have been able to live a fulfilling life because of the relationships I have built.

REFERENCES

American Speech-Language-Hearing Association. (1983). Language (definition). *ASHA, 25,* 44.

Bishop, D. V. (October 2006). What causes specific language impairment in children? *Current Directions in Psychological Science, 15*(5), 217–221.

Bishop, D., & Norbury, C. F. (2008). Speech and language impairments. In A. Thapar, Sir M. Rutter, D. Bishop, D. Pine, S. M. Scott, J. Stevenson, E. Taylor, (Eds.), *Rutter's child and adolescent psychiatry*. Oxford: Wiley-Blackwell (pp. 782–801).

Bittman, M., Rutherford, L., Brown, J., & Unsworth, L. (2012). Digital natives? New and old media and children's language acquisition. *Family Matters, 91,* 18–26.

Boroditsky, L. (2011). How language shapes thought. *Scientific American, 304*(2), 62–65.

Branson, D., & Demchak, M. (2009). The use of augmentative and alternative communication methods with infants and toddlers with disabilities: A research review. *AAC: Augmentative & Alternative Communication, 25*(4), 274–286.

Camaioni, L., Aureli, T., Bellagamba, F., & Fogel, A. (2003) A longitudinal examination of the transition to symbolic communication in the second year of life. *Infant and Child Development, 12,* 1–26.

Christiansen, C., and Townsend, E. (2010). *Introduction to occupation: The art and science of living* (2nd ed.). New Jersey: Pearson.

de Lange, C. (2012). My two minds. *New Scientist, 214*(2863), 30–33.

Goode, T. D., Jones, W., Dunne, C., & Bronheim, S. (2007). *And the journey continues.... Achieving cultural and linguistic competence in systems serving children and youth with special health care needs and their families.* Washington, DC: National Center for Cultural Competence, Georgetown University Center for Child and Human Development.

Hulit, L. M., & Howard, M. R. (2005). *Born to talk: An introduction to speech and language development, 4th edition.* New York: Macmillan.

Marinova-Todd, S. (2012). "Corplum is a core from a plum": The advantage of bilingual children in the analysis of word meaning from verbal context. *Bilingualism: Language & Cognition, 15*(1), 117–127.

Martin, B. (2012). Coloured language: Identity perception of children in bilingual programmes. *Language Awareness, 21*(1/2), 33–56.

Matlock, T., Ramscar, M., & Boroditsky, L. (2005). On the experiential link between spatial and temporal language. *Cognitive Science, 29*(4), 655–664.

National Institutes of Health, National Institute on Deafness and Other Communication Disorders (NIH NID). (2009). *Autism and Communication.* Retrieved from http://www.nidcd.nih.gov/health/voice/pages/communication-problems-in-children-with-autism-spectrum-disorder.aspx

National Institutes of Health, National Institute on Deafness and Other Communication Disorders (NIH NID). (2011a). *American Sign Language.* Retrieved from http://www.nidcd.nih.gov/health/hearing/pages/asl.aspx

National Institutes of Health, National Institute on Deafness and Other Communication Disorders (NIH NID). (2011b). *Speech and Language Developmental Milestones.* Retrieved from http://www.nidcd.nih.gov/health/voice/pages/speechandlanguage.aspx

National Institutes of Health, National Institute on Deafness and Other Communication Disorders (NIH NID). (2011c). *Cochlear implants.* Retrieved from http://www.nidcd.nih.gov/health/hearing/pages/coch.aspx

National Joint Committee for the Communicative Needs of Persons with Severe Disabilities. (1992). Guidelines for meeting the communication needs of persons with severe disabilities. *American Speech and Hearing Association, 34*(Suppl. 7), 2–3.

Nelson, L. H., White, K. R., & Grewe, J. (2012). Evidence for website claims about the benefits of teaching sign language to infants and toddlers with normal hearing. *Infant & Child Development, 21*(5), 474–502.

Owens, R. (2011). *Language development: An introduction* (8th ed.). Boston: Allyn & Bacon.

Owens, R., Metz, D. E., & Haas, A. (2000). *Introduction to communication disorders: A life span perspective.* Boston: Allyn and Bacon.

Paul, R. (2001). *Language disorders from infancy through adolescence: Assessment and intervention* (2nd ed.). St. Louis: Mosby.

Pizer, G., Walters, K., & Meier, R. P. (2007). Bringing up baby with baby signs: Language ideologies and socialization in hearing families. *Sign Language Studies, 7*(4), 387–430.

Prewitt-Freilino, J., Caswell, T. T., & Laakso, E. (2012). The gendering of language: A comparison of gender equality in countries with gendered, natural gender, and genderless languages. *Sex Roles, 66*(3/4), 268–281.

Rowland, C. (2011). *Communication Matrix.* Retrieved from http://www.communicationmatrix.org/

Scott, J., & Marshall, G. (2009). *A dictionary of sociology (Oxford dictionary of sociology).* Oxford University Press, USA.

Sundberg, M., & Partington, J. (2010). *Teaching language to children with autism or other developmental disabilities.* AVB Press; re-edited 1998 Edition (v.7.2, July 1, 2010).

Topia, M., & Hocking, C. (2012). Enabling development and participation through early provision of augmentative and alternative communication. *New Zealand Journal of Occupational Therapy, 59*(1), 24–30.

Wagner, R. K., Muse, A. E., & Tannenbaum, K. R. (2007). *Vocabulary acquisition: Implications for reading comprehension.* New York: The Guilford Press.

Winawer, J., Witthoft, N., Frank, M. C., Wu, L., Wade, A. R., & Boroditsky, L. (2007). Russian blues reveal effects of language on color discrimination. *Proceedings of the National Academy of Sciences of the United States of America, 104*(19), 7780–7785.

World Health Organization. (2001). *ICF: International Classification of Functioning and Disability.* Geneva, Switzerland: World Health Organization.

Zipke, M. (2008). Teaching metalinguistic awareness and reading comprehension with riddles. *The Reading Teacher, 62*(2), 128–137.

Zucker, T. A., Cabell, S. Q., Justice, L. M., Pentimonti, J. M., & Kaderavek, J. N. (2013). The role of frequent, interactive prekindergarten shared reading in the longitudinal development of language and literacy skills. *Developmental Psychology, 49*(8), 1425–1439. doi:10.1037/a0030347

CHAPTER 6

Mental Functions and Learning across the Life Span

Anne Cronin, PhD, OTR/L, FAOTA,
Associate Professor, Division of
Occupational Therapy, West Virginia
University Morgantown, West Virginia

Objectives

Upon completion of this chapter, readers should be able to:

- Discuss ICF definition of mental functions and how this definition relates to the aspects of cognition typically seen in the psychology and rehabilitation literature;

- Describe embodied cognition and embodied learning while reflecting on how people with cognitive impairments may best be supported to develop cognitive skills;

- Offer clinical examples of disorders in consciousness and orientation functions, and differentiate these from disorders in sleep functions;

- Compare the older Chess and Thomas categorization of temperament types with the newer approach Rothbart developed;

- Discuss the distinctions between the psychological, physiological, and social theories of intelligence;

- Explain what is meant by metacognitive knowledge, and offer clinical examples or disorders associated with deficits in this area;

- Categorize the aspects of metacognitive process in terms of their function in the performance of a complex task, such as cooking a meal;

- Compare implicit and explicit long-term memory storage, and discuss how difficulties in these areas might manifest in a clinical population; and

- Describe social learning and affordances in the context of human development and skills acquisition.

Key Terms

affordance

associative learning

attention

body image

calculation functions

consciousness

declarative learning

dementia

embodied cognition

emotional functions

energy and drive functions

executive functions

experience of time and self functions

global mental functions

global psychosocial functions

intellectual functions

long-term memory

mental functions of language

mental functions of sequencing
    complex movements

metacognition

metacognitive knowledge

metacognitive process

nonassociative learning

orientation functions

perceptual functions

procedural learning

process skills

psychomotor functions

purposeful sensory experience

sensorimotor praxis (motor planning)

sensory perceptual memory

situated learning

sleep functions

social learning

somatic awareness

specific mental functions

thought functions

use-dependent brain plasticity

working memory

CASE 1

Margie

Margie is 73 years old and has mid-stage Alzheimer's disease. Margie was formerly a practical nurse and a homemaker. She currently lives with Tom, her husband of 52 years. Tom has a heart condition and has had increasing difficulty supervising and keeping up with Margie by himself. Margie has always enjoyed walking and was an avid bird-watcher. Unfortunately, now, the walking has turned into wandering and Tom has had to call for help in finding her on several occasions. When he tried to keep her in the house, Margie often became agitated and would lash out at Tom.

After consultation with her physician, Tom has enrolled Margie in an adult day treatment program. In the day treatment program, a PT, OT, and SLP were involved in the assessment of Margie's functional status. It was determined that Margie could follow one-step directions, and could perform multistep tasks (such as folding the laundry) that were familiar to her. Margie had limited ability to learn new tasks and was often forgetful, needing prompting to stay on tasks that she had chosen for herself. Margie demonstrated problems sequencing ADL tasks like dressing and bathing. She is very social and interested in other people. Her receptive and

Continues

Case 1 *Continued*

expressive language continues to be good, although she is not well oriented to time and place. She cannot remember her address or her phone number, and does not remember to bring a cell phone with her when she "goes for a walk." Margie has poor balance and sometimes expresses a fear of falling during routine activities. Margie walks well and has moderate physical endurance. She does not always use available grab bars and demonstrates poor safety awareness in her motor skill performance, making her a fall risk.

Continues on page 118

INTRODUCTION

The term *cognition* is an inclusive term for a group of distinct mental processes that includes a wide range of functions such as attention, memory, perception, understanding, and thought. Cognitive activity of all types takes place in the context of a real-world social and physical environment, and inherently involves perception and action (Wilson, 2002). Cognition is not an isolated brain function, but a complex process that includes a constant use of communication, language, personal experience, and cultural information. The information flow between mind and world is continuous, and human thinking, decision making, and learning are all impacted by our environmental situations. This chapter introduces many terms associated with cognition, both those specific to the ICF consideration of cognition and learning, and those rehabilitation professionals commonly used. Later in the text, these aspects of cognition will be further developed as they relate to periods of human development and functional performance.

The International Classification of Functioning, Disability and Health (ICF) uses the term *mental functions* for many functions that we traditionally consider cognition. The ICF definition of mental functions is "the psycho-physiological functions that encompass thought, intellect, information processing, emotions, and behaviors, all of which are critical to daily functioning" (Vroman & Arthanat, 2012, p. 1). The ICF divides mental functions into two categories: *global mental functions*, which are underlying, largely unconscious functions that regulate arousal and mental state; and *specific mental functions,* which are conscious thought and the role of cognition in behavior and communication.

Mental functions are integral to all aspects of human development, performance, and function. **Figure 6-1** illustrates the relationship between mental functions and the other aspects of activities and participation described in the ICF. Since the groundbreaking work of Piaget, scientists have studied and developed theories about the nature of human cognition. Increasingly, neuroscience has been replacing theoretical science in the study of cognition and learning. In spite of the growing knowledge base, Piaget's assumptions about the development of cognition and his hierarchy of mental

values continue to be widely accepted today (Thelen, 2000). Of particular importance to the study of human development is Piaget's premise that the fully mature human mind emerges from early perception and action. Thelen supports this premise but, in light of modern scientific understanding, comments, "I want to question the equally pervasive acceptance of Piaget's assumption that the end point of development is increasingly abstract reasoning, formal logic, or elaborated knowledge structures and that, as a consequence, perceiving and acting become mere bystanders. I instead argue for the grounding of mental activity in continually perceiving the world and acting in it, not just in the initial state but throughout life" (2000, p. 4). Thelen's work has been important to both physical and occupational therapists working with young children, as she emphasizes the need for early movement and active participation to support early cognitive development.

The study of cognition and learning has been addressed in many scientific disciplines coming from many philosophical and theoretical backgrounds. In this chapter, we will be considering cognition in terms of the *embodied mind thesis* espoused by Thelen and Smith (1994). **Embodied cognition**, an outshoot of this thesis, is the construct that active movement and physical "doing" influences our cognition, just as the mind influences bodily actions. Scientists studying embodied cognition emphasize that the mind is not only connected to the body but that the body also influences the mind. Not only does embodied cognition address learning that takes place in the same context in which it applies, but it also has relevance to the learning of abstract concepts that extend beyond the learning situation (Wilson, 2008). Embodied cognition allows infants to analyze a specific goal and then to form intentional strategies to reach that goal. An observant infant learns that by reaching for his father's cookie, he can usually get a bite. Similarly, through lived experience, he learns that some of the things his father eats are good (like the cookie) and some are not as tasty. Through this process, infants analyze, set goals, evaluate outcomes, and choose the conditions under which to repeat a behavior. From the experience of embodied cognition, occupations emerge. This includes the emergence of habits and routines that will serve as the foundation for individuals' lifestyle.

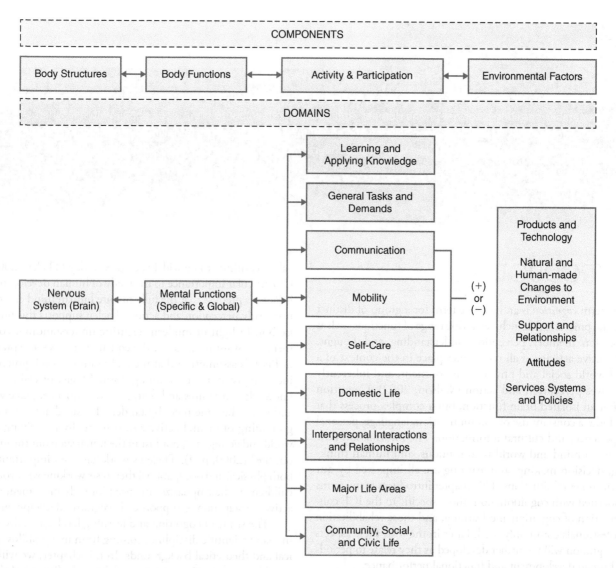

Figure 6-1   The interrelationship of the ICF mental function domain with activity, participation, and environmental factors based on Vromna, K. & Arthanat, S. (2012). ICF and Mental Functions: Applied to Cross Cultural Case Studies of Schizophrenia. In J. H. Stone and M. Blouin (eds), Internatial Encyclopedia of Rehabilitation. Retrieved from http://cirrie.buffalo.edu/encyclopedia/en/article/308

TERMINOLOGY OF THE ICF

This chapter will offer readers current terminology applied to the study of mental functions; an introduction to cognitive neuroscience principles including embodied cognition; as well as an insight into the reciprocal influences of culture, communication, and environment on cognition and learning. As with earlier chapters, the study of cognition and learning has its own distinctive vocabulary. Because the ICF categories of mental functions differ somewhat from the familiar terms *cognition* and *learning,* a detailed introduction to the ICF language is offered for readers.

Global mental functions as described in the ICF underlie the other mental activities and most typically operate below the level of personal awareness (World Health Organization, 2001). These functions are crucial to all human activity and, although often overlooked, are important predictive

factors in rehabilitation outcomes. Specific mental functions are usually conscious intentional acts such as problem solving, language, and calculation. These mental functions are also more overt and more directly related to everyday performance skills. For these reasons, specific mental functions tend to be the focus of both research and intervention strategies in the fields of health and human learning (World Health Organization, 2001).

GLOBAL MENTAL FUNCTIONS

Global mental functions are subtle and often taken for granted. **Figure 6-2** illustrates the ICF process of consciousness, orientation, intellectual functions, global psychosocial functions, temperament and personality, energy and drive functions, and sleep functions (World Health Organization, 2001). The global mental functions are illustrated graphically in **Figure 6-2**.

Consciousness Functions	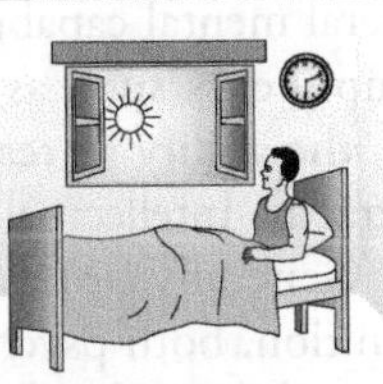	General mental functions of the state of awareness and alertness, including the clarity and continuity of the wakeful state.
Orientation Functions	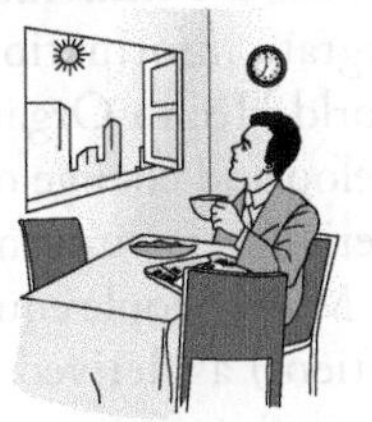	General mental functions of knowing and ascertaining one's relation to self, to others, to time, and to one's surroundings.
Intellectual Functions	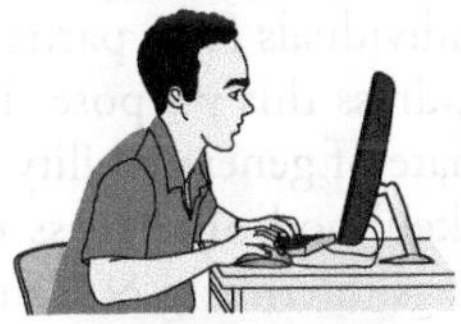	General mental functions, required to understand and constructively integrate the various mental functions, including all cognitive functions and their development over the life span.
Global Psychosocial Functions	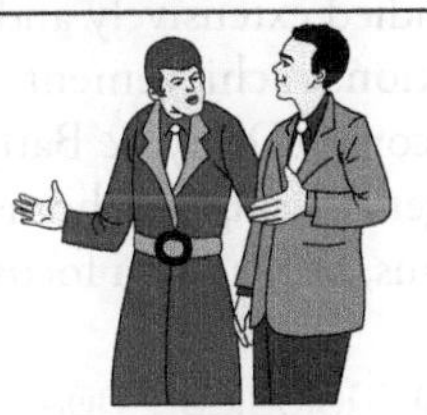	General mental functions, as they develop over the life span, required to understand and constructively integrate the mental functions that lead to the formation of the interpersonal skills needed to establish reciprocal social interactions, in terms of both meaning and purpose.
Temperament and Personality Functions	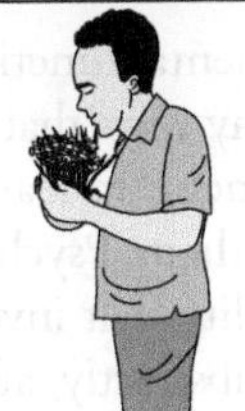	General mental functions of constitutional disposition of the individual to react in a particular way to situations, including the set of mental characteristics that makes the individual distinct from others.
Energy and Drive Functions	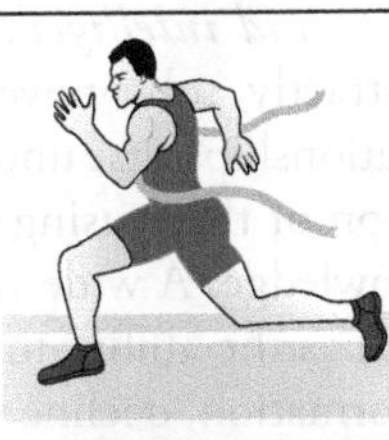	General mental functions of physiological and psychological mechanisms that cause the individual to move toward satisfying specific needs and general goals in a persistent manner.
Sleep Functions	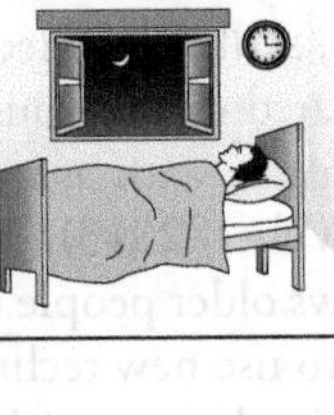	General mental functions of periodic, reversible and selective physical and mental disengagement from one's immediate environment accompanied by characteristic physiological changes.
Global Mental Functions, Other Specified and Unspecified		

Figure 6-2   This diagram offers a summary of ICF global mental functions.

Source: International Classification of Functioning, Disability, and Health

Consciousness Functions

The first of these functions, **consciousness** is a state of awareness and alertness that includes an individual's ability to sustain a wakeful state (World Health Organization, 2001). Consciousness is sentience, the state of being aware of one's own existence (Wilcock, 2006). Consciousness is required for all other mental functions to occur. In rehabilitation settings, clinicians are taught to assess consciousness by observing a client's arousal and responsiveness. Coma is considered a disorder of consciousness, and a continuum of coma states range from disorientation, through delirium, loss of meaningful communication, and finally to a true vegetative state. Both occupational and physical therapists provide care for people who are fully conscious, as well as people who are at all levels of coma. The diagnosis of dementia reflects a moderate deterioration of consciousness, and some types of seizures can lead to a transient interruption in consciousness (Bernat, 2006).

Orientation Functions

Orientation functions reflect an awareness of one's relation to self, to others, to time, and to place. Orientation is an expected baseline for reasoning. Disorientation can be caused by things as varied as personal distress, medications, illness, and injury. Orientation functions develop in early childhood. In the first year of life, infants develop an awareness of themselves as distinct and unique. As the infants come to be self-aware, they also begin to name others in their immediate environment. Time orientation develops slowly over the first several years of life, but by age 6, most children can clearly describe time as it is measured and valued in their own cultural context. This includes naming days of the week, months, seasons, and the temporal sequence of events during a routine day. Orientation to place is the last to develop, and is dependent on an abstract understanding of space and of place-names stored in memory. Orientation to place is the most sophisticated of the basic types of orientation, and often the first to be lost following an injury or illness. In the case of Margie that opens this chapter, Margie is oriented to self. She knows who she is, but she is only generally oriented to place and time. Margie knows the name of her hometown, but does not consistently remember her home address or the name of the day treatment program. Margie looks at the newspaper frequently during the day to remind herself of the day of the week, and relies on events, such as meals or the arrival of Tom to pick her up to help her stay oriented to time of day. Loss of orientation functions can lead to significant safety and daily function limitations.

Intellectual Functions

Intellectual functions are those skills required for individuals to understand and constructively integrate information from all types of mental function (World Health Organization, 2001). For our purposes, intellectual functions are a very general mental capability that includes a composite of subcomponents such as verbal reasoning, visuomotor abilities, the ability to reason, plan, solve problems, and think abstractly. Intellectual functions also include process skills.

Generally, intellectual functions are those aspects of cognition, both psychological and social function, that are required for individuals to understand and constructively integrate information from all types of mental functions (World Health Organization, 2001). Intellectual functions develop and change over the life span and are influenced by experience, environmental contexts, and learning.

Many people equate intelligence with "IQ" (intelligence quotient) as derived from a standard test, but intelligence is a relative concept. Tests of intelligence are developed by individuals for a particular purpose and are constructed to address this purpose. Intelligence tests offer a global estimate of general ability that can be useful in projecting the likelihood of success in academic and employment settings (Sternberg & Kaufman, 2011). "IQ" scores have been studied extensively and found to be stable predictors of educational achievement, special needs, job performance, and income (Deary & Batty, 2007). The measurement of intelligence using psychometric tests is important in many situations, but is not a focus of this discussion.

Psychological Approaches to Intelligence

The mental functions of individuals differ from one another in many ways that influence their ability to adapt to their environment, to learn from experience, and to solve problems facing them. Psychologists consider intelligence to be a mental capability that involves the ability to reason, solve problems, think abstractly, and learn. In the psychology literature, there is a distinction between fluid and crystallized intelligence.

Fluid intelligence is the ability to think and reason abstractly, solve novel problems, and identify patterns and relationships that underpin these problems and the extrapolation of these using logic rather than relying on acquired knowledge. A wide range of fluid intelligence capabilities, such as the ability to generate, transform, and manipulate information, decline with age.

Crystallized intelligence is the ability to utilize information, skills, knowledge, and experience that you have accumulated throughout your lifetime. Crystallized intelligence increases with age and experience (Li, Baldassi, Johnson, & Weber, 2013). This dichotomy in forms of intelligence allows older people to be both wise and challenged in learning to use new technology devices.

In the case of Margie, it was noted that she could perform multistep tasks (such as folding the laundry) that were familiar to her. In these tasks, Margie relies on crystallized intelligence. She fully understands these tasks and no longer needs to think through the steps. It was also noted that Margie had limited ability to learn new tasks. When in a novel situation, Margie was unable to identify the important steps to the task, the tools needed, or the sequence of steps needed to successfully manage the activity. Difficulties like these reflect impairment in fluid intelligence. Impairments in fluid intelligence are common in many conditions involving impaired mental functions.

Process skills are intellectual functions that rely on fluid intelligence to allow the transfer and adaptation of previously learned tasks to novel or altered situations. Another type of fluid intelligence that often diminishes with aging is working memory. **Working memory** is the ability to hold information in the mind to do verbal and nonverbal reasoning tasks (Sternberg & Kaufman, 2011). In **Figure 6-3**, the woman is trying to follow written instructions to build furniture. She may be having difficulty with working memory as she tries to translate the verbal message into actions.

Physiological Approaches to Intelligence

A physiological approach to intelligence has emerged with the recent advances in neuroscience. This approach is focused on understanding the biological basis that underlies intelligence. The two major foci in research have been in the study of brain efficiency and plasticity. Neuroplasticity was defined earlier in the text as the intrinsic lifelong capacity of the brain for reactive change in behavioral flexibility. Jung and Haier (2007) reviewed 37 imaging studies, and proposed that intelligence is related not so much to brain size or a particular brain structure,

but instead to how efficiently information travels through the brain. These scientists have developed an approach to the study of intelligence called the *parieto-frontal integration theory (P-FIT)* that is based on positron emission tomography and EEG studies (Colom et al., 2009). The P-FIT identifies a brain network related to the integration of information across various parts of the brain. As the name of the approach suggests, the focus of this research involves areas in the frontal and the parietal lobes. Although the P-FIT model has not yet been helpful in understanding the changes in intelligence across the life span, it has offered valuable insight into our understanding of working memory and fluid intelligence.

Another physiological approach, the neural plasticity model of intelligence is built upon the concept that intelligent individuals have a brain that productively changes in response to the environments and experiences (Garlick, 2003). In this model differences in intelligence are due to inherent differences in brain plasticity, the brain's capacity for neural adaptation. In this conception, the most highly intelligent individuals have "dynamic neural networks that alter their composition in order to accommodate task demands" (Sternberg & Kaufman, 2011, p. 66). Most of the research related to this approach has been done using animal models, but the approach has influenced trends in education and in therapy.

Neuroplasticity-based training concepts have been successfully used to address cognitive difficulties associated with schizophrenia (Sacks et al., 2013) and with autism spectrum disorders (Dawson, 2008). Associated with this research is a growing understanding of **use-dependent brain plasticity**, which refers to the capacity of the brain to remodel itself based on the activity patterns and environmental demands on the individual. Use-dependent brain plasticity plays a major role in the recovery of function after injury to the brain and helps explain patterns of cognitive changes associated with aging (Draganski & Kherif, 2013).

Social Approaches to Intelligence

In the social approaches to intelligence, intelligence is viewed as the end product of a "complex dynamic system involving interactions between mental processes, contextual influences, and multiple abilities that may or may not be recognized in an academic setting" (Sternberg & Kaufman, 2011, p. 67). It is from researchers exploring the social approaches to intelligence that recent work in describing not a single intelligence, but multiple intelligences, arises. Sternberg (2005) has proposed a *triarchic theory of successful intelligence,* offering three interacting aspects that result in intelligence. These aspects of intelligence are described as wisdom, intelligence, and creativity. Sternberg's model has been effective in helping to understand the development of cognition and the cognitive skills needed for mastery in aspects of daily human performance.

Gardner (2006) also sees intelligence as having many aspects. He reports that all humans have at least eight distinct intelligences. In his *Theory of Multiple Intelligences,*

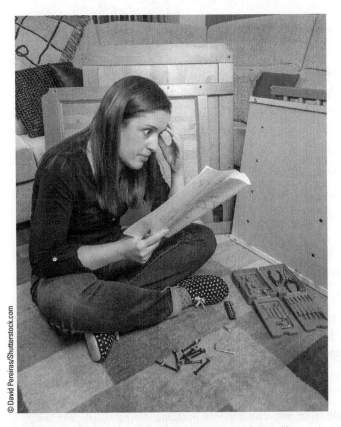

© David Pereiras/Shutterstock.com

Figure 6-3 This woman is challenged by the need for working memory to hold verbal information in mind while she tries to put together furniture.

Gardner defines an intelligence as "the ability to solve problems, or to create products, that are valued within one or more cultural settings" (Gardner, 1993, p. x). Gardner's theory has gained much popular attention because it appeals intuitively to those who recognize skills and abilities in people around them who perhaps did not do well in traditional schooling. Gardner's theory has been embraced by many as a tool to enhance teaching and promote learning. For students of human development, it is important to understand intelligence as a fundamental ability to perform successfully in society. **Table 6-1** presents the seven types of learning styles described by Gardner. The use of multiple learning styles and multidimensional teaching strategies are valuable tools in clinical practice.

Although the three approaches to intelligence described in this chapter—the pyschologic, the physiological, and the social—are very different, each approach leads to research that better informs us about human function. It is believed that as the research continues and new technologies for studying the brain emerge, these three approaches will become more integrated (Sternberg & Kaufman, 2011).

Intelligence in a Global Perspective

Consistent with the idea of embodied cognition, culture influences the contents of cognition, especially the domains of perception and memory (Wilson, 2010). Additionally,

---

TABLE 6-1   Gardner's Learning Styles Reflecting Multiple Intelligences

Linguistic Learner
- Likes to read, write, and tell stories.
- Is good at memorizing names, places, dates, and trivia.
- Learns best by saying, hearing, and seeing words.

Logical/Mathematical Learner
- Likes to figure things out, ask questions, and explore patterns and relationships.
- Is good at math, reasoning, logic, and problem solving.
- Learns best by categorizing, classifying, and working with abstract patterns/relationships.

Spatial Learner
- Likes to draw, build, design, and create things, and to play with machines.
- Is good at imaging things, sensing changes, solving mazes/puzzles, and reading maps and charts.
- Learns best by visualizing, dreaming, and working with colors/pictures.

Musical Learner
- Likes to sing, hum tunes, listen to music, play an instrument, and respond to music.
- Is good at picking up sounds, remembering melodies, noticing pitches/rhythms, and keeping time.
- Learns best by rhythm, melody, and music.

Bodily/Kinesthetic Learner
- Likes to move around, touch, and use body language.
- Is good at physical activities.
- Learns best by interacting with space and processing knowledge through bodily sensations.

Interpersonal Learner
- Likes to talk to people and join groups.
- Is good at understanding people, organizing, communicating, manipulating, and mediating conflicts.
- Learns best by sharing, comparing, relating, cooperating, and interviewing.

Intrapersonal Learner
- Likes to work alone and pursue own interests.
- Is good at understanding self, focusing inward on feelings/dreams, following instincts, pursuing interests/goals, and being original.
- Learns best by working alone, doing individualized projects, using self-paced instruction, and having own space.

the highly focused crystallized intelligence skills valued in education in North America may not be useful to children learning to function in challenging social and economic conditions. For example, traditional educational models are often unsuccessful in preparing low-income urban children for either the workplace or higher education opportunities.

The views presented in this chapter draw from the western European tradition. What intelligence is, is perceived differently based on cultural traditions and values. Greenfield and Suzuki (1998) observed that "cultures define intelligence by what is adaptive in their particular niche" (p. 82). Tippeconnic and Tippeconnic (2012) noted that many educational institutions for Native American students are effectively using tribal values as a way to provide an overall framework to teaching, learning, research, and governance. This approach does not redefine intelligence, but frames the academic process in a manner that is more meaningful and more applicable to the learners.

Impairments in Intellectual Functions

Intellectual impairments can be developmental, as seen in an infant born with Down syndrome; it can be the result of brain pathology, as seen following a traumatic head injury or brain tumor; or it can be as a result of disease, as in the case of Alzheimer's dementia.

Dementia is a disease state, not simply forgetfulness, in which both memory and cognitive abilities deteriorate over time. It affects memory, thinking, language, judgment, and behavior. In most cases the onset of dementia is insidious and unrecognized by individuals or their loved ones until the condition has advanced. Most types of dementia are nonreversible (degenerative). *Alzheimer's disease,* used in the case example of Margie, is the most common type of dementia (A.D.A.M. Medical Encyclopedia, 2011).

In considering adults who lose mental function, the terms *vulnerable* and *maintained abilities* are used to help understand patterns of impairment (Sternberg, Lautrey, & Lubart, 2003).

Vulnerable abilities are those most likely to decrease or diminish with advancing age. The most significant of the vulnerable abilities are spatial reasoning, perceptual speed, short-term memory, visual processing, and processing speed. These abilities include many process skills that assist in managing and modifying tasks in progress. The loss of vulnerable abilities is common in the elderly, but it is also noted following traumatic brain injury or as a secondary effect of severe illness. The slowed performance of ADLs common to the elderly is in part due to a decline in process skills.

Maintained abilities include cultural and academic knowledge, verbal comprehension, vocabulary, number facility, and fluency of retrieval from long-term memory. Maintained abilities typically include habits. Habits, as defined earlier in this text, are behaviors so ingrained in activity and context that they are performed without conscious thought. Habits "support performance in daily life

and contribute to life satisfaction" (AOTA, 2014, p. 623). These abilities are typically maintained and do not diminish with age. For this reason, in the case of Margie, she is still quite independent in eating, dressing, and toileting. All three of these are complex multistep tasks, but tasks that had become habits and no longer required cognitive focus to complete. Ingrained habit patterns support previously learned behaviors in the presence of appropriate cues. Vulnerable abilities, like fluid intelligence, are more likely than maintained abilities to be impacted by brain injury or disease (Sternberg, Lautrey, & Lubart, 2003).

Global Psychosocial Functions

Global psychosocial functions is the term used in the ICF to describe the essential mental abilities that allow individuals to integrate aspects of social experience, personality, and emotions to provide a foundation for the formation of interpersonal skills. People with difficulty in this area might show poor attention to social stimuli and be less likely to respond to their own name. Skill deficits of this type are common in people with autism spectrum disorders. Common early signs of psychosocial skill deficits seen in young children with autism are poor eye contact, poor turn taking in communication and in play, and an inability to interpret paralanguage.

Temperament

Temperament was first discussed in Chapter 3 of this text and is "the constitutional disposition of the individual to react in a particular way to situations" (World Health Organization, 2001, p. 42). Temperament is a collection of inborn differences between individuals that is closely associated with personality. It has been widely studied, beginning with the work of Thomas, Chess, Birch, Hertzig, and Korn (1963) in their New York Longitudinal Study (NYLS). Many other researchers have added to the literature about temperament, but the characteristics of temperament described in the NYLS and shown in **Table 6-2** continue to be the most widely tested in clinical and educational settings (Carey & McDevitt, 1995).

No one classification system for temperament has been determined to be the most useful. The classifications presented in **Table 6-2** are the most widely used. Any of the nine characteristics listed in **Table 6-2** that is extremely low or extremely high can be problematic for individuals. Further study of temperament has introduced the idea of "temperament risk factors." These are "any temperament characteristic predisposing a child to a poor fit (incompatible relationship) with his or her environment, to excessive interactional stress, and conflict with caretakers" (Cary & McDevitt, 1995, p. 13).

More recently, Rothbart (2007) described temperament as the individual personality differences seen in early childhood that are present prior to the development of

TABLE 6-2   Temperament Categories and their Characteristics

Temperament	Characteristics
Activity Level	A measure of physical motion during sleep, eating, play, dressing, bathing, and so forth.
Rhythmicity	The regularity and predictability of basic physiologic functions, such as hunger, sleep, and elimination.
Approach/Withdrawal	The nature of the individual's initial responses to new stimuli—people, situations, places, foods, toys, procedures.
Adaptability	The ease or difficulty with which reactions to stimuli can be modified; the individual's ability to accommodate the unexpected.
Intensity	The energy level of responses, regardless of quality or direction. This is how intellectually or emotionally focused the individual is; it does not relate to physical activity.
Mood	The amount of pleasant and friendly or unpleasant and unfriendly behavior in various situations; the individual's typical affect.
Persistence/Attention Span	The lengths of time particular activities are pursued by a child; how long a child will work at a given task.
Distractibility	The effectiveness of extraneous environmental stimuli in interfering with ongoing behaviors.
Sensory Threshold	The amount of stimulation, such as sounds or light, necessary to evoke discernible responses in the child.

Web Questionnaires on Temperament

- An Image of Your Child: Discover Your Child's Temperament Style (infants-toddlers) (from The Preventive Ounce) at http://www.preventiveoz.org/image.html
- The Keirsey Temperament Sorter II (from The Keirsey Web Site) at http://www.advisorteam.com/temperament_sorter/register.asp?partid
- Myers-Briggs Personality Type (from Know Your Type) at http://www.knowyourtype.com/
- Personality Compass (from Personality Compass) at http://www.personalitycompass.com/

Adapted from Cary & McDevitt, 1995; Web resources. Reference Crediting: Carey, T., & McDevitt, S. (1995). Coping with children's temperament: A guide for professionals. New York: Basic Books.

higher cognitive and social aspects of personality. Rothbart's approach differs from the earlier Chess and Thomas definition in that she does not attempt to label individuals into typologies; rather she focuses on biologically based individual traits that are influenced over time by experience. In this conception, temperament is reflected in individual differences in self-regulation and reactivity (Rothbart & Bates, 2006). The first of Rothbart's dimensions, *surgency/extraversion,* includes positive anticipation, impulsivity, high activity levels, and sensation seeking. The second dimension, *negative affect*, includes fear, frustration, sadness, discomfort, and anger. The final dimension, *effortful control,* includes the intentional control of attention, the ability to inhibit impulses, and perceptual sensitivity (Rothbart, 2007).

Dimensions of temperament have been studied over time and found to be stable within individuals. This means that the temperament displayed at 5 years of age is likely to be the temperament displayed by the same individual in adulthood. The main focus of the study of temperament has been in early identification and prediction of children who are vulnerable or at risk for developmental challenges (Bijttebier & Roeyers, 2009).

Energy and Drive Functions

Energy and drive functions, as described in the ICF, include the physiological and psychological mechanisms that result in an individual's energy level, motivation, appetite, craving (including craving for substances that can be abused), and impulse control (World Health Organization, 2001). There is both a physiological and a cognitive component to energy and drive functions. Motivation is an intrinsic cognitive drive toward action and is believed to be a key component in human occupation. The stronger the motivation individuals have for an occupation, the more likely they are to fully engage in that occupation. Motivation can be intrinsic or extrinsic. Certainly motivation, whether it is an intrinsic motivation to improve or an external motivation to be discharged from the hospital, is a primary predictor of a successful outcome in therapy (Gasser-Wieland & Rice, 2002; Ng & Tsang, 2002).

Sleep Functions

Sleep functions are the periods of mental disengagement from one's immediate environment accompanied by characteristic physiological changes. This disengagement is reversible; an individual can wake and regain alertness, and he or she can choose when to sleep or to be awake. Sleep is an important daily life function, but it is not typically considered an occupation because the individual is passive rather than active during sleep. Sleep and dreaming during sleep have been associated with physical health including immune system function and stress recovery (Wells & Vaughn, 2012). People who cannot control sleep may have functional impairment caused by this lack of control. Insomnia is associated with increased accidents and errors in the workplace, diminished academic performance in students, and increased substance abuse (Wells & Vaughn, 2012). Narcolepsy is a condition characterized by sudden, uncontrolled bouts of sleep. These can occur without warning and make many ordinary tasks, like driving a car, life threatening.

SPECIFIC MENTAL FUNCTIONS

Specific mental functions, the term used in the ICF for thoughts and intentional acts of reasoning and planning, is not widely used in the psychology and rehabilitation literature. The specific mental functions described in the ICF are attention and perceptual functions, memory functions, psychomotor functions, emotional functions, thought functions, higher-level cognitive functions, mental functions of language, calculation functions, the mental function of sequencing complex movements, and experience of self and time functions (World Health Organization, 2001).

Attention and Perception

Attention is defined in the ICF as a specific mental function that involves focusing on a stimulus or internal experience for a required period of time. Attention is central to many of the specific mental functions as it serves to maintain a general readiness to respond, determines the threshold for response to a stimulus, and selects appropriate stimuli from all possible sensory inputs (Levy, 2011). The determination of what to attend to and when to attend is based on both memories and real-time perceptual input. **Somatic awareness** is an aspect of attention that focuses on information about the state of the body (touch, pressure, temperature, pain, and so on).

Perceptual functions include recognizing and interpreting sensory stimuli from all sensory systems, both individually and in combination. Our perception of what we see comes from our experience and exposure of it.

All perception involves signals in the nervous system that can come from any sensory system. Perception is not a passive receipt of sensory signals, but is shaped by learning, memory, and expectation (Bernstein, 2010). Perception involves a two-way consideration of information from the cortex (memories) and the sensory system (input). In infancy and early childhood, sensory inputs are gathered and stored in memory. In this way, low-level information is used to build up higher-level information (that is, shapes for object recognition). In adults, the analysis is more "top-down" processing, where knowledge helps define sensations but also shape expectations. An example of this is how the smell or sight of a food creates expectations about the taste of the food.

Memory Functions

Memory functions include registering and storing information and retrieving it as needed by the individual (World Health Organization, 2001). Memory doesn't necessarily mean memorizing something. Memory can be explicit, conscious memory that can be recalled intentionally, or it can be implicit, memories that are recalled unconsciously. Implicit memories develop first, early in infancy. Explicit memory skills develop throughout the life, beginning in the preschool years (Feldman, 2011). We remember how relevant it is to us, and decide if it's worth remembering. The cognitive information processing model characterizes memory as a recursive process with three stages. This is illustrated in **Figure 6-4**. In considering this model, readers should note that memory can fail at any of the three stages, and that the process of memory is closely intertwined with the process of learning. For this reason, people with memory deficits nearly always also have learning deficits.

As illustrated in **Figure 6-4**, **sensory perceptual memory** is the first step in the process of memory. Sensory perceptual memory is fleeting, lasting no more than four to five seconds after the stimulus is withdrawn. The importance of this stage is that it allows for the perceptual analysis that filters information deemed unimportant and moves forward information deemed as important. People who have difficulty with sensory perceptual memory do not remember spoken directions, or whether they have already added the last ingredient while cooking. Immediate memory is the ability to remember and act on information immediately preceding the present need for the information.

Perceptual filtering uses long-term memories as a guide. Considering this, it becomes clear why the attentional skills of infants are very poor: They have poor initial filters. This also explains why there are cultural differences in responses to environmental input. Something that is crucially important in one cultural context, like the spatial arrangement of furniture, may be meaningless in another. It is memory that holds the cultural knowledge and uses it as a filter.

Short-term/working memory includes both primary memory and working memory (Levy, 2011). *Primary memory* refers to the amount of information that individuals can

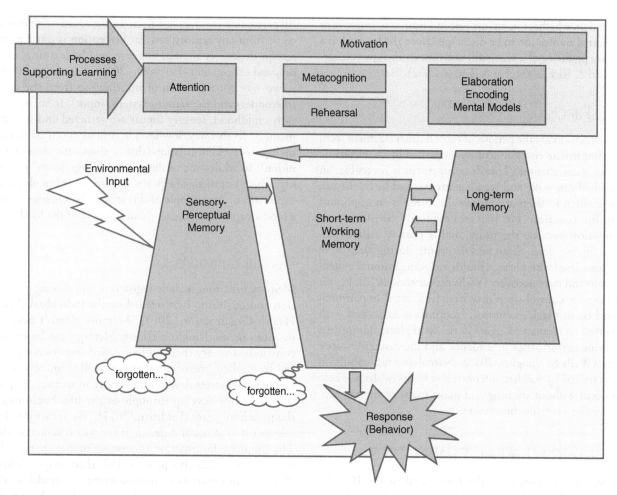

Figure 6-4   Cognitive Information Processing Model

assimilate and be able to recall immediately. Primary memory produces a temporary memory store of around a 30-second duration from which information is lost if not consolidated into long-term memory (World Health Organization, 2001).

Working memory actively holds information in the mind to do verbal and nonverbal tasks such as reasoning and comprehension, and to make it available for further information processing (Becker & Morris, 1999). Working memory capacity is an important consideration in the quality and effectiveness of all other aspects of the specific mental functions, especially metacognitive functions (Levy, 2011). It is as part of working memory that the initial processing incoming information occurs, transferring information to long-term memory and retrieval of information from long-term memory. The amount of work imposed on working memory in the process of learning a new task is called *cognitive load.*

Figure 6-4 illustrates the dual role of short-term/working memory as a filter that can result in an immediate response, can result in a new long-term memory, or both results can occur in response to the same stimulus. People with poor short-term/working memory forget conversations and where they left things around the house, though they are usually able to use immediate information and act

on it. Short-term memory influences the performance of many important daily tasks, because it is needed to assist in performing desired action sequences without interruption until the task is completed. This aspect of short-term memory is called *temporal sequencing* in the *Occupational Therapy Practice Framework* (AOTA, 2014).

Long-term memory is described by Levy (2011) as "the permanent, apparently limitless, component of the information processing system" (p. 104). Long-term memory permits the long-term storage of information from short-term memory and both autobiographical memory for past events and semantic memory for language and facts (World Health Organization, 2001). Cognitive information processing theory indicates that long-term memories are divided into explicit and implicit memory stores. *Explicit memory* is the conscious, intentional recollection of previous experiences and information that allows us to remember daily things like the time and place for college classes and also allows us to remember episodes from our childhood. Explicit memory is what we use when we consciously try and remember something.

Implicit memory is a type of memory in which previous experiences aid in the performance of a task without conscious awareness or intent to remember any of these previous experiences (Levy, 2011). Implicit memory allows people to remember how to tie their shoes or ride a bicycle without consciously thinking about these activities. In people with dementia, explicit memory may be significantly impaired, while a person continues to have functional implicit memory. This is seen in ordinary daily tasks like eating with a spoon. A person with dementia may sit at the table in front of her meal and not attend to the meal or initiate self-feeding. When a spoon is placed in her hand, and movement is prompted, the same individual may be able to effectively scoop food, carry it to her mouth on a spoon, take the bite, and return the spoon for another scoop of food. The memory of the procedure of self-feeding remains although the orientation to the task and the ability to initiate the task is impaired.

Psychomotor Functions

Psychomotor functions are the mental functions of control over physical and motor skills. These control functions include the ability to originate (plan) and initiate (begin) movements, monitor and adapt or adjust motions in progress, perform learned tasks automatically without conscious direction, and pace, limit, or end movement based on activity demands (World Health Organization, 2001). Psychomotor skills allow individuals to drive an automobile while listening to a conversation. All of the basic control involved in driving a car is subconscious, unless challenging road conditions occur. Psychomotor mental functions underlie many functional limitations following brain injury or disease. Some disabilities associated with impaired psychomotor control are psychomotor retardation (very slow movement responses), agitation (excess movement without direction), posturing/catalepsy (spontaneous maintenance of postures), echopraxia/echolalia (mimicking of another's movements/speech), and stereotypy (repetitive, nondirected motor activity). These types of disorders are associated with conditions of significant mental impairment such as autism and schizophrenia.

Emotional Functions

Emotional functions include those specific mental functions related to feelings, or the affective reactions of individuals (World Health Organization, 2001). These functions include not only emotions, but also the mental regulation of the appropriateness and degree of the emotion within an individual's social and environmental context. Emotions such as sadness, happiness, love, fear, anger, hate, tension, anxiety, joy, and sorrow are a part of a healthy human repertoire. The ability to appropriately assign and regulate these emotions within reasonable contexts is a mental function. Difficulty in this area includes disabilities like lability (poor regulation) of emotion and flattening of affect. These types of disorders are associated with human conditions like depression (mood disorders) and may be a temporary or a persistent problem.

Thought Functions

Thought functions, the ideas and imaginings of individuals, are recognized as the source of creativity and individuality in problem solving. The category of thought functions is broad, including many aspects of thinking such as the pace, control, and content of thought. Thought functions include both goal-directed thought functions and non-goal-directed thought functions such as daydreaming. Common disorders of thought functions seen in rehabilitation settings are flight of ideas, thought block, incoherence of thought, delusions, obsessions, and compulsions.

Higher-Level Cognitive Functions

Complex goal-directed behaviors such as decision making, abstract thinking, planning, problem solving, carrying out plans, mental flexibility, and deciding which behaviors are appropriate under what circumstances are described in the ICF as higher-level cognitive functions. In rehabilitation, these same abilities are more typically called metacognition or executive functions.

Metacognition is an important higher-level cognitive function that involves complex goal-directed thinking that allows us to plan, organize, execute, and evaluate our day-to-day activities. The term *metacognition* literally refers to the act of thinking about thinking, or the cognition of cognition. Although the terminology used in the ICF differs from that used in neurocognitive research, the specific mental functions of thought and perceptual functions are consistent with Katz and Maeir's (2011) description of metacognitive knowledge.

Metacognitive knowledge is what individuals know about themselves and others in terms of self, task, and problem solving. Common disorders of metacognitive knowledge seen in rehabilitation settings manifest as deficits in awareness. Unawareness problems include explicit verbal denial of deficits, or lack of awareness of a limb or a body side, as is seen in left-side neglect (Prigatano, 2010).

Metacognitive process is described by Katz and Maeir (2011) as the regulation of thought and control of thoughts. The rehabilitation literature calls the specific aspects of metacognitive process "executive functions." **Executive functions** are those cognitive abilities that enable individuals to respond to novel situations or unexpected challenges. These include multifactor goal-directed behaviors such as decision making, abstract thinking, planning and carrying out plans, mental flexibility, and deciding which actions to use in any given situation. Executive functions also include those capacities that are essential for directed, efficient participation in activities (Lezak, Howieson, Bigler, & Tranel, 2012). Lezak and colleagues (2012) identify four subcategories of executive function: volition, planning, purposive action, and effective performance. **Table 6-3** describes each of these four subcategories. Some of the terms used in **Table 6-3** may not be familiar. In this context, *organization* involves monitoring

TABLE 6-3 Aspects of Executive Function

Volition	Self-awareness, initiation, motivation.
Planning	The identification and organization of the steps and elements needed to carry out a goal. This includes sustained attention, impulse control, memory, abstraction, mental flexibility to consider alternatives, and the ability to choose between options.
Purposive Action	The ability to self-regulate actions and the ability to translate an intention into a plan of action. This includes the initiation, maintenance, alteration, and cessation of a sequence of events.
Effective Performance	This includes the ability to monitor, detect errors, self-correct, and to regulate the intensity and tempo of a performance.

Adapted from Katz and Maeir, 2011 p. 23. Reference Crediting: Katz, N. & Maeir, A. (2011). Chapter 2: Higher-level Cognitive Functions Enabling Participation: Awareness and Executive Functions. In Katz, N. (ed.). Cognition, occupation and participation across the lifespan: neuroscience, neurorehabilitation and models of intervention in occupational therapy, 3rd edition. Bethesda, MD: American Occupational Therapy Association.

something with complex features and coordinating the parts into a workable whole. This is the mental function involved in developing a method of proceeding or acting (World Health Organization, 2001).

Organization can be task-specific—as in setting out all the tools needed for a task before beginning the task, or temporal, as in ordering a task sequence logically from beginning to end. Organization can also be spatial, as in gathering and logically positioning tools and materials for a particular task.

Initiation is the ability to start something. People who have difficulty with initiation will know that they need to start a task, know how to do the task, want to do the task, and still sit there without starting. If these individuals are told, "Start now," they can proceed normally, until they change activities or need to stop and then start again. Initiation is considered an aspect of temporal organization in the *OT Practice Framework* (AOTA, 2014). Functionally, they should be able to self-initiate a desired task and should be able to change to a new task step without hesitation or prompting by another.

Abstraction is the mental function of considering something as a general idea, quality, or characteristic (World Health Organization, 2001). This mental function allows individuals to consider new or novel solutions to problems. Abstraction is also a creative process that allows for alternative plans of action and is therefore related to both problem solving and cognitive flexibility. These three domains—abstraction, problem solving, and cognitive flexibility—are typically considered separately but are difficult to separate in functional daily tasks, like home repair or information processing.

Cognitive flexibility is the ability to switch behavioral response according to the context of the situation, the ability to consider alternatives and change strategies or approaches to a problem. Cognitive flexibility allows for deviation and the consideration of alternatives in daily activities. For example, although a project's instructions state that a carpenter should use nails to hold his materials together, he may decide instead to use screws when he finds no nails in his toolbox. He has

appropriately chosen another strategy to complete the task rather than discontinuing it because of a technical problem.

Mental Functions of Language

There are many complex thought processes associated with human language. Chapter 5 introduced language as a set of shared rules that allow people to express their ideas in a meaningful way. Language is inherently abstract in that it involves recognizing and using signs and symbols. The specific **mental functions of language** described in the ICF are recognizing and using signs, and recognizing and using symbols as they relate to a language (World Health Organization, 2001). As the mental function on thinking about thought is called metacognitive reasoning, the mental function of thinking about language is also called *metalinguistic reasoning* in the rehabilitation literature.

The mental functions of language include all of the receptive language and coding/decoding of spoken, written or other forms of expressive language. The earlier chapter on communication (Chapter 5) introduced the abstraction of writing as a set of symbols that needed to be cognitively decoded. Impairments in metalinguistic reasoning will lead to impairments in seemingly physical tasks such as handwriting and performing tasks that require specific responses to abstract language cues. Metalinguistic reasoning deals with the relation between language and other cultural factors in a society that allows language users to accommodate special listener (or reader) needs (Bialystok & Ryan, 1985).

Calculation Functions

Comparable to the preceding discussion of language, arithmetic is also inherently abstract in that it involves recognizing and using signs and symbols. **Calculation functions** are described in the ICF as determination, approximation, and manipulation of mathematical symbols and processes

(World Health Organization, 2001). Although physical and occupational therapists may not immediately see how this particular area of mental functions relates to their practice, many of the strategies we use to support a client's return to function involves simple counting, addition, and/or subtraction. Home exercise programs, for example, nearly always involve counting repetitions of an exercise, often a complex repetition such as "perform three sets of ten, twice daily." For people hoping to function independently in the community, calculation functions are central to their ability to manage their finances. A client with a deficit in calculation functions may need more tangible tools to keep track of activities rather than mathematical calculations.

Mental Functions of Sequencing Complex Movements

The **mental function of sequencing complex movements** is defined in the ICF as the mental aspect of sequencing and coordinating complex, purposeful movements (World Health Organization, 2001). This includes the ability to ideate what the movement should do, how it should happen, and what the outcome of the movement should be. In the rehabilitation community, this ability is called *motor planning,* motor praxis, or most typically *sensorimotor praxis.* **Sensorimotor praxis** is the ability of the brain to conceive, organize, and carry out a sequence of unfamiliar actions (Golisz & Toglia, 2003). Sensorimotor praxis underlies successful performance of many motor tasks that include a challenging cognitive component such as dressing, excelling at sports, and driving a motor vehicle. The terms *dyspraxia* and *apraxia* reflect disorders in the mental functions of sequencing complex movements. Dyspraxia means disordered motor planning, and is often seen in children. Conditions like developmental coordination disorder and dyspraxic syndrome reflect this type of disorder. Apraxia means that motor planning is almost absent. Apraxia is sometimes seen following a head injury or cerebral vascular accident.

Experience of Self and Time Functions

The **experience of self and time functions** are specific mental functions related to the awareness of one's identity, one's body, one's position in the reality of one's environment, and of time (World Health Organization, 2001). This includes the cognitive skill of body image.

Body image is the awareness of one's body and representations of it. Disorders in this area of function are conditions involving thought disorders like schizophrenia and anorexia.

Experience of time functions include the subjective experience of the meaning of time, and the perception of both the length and passage of time. The awareness of time improves from early childhood as children's attention and short-term memory capacities develop. For children to gauge the time required for a task, they must both attend to it and

process a stream of time data without losing concentration. For this reason, individuals with attention deficit/hyperactivity disorder may find it hard to gauge time correctly (Droit-Volet, 2013). Emotion also impacts the subjective perception of time. Droit-Volet (2013) notes that showing a subject a threatening stimulus produces a temporal lengthening effect compared to a nonthreatening stimulus.

LEARNING AND APPLYING KNOWLEDGE

The process of learning, applying knowledge to daily activities and challenges, solving problems, and making decisions falls under the category of activities and participation in the ICF classification system (World Health Organization, 2001). Although the ICF lists primarily categories of academic learning, learning occurs in all arenas of human function. Situated learning, social learning, and motor learning are of particular interest for health professionals.

SITUATED LEARNING

Situated learning is learning that occurs through purposeful sensory experiences in the context that the learned behavior is needed. Situated learning is one of the earliest and most basic cognitive strategies for acquiring specific skills (Lave & Wenger, 1990). As noted in the case of Margie introduced earlier in this chapter, new learning and problem solving in novel situations are difficult for her. Although learning of all types may be impaired, Margie is more likely to be able to learn a specific task in the context in which it is needed versus learning in one setting and applying it to another situation. For example, Margie can learn to check her email on one computer system, but will be at a loss to do the same task on a different computer, even though the format and interface are the same.

The ICF categories, now more than a decade old, do not fully encompass the current state of understanding of the environmental and contextual influences on learning that will be presented here. Mental functions are grounded in mechanisms—that is, mechanisms of sensory processing and motor control—that evolved from interaction with the environment. This is best shown with infants or toddlers. Children utilize skills and abilities they were born with, such as sucking, grasping, and listening, to learn more about the environment. The skills are broken down into five main categories that combine sensory with motor skills, sensorimotor functions. The five main skills are:

1. *Mental imagery,* visualizing something based on your perception of it, when it is not there or is not present. An example of this would be having a race. You are all excited and full of adrenaline and you take a moment and you can actually see yourself winning the race.

2. *Working memory,* the ability to hold information in the mind to do verbal and nonverbal reasoning tasks.

3. *Episodic memory,* a category of long-term memory involving the recollection of specific events, situations, and experiences.

4. *Implicit memory,* information that you remember unconsciously and effortlessly.

5. *Reasoning and problem solving,* or having a mental model of something that will increase problem-solving approaches.

Purposeful Sensory Experience

Any intentional use of the senses to gain information is a **purposeful sensory experience**. These experiences form the foundation for learning. *Watching* is the purposeful use of vision to intentionally experience something, such as watching a television show or a classroom demonstration. Similarly, *listening* is using the sense of hearing intentionally to experience auditory stimuli, such as listening to music or a lecture. Purposeful sensory experiences include any use of the body's senses intentionally to experience stimuli, and include the acts of touching and feeling textures, tasting sweets, or smelling flowers (World Health Organization, 2001). In the viewpoint of learning theorists, sensory perception involves not only translating inputs into symbolic representation in the brain, but also integrating these inputs based on the properties of the environment within which they are perceived (Wilson & Peterson, 2006).

Situated learning involves action, and facts and rules learned through this method are embedded in social and environmental contexts. In the situated learning process, memory is seen as an interaction with the world, bounded by meaningful situations (Young, Kulikowich, & Barab, 1997). In this type of learning, individuals directly perceive and interact with the environment, and do not need memory in the form of stored symbolic representations. For this reason, situated learning is often a valuable tool in rehabilitation settings where the clients may have memory or cognitive impairments. Learning through doing, in the real-life context within which the activity should occur, is the best way to support skills acquisition. The significant limitation to this approach is that the learning acquired in a specific situation may not generalize to new contexts (Young, 2004).

Basic Learning

There are many common and widely used learning strategies, such as those included in the ICF: copying, rehearsing, learning to read, learning to write, and learning to calculate. How and how effectively individuals learn is based on many things, not just the environment or the learning strategies employed. An **affordance** is a perceived or actual property of a thing or situation that determines just how the thing could be used or the situation managed to support learning

(Norman, 1988). For example, a spoon is for scooping and transporting foods, and therefore affords eating. In the case of a person like Margie, who has impaired problem solving, the affordances of the task or situation can help her remain at least partially functional. She can respond to cues such as the placement of furniture to help her know where to sit, or the resemblance of a tool to a familiar tool, such as different types of brushes, to give her cues on how to use the objects.

Acquiring Skills

Learning is a product of interaction that results in acquiring new, or modifying existing, knowledge, behaviors, skills, or values. Learning utilizes body functions and affordances with an intentional focusing of attention on stimuli of interest. Learning is often intentional and the result of focused individual effort, but it can also occur as a result of habituation. There is evidence that even prenatally, human learning can result from habituation (James, Spencer, & Stepsis, 2002).

In the neonate, learning is largely sensory based and nonassociative, meaning it does not rely on memory or prior experiences to associate a stimulus with a sensory experience. With repeated experience of a stimulus, individuals habituate to it (decide that it is unimportant and no longer respond) or sensitize to it (recognize the stimulus as important and alert to it) (Bouton, 2007). **Nonassociative learning** is important in learning physical and motor skills. This type of learning can result in both transient and long-term modulation at the synaptic level and is important in rehabilitation of movement disorders.

Associative learning, which emerges in infancy, is a type of learning based on the assumption that ideas and experiences reinforce one another and can be linked to enhance the learning process. In associative learning, individuals learn to predict relationships and draw on long-term memory to make associations. Several types of associative learning have been identified. These are learning based on classical conditioning and operant conditioning, as well as declarative learning and procedural learning (Bouton, 2007).

Learning Stages

As we practice any new skill, we get faster at it, and it takes less memory and conscious effort to recall and perform. These qualitative changes are characterized by different stages in learning. Learners work out what information is relevant and what is not relevant and then break down the task into subtasks and individual actions.

The first stage in learning is the *cognitive stage.* During this stage the person uses primarily declarative learning. **Declarative learning** is learning that individuals are conscious of and make an effort to support. This type of learning predominates as individuals attempt a new skill at any age. Declarative learning requires both awareness of and attention to the task. The early phase of learning deals with behaviors shaped by declarative knowledge (facts and propositions). During this stage the learner is more concerned about what to do rather than how to do it. The next stage in learning is the *associative stage*. This stage is predominated by **procedural learning**, with little conscious processing required. The learner is concerned with performing and refining skills, and decisions about what to do become more automatic. Here, thinking about what you are doing can actually be disruptive to the smooth performance of a skill learned in this stage. This phenomenon, "paralysis by analysis," is a common feature of sport and athletic training. For instance, it is difficult to drive a car while explaining to someone else exactly what you are doing. The final stage in learning is the *autonomous stage*. At this stage the individual can complete the task automatically without having to think about it. Procedural knowledge is what we use when we have practiced until the task is automated. Here the procedures and the conditions that call for their use were learned in the declarative phase. The task no longer is inferred from declarative knowledge each time it is performed. Instead, the goal to drive the car home triggers a whole sequence of actions in an interface without having to think about each step explicitly.

MOTOR LEARNING

Motor learning occurs much like other learning, but is of particular interest to occupational and physical therapists. Motor learning involves basic motor skill acquisition (for example, learning to walk), the calibration of movements (learning to hold a juice box lightly so the liquid does not squirt out), and refining the smoothness and accuracy of movements as individuals seek expertise in any motor skill. **Figure 6-5** shows a young ballerina learning to dance in the formal ballet style that requires systematic training and practice. Motor skill alone is not adequate to achieve the level of control needed for this task. Motor learning includes thinking about movement, the desired goal, and the detection of errors in the process of moving in a combination of physical movement and cognitive analysis. When an individual learns a skill, such as dancing in toe shoes, practice and active movement are obviously involved. In the course of practicing, the individual receives information about how the task is progressing. That information is feedback, the sensory information that is available as a result of movement. Motor learning itself cannot be measured, but only inferred from motor performance. There are several classic theories of motor learning. These theories are discussed in Chapter 3 with other theoretical approaches to developmental and functional performance.

SOCIAL LEARNING

Social learning refers to the acquisition of behaviors within a social context that can take place at any stage in life. It includes a broad scope of learning contexts including the learning that takes place through social interaction between peers, and learning that is societal in scale. Social learning is also called *observational learning*. This type of learning begins with sensory attention (looking, listening, touching) to the actions

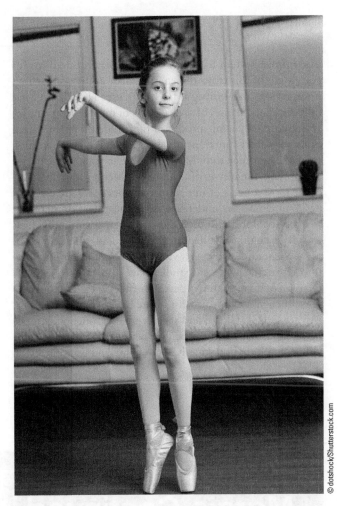

Figure 6-5   This young girl has been cognitively engaged in motor learning as she works to gain skill in dancing in her new ballet shoes. Competence in this challenging motor task can only develop with mental as well as physical effort.

or experiences of others, followed by imitation. Individuals are active in choosing models for social learning, and a model may present either socially positive or negative behavior (Ormrod, 2011). For example, a mother may model food preparation for her daughter. This modeling involves the process skills of knowledge (learning use of tools and techniques), temporal organization, and organizing space and objects. In addition to the task-performance skills, parental cooking instruction also models personal and social roles and routines. As a result of such parental modeling, a common experience of new partners is the awareness that the other person does not do something "right." For example, placing clean drinking glasses upside down on a shelf is "right" because it is how the behavior of putting glasses away was first modeled. The models for social learning usually come from one of three sources: a live model, verbal instruction, or through social media like television or the Internet (Ormrod, 2011).

Vicarious learning, or the process of learning from other people's behavior, is a central idea of social learning theory. This explains how individuals can witness observed behaviors of others and then reproduce (or avoid) the same actions.

SUMMARY

The human system has a vast and complex mechanism for taking in stimuli from the environment and then sorting, interpreting, and storing it for future use. This chapter has introduced the names of several types of mental functions involved in the dynamic process of human development. Each of these mental functions develops and interacts beginning prenatally so that individuals are able to make productive use of their time by early adulthood. Mental functions underlie most aspects of human performance and are essential as a foundation for understanding human development but also as a tool for health professionals working with individuals who have cognitive differences. Optimal cognitive development has traditionally been viewed as a priority for intervention research, but recent studies have also suggested that a focus on optimal cognitive development over the life course to prevent cognitive impairment in late life is equally important (Anstey, 2014). Global and specific mental function components interact with the specific characteristics of each individual, resulting in distinctive personality and learning styles. These learning styles represent intrapersonal characteristics and are important to successful interpersonal functioning.

Cognition and cognitive skills build with the maturation of individuals. Although evidence of learning can be elicited prenatally, the abilities of young children remain restricted by their level of nervous system development. Typical age-related cognitive achievement in childhood will be included in the chapters of these age groups. Learning is greatly influenced by opportunity and experience in the environment, including the roles modeled and the cultural context. In adulthood, learning continues to occur, but in a more selective and specialized way. That is, learning occurs when a specific behavior is used that was observed or tried previously that resulted in some outcome. If the outcome is perceived as positive, individuals will use that behavior again. If the outcome is perceived as negative, the behavior is likely to be suppressed. Learning is more than the gaining of academic skills. It can be of many types, including sensory, motor, interpersonal, intrapersonal, social, and cultural.

CASE 1

Margie Continued . . .

With team-based intervention, Margie is likely to be able to remain with Tom in her familiar home environment for an extended time. The OT has focused on adapting the home environment, and reorganizing and simplifying tasks. Tom has been given support in understanding his wife's condition as well as ideas for home modification that will support both his wife's and his own independent function in their home. The PT has enrolled Margie in a dance class that is aimed at providing pleasurable exercise and improving her balance. This activity will reduce Margie's fall risk and hopefully give her enough physical activity to reduce her tendency to wander from home.

In the day treatment center, Margie's therapy is conducted by a certified occupational therapy assistant (COTA) and a physical therapy assistant (PTA). In this setting, Margie is actively involved in exercise programs and in activities to support her continued participation in ADLs. Although Margie's condition is progressive, and further deterioration is inevitable, supportive therapies can help her more fully participate in self-care, leisure, and community activities to enhance her quality of life while reducing the burden on Tom, her caregiver.

Guiding Questions

Some questions to consider:

1. Margie needs constant supervision for safety, do you think she would be better off in a residential facility like a nursing home? Why or why not?
2. Research shows that engagement in pleasant sensory-rich experiences, such as interactions with familiar, liked animals (dogs and cats) or music, can offer people with dementia positive experiences and help reduce distress. Have you seen these types of strategies used in your clinical experiences?

CASE 2

Eva

Eva, 33, was recently discharged from the hospital to home following surgery to remove a bone cancer (osteosarcoma) at the proximal femur, and a portacath was installed in her chest for chemotherapy. At this time Eva is independent in eating, upper-body dressing. and basic grooming, although she needs some assistance with bathing and toileting. Since the start of chemotherapy, Eva has had little appetite and she fatigues easily.

Eva and her husband live on a small farm. Her husband works as a bank manager and works a typical 40-hour week. She has two daughters, ages 6 and 9, who attend school during the day and help Eva in the mornings and evenings. Before her cancer developed, Eva was a very active equestrian. She enjoyed hunting, gardening, needlepointing, and taking care of her horses and dogs. Since her hospitalization, Eva's daughters have taken over the feeding of the horses and the two family dogs. Her husband has hired a teenager from the community to perform the more strenuous animal care in the evenings.

Eva takes a long time to complete most tasks, and continues to complain of pain in the left hip during activity. Eva is also experiencing "chemo brain." Although her chemotherapy has been completed, she still sometimes finds she has trouble concentrating, a short attention span, and a tendency to "space out." She takes a long time to finish most tasks due to disorganized, slower thinking and processing.

During the day Eva is home alone except for her home health providers (including PT and OT). Her daughters get her set up in the recliner, with snacks and drinks before leaving for school. Eva often remains there until they return from school, even though she is safe to walk using a rolling walker. When asked, Eva always says that she "meant to" get up and do things. When the OT and PT put together a daily "to-do" list of physical activities that included walking out to get the mail and going outside to throw the ball for the dogs, Eva did not remember the list without someone reminding her to look at it. Even then, she needed someone with her to keep her on task during her therapy activities.

Assessment of cognitive functions indicated deficits in working memory and in the executive functions of initiation, temporal sequencing, and persistence in task performance. Eva started a cognitive training program with her OT, and with the support of Eva's family, her smartphone was programmed with alarms to prompt her in daily therapy activities. Eva's daughters encouraged her, and left "surprises" for her in the mailbox and on the back porch to encourage her independent movements. It became a game for them to come home from school and see how many of their surprises she had found.

As Eva began to move around more during the day, her strength quickly returned. Her "to-do" list was expanded to include a trip up and down the stairs and a trip out to the barn. Throughout the time she was receiving chemotherapy, Eva had periods of confusion and fatigue, but the cognitive therapy and the use of timers and alerts allowed her to keep up her activity level and regain her physical strength. Over time Eva was able to participate in activities at her daughters' school and to begin riding her horse again. Eva's chemotherapy extended over a period of six months, and after her cognitive problems were addressed, Eva was able to maintain a high enough physical activity level to allow her to do the things that were important to her.

Continues

Case 2   *Continued*

Guiding Questions

Some questions to consider:

1. It is common to think of cognitive problems and problems of the elderly. Eva has survived a life-threatening illness but continues to have difficulty participating due to changes in her cognition. Can you think of other reasons that a young adult may have cognitive impairments that limit participation in daily occupations?
2. Chemotherapy-induced cognitive impairments may be significant, but for many people they resolve over time. In the case of Eva, do you think that she would have been better off just waiting to see if it got better, or was it better to invest the time and money in treatment? Explain your reasoning.

Speaking of
Making a Difference

GARTH GRAEBE, OTR, OCCUPATIONAL THERAPIST

Jenny, a 40-year-old female, came to our clinic with a complaint that she was having difficulty keeping up at work. A few months ago she had been injured in a skiing accident. She suffered a concussion and lost consciousness for a few minutes. She returned to work after taking two weeks off to recuperate due to severe headaches, which eventually lessened. She now complains of headaches at the end of her workday, and stated that she does not usually have them on the weekends. Jenny works as a receptionist for a busy insurance agency. Her duties include answering the phone, greeting customers, and typing letters. She stated that when multiple phone lines ring, she typically answers all of them first and then transfers the calls to the appropriate person. Lately she has been having great trouble remembering which call is for whom. She also stated that when customers are waiting to see the executives, she often forgets who they are waiting for.

Additionally she has noticed that she is having a lot of difficulty staying on task with her typing. If she is interrupted by the phone or a customer, she has a great deal of difficulty finding the place where she left off. She is concerned that she may be at risk for losing her job as she has been reprimanded several times for her mistakes. She is single and lives alone in an apartment in the city. She denied any functional difficulties at home or in the community at large. I performed a standardized, continuous performance test of attention with Jenny, and was able to identify deficits with selective and divided attention, immediate memory, and generally slow mental processing speed. During the evaluation, I also noted that she became overly anxious when she would make a mistake. She indicated that she is often anxious at work and that her anxiety has gotten worse lately. Occupational therapy treatment included computerized cognitive exercises, compensatory techniques to aid her memory, and education in relaxation techniques to help her manage her anxiety.

Jenny came for treatment two times per week for five weeks. To help her at work, a small dry erase board with the names of the executives on labels was used to help her remember the phone lines and customers. When calls

Continues

Speaking of   *Continued*

came in, she would write the line number under the executive's name. In like manner, she would write the names of visitors under the executive's names as well. Once the calls were transferred and the visitors attended to, she would erase her notations. To help her with her typing, a typing stand with a movable placeholder was recommended. She was instructed to move the placeholder after each paragraph was typed.

Her computerized cognitive training consisted of working memory, processing speed, visual scanning, and visual attention exercises. The exercises were graded to her current level and then gradually increased in difficulty and speed. She reported that the compensatory techniques were immediately helpful, and she only occasionally made mistakes when she would either forget to write on the board or forget to erase it. At the end of the third week, she noticed that she no longer needed the placeholder on the typing stand and that her typing speed and accuracy had increased though she still had some difficulty and would become confused during especially busy times. At the end of week five, she was no longer using the dry erase board, and although she still got "a little anxious" when the pace picked up, she would use the relaxation techniques and was able to cope much better. Smiling, she stated that her boss told her she was doing a "fine job."

To most people, Jenny did not seem to have a problem, but if Jenny lost her job, she would have had few options to move forward. Also, Jenny had lost her confidence and was anticipating failure in every task. Although the focus of OT was to get her back to work, she also reported that she felt better about herself and relaxed more. People like Jenny help me see how important my work can be in the lives of some people.

REFERENCES

A.D.A.M. Medical Encyclopedia. (2011). *Dementia*. PubMed Health, U.S. National Library of Medicine. Retrieved from http://www.ncbi.nlm.nih.gov/pubmedhealth/PMH0001748/.

American Occupational Therapy Association (AOTA). (2014). *Occupational therapy practice framework: Domain and process* (3rd ed.). Bethesda, MD: AOTA Press.

Anstey, K. J. (2014). Optimizing cognitive development over the life course and preventing cognitive decline: Introducing the Cognitive Health Environment Life Course Model (CHELM). *International Journal of Behavioral Development, 38*(1), 1–10.

Becker, J., & Morris, R. (1999). Working memory. *Brain and Cognition, 41*, 1–8.

Bernat, J. (2006). Chronic disorders of consciousness. *Lancet, 367*(9517), 1181–1192.

Bernstein, D. (2010). *Essentials of psychology* (5th ed.). Independence, KY: Wadsworth Publishing.

Bialystok, E., & Ryan, E. (1985). Toward a definition of metalinguistic skill, *Merrill-Palmer Quarterly, 31*(3), 229–251.

Bijttebier, P., & Roeyers, H. (2009). Temperament and vulnerability to psychopathology: Introduction to the special section. *Journal of Abnormal Child Psychology: An Official Publication of the International Society for Research in Child and Adolescent Psychopathology, 37*(3), 305–308.

Bouton, M. E. (2007). *Learning and behavior: A contemporary synthesis*. Sinauer MA: Sunderland.

Carey, T., & McDevitt, S. (1995). *Coping with children's temperament: A guide for professionals*. New York: Basic Books.

Colom, R., Haier, R. J., Head, K., Alvarez-Linera, J., Quiroga, M., Shih, P., & Jung, R. E. (2009). Gray matter correlates of fluid, crystallized, and spatial intelligence: Testing the P-FIT model. *Intelligence, 37*(2), 124–135.

Dawson, G. (2008). Early behavioral intervention, brain plasticity, and the prevention of autism spectrum disorder. *Development And Psychopathology, 20*(3), 775–803.

Deary, I. J., & Batty, G. D. (2007). Cognitive epidemiology. *Journal of Epidemiology and Community Health, 61*(5), 378–384.

Draganski, B., & Kherif, F. (2013). In vivo assessment of use-dependent brain plasticity—Beyond the "one trick pony" imaging strategy. *Neuroimage, 73*, 255–259.

Droit-Volet, S. (2013). Emotion and magnitude perception: Number and length bisection. *Frontiers in Neurorobotics, 7*, 24. Retrieved from http://www.frontiersin.org/Journal/10.3389/fnbot.2013.00024/full

Feldman, R. (2011). *Child development* (6th ed.). Upper Saddle River, NJ: Prentice Hall.

Gardner, H. (1993). *Frames of mind: The theory of multiple intelligences* (10th anniversary ed.). New York: Basic Books.

Gardner, H. (2006). *Multiple intelligences: New horizons.* New York: Basic Books.

Garlick, D. (2003). Integrating brain science research with intelligence research. *Current Directions in Psychological Science, 12,* 185–189.

Gasser-Wieland, T., & Rice, M. (2002) Occupational embeddedness during a reaching and placing task with survivors of cerebral vascular accident. *OTJR: Occupation, Participation, and Health, 22,* 153–160.

Golisz, K. M., & Toglia, J. P. (2003). Cognitive perceptual evaluation. In E. B. Creapeau, B. Schell, & E. Cohn (Eds.), *Willard and Spackman's occupational therapy* (10th ed.). Philadelphia: Lippincott.

Greenfield, P. M., & Suzuki, L. K. (1998). Culture and human development: Implications for parenting, education, pediatrics, and mental health. In W. Damon (General Ed.) & I. E. Sigel & K. A. Renninger (Vol. Eds.), *Handbook of child psychology: Vol. 4. Child psychology in practice* (5th ed.). New York: Wiley.

James, D., Spencer, C., & Stepsis, B. (2002). Fetal learning: A prospective randomized controlled study. *Ultrasound Obstetrics and Gynecology, 20*(5), 431–38.

Jung, R., & Haier, R. (2007). The Parieto-Frontal Integration Theory (P-FIT) of intelligence: Converging neuroimaging evidence. *Behavioral and Brain Sciences, 30*(2), 135–154.

Katz, N., & Maeir, A. (2011). Chapter 2: Higher-level cognitive functions enabling participation: Awareness and executive functions. In N. Katz (Ed.), *Cognition, occupation and participation across the life span: Neuroscience, neurorehabilitation and models of intervention in occupational therapy* (3rd ed.). Bethesda, MD: American Occupational Therapy Association.

Lave, J., & Wenger, E. (1990). *Situated learning: Legitimate peripheral participation. Cambridge,* UK: Cambridge University Press.

Levy, L. (2011). Chapter 6 Cognitive information processing. In N. Katz (Ed.), *Cognition, occupation and participation across the life span* (3rd ed., pp. 93–115) Bethesda, MD: AOTA Press.

Lezak, M., Howieson, D., Bigler, E., & Tranel, D. (2012). *Neuropsychological assessment* (5th ed.). New York: Oxford University Press.

Li, Y., Baldassi, M., Johnson, E. J., & Weber, E. U. (2013). Complementary cognitive capabilities, economic decision making, and aging. *Psychology and Aging, 28*(3), 595–613.

Ng, F., & Tsang, H. (2002). A program to assist people with severe mental illness in formulating realistic life goal. *Journal of Rehabilitation, 16*(4), 59–66.

Norman, Donald (1988). *The design of everyday things.* New York: Basic Books.

Ormrod, J. E. (2011). *Human learning* (6th ed.). Upper Saddle River, NJ: Prentice-Hall.

Prigatano, G. (2010). *The study of anosognosia.* New York: Oxford University Press.

Rothbart, M., & Bates, J. (2006). Temperament. In N. Eisenberg, W. Damon, & L. M. Richard (Eds.), *Handbook of child psychology: Vol. 3, Social, emotional, and personality development* (6th ed.; pp. 99–166). Hoboken, NJ: John Wiley & Sons Inc.

Rothbart, M. (2007). Temperament, development, and personality. *Current Directions in Psychological Science, 16*(4), 207–212.

Sacks, S., Fisher, M., Garrett, C., Alexander, P., Holland, C., Rose, D., & . . . Vinogradov, S. (2013). Combining computerized social cognitive training with neuroplasticity-based auditory training in schizophrenia. *Clinical Schizophrenia & Related Psychoses, 7*(2), 78–86A.

Sternberg, R. (2005). The WICS model of giftedness. In R. J. Sternberg & J. E. Davidson (Eds.), *Conceptions of giftedness* (2nd ed., pp. 327–342). New York: Cambridge University Press.

Sternberg, R., & Kaufman, S. (2011). *The Cambridge handbook of intelligence.* New York: Cambridge University Press.

Sternberg, R., Lautrey, J., & Lubart, T. (Eds.). (2003). *Models of intelligence: International perspectives.* American Psychological Association, Washington DC.

Thelen, E. (2000). Grounded in the world: Developmental origins of the embodied mind. *Infancy, 1*(1_, 3–28).

Thelen, E., & Smith, L. (1994). *A dynamic systems approach to the development of cognition and action.* Cambridge, MA: MIT Press

Thomas, A., Chess, S., Birch, H., Hertzig, M., & Korn, S. (1963). *Behavioral individuality in early childhood.* New York: New York University Press.

Tippeconnic, J., & Tippeconnic Fox, M. (2012). American Indian tribal values: A critical consideration in the education of American Indians/Alaska Natives today. *International Journal of Qualitative Studies in Education (QSE), 25*(7), 841–853.

Vroman, K., & Arthanat, S. (2012). ICF and mental functions: Applied to cross cultural case studies of schizophrenia. In J. H. Stone & M. Blouin (Eds.), *International encyclopedia of rehabilitation.* Retrieved from http://cirrie.buffalo.edu/encyclopedia/en/article/308

Wells, M., & Vaughn, B. V. (2012). Poor sleep challenging the health of a nation. *Neurodiagnostic Journal, 52*(3), 233–249.

Wilcock, A. (2006). *An occupational perspective of health* (2nd ed.). Thorofare, NJ: SLACK Incorporated.

Wilson, M. (2002). Six views of embodied cognition. *Psychonomic Bulletin and Review, 9,* 625–636.

Wilson, M. (2008). How did we get from there to here? An evolutionary perspective on embodied cognition. In P. Calvo & T. Gomila (Eds.), *Directions for an embodied cognitive science: Towards an integrated approach.* Elsevier.

Wilson, M. (2010). The re-tooled mind: How culture re-engineers cognition. *Social Cognitive and Affective Neuroscience, 5*(2–3), 180–187.

Wilson, S. M., & Peterson, P. L. (2006). *Theories of learning and teaching: what do they mean for educators?* Washington, DC: National Education Association.

World Health Organization. (2001). *ICF: International classification of functioning and disability.* Geneva, Switzerland: World Health Organization.

Young, M. (2004). An ecological psychology of instructional design: Learning and thinking by perceiving-acting systems. In D. H. Jonassen (Ed.), *Handbook of research for educational communications and technology* (2nd ed.). Mahwah, NJ: Erlbaum.

Young, M. F., Kulikowich, J. M., & Barab, S. A. (1997). The unit of analysis for situated assessment. *Instructional Science, 25*(2), 133–150.

CHAPTER 7

Environmental Contexts

Anne Cronin, PhD, OTR/L,
Associate Professor,
Division of Occupational Therapy,
West Virginia University, Morgantown,
West Virginia With contributions by
Ingrid M. Kanics, OTR/L,
Kanics Inclusive Design Services, LLC

Objectives

Upon completion of this chapter, readers should be able to:

- Understand the complex relationship between environmental contextual factors and occupation for individuals of all ages;

- Define universal design and its importance in both physical and electronic access for people with differing abilities;

- Define the environmental contexts identified by the ICF that are presented in this chapter;

- Differentiate and offer examples of accessibility and negotiability in the environmental contexts;

- Describe the relationships among attitudes, roles, and habits; and

- Discuss the implications of technology for expanding environmental access.

Key Terms

accessibility

ageism

aging in place

animal-assisted therapy (AAT)

assets

attitudinal environment

attitudinal racism

client-centered care

elder cottage housing
    opportunities (ECHO)

HomeFit

inclusive design

malingering

mixed-use development

negotiability

physical environment

products and technology

Rebuilding Together

retirement community

routine

service animal

sick role

sustainability

universal design (UD)

virtual environment

visitability

CASE 1

Trina

Trina (aged 56) has Down syndrome and had been living with her mother until last year. Trina had lived in the same city neighborhood since she was very small, and she knew most of the shopkeepers near her home. When Trina's mother died, she was moved into her sister's home. Trina had very firmly set routines; she woke up early every morning, took a shower, and had breakfast. Her sister encouraged these routines because they gave Trina comfort and added structure to her day. The routines centered around typical mealtimes, and at these times Trina did well. Outside of these routines, Trina was unable to function well. Trina had done much of the routine housework while she lived with her mother, and was well able to manage these tasks. When she had finished her chores, Trina often went out for a walk. She had a walking route that was about a mile long, which was peppered by friendly shopkeepers. She would walk and visit, and sometimes stop for a snack on her daily jaunts.

In her sister's house, Trina became restless and paced through the house or the yard. She wanted to "help" but was seldom able to complete a task without some supervision. Now, every time she passed the dishwasher or the laundry room, she checked to see what needed to be done, until it seemed like an obsession. Unfortunately, the machines were different and the family needs were different, and Trina had trouble adjusting to these changes.

In her mother's home Trina had been able to manage so well that her cognitive and physical impairments were hardly noticeable to people outside of the family. In her sister's home Trina demonstrated difficulties in problem solving, memory, physical endurance, and balance. She had difficulty not only with the use of different home appliances, but also because she had difficulty with the layout of the house. The house had two flights of stairs and a sunken living room. Trina did not always look carefully where she was walking and had tripped over shoes left near the front door and on the stair down into the living room.

Trina enjoyed living with her sister and her nieces (both school-aged), but because her sister worked and the girls went to school, Trina was often home alone. She had seldom been home alone before, and was now fearful when left alone in her sister's home.

In the move to her sister's house, Trina had left a busy urban setting and was now in the suburbs. She must rely on someone to drive her everywhere, and she has no opportunity to interact socially with anyone but her immediate family. Trina is happy to be with her sister but is lonely and is more dependent in everyday function than she has been since she was a young child.

Continues on page 140

INTRODUCTION

With the ICF document, the international community has made a strong statement that function and participation are not simply based on features intrinsic to an individual, but that complex external factors are integral to determining functional capacity and health. We are considering the concept of environmental contexts broadly in this chapter, looking at influences of the physical environment, social environments, and attitudinal environments on human occupation. Contextual factors provide resources that support or inhibit a client's performance. Some examples of contextual factors are presence of a willing caregiver, the delivery of services (for example, limits placed on length of intervention in an inpatient hospital setting), and access to the Internet. The ICF description of the environmental contexts in which people live and conduct their lives argues that factors "external to individuals can have a positive or negative influence on the individual's participation as a member of society, on performance of activities of the individual, or on the individual's body function or structure" (World Health Organization, 2001, p. 22). Although issues of environment may seem secondary to busy health professionals, these issues impact health and human function in a myriad of ways, both global and local. Schrecker (2012) comments on global concerns when he notes that "the world economy is entering an era of multiple crises, involving finance, food, security, and global environmental change" (p. 557). The world issues Schrecker mentioned also appear locally. Limited access to drinking water had been cited for years as a global health concern. Although this concern does not often touch residents of the United States, as this text was being written, a 10,000-gallon chemical spill contaminated drinking water for West Virginia residents, leaving them without safe drinking water on tap for weeks. This isolated chemical spill closed schools and businesses. The spill also caused severe problems in hospitals and nursing homes that needed to care for people with health challenges.

A healthy community environment "encompasses aspects of human health, disease, and injury that are determined or influenced by factors in the overall environment. Examining the interaction between health and the environment requires studying not only how health is affected by the direct pathological impacts of various chemical, physical, and biologic agents, but also by factors in the broad physical and social environments, which include housing, urban development, land use, transportation, industry, and agriculture" (CDC, 2010).

In this chapter, we will focus on the three types of external environmental factors described in the ICF: (1) natural environment and human-made changes to the environment; (2) products and technology: and (3) support and relationships, attitudes, services, systems, and policies (World Health Organization, 2001).

NATURAL ENVIRONMENT AND HUMAN-MADE CHANGES TO THE ENVIRONMENT

The **physical environment** includes both the natural and man-made features of the physical space people occupy. The natural environment includes physical features of the outdoor environment such as landforms, and climatic features such as seasonal variations and unexpected natural events (hurricanes, earthquakes, and so on). Characteristics of the physical environment influence what occupations people engage in as well as how and why they engage in them. People living in tropical climates often organize their meals and daily routines to allow for an early afternoon break or quiet time, the "siesta" during the heat of the day. Similarly, in very cold climates, going to work may take extra time and preparation in the winter months. This includes extra layers of clothing and perhaps the need to clear snow and ice from pathways or vehicles.

Human-made changes to the environment include any alterations in the natural environment, caused by people that result in the disruption of people's day-to-day lives. Examples of this include the displacement of people due to wars, and water or air pollution. Although the concept has become highly politicized, a consensus of international science organizations affirm that "warming of the climate system is unequivocal, as is now evident from observations of increases in global average air and ocean temperatures, widespread melting of snow and ice, and rising global average sea level" (Intergovernmental Panel on Climate Change, 2007). Although climate change will not be the focus of this chapter, the major public health crises projected for the 21st century, food production and financial security, are directly related to global climate change a human-made change to the environment (Schrecker, 2012).

The physical environment has a pervasive influence on all human activities and participation. For example, features of the physical environment can influence such diverse things as the rate of child development (Maleta, Virtanen, Espo, Kulmala, & Ashorn, 2003), mother-child dynamics (Olson & Esdaile, 2000), the ability to engage in productive paid work (Bootes & Chapparo, 2002), and the possibility of becoming independently mobile (Jones, McEwen, & Hansen, 2003). Bonnefoi and colleagues (2010) identified environmental toxicology (the study of toxins in the environment), risk assessments of sensitive populations, the aging of world populations, and improved science-driven regulatory and policy frameworks as the most crucial public health issues through 2020. Whether impacted in their ability to address the needs of clients, as in the water crisis in West Virginia, or in an increase in environmentally influenced health conditions, all health care providers will be impacted by the influence of the physical environment in their practice.

The term **sustainability** refers to the potential for the creation and maintenance of conditions under which humans and nature can exist in productive harmony (Environmental Protection Agency, 2014). Increasingly, the concept of sustainability is being incorporated into health care practices and clinical reasoning. In health care, the concept of sustainability is translated both into conservation of resources and into leadership priorities in promoting healthy values. Sustainability should also be considered in planning interventions for clients. Home exercise programs that are embedded in the features available in the individuals' home environment and that are consistent with daily occupational needs are more likely to be sustainable, used consistently by clients over time, than standard programs that do not reflect the individuals' environmental context.

PHYSICAL GEOGRAPHY

Shumway-Cook and colleagues (2003) report that mobility disability results, in part, from avoidance of physically challenging features within the environment. For example, people living in a mountainous terrain will have different mobility challenges than do people living on an open plain. Issues of terrain are common in the authors' home state of West Virginia. The beautiful and rugged environment is much admired for adventure sports, and for adventurous children, as illustrated in **Figure 7-1**, but it is very limiting for wheelchair users.

Although there are adventurous people who try mountain climbing, boating, and skiing in spite of their wheelchairs, people more typically feel discouraged rather than challenged by obstacles (Shumway-Cook et al., 2003). On a less dramatic scale, people living in rural areas may be unable to use motorized scooters or power wheelchairs safely, although their urban counterparts will find these tools invaluable. Trina, in moving to her sister's home, was challenged by the physical geography. Her sister lived in a subdivision consisting of single-family homes with no stores in walking distance. Like people in many

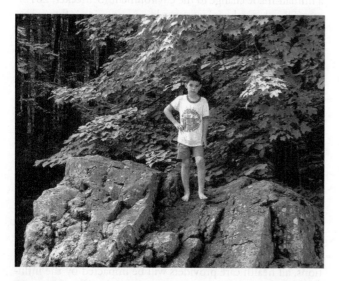

Figure 7-1 Physical terrain provides a fun challenge for this boy, but can pose insurmountable obstacles for people with mobility impairments.

American suburbs, Trina did not have access to public transportation and found that she could not engage in leisure activities that she had previously enjoyed.

Population density can influence the availability of services and the perception of security. In suburbs with single-family houses on large lots, population density may be too low to support a public transportation system and can isolate nondrivers like Trina. Similarly, elderly people in a rural area where housing is scattered and not organized into housing developments may have no close neighbor and feel isolated. People living in densely populated urban areas are likely to have good access to public transportation, stores, recreation, and health care services, but also have the added challenge of a high crime rate. These examples offer further insight into how environmental contexts influence daily occupations.

CLIMATE AND NATURAL EVENTS

Climate is another physical feature that can greatly impact function. People living in cold climates will have the health and mobility challenges that extreme weather, ice, and snow pose. Retired people with the financial means to relocate during the winter months are called "snowbirds" as they annually migrate to warmer climates. Extreme temperatures, both hot and cold, can be a health risk for people with cardiovascular and respiratory limitations. In the United States, every summer, some older people die in urban areas due to complications secondary to extreme heat conditions.

Earthquakes, floods, and volcanoes are listed as aspects of the natural environment by the ICF model. For therapists, this seems far beyond our scope of consideration, but in fact it can easily become a variable in intervention planning. For example, along the Mississippi River, there are occasional severe floods. These floods cause obvious immediate problems but also cause lasting problems in the form of contaminated wells, damaged structures, increased insect populations, and mildew inside living structures. This type of natural event can leave people who have managed independently for years suddenly needing support for ordinary ADLs and IADLs. Frail elderly people who have been managing marginally may be forced out of their homes if accommodation cannot be made.

When climate events are catastrophic, the results to human activity and participation are likely to include occupational deprivation, a concept first introduced in Chapter 4 of this text. In the case of a severe earthquake or weather-related catastrophe, people's lifestyles will be disrupted. That disruption may be temporary, resolving over time, or it may be persistent. Following the 2004 tsunami in the Indian Ocean, people living in coastal communities, especially those who earned a living from fishing, were deprived of their livelihood, and their daily occupations were profoundly changed.

Occupational and physical therapists have a role in their community in helping people plan for common climate challenges in their communities. Whether teaching ergonomic strategies for snow removal or assuring that people have an emergency call system in case of a fall, clinicians respond to challenges posed by the natural environment. Many individual therapists volunteer with regional agencies to assist with disaster relief efforts. This role is very important as most emergency response teams are poorly prepared to deal with people with physical or cognitive disabilities.

HUMAN-CAUSED EVENTS

Likewise, human disruptions of the natural environment can disrupt people's day-to-day lives. Urban dwellers who have had the experience of being blocked in their driveways because of snow left behind by city snow removal teams will understand this. Similarly, people may be required to evacuate from their homes when the government perceives a threat, such as a wildfire or toxic pollution. Disruptions in familiar routines and removal from familiar environments can cause distress and sometimes disorientation.

On a larger scale, human events may cause people to be displaced or homeless. The Fukushima Daiichi nuclear disaster in 2011 resulted in the sudden evacuation and long-term relocation of more than 1,500 people. People all over the world are also refugees from areas experiencing war or civil unrest. Refugees of all types face significant health problems, both in the separation from their usual service providers and sources of medications, but also in the additional distress and housing challenges caused by the relocation (Weine, 2011). The role of physical and occupational therapists in response to human-caused events is similar to that described earlier in response to climatic and natural events. Helping people, especially people with disabilities, manage in the face of environmental challenges can be a valuable service for the community.

HOUSING

Poor housing can cause or contribute to many preventable diseases and injuries, such as respiratory, nervous system and cardiovascular diseases and cancer. Similarly, pollution and lack of green spaces and mobility options poses potential health risks. The Centers for Disease Control and Prevention has emphasized that more than housing needs to be addressed in building healthy communities. Many communities grow and expand without central planning. The poorly planned growth around cities that fails to consider regional implications is called *urban sprawl*. Traits associated with the concept of sprawl include the disappearance of farmland, fields, and natural woodland as cities expand outward and consume once rural or natural areas, as well as large tracts of land converted into housing, commercial enterprises, or paved parking lots and widespread strip commercial development along major transportation corridors (Perdue, Stone, & Gostin, 2003).

In patterns of urban sprawl, automobiles become the primary means of transportation, because there is no coordinated or planned public transportation infrastructure. This results in extensive road construction to accommodate automobiles, increased traffic congestion, poor air quality, contaminated water and land, and scarce affordable housing. Although parking lots are a common feature in urban sprawl, sidewalks for pedestrians and bicycle lanes for non-car users are often rare. As a result, there is less safety for pedestrians, bicyclists, and automobile occupants (CDC, 2010).

Urban sprawl has been a particular problem for the elderly who are limited in their ability to maintain and drive an automobile. Mixed-use developments are a growing trend to counteract the negative effects of urban sprawl. A **mixed-use development** is the use of a building, set of buildings, or neighborhood for more than one purpose. Mixed-use development provides a range of commercial and residential unit sizes and options. Unlike modern suburban developments that include housing but do not include stores or other businesses, mixed-use developments have housing, services such as shopping, and customer services businesses (such as hairdressers and laundry services), recreational facilities, and public transportation options. When people live in mixed-use developments and when they have access to reliable public transportation, they tend to walk more and their health improves (MacDonald, Stokes, Cohen, Kofner, & Ridgeway, 2010; Mumford, Contant, Weissman, Wolf, & Glanz, 2011).

Mixed-use developments are a trend that is aimed at making communities more livable. Other trends focus more on the elderly as a growing population of people with special housing needs. Some of these trends include retirement communities and Elder Cottage Housing Opportunities. A **retirement community** is a residential development designed for older adults who are generally able to care for themselves. Typically these are age-restricted or age-qualified communities, and the community offers shared services or amenities such as meal preparation and maid services. These communities have been very successful in addressing the needs of elders, but are available only to those elders with good financial resources, as they require a substantial monthly payment to the community in addition to the cost of renting (or purchasing) the housing unit. In a study exploring the environmental factors associated with a positive response to retirement communities. Nathan, Wood, and Giles-Corti (2013) identified three valued aspects that support active living. These are a positive social environment within the community, services and facilities that are provided in the village, and the presence of suitable pedestrian infrastructure.

The **Elder Cottage Housing Opportunities (ECHO)** trend started in Australia and involves the installation of a temporary, manufactured home, which can be added as a separate structure on the same property as a single-family home belonging to an adult child or another relative. The ECHO approach, although still expensive, is less costly than a move to a retirement community. The initial purchase and installation of the cottage is a large one-time cost, but after it is installed, the unit is cost-effective. In these cases the older adult continues to live independently, but has ready access to family for support.

VIRTUAL ENVIRONMENTS

An increasingly important environment for function is the **virtual environment**, an environment in which individuals interact by means of electronic media (American Occupational Therapy Association, 2014). Although many people think of virtual environments as a sort of playground for the young, half of American adults ages 65 and older are online (Zickuhr & Madden, 2012). Occupations that once involved physical travel, such as shopping, can now be done online, with goods delivered to your home. Virtual environments have also led to the expansion of some occupations. The explosive growth in blogging, or keeping a public online diary, has become a valued and respected occupation in contemporary society. For some individuals, blogging has led to publication of their written work in traditional print media. Communication technologies such as email, video chat software, and text messaging can be enablers for those aging in place. Older adults are also avid cell phone users, and one in three online seniors use social networking sites such as Facebook, LinkedIn, or Pinterest (Zickuhr & Madden, 2012). This increasingly widespread use of communication technologies can have a beneficial effect for many people, especially seniors, keeping them socially linked to loved ones even when they are not physically able to travel or visit regularly.

PRODUCTS AND TECHNOLOGY

The ICF category of **products and technology** refers to physical items that people come in contact with while completing their daily activities. Products and technology are central to the practice of occupational and physical therapists as they work to enhance the function of their clients. These items can include fundamental needs like food and medications or complex items such as regional land-use policies, including the design, planning, and development of space. Some selected subtypes of products and technologies are presented in **Table 7-1** with a discussion of limitations in clinical application.

As rehabilitation specialists, we tend to think of specialized adaptations, but products and technology also relate to ordinary everyday items. For example, the ability to don and doff items of clothing is an important developmental milestone for children. As children gain control over their lives, this is often expressed by their ability to shed their clothing on their own. As their motor, visuospatial, and cognitive skills develop, they master the ability to choose and don their own clothing. The skills developed and necessary for this major landmark can vary widely between cultures. The skills necessary for preschool children to don the typical American clothing items of jeans, shirt, socks, and

---

TABLE 7-1   Selected Subtypes of ICF Products and Technologies

Product	ICF Definition (World Health Organization, 2001)	Example of Limitation
Products or substances for personal consumption	Any object or substance gathered, processed, or manufactured for ingestion, including food and medicines	Limitations affect social function. An adolescent who has cerebral palsy and limited abilities to chew and swallow will not be able to participate in class pizza parties.
Products and technology for personal use in daily living	Equipment, products, and technologies used by people in daily activities	Limitations may be culturally influenced. A child who cannot manage eating utensils may be socially limited in a Western culture, where this is not accepted; however, in a Pakistani culture, this would be acceptable.
Products and technology for personal indoor and outdoor mobility and transportation	Equipment, products, and technologies used by people in activities of moving inside and outside buildings	Limitations may be environmentally determined. Many shopping malls now offer rental of motorized scooters for people with limited mobility. These devices would not be equally useful in a street market with curbs, uneven pavement, and gravel paths.
Products and technology for communication	Equipment, products, and technologies used by people in activities of sending and receiving information	Limitations influence ability to communicate. Telephone access to emergency rescue systems is widely available. People with speech or hearing impairments will not be able to use this safety program.
Products and technology for employment	Equipment, products, and technology used for employment to facilitate work activities	Limitations may impact ability to perform employment tasks. Traditional storage and filing cabinets are not accessible to people who cannot stand.

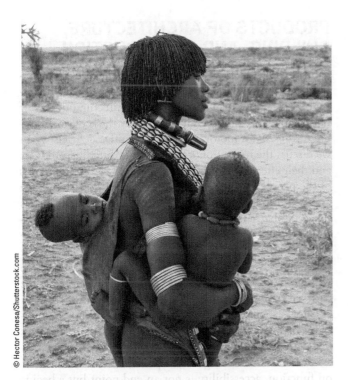

© Hector Conesa/Shutterstock.com

Figure 7-2   The ADL skills these young boys need will be complex, but very unlike the skills needed by average American children.

shoes may be quite unnecessary for these young Ethiopian children pictured in **Figure 7-2** to function in their own social and cultural environment.

Independence in the process of daily ADLs is a source of personal challenge and pride in the preschool years. As individuals move into late adulthood and experience motor and visual changes associated with natural aging, the experience of dressing oneself can once again gain significance. Independence in ADLs is a key factor in determining the ability of older individuals to continue living independently. As shown in **Figure 7-3**, the

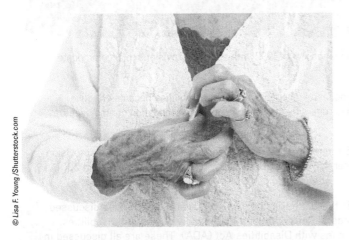

© Lisa F. Young/Shutterstock.com

Figure 7-3   This older woman has rheumatoid arthritis in her hands, which makes buttoning very difficult. She may choose a different product, such as a top that pulls over her head, or an assistive technology device, such as a button hook to address this limitation.

buttons, snaps, and zippers that challenged a 4-year-old with poor motor skills can once again become challenging as difficulties with sensory and motor changes associated with aging or an age-related disease like arthritis change the function of older individuals. Often older people alter their wardrobe choices to increase his independence. These changes can include the use of elastic-waist skirts and pants, pullover versus button-down tops, and loafers or slip-on shoes versus tennis shoes.

Older individuals from a different culture might find the changes associated with aging challenging in different ways. For example, there are many different types of toilets in the world. The need to use a toilet that is not inside the home may be very challenging for older adults with mobility problems. Similarly, toilets that are intended to be used while standing may be unmanageable for people with weakness or arthritis pain.

ASSETS

Assets are "products or objects of economic exchange such as money, goods, property, and other valuables which an individual owns or to which he or she has rights of use" (WHO, 2001, p. 98). Children are often raised within the asset boundaries set by their parents or caretakers. An *asset boundary* may be something simple such as access to food during nonmeal times, or it may be something more complex such as money that in turn can provide access to an education.

The amount of assets possessed by parents can either facilitate or inhibit development of children or the function of older persons. In Trina's case, introduced at the beginning of this chapter, Trina's family has adequate assets to care for her. In living with her mother, Trina's need for supervision and care were balanced by her need to contribute to household maintenance. Although Trina was dependent on her mother, she was also able to provide valuable supports for her mother as she aged. Trina's sister was able to provide housing for Trina, but the physical and social characteristics of the sister's home inhibited Trina's independent function.

Children raised in poverty have decreased opportunities in terms of access to education and health care as compared with children raised in affluent environments. The true impact this has on the development of children, though, is a complicated equation in which the society's values, supports, and political environment must be included. In Chapter 4 of the text, the concept that there can be a "culture" and the impact of poverty on lifestyle is introduced.

Research consistently shows that both physical and mental health are associated with socioeconomic status (SES). Low SES and low levels of educational achievement were both associated with increased morbidity (Hosseinpoor, Williams, Itani, & Chatterji, 2012). Low-income individuals are two to five times more likely to suffer from a diagnosable mental disorder than those in the top SES bracket (Stansfeld, Clark, Rodgers, Caldwell, &

Power, 2011). Within families, economic hardship can lead to marital distress and disrupted parenting that in turn may increase mental health problems among children, such as depression, substance abuse, and behavior problems (Conger, Conger, & Martin, 2010).

Lack of assets in early childhood, which results in a less than optimal developmental outcome, is a key aspect in the perpetuation of the culture of poverty. The effect of assets on development and aging is often tempered or worsened by the effects of other environmental factors such as support and relationships, attitudes, and services, systems, and policies. Therapists generally underestimate the effects of the physical environment on health and social participation. Physical environments that provide access and opportunity for participation were found to be conducive to fostering occupational performance (Rebeiro, 2001).

As individuals age, assets continue to affect aging and the experience of older individuals. In most societies, aging is associated with a decrease in income as individuals pass from workers to retired people, or as changes in motor, visual, and cognitive systems dictate a change in employment. This loss of monetary assets has a direct effect on health and wellness in the aged population. Seniors who have collected greater assets during their life have more flexibility to pick and choose where and how they want to live during retirement than seniors who were unable to accumulate financial assets as working individuals. Frail, disabled, and widowed elders who live alone are more likely to have limited assets and report more depression, loneliness, and sleep problems. Hays and George (2002) report that these same widowed elders "use more formal home-care services; have less access to help in emergencies; and are at greater risk of unstable living arrangements and of institutionalization compared to similar elders living with others" (p. 284).

PRODUCTS OF ARCHITECTURE, BUILDING, AND CONSTRUCTION

Most architecture and buildings are designed for average-sized adults with normal motor, cognitive, and sensory perceptual function. The fixtures and architectural details of most settings are not intended for use by those of small stature or those with motor, visual, or cognitive deficits. When we discuss the impact of architectural or building products and their effects of development, we need to think in terms of the people using them and the activities for which they are used. Providing **accessibility** in an environment means removing barriers that prevent people with activity limitations from using services, products, and information available in that environment. Many access-related technologies have become prevalent because they assist all people, not just those with limitations. Some of these common access features are curb-cut ramps along sidewalks, the bell that chimes when an elevator is about to arrive, and the door that opens automatically on your approach. **Table 7-2** lists the government laws mandating accessibility in several countries.

When considering the impact of the environment on function, accessibility is not an end point but a beginning. A subcategory of accessibility is **negotiability**, which is the ability to access a feature of the environment and use it for its intended purpose in a manner acceptable to the person. Negotiability is more than the ability to move around objects within the environment, but the ability to move within the environment AND interact meaningfully within it. A common assignment given to college students studying the impact of disability is to go through their own community and check accessibility. It is not uncommon to find parking lots with designated wheelchair parking, but no snow removal on the path from the lot to the building.

TABLE 7-2	Examples of Government Laws Mandating Accessibility
Australia	Australia passed the Disability Discrimination Act of 1992 with specific provisions to accommodate people with disabilities.
Canada	The Policy on the Provision of Accommodation for Employees with Disabilities became effective July 1, 1999, and outlines responsibilities regarding the employment accommodation of employees with disabilities.
United Kingdom	The Disability Discrimination Act 1995 refers to accessibility in employment issues and the provision of goods, facilities, and services. Another act, the Special Educational Needs and Disability Act 2001, extends this act to schools.
United States	Legislation relating to accessibility in the United States involves several laws. Those discussed in this text are Section 508 of the Federal Rehabilitation Act, the Individuals with Disabilities Education Act (IDEA), and the Americans with Disabilities Act (ADA). These are all discussed in more detail in Chapter 21.

Adapted from World Health Organization, 2001. Reference Crediting: World Health Organization. (2001). ICF: International classification of functioning and disability. Geneva, Switzerland: World Health Organization.

Shoppers often find that the stores are physically accessible, but that items to be purchased are stored on shelves far outside of the wheelchair users' reach. An example of a negotiability limitation is illustrated in **Figure 7-4**. This playground structure was built with a long access ramp so that a child in a wheelchair could access the structure. Unfortunately, the grass lawn in front of the ramp is not easily accessible, nor are the slides that are the prominent feature of the play structure.

For users with impairments, barriers to accessibility are myriad. **Table 7-3** presents some of the typical barriers encountered by people using a wheelchair. Examples are given for entering a building, for kitchen areas, and for school. There are as many other possible barriers as there are occupational environments.

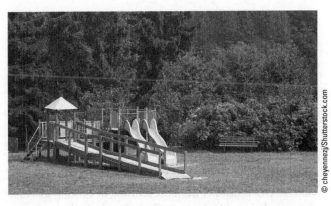

Figure 7-4 This play area may be accessible, but it is not negotiable. Children needing the wheelchair ramp to access the structure will have difficulty traversing the uneven grass lawn to get to the structure.

TABLE 7-3 Typical Barriers Encountered by People Using a Wheelchair	
Entering a Building	
Parking	Space too narrow to permit transfer to a wheelchair.
	Space not level.
	Curb or step to be negotiated.
	Parking meter out of reach.
Approach	Street between parking space and building entrance.
	No curb-cut or traffic light at crossing.
	No snow removal.
	Step between sidewalk and entrance to be negotiated.
Entrance	Doors too narrow for wheelchair.
	Distance between outer and inner door too short to negotiate in wheelchair.
	Excessive force needed to operate doors.
Household Kitchens	
Room layout	Small "alley" style layout does not allow for wheelchair negotiability.
	Appliances poorly located for negotiability.
	Appliance doors open downward and block access to interior of appliance.
	Sinks too high for wheelchair users.
	Appliance and light switches high on wall, requiring one to reach across countertop or cooking surface.
	Storage areas too high.
	Cabinets and cooking areas reached only by parking wheelchair parallel to area.
Schools	
Lecture areas	No level station for wheelchair.
	No writing surface to accommodate person in a wheelchair.
	Aisles too steep or too narrow.
	Internet hookups and electric outlets placed in fixed station where wheelchair user cannot work.
Campus	Storage lockers with combination locks above eye level.
	Travel between buildings involves steps, steep ramps, and delayed snow removal.
	Accessible transportation and parking limited.
	Crowded hallways difficult to negotiate in allotted time.
	Water fountains and pay phones out of reach.

Universal design (UD) refers to a philosophical approach to planning and design that focuses on producing buildings, products, and environments that are inherently accessible to both people without disabilities and people with disabilities. Curb cuts or sidewalk ramps, essential for people in wheelchairs but also used by all, are common examples.

Internationally, the concepts of UD have taken hold in both commercial and residential design. UD involves the efforts of surveyors, architects, planners, engineers, and facilities managers, as well as health care and rehabilitation professionals. UD is distinct from the refitting of existing spaces in that it is designed from the ground up to be inclusive.

Seven principles were defined to provide guidance for those designing inclusive environments and products for those with varying abilities. These principles are presented in **Table 7-4**. The UD movement has continued to grow internationally to become the basis for better design in countries beyond the United States.

Concepts of universal design (UD) accessibility and negotiability are equally applicable to the virtual environment and to the physical environment. UD for the Internet is "making sure that the presentation of content on the Internet and the design of Internet technology is flexible enough to accommodate the needs of the broadest range of users possible, regardless of age, language, or disability"

TABLE 7-4   Universal Design Principles Table

Principle	Intent	Guidelines
Equitable Use	The design is useful and marketable to people with diverse abilities.	• Provide the same means of use for all users: identical whenever possible, equivalent when not. • Avoid segregating or stigmatizing any users. • Provisions for privacy, security, and safety should be equally available to all users. • Make the design appealing to all users.
Flexibility in Use	The design accommodates a wide range of individual preferences and abilities.	• Provide choice in methods of use. • Accommodate right- or left-handed access and use. • Facilitate the users' accuracy and precision. • Provide adaptability to the users' pace.
Simple and Intuitive Use	Use of the design is easy to understand, regardless of the users' experience, knowledge, language skills, or current concentration level.	• Eliminate unnecessary complexity. • Be consistent with user expectations and intuition. • Accommodate a wide range of literacy and language skills. • Arrange information consistent with its importance. • Provide effective prompting and feedback during and after task completion.
Perceptible Information	The design communicates necessary information effectively to users, regardless of ambient conditions or the users' sensory abilities.	• Use different modes (pictorial, verbal, tactile) for redundant presentation of essential information. • Provide adequate contrast between essential information and its surroundings. • Maximize "legibility" of essential information. • Differentiate elements in ways that can be described (i.e., make it easy to give instructions or directions). • Provide compatibility with a variety of techniques or devices used by people with sensory limitations.
Tolerance for Error	The design minimizes hazards and the adverse consequences of accidental or unintended actions.	• Arrange elements to minimize hazards and errors: most used elements, most accessible; hazardous elements eliminated, isolated, or shielded. • Provide warnings of hazards and errors. • Provide fail-safe features. • Discourage unconscious action in tasks that require vigilance.

Continues

TABLE 7-4	Universal Design Principles Table	*(continued)*
Low Physical Effort	The design can be used efficiently and comfortably and with a minimum of fatigue.	• Allow users to maintain a neutral body position. • Use reasonable operating forces. • Minimize repetitive actions. • Minimize sustained physical effort.
Size and Space for Approach and Use	Appropriate size and space is provided for approach, reach, manipulation, and use regardless of users' body size, posture, or mobility.	• Provide a clear line of sight to important elements for any seated or standing users. • Make reach to all components comfortable for any seated or standing users. • Accommodate variations in hand and grip size. • Provide adequate space for the use of assistive devices or personal assistance.

Adapted from Joines & Valenziano, 1998. Reference Creditng: Joines, S. & Valenziano, S. (1998). The Universal Design File: Designing for People of All Ages and Abilities, Revised Edition. NC State University, The Center for Universal Design. Retrieved from http://design-dev .ncsu.edu/openjournal/index.php/redlab/article/viewFile/102/56

(Burks & Waddell, 2001). With the increasing use of Internet-based resources for health literacy, social interaction, and basic communication, this is an important aspect of universal design for the 21st century.

In the commercial realm, the Global Universal Design Commission (GUDC), Inc., is an international group who "is currently developing UD voluntary consensus standards for commercial buildings, which will expand access to buildings for all people, regardless of physical stature and varying abilities. The approved UD standards will guide corporations and government entities in the creation of barrier-free facilities, providing diverse users with access to commerce, public services, entertainment and employment opportunities" (GUDC, 2009). An example of how these principles have been applied by government is the Smart Home Program of the Department of Housing and Public Works of Queensland, Australia. This program includes universal design principles as a key leg in their "social sustainable model" within their "triple bottom line model" to design better sustainable homes throughout that region of Australia (Queensland Department of Public Works, 2008).

In the United Kingdom, the Commission for Architecture and the Built Environment (CABE) has taken the ideas of universal design even further to develop the five guiding principles of **inclusive design**. These principles strive to create places for everyone regardless of age and ability. These principles are presented in **Table 7-5**.

Inclusive design emphasizes the role of individuals with a disability in the design process. This approach is intended to increase equity in access to services and resources and is intended to enhance the experience of all users, not just users with disabilities.

Table 7-6 offers a specific set of guidelines for UD in housing, which reflects the UD principles listed earlier.

TABLE 7-5	Guiding Beliefs of Inclusive Design

1. Inclusive design places people at the heart of the design process.

2. Inclusive design acknowledges diversity and difference.

3. Inclusive design offers choice where a single design solution cannot accommodate all users.

4. Inclusive design provides for flexibility in use.

5. Inclusive design provides buildings and environments that are convenient and enjoyable to use for everyone.

Adapted from Commission for Architecture and the Built Environment, 2006. Reference Crediting: Commission for Architecture and the Built Environment (CABE) (2006). The principles of inclusive design. Retrieved from http://webarchive .nationalarchives.gov.uk/20110118095356/ http://www.cabe.org.uk /files/the-principles-of-inclusive-design.pdf

The UD concepts recommend that all new housing be built within the UD standards, a practical approach for existing homes and businesses is to upgrade to a standard that would allow people with a physical impairment to visit comfortably.

Visitability is a national trend to design and building of both individual homes and businesses so that they are easy to access regardless of one's physical abilities. This concept requires that a family home meet the following three requirements: (1) have at least one zero-step entrance; (2) have doorways with a minimum of 32-inch clearances; and (3) have at least one bathroom on the main floor that is wheelchair accessible (Visitability, 2010). Most therapy outpatient clinics are designed to be visitable. They are

TABLE 7-6   Home Features and Products Using Universal Design

No-step entry	A step-free entrance into your home lets everyone, even those who use a wheelchair, enter the home easily and safely.
Single-floor living	Having a bedroom, kitchen, full bathroom with plenty of maneuvering room, and an entertainment area on the same floor.
Home entry	A covered entryway protects you and your visitors from rain and snow while searching for keys or waiting for entry.
Wide doorways	Doorways at least 36 inches wide allow the movement of both wheelchairs and large pieces of furniture or appliances through your home.
Wide hallways	Hallways that are 42 inches wide and free of hazards or steps let everyone and everything move in, out, and around easily.
Reachable switches	Light switches that are from 42 to 48 inches above the floor, and electrical outlets 18 to 24 inches off the floor can be reached even if you are seated.
Easy-to-use handles and switches	Lever-style door handles and faucets, and rocker light switches, make opening doors, turning on water, and lighting a room easier.
Bathroom features	Low or no-threshold stall showers with built-in benches or seats and nonslip floors, bathtubs, and showers provide accessibility.

Adapted from AARP, 2009. Reference Crediting: American Association of Retired Persons (AARP), (2009). Accessible Remodeling What Is Universal Design? The basics of building homes for the safety, comfort and convenience of everyone. Retrieved from http://www.aarp .org/home-garden/home-improvement/info-09-2009/what_is_universal_design.html

generally accessible to people who are wheelchair users, but the storage of materials may not be designed to accommodate a therapist who is a wheelchair user. Universal design principles are considered in this case, but the design assures access rather than true negotiability by a therapist who is a wheelchair user.

Most adults would prefer to remain in their home of choice as long as possible. In fact, 90 percent of adults over the age of 65 report that they would prefer to stay in their current residence as they age (Kochera, Straight, & Guterbock, 2005). Designing homes that will allow people to stay in their home as their abilities change is a component of the UD movement. Beyond UD, the consideration of the whole community and the options for retrofitting existing housing to meet the needs of the elderly is good for the community, the elderly, and reduces the cost of care for older people who would otherwise have to move into a nursing home. The Centers for Disease Control and Prevention (2010) defines **aging in place** as "the ability to live in one's own home and community safely, independently, and comfortably, regardless of age, income, or ability level." Older adults want to remain in their own homes or communities and continue to participate in community life. The degree to which older adults are able to do this is determined, in part, by how communities are designed (Farber & Shinkle, 2011). When older people can no longer manage in their own homes, they often join the home of one of their children or another extended family member. In fact, one-third of American households are home to one or more residents 60 years of age or older (Pynoos, Caraviello, & Cicero, 2009).

There are many approaches to supporting aging in place. One of these is offering education and physical support in helping people modify their homes to meet their changing needs as they age. Community organizations such as Rebuilding Together and the National Aging in Place Council work with community members to help them modify their homes so that they can continue to live in their home environments and communities. **Rebuilding Together** is a nonprofit organization providing critical home repairs, modifications, and improvements for America's low-income homeowners. The National Aging in Place Council is a senior support network that was founded on the belief that an overwhelming majority of older Americans want to remain in their homes for as long as possible, but lack awareness of home- and community-based services that make independent living possible. This group has a network of professionals from the private, public, and nonprofit sectors who can help elders plan for future housing and care needs.

An initiative that focuses on public education rather than local volunteerism is the **HomeFit** program developed by the American Association of Retired Persons and the American Occupational Therapy Association. The *AARP HomeFit Guide* is available for free through the Internet and includes a checklist to help older people assess the livability of their home, reviews universal design principles, includes home safety checklists, makes recommendations for home maintenance by season, and offers home energy tips (AARP, 2012). This exemplary program offers not only recommendations for home modifications but also guidance about home maintenance and energy conservation that can help elders remain in their home in important, often overlooked ways.

SUPPORT AND RELATIONSHIPS

Support and relationships in the ICF document refers to "people or animals that provide practical physical or emotional support, nurturing, protection, assistance, and relationships to other persons, in their home, place of work, school or at play, or in other aspects of their daily activities" (World Health Organization, 2001, p. 12). *Relationships* include immediate family, extended family, friends, acquaintances, peers, colleagues, neighborhood and community members, people in positions of authority, and people in subordinate positions. The effect these relationships have on the development and aging of individuals differs according to the varieties of possible relationships that may exist.

Human relationships will be discussed in the context of development in each of the life span chapters, and so will not be addressed in detail here. One human relationship that we will consider here is the category described in the ICF as "Health Professionals." This is a broad category that includes all service providers working within the context of the health system, including physicians, nurses, physical therapists, occupational therapists, and speech therapists (World Health Organization, 2001).

Health professionals are expected to demonstrate respect for their clients as unique individuals and provide high quality care that is consistent with the desires and values of the client. This focus on the individual is supported as evidence-based practice medicine in that a good outcome must be defined in terms of what is meaningful and valuable to the individual person. This approach is called **client-centered care**. Often the terms *client-centered care* and *patient-centered care* are used synonymously. This approach to health care focuses on interactions between clients and health care professionals that are both respectful and responsive to individual client preferences, needs, and values. Client-centered care approaches ensure that client values guide all clinical decisions (Institute on Medicine, 2001).

As therapists and health care providers, we have a privileged relationship and a responsibility to recognize the potential influence we may have in an individual's pursuit of functional performance. Townsend (2003) reflects on the social and ethical responsibilities of therapists in their role as authority figures. In the many decisions we as therapists guide, we have a responsibility to weigh our expectations and responsibilities as we offer advice. In the case of an aging father newly confined to a wheelchair for mobility, therapists will feel pressure to be cost-effective, but a standard-type wheelchair may be difficult for a client with poor upper-body strength or an active lifestyle to manage. Our responsibility in client-centered practice is to learn about people's lifestyle and expectations for independent mobility as they consider types of wheelchairs and other such equipment.

DOMESTICATED ANIMALS

Domestic animals are listed as a form of support and relationships in the ICF. In this category, any animals that provide physical, emotional, or psychological support, such as pets (dogs, cats, birds, and so on) and animals for personal mobility and transportation are included. In this discussion, we will consider domesticated animals as companions, as they are involved in animal-assisted therapies.

Domestic animal companions are important to many people, and there have been many conflicting studies about the impact of companion animals on health and well-being. In a recent study, Winefield, Black, and Chur-Hansen (2008) report that when looking at a large sample, pet ownership does not impact an individual's physical health either positively or negatively. Many other studies have been more positive about the impact of pets. McConnel and colleagues (2011) report that there is correlational evidence that pets may help individuals facing significant life stressors, such as loss of a loved one or a serious illness. These authors found that pet owners fared better on well-being (for example, greater self-esteem, more exercise) and that they were, in some cases, less fearful. The authors found that pets did provide emotional support and that the support that pets provided complements rather than competes with human sources of support. Pets can serve as important sources of social support for some people, and they provide many positive psychological benefits for their owners.

Animal-assisted therapy (AAT) is a type of therapy that involves animals as a form of intervention or support for people with social, emotional, or cognitive impairments. Many occupational and physical therapists use this approach to therapy. Animals (most typically dogs) can be used in a variety of settings such as prisons, nursing homes, schools,

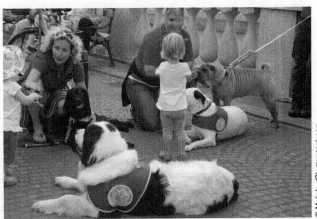

Figure 7-5 Therapy dogs are selected to be calm and tolerant of handling. Dogs trained as therapy dogs may be used as both physical and mental health supports.

and hospitals (Fine, 2010). Animals must be trained before use in therapy so that their behavior is regulated and so that they will respond to instructions. **Figure 7-5** shows a public event in which trained "therapy dogs" interact with young children.

Therapy animals offer emotional support and can be motivational in therapy sessions. Therapy animals, even registered and trained therapy animals, are not legally defined as "service" animals. **Service animals** are working animals trained to perform specific tasks relating to their owners' disability. *Assistance dogs* are the most common type of service animal. There are three types of assistance dogs: *guide dogs* are for the blind and visually impaired; *hearing dogs* are for the deaf and hard of hearing; and *service dogs* are for people with disabilities other than those related to vision or hearing. Trained service animals can "hear alarms, telephones, and doorbells for people who are deaf. They guide people with vision impairments, pick up things for people with mobility limitations, or pull a wheelchair for manual chair users who experience fatigue at the end of the day, or do not have quite the strength necessary for hills" (Albrecht, Seelman, & Bury, 2001, p. 716). A fairly recent addition to the service dog genre are service dogs for people with mental health or behavioral challenges. As detailed in **Table 7-7**, *certified autism service dogs* are trained to increase safety levels, improve socialization, and suppress behavioral outbursts. Service dogs are also trained to assist veterans with anxiety-related problems such as post-traumatic stress disorder.

In most countries in the world, disabled individuals with assistance dogs are guaranteed legal access to all places of public accommodation, modes of public transportation, recreation, and other places to which the general public is invited (Assistance Dogs International, 2012). The biggest limitation associated with service animals, in general, is the cost of training them. Albrecht, Seelman, and Bury (2001) also remark that programs to train these animals are only available in the wealthiest countries, and access to the animals

requires a period of one-to-one training with the animal, often in a distant community. For these reasons, even in wealthy countries, the use of service animals is fairly limited.

ATTITUDES

Attitudes as an environmental consideration—that is, **attitudinal environment**—relates to observable consequences of customs, practices, ideologies, values, norms, factual beliefs, and religious beliefs (World Health Organization, 2001). Attitudes influence individual behavior and social life at all levels, including some unconscious levels. As students in the health professions, you probably consider yourself to have an open and positive attitude toward people with activity limitations. Yet the popular culture of magazines, movies, and the Internet provide many not-so-subtle messages about people who function differently. **Figure 7-6** pictures a man with Down syndrome in middle adulthood. In searching for a photo to illustrate this text, the authors were surprised to find many Internet images of people with Down syndrome in the preschool years but few images of adult or aging people with Down syndrome. Why? This difference in availability in images is not the case for typically developing children. Do people, like Trina, with Down syndrome lose their appeal or become embarrassing as they age? This is an example of a societal attitude that is not evident to casual observers.

Auslander and Gold (2000) analyzed the portrayal of people with disabilities in popular press materials in both Canada and Israel. These authors found that people with physical disabilities received the most positive media attention in both countries. Interestingly, mental health disabilities were second on the list, with people with developmental disabilities coming in last in terms of both the frequency and tone of media attention. These authors emphasize, "The press has an important role in

---

TABLE 7-7   Benefits of Certified Service Dogs for Autism

Increase Safety Levels: Children with autism have a high tendency to bolt and have no concept of danger. The dogs can be tethered to a child and trained to take commands from the parent. When a child goes to run, the dogs are given a "halt" command, anchoring the child from going any farther than the tether allows.

Improve Socialization: When individuals see a child with a certified service dog, it sparks interest and questions that engage the child and encourages the child to talk about their dog.

Suppress Behavioral Outbursts: Individuals with autism have a difficult time transitioning to new environments and often experience sensory overload. Their certified service dog remains a constant in their life and allows them to focus on their dog as opposed to their environment, which often assists with suppressing behavioral issues. The dog also acts as a tactile distraction to redirect a child to a more positive behavior.

Adapted from National Service Dogs, 2012. Reference Crediting: National Service Dogs. (2012) Certified Service Dogs for Autism. Retrieved from http://www.nsd.on.ca/programs/certified-service-dogs-for-autism/

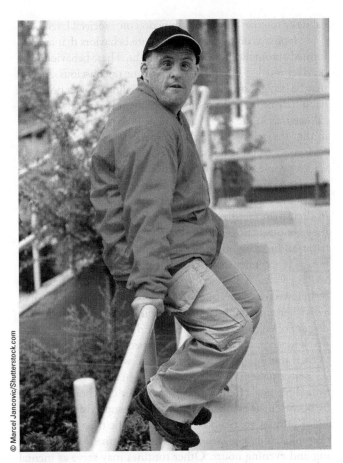

© Marcel Jancovic/Shutterstock.com

Figure 7-6 People with developmental disabilities mature and move into adult roles and lifestyles and are able to function well in a variety of environmental contexts. In some cases, the attitudinal environment may be more limiting for these people than the physical environment.

reflecting and shaping public attitudes. In many ways media coverage reinforces negative attitudes toward people with disabilities, particularly those with psychiatric and developmental disabilities" (Auslander & Gold, 2000, p. 430).

ROLES

A role is a culturally prescribed pattern of behavior. Some roles carry rights and responsibilities. An example of this would be the right of a parent to set rules, and the responsibility of a parent to provide food and safe housing for their child. Specific life roles will be discussed in the life span chapters of this text, in relation to the period in the life span in which they are considered normative. There are other societal roles that are influenced by cultural expectations and impact an individual's everyday function within a society. Through our cultural experiences, we gather information about what roles we should adopt and what roles we should avoid. In addition we may come to believe that some roles are not available to us based on gender, disability, or racial background. Royeen and Crabtree (2006) describe **attitudinal racism** as actions based on a set of stereotypical assumptions, feelings, beliefs, and attitudes about or toward a group of people that influences the roles they are able or expected to assume in society.

Ageism is a specific type of attitudinal racism that involves discriminating against individuals or groups because of their age. An example of this might be the assumption that all older people in a skilled nursing facility are either hearing impaired or senile, and it is necessary to talk slowly and loudly to them in a childlike manner. *Sexism* is another form of attitudinal racism that may be more familiar. Sexism may be overt, or it may be less obvious as in the case of a young, attractive female with fibromyalgia demonstrating weakness and fatigue in a clinic setting. A *sexist* therapist might assume that she is being a drama queen and is seeking attention in pretending to be sicker than she is, and not considering that there might be reasonable accommodations that might ease her distress.

Another example of attitudes toward specific social roles was first described by Talcott Parsons (1951). Parsons defends that in society there are sanctioned ways for an ill person to behave, to receive social support for illness and disability. In assuming a *sick role,* people can be held in sympathy and therefore be free from blame for their condition. Within this conception, a person who is sick is released from daily role expectations, and is given a new set of sick role expectations. The **sick role** is a distinct role, a socially recognized way of behaving when you are ill. This role affords sick people certain rights: (1) the exemption from normal social roles, and (2) an absence of blame for their condition. Sick people are given special support and attention, as long as they maintain the social obligations associated with the sick role. These obligations are that the sick people should be actively trying to get well and that they should seek competent help and cooperate with the treatment.

If you have a fever, are flushed, and are coughing in your workplace, you are likely to be identified as "sick" and sent home to recuperate. While you remain sick, you do not have to go to work, take care of your household, and meet your social commitments. You are welcome to stay in bed, wear your pajamas all day, and look pitiful. In fact, you are afforded special care and privileges. Your friends may bring you soup or medicines, and offer condolences. The sick role provides an example of societal-level opinions and beliefs that are reflected in family, teachers, roommates, employers, and other community members about how a person should behave if she is to be given respite from performing her expected roles. People with emotional distress or cognitive impairment are less likely to be afforded the sick role because they don't look or act sick.

Parsons also notes that "the privileges and exemptions of the sick role may become objects of a 'secondary gain,' that the patient is positively motivated, usually unconsciously, to secure or to retain" (Parsons, 1951, p. 439). In health care settings this is called **malingering**. People who malinger enjoy exemption from work and social demands, and either exaggerate their disability or fail to follow through on intervention strategies aimed at returning them to the workforce.

Another widely held societal attitude is the value of a strong "work ethic." Work, especially paid work, is highly valued in American culture. The role of worker is highly valued. People who engage in unpaid work, like housework and child care, may be less valued even though they are equally productive. Because of this, people who leave paid-work positions because of activity limitation or to provide caregiving support may feel devalued and perceive a loss of status.

Mothers and "mothering" is also a socially constructed role. Expectations about what describes an effective mother vary even within a population group. In the United States, there is an expectation that mothers will remain intimately involved in their children's daily activities, organizing "playdates," enrolling their children in an activity, supporting athletic and other social pursuits to fill their children's time. Mothering is put on a pedestal as a core building block of society, yet mothers are often isolated and have limited fiscal resources. Mothers of children who have activity limitations, especially activity limitations like attention deficits that do not conform to the "sick role," are openly criticized and marginalized. Cronin (2003) found a consistent pattern of discord and lack of support from both school and health care providers reported by mothers of children with attention deficit disorder.

Fitzgerald (1997) reports, "Science, bureaucracy, and organized religion have played an important role in shaping the construction of disability—as the broken, incomplete and imperfect self, as the case requiring management, and as the object of pity and charity" (p. 407). When students select careers in health professions, they often comment that they "really want to help people." This is a positive, socially endorsed value. The desire to help people can be generous and adaptable, but it also can be based in the belief that people who are different are in some way unfortunate and worthy of charity.

Echoing the stance of the national disability rights movement, Fitzgerald (1997) notes that "concepts such as the medical model of disability and the evolving genetic model of disability have shaped the way in which we construct disability and, consequently, the way in which we treat people with disability—through isolation, segregation, and elimination" (p. 407). The client-centered approach to intervention is a movement away from this traditional "helping" ideal and should help people new to these professions challenge their own thinking in their approaches to people in their professional practice.

HABITS AND ROUTINES

Within the ICF model, *attitudes* include "customs, practices, rules, and abstract systems of values and normative beliefs that arise within social contexts and that affect or create societal and individual practices and behaviors, such as social norms of moral and religious behavior or etiquette; religious doctrine and resulting norms and practices; norms governing rituals or social gatherings" (World Health Organization, 2001, p. 192). Chapter 4 of this text deals extensively with culture and cultural issues. What remains to be covered are customs in the form of habits or routines that impact function on a societal level.

Habits, as noted in Chapter 6, are behaviors that are performed automatically and with thought. These behaviors have been repeated so often that they become unconscious. A habit may be benign, such as nodding and smiling to greet people. A habit may be based on some strong physiologic or psychological need, as in the case of addiction. Habits can be beneficial, in that they allow us to focus our thoughts elsewhere while performing routine tasks. Habits can protect function as well. Older people with dementia can often continue to perform familiar ADLs because the tasks have become habitual. This is one of the reasons why older people are often more functional in their own familiar environments than they appear when they are hospitalized. Habits can be destructive as well. The habit of directing questions and conversations only to members of one gender can alienate the other gender.

A **routine** is a prescribed, detailed sequence of actions to be followed regularly, one that is customary to an individual or a social group. Routines like a morning shower or walking the dog are often mechanically performed procedures or activities that add shape to the day. Although people do not often think of their routines, they often miss them when they can no longer perform them. People who have been in the hospital, even for a short stay, often luxuriate when they can shower on their own, with their own things, and without supervision.

Routines are often linked to a specific time of day—for example, ADL routines are usually performed in the morning and evening hours. Other routines may serve as mental or physical reprieves from work. The afternoon "teatime" is a good example of a healthy break from desk work. When working with clients, an excellent therapy strategy is to build health-promoting behaviors into routines, so that clients will be able to continue the behaviors when they no longer have therapy support. Routines can also be customs, such as morning tea or participation in activities within a faith community.

SERVICES, SYSTEMS, AND POLICIES

The ICF addresses many services, systems, and policies that affect function. Before moving forward in the discussion of how these things affect development and aging, it is important to differentiate the terms. The ICF defines *services* as "services that provide benefits, structured programs, and operations, in various sectors of society, designed to meet the needs of individuals." *Systems* are "administrative control and organizational mechanisms, and are established by governments at the local, regional, national, and international levels." *Policies* are "constituted by rules, regulations, conventions, and standards established by governments at the local, regional, national, and international levels, or by other recognized authorities" (World Health Organization, 2001, p. 192).

Within the American government structure, policies are the legislative actions taken by the federal, state, or local governments to meet perceived needs. Chapter 21 in this text will extensively review services, systems, and policies

TABLE 7-8	Housing Policies within the ICF Categories of Services, Systems, and Policies

ICF Category	Housing
Policy	*Home Equity Conversion Mortgages* for seniors are an example of an alteration to mortgage laws to aid those who have equity in their homes and can pay that equity back into a mortgage so that they can afford to stay in their home.
Systems	U.S. Department of Housing and Urban Development Local governmental zoning boards Local utility boards
Services	Federal: Public housing is available in the United States to provide decent and safe rental housing for eligible low-income families, the elderly, and people with disabilities.
	Private: Local real estate developers building mixed-used housing developments.
	Private: Local charities such as Rebuilding Together offer volunteer support to provide home modifications for needy elders.
	Private: Families choose to install an ECHO unit next to their family home to provide a supported home for an older family member.

impacting participation and function in the United States. For this chapter, we will introduce some examples about how policies shape the environmental context for individuals.

Housing Laws and Options

Earlier in the chapter, we discussed some specific housing challenges and options for people as they age. Housing is part of a social infrastructure that is highly regulated at both national and local levels. **Table 7-8** illustrates examples of the multiple levels of services, systems, and policies considered in the ICF framework in the specific context of housing. Broad population-based policy decisions can have important impacts on individuals. For example, although a family might find an ECHO unit the best approach for meeting their needs, local zoning laws may prohibit the installation of this type of temporary housing in an established residential area.

Driving and Driver Licenses

Another important area of function that is greatly impacted by aging is driving. Griffin (2004) reports that "older drivers are more likely than drivers in their thirties, forties, or fifties to be involved in traffic crashes, and they are more likely to be killed in traffic crashes. The number of Americans 65 years of age and older is expected to double between 2000 and 2030. Americans are living longer and driving longer. Together these trends suggest that the number of older drivers killed on U.S. streets and highways will grow" (p. 7).

At this time, 28 states have special requirements for older people renewing their driver's licenses. For example, in California, younger drivers with good driving records may automatically renew their license, but anyone over 70 must take both a written test and eye exam at a state office to renew. When older adults renew their license, they may be required to take a physical driving test at the discretion of a Department of Motor Vehicles employee, if some kind of lack of ability or diminished ability to drive is suspected.

Currently, few elders lose their licenses before being involved in a serious accident. There have been several consumer education, caregiver education, and public awareness campaigns developed to help provide older drivers with information and support in driving safely for as long as possible, and recognizing when to surrender their driving privileges. Health care professionals can do much to support older people and help them understand their own abilities and limitations with regard to driving. For many older people, such as the woman pictured in **Figure 7-7**, driving is

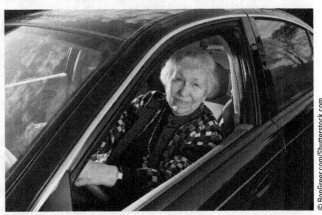

Figure 7-7   For this 86-year-old woman, driving her car is an important daily occupation.

the only way they have to get food, medications, and other personal needs. In addition, driving may be the only access they have to social and faith communities that are important to them. No state has yet set an official upper age limit on people eligible to have a driver's license, but it is a topic that will gain increasing attention in the upcoming years.

SUMMARY

Although recognition of the many aspects and influences of environmental factors on human function predated the ICF model, these factors have never before received sufficient focus by either health care providers or policy makers. Aspects of the environment are also addressed in the discussions of culture and policy.

Although it is more comfortable to look within the scope of your professional experience to define roles and prescriptive strategies for interacting with clients and families, effective clinicians will consider the context and perspective of their consumers and be adaptable to best serve the needs of those people and their families.

CASE 1
Trina . . . Continued

Trina's sister wanted so see Trina return to her prior level of independent function and allow her to feel useful and valued in the family. She found that taking pictures and making visual schedules showing Trina how to operate the washing machine and dishwasher allowed Trina to regain some of her previous tasks in the home. To address Trina's balance and endurance problems, motion-sensitive lighting was placed throughout the main part of the house, so that if Trina began to wander at night, she could clearly see where she was going. Enlisting Trina's nieces as helpers, Trina learned to use a cell phone and to exercise using a video-gaming system. The girls found a dance-based exercise program that they enjoyed and encouraged Trina to "dance" with them. With a little exploration of the community, Trina's sister found that the local senior center had a van that would pick people up from their homes and bring them to the senior center for recreational programs. Before long, Trina had established a routine of getting ready for school with her nieces. Shortly after the girls were picked up by their school bus, Trina got on the van for the senior center. She stayed at the senior center through lunch and then returned home. This routine allowed Trina to engage socially and remain in a supervised environment while the other family members were out of the home. Although the change in environment was distressing for Trina at first, by exploring modification of the home environments and incorporating existing community resources, Trina was able to regain her independence and build valued social activities.

Guiding Questions
Some questions to consider:

1. When Trina lived in the city, her mother had helped her build relationships with several local business people. This gave Trina a unique developmental niche in her community. Describe how the environment can serve as a development niche for adults with intellectual impairments like Trina.
2. From her nieces, Trina gained access to virtual environments—new communication and entertainment options. Explore the web and your favorite "app store" to find "apps" for visual schedules of communication tools that could be used by adults like Trina who could not read.

CASE 2

Tanner and Katie

Tanner and his wife Katie are both veterans. Tanner had a traumatic brain injury (TBI) from serving in Afghanistan and suffers from what the Army calls "polytrauma." In addition to his TBI, Tanner had his left leg amputated above the knee and has chronic back pain. Katie has a condition called post-traumatic stress disorder (PTSD). Tanner wears a prosthetic, but feels conspicuous when he goes out. After his combat experience, he feels that he does not fit in and that he and "civilians" have little in common. Katie prefers to be in quiet places. She does not like loud noises or crowds as these things trigger painful memories and flashbacks. Both Tanner and Katie returned to civilian life uncomfortable and unwilling to participate in community life. They became increasingly isolated and unhappy.

With the emotional and fund-raising support of family, friends, church, and the Veterans Administration, Tanner and Katie were able to train with the *National Service Dog* organization. Here, Tanner says they "made a new best friend, our lovely chocolate Labrador retriever named Lacy." Since Lacy joined their family, Katie and Tanner have begun to look beyond their immediate problems and to enjoy the moment. Tanner remarked that Lacy has "filled our lives with giggles and surprises."

Lacy is trained to recognize Katie's "tells" and gives her a gracious way out of a situation before hitting full panic. Throughout the day, Lacy offers social support through friendly "nudges" and grounding looks when her sympathetic nose rests on a quivering knee in a friendly "visit."

Since their discharge from the army, Tanner and Katie have drifted along with little routine to their days. The care of a dog has added structure and meaning to their days. It has also helped them focus on Lacy's needs rather than on their own. Tanner has been in charge of making sure Lacy gets regular exercise, and through the process of walking her daily, his own walking and his pain management have improved dramatically.

Both Tanner and Katie found that it was easier to think about going out socially once they had Lacy. Not only could Lacy help them know when to exit a situation, people were curious about her, and she offered a focal point for conversations that was not threatening. After attending church with Lacy the first time, Katie commented that she was no longer a person with a problem, but now was a person with a dog—such an easy fix for such a complex issue.

Guiding Questions

Some questions to consider:

1. As veterans, Tanner and Katie face a challenging attitudinal environment—in part because the conflict in which they served was not popular with civilians and because they had important experiences that were far outside the experience of civilians. What other social and attitudinal supports might help this couple reintegrate into their community?
2. Tanner will need ongoing physical therapy as he adjusts to his prosthesis and works to increase his endurance when walking. Tanner is trained as an electrician. What sort of environments is Tanner likely to face as he returns to work? What other types of mobility would an electrician need in his regular workday?

Adapted from National Service Dogs. (2012a) "Diane, Jim & NSD Lady – Skilled Companion Dog for Veterans Team". Retrieved from http://www.nsd.on.ca/about/testimonials/

Speaking of
Barriers

MARYBETH MANDICH, PT, PhD,
PEDIATRIC PHYSICAL THERAPIST

There is a song about West Virginia that refers to the majestic and grand West Virginia hills. Well, majestic and grand they may be to some, but to others with disabilities, they are real barriers. Some years ago, I was asked by the mother of a teenage girl with spina bifida to serve as an outside expert on a case involving the local school system. The situation was that this young lady was fairly independent in mobility, especially using her manual wheelchair. However, when the girl entered high school, she was confronted with a new physical barrier. The high school was built as a campus arrangement, with different buildings for different activities and classes. Unfortunately, the cafeteria was a great distance from the classroom. The walkway between buildings was paved, but not covered, and the terrain was very hilly, typical of West Virginia. This created a natural physical barrier. Initially, the young woman valiantly tried to propel her wheelchair to the cafeteria. However, she was always late for lunch and consequently late in returning to her classroom. The school imposed a solution to this problem. They said the girl had to stay in the classroom each day, and someone would bring her a lunch tray.

Congratulations…the physical barrier was conquered! However, another barrier was created—a social one. Any of us who have lived through high school know how important lunchtime is. It's a time to visit with friends who may not share your classes. It's a time to gossip and flirt and cram for quizzes. In the long run, it was the social, not the physical, barrier that presented a bigger obstacle to this young woman.

At this point, the concept of reasonable accommodation came in. I believe it was a reasonable accommodation to allow this young lady to leave for the cafeteria early, get her lunch before the crowds came, and still be able to fully participate in lunchtime with her classmates and peers. In bad weather, the option to remain in the classroom could be presented to the girl. That was my "expert" (or commonsense) recommendation. But the school resisted—now presenting an attitudinal barrier. Eventually, by threatening to take the case to the courts, the mother was able to get the school system to agree to the reasonable accommodation. But it was quite a battle for all of us, not least for the young lady.

Barriers people with disabilities encounter are sometimes obvious and sometimes subtle. Even in this simple story of one person, multiple barriers are present. Some of the barriers are not created by people, but some of them are. I think it's our job to be social activists, to be conscious of barriers of all types, and to be vigilant in eliminating or minimizing their impact on quality of life for our clients.

REFERENCES

Albrecht, G., Seelman, K., & Bury, M. (2001). *Handbook of disability studies.* Thousand Oaks, CA: Sage Publications.

American Association of Retired Persons (AARP). (2009). *Accessible remodeling: What is universal design? The basics of building homes for the safety, comfort and convenience of everyone.* Retrieved from http://www.aarp.org/home-garden/home-improvement/info-09-2009/what_is_universal_design.html

American Association of Retired Persons (AARP). (2012). *AARP HomeFit guide: Make your house a home—for life.* Retrieved from http://www.aarp.org/home-garden/livable-communities/info-07-2011/aarp-home-fit-guide-aging-in-place.html

American Occupational Therapy Association. (2014). *Occupational Therapy Practice Framework: Domain and process* (3rd ed.). Bethesda, MD: AOTA Press.

Assistance Dogs International. (2012). *About assistance dogs.* Retrieved from http://www.assistancedogsinternational.org/aboutAssistanceDogs.php

Auslander, G., & Gold, N. (2000). Media reports on disability: A binational comparison of types and causes of disability as reported in major newspapers. *Disability and Rehabilitation, 21,* 420–431.

Bonnefoi, M. S., Belanger, S. E., Devlin, D. J., Doerrer, N. G., Embry, M. R., Fukushima, S., &... van der Laan, J. (2010). Human and environmental health challenges for the next decade (2010-2020). *Critical Reviews in Toxicology, 40*(10), 893–911.

Bootes, K., & Chapparo, C. (2002). Cognitive and behavioral assessment of people with traumatic brain injury in the work place: Occupational therapists' perceptions. *Work, 19*(3), 255–268.

Burks, M., & Waddell, C. (2001). *Universal design for the Internet.* Internet Society. Retrieved from http://www.isoc.org/briefings/002/

Centers for Disease Control and Prevention (CDC). (2010). Healthy Places terminology. Retrieved from http://www.cdc.gov/healthyplaces/terminology.htm

Commission for Architecture and the Built Environment (CABE). (2006). *The principles of inclusive design.* Retrieved from http://webarchive.nationalarchives.gov.uk/20110118095356/http:/www.cabe.org.uk/files/the-principles-of-inclusive-design.pdf

Conger, R., Conger, K., & Martin, M. (2010) Socioeconomic status, family processes, and individual development. *Journal of Marriage & Family, 72,* 685–704.

Cronin, A. (2003). Mothering a child with a hidden disability. *American Journal of Occupational Therapy, 58(1),* 83–92.

Environmental Protection Agency. (2014). *What is sustainability?* Retrieved from http://www.epa.gov/sustainability/basicinfo.htm

Farber, N., & Shinkle, D. (2011). *Aging in place: A state survey of livability policies and practices.* AARP Public Policy Institute. Retrieved from http://www.aarp.org/home-garden/livable-communities/info-11-2011/Aging-In-Place.html

Fine, A. (2010). *Handbook on animal-assisted therapy, Third Edition: Theoretical foundations and guidelines for practice.* Academic Press.

Fitzgerald, J. (1997). Reclaiming the whole: Self, spirit and society. *Disability and Rehabilitation, 19,* 407–413.

Global Universal Design Commission, Inc. (2009). *IDeA Center for Inclusive Design and Environmental Access.* Retrieved from http://www.ap.buffalo.edu/idea/projects/index.asp

Griffin, L. (2004). *Older driver involvement in injury crashes in texas 1975–1999.* AAA Foundation for Traffic Safety. Retrieved from http://newsroom.aaa.com/wp-content/uploads/2011/09/OlderDriverInvolvementInInjuryCrashes.pdf

Hays, J., & George, L. (2002). The life-course trajectory toward living alone: Racial differences. *Research on Aging, 24*(3), 283–307.

Hosseinpoor, A., Williams, J., Itani, L., & Chatterji, S. (2012). Socioeconomic inequality in domains of health: Results from the World Health Surveys. *BMC Public Health, 12*(1), 198–206.

Intergovernmental Panel on Climate Change. (2007). Climate Change 2007: Working Group I: The physical science basis. *Direct observations of recent climate change.* Retrieved from http://www.ipcc.ch/publications_and_data/ar4/wg1/en/spmsspm-direct-observations.html

Institute on Medicine. (2001). *Crossing the quality chasm: A new health system for the 21st century.* Retrieved from http://www.iom.edu/Reports/2001/Crossing-the-Quality-Chasm-A-New-Health-System-for-the-21st-Century.aspx

Joines, S., & Valenziano, S. (1998). The Universal Design File: Designing for people of all ages and abilities (rev. ed.). NC State University, The Center for Universal Design. Retrieved from http://www.google.com/url?sa=t&rct=j&q=&esrc=s&source=web&cd=1&ved=0CCAQFjAA&url=http%3A%2F%2Fwww.certec.lth.se%2Ffileadmin%2Fcertec%2FKirre%2F102-154-1-PB.pdf&ei=gNn8U4uvJqPjsAT3_IC4Dw&usg=AFQjCNErChoDwg6bX7zRwrWWTdXtg5lCpA&sig2=cAVioWPS32h6OL6_yBIj_A.

Jones, M., McEwen, I., & Hansen, L. (2003). Use of power mobility for a young child with spinal muscular atrophy. *Physical Therapy, 83*(3), 253–262.

Kochera, A., Straight, A., & Guterbock, T. (2005). Beyond 50.05: A report to the nation on livable communities—Creating environments for successful aging. Washington. DC: American Association of Retired Persons.

Maleta, K., Virtanen, S. M., Espo, M., Kulmala, T., & Ashorn, P. (2003). Seasonality of growth and the relationship between weight and height gain in children under three years of age in rural Malawi. *Acta Paediatrics, 92(4),* 491–497.

MacDonald, J., Stokes, R., Cohen, D., Kofner, A., & Ridgeway, G. (2010). The effect of light rail transit on body mass index and physical activity. *American Journal of Preventative Medicine, 39,* 105–112.

McConnel, A. R., Brown, C. M., Shoda, T. M., Stayton, L. E., & Martin, C. E. (2011). Friends with benefits: On the positive consequences of pet ownership. *Journal of Personality & Social Psychology, 101*(6), 1239–1252.

Mumford, K., Contant, C., Weissman, J., Wolf, J., & Glanz, K. (2011). Changes in physical activity and travel behaviors in residents of a mixed-use development. *American Journal of Preventative Medicine, 4,* 504–507.

Nathan, A., Wood, L., & Giles-Corti, B. (2013). Environmental factors associated with active living in retirement village residents: Findings from an exploratory qualitative enquiry. *Research on Aging, 35*(4), 459–480.

National Aging in Place Council. (2012). *Our mission.* Retrieved from http://www.ageinplace.org/about_us/our_mission.aspx

National Service Dogs. (2012a). *Certified service dogs for autism.* Retrieved from http://www.nsd.on.ca/programs/certified-service-dogs-for-autism/

National Service Dogs. (2012b). Diane, Jim & NSD lady—Skilled companion dog for veterans team. Retrieved from http://www.nsd.on.ca/about/testimonials/

Olson, J., & Esdaile, S. (2000). Mothering young children with disabilities in a challenging urban environment. *American Journal of Occupational Therapy, 54*(3), 307–314.

Parsons, T. (1951). *The social system.* England: RKP.

Perdue, W., Stone, L., & Gostin, L. (2003) The built environment and its relationship to the public's health: The legal framework. *American Journal of Public Health, 93*(9), 1390–1394.

Pynoos, P., Caraviello, R., & Cicero, C. (2009). Lifelong housing: The anchor in aging-friendly communities. *GENERATIONS—Journal of the American Society on Aging, 33,* 26–32.

Queensland Department of Public Works. (2008). Smart and sustainable homes design objectives. Retrieved from http://www.hpw.qld.gov.au/SiteCollectionDocuments/SmartHousingDesignObjectives08.pdf

Rebeiro, K. L. (2001). Enabling occupation: The importance of an affirming environment. *Canadian Journal of Occupational Therapy, 68*(2), 80–89.

Rebuilding Together. (n.d.). *What we do.* Retrieved from http://rebuildingtogether.org/whatwedo/

Royeen, M., & Crabtree, J. (2006) *Culture in rehabilitation: From competency to proficiency.* Upper Saddle River, NJ: Pearson Prentice Hall.

Schrecker, T. (2012). Multiple crises and global health: New and necessary frontiers of health politics. *Global Public Health, 7*(6), 557–573.

Shumway-Cook, A, Patla, A. E., Stewart, A., Ferrucci, L., Ciol, M. A., & Guralnik, J. M. (2002). Environmental demands associated with community mobility in older adults with and without mobility disabilities. *Physical Therapy, 82*(7), 670–681.

Stansfeld, S., Clark, C., Rodgers, B., Caldwell, T., & Power, C. (2011). Repeated exposure to socioeconomic disadvantage and health selection as life course pathways to mid-life depressive and anxiety disorders. *Social Psychiatry & Psychiatric Epidemiology, 46*(7), 549–558.

Townsend, E. (2003). Reflections on power and justice in enabling occupation. *Canadian Journal of Occupational Therapy, 70*(2), 74–87.

Visitability. (2010). *Housing that builds in freedom.* Retrieved from http://www.visitability.org/

Weine, S. (2011). Developing preventive mental health interventions for refugee families in resettlement. *Family Process, 50*(3), 410–430.

Winefield, H. R., Black, A., & Chur-Hansen, A. (2008). Health effects of ownership of and attachment to companion animals in an older population. *International Journal Of Behavioral Medicine, 15*(4), 303–310.

World Health Organization. (2001). *ICF: International classification of functioning and disability.* Geneva, Switzerland: World Health Organization.

Zickuhr, K., & Madden, M. (2012). *Older adults and Internet use.* Pew Internet and American Life Project. Retrieved from http://www.pewinternet.org/Topics/Demographics/Seniors.aspx?typeFilter=5

PART 2

Life Stage
Characteristics

CHAPTER 8

Prenatal Development

Elsie R. Vergara, ScD, OTR, FAOTA,
Occupational Therapy Program,
Department of Rehabilitation
Sciences, Sargent College,
Boston University Boston,
Massachusetts
and

Mary Beth Mandich, PT, PhD,
Professor and Chairperson,
Division of Physical Therapy,
West Virginia University, Morgantown,
West Virginia

Objectives

Upon completion of this chapter, readers should be able to:

- Identify the three classic periods of prenatal development—germinal (pre-embryonic), embryonic, and fetal—and the postconceptional ages covered within each period;

- Describe the various classification systems used for monitoring the developmental progression of embryos and fetuses;

- Describe the developmental changes that occur in growing humans from conception to birth across the various body systems;

- Identify the main factors and critical, or sensitive, periods associated with atypical development, including multiple gestation, genetic alterations, congenital anomalies, and developmental disabilities; and

- Identify and discuss contemporary issues related to embryonic development, including the use of reproductive technologies and stem cells.

Key Terms

behavioral state	fetal viability	pluripotent stem cells
blastocyst	germinal (pre-embryonic) period	polyhydramnios
cephalocaudal	gestational (menstrual) age	postconceptional age
chondroskeleton	mesenchymal cells	proximodistal
critical period	mesoderm	teratogen
ectoderm	neural plate	trimester system
embryonic period	notochord	trophoblast
endoderm	oligohydramnios	vascularization
epiblast	organogenesis	very low birth weight (VLBW)
fetal period	ossification	

INTRODUCTION

Prenatal development provides the foundation for development throughout the life span. Although this chapter does not represent a specific clinical population, it does prepare clinicians to understand and apply sound clinical reasoning to developmental differences throughout the life span. Understanding basic embryology prepares clinicians to understand birth defects and a variety of atypical physiological patterns as diverse as cystic fibrosis and cancer.

The ICF classification system was not intended to be applied prenatally, but in an effort to integrate this information with the subject of rehabilitation, we will use the classification system introduced in Chapter 1 as an organizing framework for discussing the prenatal period. The prenatal time period, from conception until birth, is the most rapid period of structural and functional change in the human life span. During the first eight weeks following conception, the body structures of all systems are formed. The remainder of the prenatal period is characterized by structural maturation and refinement, as well as the activation of functions across pertinent body systems. *Fetus* is the term used for developing humans after the 8th week (from birth to the 8th week, the developing human is called an *embryo*). Although rehabilitation therapists are not typically involved with embryos or fetuses in utero, they often work with pregnant women and with newborn infants. Moreover, rehabilitation therapists who work in neonatal intensive care units may encounter infants who have a history of birth as early as 22 weeks of gestation whose developmental patterns in many ways resemble fetuses approaching the last trimester of prenatal development. A strong knowledge base of prenatal development is crucial to understanding many of the diseases, impairments, and developmental differences in children, as well as the behavioral patterns of premature infants. Finally, there is neurobehavioral continuity between prenatal and postnatal development, such that it is important to understand birth as a life event rather than the beginning of the structure-function dimension (Stanojevic et al., 2011).

OVERVIEW OF PRENATAL DEVELOPMENT

Despite the lack of consensus about the beginning of human life or the ethicality of abortion or genetic research, there is considerable agreement that development of a human embryo conceived through natural means begins shortly after fertilization has occurred, within 12 to 24 hours after the sperm penetrates the ovum (that is, egg cell). Fertilization, also called conception, is believed to be complete when the sperm and the ovum fuse into a single cell called the *zygote*. The exact moment when human life begins is less clear; however, one argument reported by Meyer (2008) suggests human life does *not* begin until approximately the 13th day after fertilization, when implantation in the uterine wall is complete. He bases this argument on the premise that, up until this time, division of the zygote into two (identical twins) is possible. Therefore, the individual life course is not specified until this time period has elapsed and the product of fertilization is destined to become a distinct individual. There is obviously significant controversy over the beginning of human life, which will be discussed further in a later section of this chapter.

Emergence of the zygote marks the beginning of the first of three prenatal periods: germinal (or pre-embryonic),[1] embryonic, and fetal. The **germinal (pre-embryonic) period** lasts approximately two weeks from conception until the unicellular zygote has implanted in the uterus. The germinal period is characterized by rapid cell division and *pluripotent cells*. **Pluripotent stem cells** are cells that are capable of differentiation into many different kinds of cells, that is, their cell lineage is not yet irrevocably determined

---

[1] Some consider this stage part of the embryonic period.

(Kim & Clark, 2014). These pluripotent cells are the *stem cells* that have received so much publicity in recent years, as there is hope these cells can be harvested and, when implanted in individuals with disease, can replace the diseased cells with healthy ones. Stem cell treatments are becoming common in the treatment of cancer and other disorders.

After the organism has been implanted in the uterine lining, it is known as an embryo, a complex multicellular organism capable of producing all of the organs and tissues of the body. The **embryonic period** extends to the end of the 8th week after conception, when all of the major body structures have been formed and the embryo has developed human characteristics, at which time it can be considered a fetus. It is the period when the developing organs are most sensitive or susceptible to the effects of toxic substances or abnormal conditions (Bruer, 2001).

The **fetal period** is the longest, extending from approximately the 9th week after conception until the moment of birth. This period involves extensive growth as well as complex structural and physiologic refinement of the tissues, organs, and systems that were formed during the embryonic period.

By the time infants are born, they will have developed all of the body structures they will ever have. Any abnormality in the structural development of an infant must have therefore occurred during the period of **organogenesis** (organ formation) in the early stages of development. Although infants' structural development essentially ends long before they are born, much of the functional development of the structures will occur throughout the entire gestational period and even after birth. This chapter will describe the normal developmental process from conception to birth, highlighting the fetal **critical periods**. Critical periods are highly sensitive periods during which developing infants are at greatest risk for congenital anomalies or developmental disabilities should the developmental process be interrupted or altered. A quick overview of the major developmental changes and milestones throughout the entire gestational period is found in **Table 8-1**.

TABLE 8-1	Major Developmental Changes and Milestones throughout Gestational Period

Period After Conception	Structural and Functional Changes During Period
0 to 4–5 weeks	• Fertilized egg descends from fallopian tube to uterus. • Early cell division occurs with formation of embryonic disk—zygote becomes an embryo. • Developing embryo attaches to uterine wall.
4 weeks 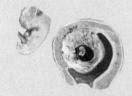	• Embryo divides into three layers of cells: ectoderm (nervous system and sense organs); mesoderm (circulatory, skeletal, and muscular systems); endoderm (digestive and some glandular systems). • Special layer of cells begins to grow into the uterine wall, where the placenta will be formed. • Special cells grow to form the amnion (water sac). • Heart tube forms; blood begins to circulate through embryonic disk tubes toward the end. • Development of neural system begins, and neural groove appears. • Intestinal tract, lungs, liver, and kidneys begin to develop. • Small buds appear on sides of body—the beginning of limbs. • By the end of this period, embryo is about 4 to 6 mm long; head is forming; body is curled.
5 to 8–9 weeks	• Bones and muscles begin to give contour to body. • Face and neck appear—human resemblance begins.
8 weeks 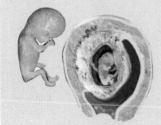	• Brain grows faster than rest of body; forehead becomes prominent as a result of proliferation of brain tissue. • Limb buds elongate; muscles and cartilage develop. • Sex organs begin to form. • Embryo grows to 30 to 50 mm in length. • Embryo becomes a fetus.

Continues

TABLE 8-1   Major Developmental Changes and Milestones throughout Gestational Period   *(continued)*

Period After Conception	Structural and Functional Changes During Period
9 to 12–13 weeks	• Fetal period begins. • Head continues to grow faster than rest of body.
12 weeks 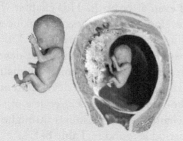	• Eyelids are fused. • Sexual differentiation becomes visible. • Buds for temporary teeth emerge. • Vocal cords appear. • Digestive system begins to function; stomach and bile secretions begin. • Kidneys begin to function; fetus urinates into the amniotic fluid. • Placenta passes waste products from infant to mother. • Bones and muscles continue to develop. • Spontaneous movements of arms, legs, shoulders, and fingers occur by end of the third month.
13 to 16–17 weeks	• Growth rate of lower parts of body accelerates. • Head size decreases proportionally from one-half to one-fourth body size.
16 weeks 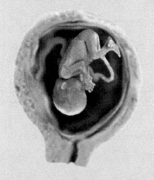	• Fetus is less curled. • Hands and feet are well formed, with fingernails. • Skin appears dark red (blood flows superficially) and wrinkled (lacks underlying fat). • Fingers may curl into flexion. • Reflexes become more active as nervous system maturation continues. • Strength of movement of arms and legs increases. • Fetus grows to 15 cm and weighs close to 300 g.
17 to 20–21 weeks	• All body structures closely resemble their final form. • Sweat glands appear and become functional.
20 weeks 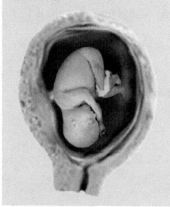	• Hair appears on scalp. • Skin continues to appear wrinkled. • Spine becomes more straight. • Spontaneous activity continues to increase. • Movements may or may not be perceived by mother. • By 21 weeks, fetus measures 19 cm (about 1 ft) and weighs 460 g (approximately 1 lb).

Continues

TABLE 8-1 Major Developmental Changes and Milestones throughout Gestational Period *(continued)*

Period After Conception	Structural and Functional Changes During Period
21 to 24–25 weeks	• Eyes are completely formed; eyelids open toward the end of this period. • Taste buds appear on tongue and mouth—more prominent than in the infant or adult.
24 weeks 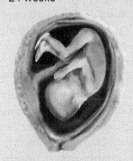	• Structures continue to grow; infant continues to gain weight. • By the end of this period, fetus is 24 cm long and weighs over 1000 g.
25 to 28–29 weeks	• Fetus is viable—may live independently, although may require temperature support. • Cerebral hemispheres cover almost the entire brain.
28 weeks 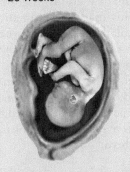	• Neonatal reflexes are fully developed. • May cry, breathe, swallow, and suck thumb. • Head hair continues to grow; body hair (lanugo) disappears. • By the end of this period, fetus is 27.5 cm long and weighs 1500 g.
28 to 32–33 weeks	• Rapid accumulation of fatty tissue occurs over the entire body. • Fat accumulation serves as insulation—fetus is better able to tolerate external temperature.
32 weeks 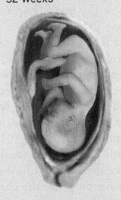	• Intrauterine crowding may decrease movement range and frequency. • Fetus can live independently without life support. • By the end of this period, fetus is 30 cm long and weighs approximately 2500 g (5 lb).
More than 32 weeks	• Fetus is fully viable; grows to 36 cm and weighs over 3500 g.

PRENATAL CLASSIFICATION SYSTEMS

Close monitoring of an infant's prenatal development is essential to assure that the fetus is growing and developing appropriately and to identify any deviations from typical patterns that may require early attention. Prenatal development is described using a variety of classification systems. Classification by menstrual, or gestational, weeks is the system most widely used by obstetricians and other clinicians to assess the maturity of an embryo or fetus and to monitor its development along the entire pregnancy. Gestational age is also used after birth to estimate various developmental and medical risk factors. A developing infant's estimated **gestational (or menstrual) age** is measured in weeks from the first day of the pregnant woman's *last menstrual period (LMP).* Use of the LMP, although convenient, overestimates the length of a pregnancy by about 2 weeks because it includes approximately 14 days between the first day of menstruation and ovulation, before fertilization occurs. Although practical and easy to calculate, estimates based on the LMP are somewhat unreliable because they depend on the woman's memory and menstrual regularity (Hadlock, 1994; Sawin & Morgan, 1996). When fertilization has occurred in vitro or is the result of artificial insemination, or in the science of embryology, gestation may be estimated based on the **postconceptional age**, which is the actual dating of the pregnancy from time of formation of the zygote, not on the LMP. A normal full-term pregnancy lasts approximately 40 weeks (280 days) from the LMP, or approximately 266 days (38 weeks) postconception or fertilization.

These two classification systems (that is, by gestational [LMP] or by postconceptional age) are used with great frequency and not always consistently; therefore, it is essential that the type of classification system used be clearly stated to avoid interpretation errors when reporting the age of a developing infant. The developmental stages presented in this chapter will be based on postconceptional age unless otherwise specified.

The most convenient classification, the **trimester system**, divides the nine months of pregnancy into three-month periods, counting from the date of the LMP. Many obstetricians and midwives use the trimester system because it is a simple method to monitor the pregnancy and explain to the parents the prenatal progression of their developing infant. Describing or monitoring a pregnancy by trimesters is criticized in the literature as a system that lacks precision and may be confusing (Sawin & Morgan, 1996). Arguments against the trimester system include issues such as (1) that the duration of a human pregnancy (40 weeks or 280 days) is not divisible by 3, thus creating confusion regarding the time span covered within each trimester; and (2) that determining the number of gestational weeks covered within a month of pregnancy is also inexact (Sawin & Morgan, 1996). Furthermore, monitoring a pregnancy by trimesters or months is somewhat artificial because it does not correspond to the embryonic or fetal milestones. Sawin and Morgan (1996) proposed a physiologically based alternate system that divides the pregnancy into four ten-week quartiles according to "natural embryonic and fetal developmental landmarks" occurring approximately every five weeks. Although somewhat more difficult to comprehend by laypeople, this system has been gaining popularity since the mid-1990s.

Embryologists use a sophisticated and discrete stage system called *Carnegie stages* to classify embryos in the first nine weeks postconception, a period roughly equivalent to the first trimester (O'Rahilly & Muller, 1987). The Carnegie system describes 23 stages of maturity of an embryo based on external physical characteristics rather than the embryo's size or age (Nishimura, Tanimura, Semba, & Uwabe, 1974; O'Rahilly & Muller, 1987; University of New South Wales, 2012). A given stage number may be assigned to embryos of slightly different ages or sizes because of individual variations in growth and physical development. This maturity estimation method is highly reliable, particularly in situations where the growth of the fetus has been compromised, such as infants with intrauterine growth retardation or infants in distress. For students interested in the "Virtual Human Embryo Project" (2014), funded by the National Library of Medicine, an atlas of embryonic development based on the Carnegie classification stages may be found at http://www.ehd.org/virtual-human-embryo.

FERTILIZATION

The egg cells or ova (plural of ovum) of a woman are formed prenatally during the fetal period. Ova are estimated to be the largest cells in the body (England, 1996). Primitive ova undergo their first cellular division prenatally, before a female infant is born. The daughter cells that result from the first meiotic division are called *primary oocytes.* They will be *haploid;* that is, they will have half the number of chromosomes of their parent cell. The primary oocytes that develop prenatally will remain inactive until near puberty, when a second meiotic division will occur (Moore, Persaud & Torchia, 2011; Nussbaum, McInnes, & Willard, 2007). The second meiotic division is similar to a regular mitosis cell division, but the dividing cells will have only half the chromosomes. Before the cells divide, each chromosome will divide into two halves, or *chromatids,* thus giving rise to new cells with the same number of chromosomes as their parent cell, the primary oocyte. The new cells will be called *secondary oocytes*. The secondary oocytes will have a total of 23 chromosomes—22 chromosomes plus the sex chromosome, which will always be an X chromosome because the woman's cells do not have a Y chromosome.

As the male approaches puberty, the primitive germ cells formed prenatally that had remained dormant for years begin to multiply, grow, and divide, becoming primary spermatocytes containing the same number of chromosomes as the primitive cells. A process similar to the meiotic division of the oocytes begins, through which the number of chromosomes in the *diploid* (double chromosome) primary spermatocyte is reduced by half. This division results in the formation of two haploid secondary spermatocytes. A second meiotic division then takes place in which each of the secondary spermatocytes further divides into two *spermatids* that will eventually become mature sperm, but the number of chromosomes is not reduced during the second division. Each resulting sperm will thus have 22 chromosomes plus the sex chromosome, but, unlike the oocyte, there will be two types of sperm, one carrying the X and the other carrying the Y chromosome.

Mature sperm are believed to be the smallest cells in the human body (England, 1996). Normal sperm have an oval-shaped head, a central section, and a flexible tail. The head carries the genetic material (that is, DNA), and the tail gives the sperm the ability to swim distances many times its size. If a sperm comes in contact with a mature oocyte and is able to penetrate it, the pronuclei of the two haploid cells will merge and the fertilized oocyte will become a unicellular diploid zygote. The type of sperm that fertilizes the ovum will determine the embryo's sex: female if the sperm carries the X chromosome and male if it carries the Y chromosome.

DEVELOPMENT OF BODY STRUCTURE IN THE PRE-EMBRYONIC (GERMINAL) PERIOD

The germinal phase begins with fertilization and formation of the zygote. A zygote is a unicellular organism that contains 46 chromosomes arranged as two pairs of 23 chromosomes—one pair coming from the mother and the other from the father. The zygote's genetic composition will be unique because it results from a combination of the genes from both parents. The father's germ cell will always determine the sex of the embryo.

A woman may sometimes release two (or even more) ova within a very short period of time. If both ova are fertilized, the woman will conceive one embryo from each fertilized ovum. The product of this conception will be fraternal, or dizygotic (two-zygote), twins—or multiples in rare cases when more than one egg is fertilized. These embryos may be of the same or different sex and may look very different from each other. In the United States, about two-thirds of twins are dizygotic, with the incidence of dizygotic twin pregnancies increasing with age of the mother (Moore, Persaud, & Torchia, 2011). The remaining one-third of the twin pregnancies result from an alteration in the division of the zygote within the first week of development. The exact mechanism by which such alterations in the division of the zygote occur is not clearly understood, but some believe that these alterations result from an incorrect encoding of the fertilized cell that signals it to become two distinct zygotes. Monozygotic twins share exactly the same genetic material because they come from the same fertilized cell. Any differences between them will be the result of environmental influences on development.

The cells of the zygote are believed to be pluripotent (a term introduced earlier); that is, any cell of the zygote can give rise to any cell of the embryo (Kim & Clark, 2014; Polifka & Friedman, 2002). Although zygote cells are pluripotent, it is believed that, after the first two weeks or by the time the zygote becomes an embryo, it will bring a patterning of information that will determine which parts of the body will emerge from its different cells (Pearson, 2002). Developing cells will be constrained to become specific cells during certain periods, induced by their neighboring cells (Bruer, 2001). Therefore, the germinal stage has received a great deal of attention in the science of in vitro fertilization and stem cell research.

THE 1ST WEEK

Germinal development begins almost instantly after fertilization (Pearson, 2002). During the 1st week of the germinal period, the unicellular zygote will become a **blastocyst**. A blastocyst is a multicellular product of conception during the 1st week in which embryonic tissue (inner cell mass) is first differentiated from extra-embryonic tissue (fetal membranes and placenta).

Within the first 30 hours, the zygote will undergo its first mitotic division, during which the maternal and paternal chromosomes will intermingle, and within 40 hours the zygote will already have four cells. A process of rapid cell division called *cleavage* will begin by the second day[2], through which the blastomere cells that will give rise to the embryo emerge. Cleavage will continue for four days after fertilization as the zygote moves downstream through the uterine tube (Graham

---

[2] There is some variability in the embryonic and fetal measurements reported in the literature. The measurements reported by (Moore, Persaud, & Torchia, 2011) are used in this chapter because of the credibility of the source.

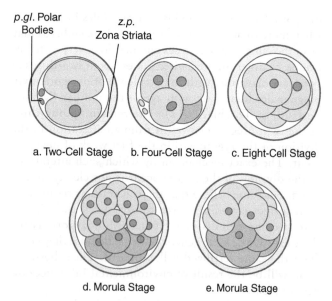

Figure 8-1 Cleavage is the rapid cell division that occurs in the days after fertilization

& Morgan, 2002). Blastomere cells will become progressively smaller with each cell division. As the zygote reaches eight to nine cells, the blastomeres will begin to organize into a compact ball of undifferentiated cells called a morula. By the 4th day[3], the morula will have approximately 32 cells arranged into an inner cell mass and an outer ring, which is surrounded by a layer of cells called the *zona pellucida*. A fluid-filled cavity will begin to form in the inner cell mass, and as fluid accumulates, the inner cell mass will separate from the outer ring, forcing the inner cell mass toward one pole. This process is illustrated in **Figure 8-1**.

The inner cell mass, consisting of about 15 percent of the pre-embryo, will become the embryoblast, the cells from which the embryo and other related tissues will emerge (Pearson, 2002). The outer ring will become the **trophoblast**—the cells that will penetrate the uterine wall and give rise to the placenta and other tissues. By the 5th day, the emerging structure will be called the blastocyst. When the blastocyst reaches the uterine cavity, it will still be about the same size as the unicellular zygote, because its dividing cells have become half the size of their parent cell with each cell division (Moore, Persaud, & Torchia, 2011).

The blastocyst will begin to "hatch" as the zona pellucida disintegrates during the two days it remains floating in the uterine cavity. Once it sheds, the blastocyst will begin to grow, because it will no longer be tightly contained by the zona pellucida (Kim & Clark, 2014; Moore, Persaud, & Torchia, 2011). The "hatched" blastocyst will begin to penetrate the uterine lining at the embryonic pole of the inner cell mass around the 6th day after fertilization. The trophoblast will grow and separate

into an inner layer and an outer mass as it becomes attached. The outer mass of the trophoblast will form tentacle-like projections that penetrate the intrauterine wall and extend toward the point of attachment of the embryonic pole. The inner layer will form the placental structures. Toward the end of the 1st week after fertilization, the outer mass will start producing enzymes that disintegrate the tissues around the implantation site, enabling the blastocyst to implant deeper into the uterine wall (Moore, Persaud, & Torchia, 2011). Pregnancy formally begins with the completion of implantation (Graham & Morgan, 2002).

Atypical implantation of the blastocyst may occur during the 1st week. The most common abnormality is implantation of the blastocyst in the inferior portion of the uterus, a condition called *placenta previa*. Premature separation of the placenta accompanied by severe bleeding often occurs when the embryo has implanted low in the uterus. Another, more serious implantation abnormality is *ectopic implantation*. In this case the blastocyst becomes implanted outside the uterus, usually in the intrauterine tubes. Tubal rupture and other serious complications from ectopic pregnancies are common and will cause severe bleeding, placing the mother's life at high risk. Other implantation abnormalities are rare (Moore, Persaud, & Torchia, 2011).

THE 2ND WEEK

The beginning of the 2nd week is characterized by rapid division and differentiation of the trophoblast, accompanied by quickly progressing implantation of the blastocyst. This process requires adequate hormonal support and the release of protein-dissolving trophoblast enzymes, which erode the tissues around the implantation site, enabling deeper penetration of the blastocyst into the uterine wall.

As implantation continues, during the first part of the 2nd week, the inner cell mass of the blastocyst will begin to form a new cavity that will be lined with a layer of cells called *amnioblasts*. Amnioblasts will form the amniotic tissues. The lining layer becomes the amnion and the cavity the amniotic cavity. The inner cell mass of the pre-embryo will reorganize into a flat, bilaminar structure of somewhat differentiated cells called the *embryonic disk*. The layer of the disc that is farthest from the amniotic cavity will form the primary yolk sac. Yolk sac cells will form a layer of connective tissue called the *extraembryonic mesoderm* that will encircle the amnion and the yolk sac. Simultaneously, many small cavities will begin to appear in the trophoblast near the embryonic pole. These cavities will begin to accumulate maternal blood, marking the beginning of what will later become the uteroplacental circulation system. By the 10th to the 12th day, a rudimentary network of arteries and veins will have formed, initiating a primitive blood circulation process that will nurture the embryonic disk.

By the 12th day, the blastocyst will have penetrated fully into the uterine wall. The trophoblast around the

[3] Ibid.

embryonic pole that will later become the placenta will begin to look like a sponge. Toward the end of the 2nd week, the primary chorionic villi of the placenta and a membrane called the *chorionic sac* will begin to be formed from the trophoblast. The chorionic sac will eventually enclose the embryo, the amniotic sac, and the yolk sac.

Completion of implantation by the end of the 2nd week marks the end of the germinal period and the beginning of the embryonic period. By this time, the embryo will have a flattened appearance with thickening of a small area of the embryonic disk. This thickened area will become the prechordal plate—the area from which the mouth and some head structures will emerge. Identification of abnormalities in the developing embryo, particularly chromosomal alterations, is becoming more available; however, the risk and reliability of some of these procedures remain questionable. Preimplantation diagnosis is a preferred alternative to prenatal (fetal) diagnosis for couples at risk for transmitting a genetic disorder (Kanavakis & Traeger-Synodinos, 2002).

DEVELOPMENT OF BODY STRUCTURE IN THE EMBRYONIC PERIOD

The embryonic period begins at the close of the 2nd week, with the embryo securely implanted in the uterine endometrium, and continues throughout the 8th week.

It is a period of active cell proliferation, migration, and differentiation resulting in the formation of nearly all the tissues and organs of the body. Development will progress from the cephalic to the caudal ends of the embryo, with head and upper trunk structures forming and becoming functional several days before lower trunk and leg structures. By the end of the 8th week, the embryo will have a human resemblance. It will have rudimentary eyes and eyebrows, ears, arm buds with hands, fingers, leg buds with feet, and toes. The embryo's head will be proportionately much larger than the rest of the body.

The embryonic period is when the developing organs are most sensitive or susceptible to the effects of toxic substances or abnormal conditions (Bruer, 2001). A **teratogen** is any agent that causes the production of physical defects in the developing embryo. **Table 8-2** lists some of the known teratogens and their effects. Teratogens may alter many processes during this period including cell migration, programmed cell death, gene expression, and tissue formation. Therefore, the embryonic period is when exposure to teratogens will be most devastating to developing embryos (Moore, Persaud, & Torchia, 2011; Sawin & Morgan, 1996). The type of anomaly that may occur from teratogen exposure is determined by gestational timing of exposure, dose, duration, and nature of the teratogen (Graham & Morgan, 2002; Polifka & Friedman, 2002). During periods of major structural formation, a teratogen is likely to have a greater impact on the system. These periods of major development are known as

TABLE 8-2 Some Known Human Teratogens	
Teratogens	**Results**
Medications	
Thalidomide	Limb reduction defects, ear anomalies
Streptomycin	Hearing loss
Tetracycline	Stained teeth, enamel hypoplasia
Valproic acid	Neural tube defects, dysmorphic facial features
Isotretinoin	Pregnancy loss, hydrocephalus, other CNS defects, small or absent thymus, microtia/anotia, conotruncal heart defects
Antithyroid drugs	Hypothyroidism, goiter
Androgens and high doses of norprogesterones	Masculinization of external female genitalia
ACE inhibitors	Renal dysgenesis, oligohydramnios sequence, skull ossification defects
Carbamazepine	Neural tube defects
Cocaine	Pregnancy loss, placental abruption, growth retardation, microcephaly
Lithium	Ebstein anomaly

Continues

TABLE 8-2 Some Known Human Teratogens *(continued)*

Teratogens	Results
Maternal Infections	
Toxoplasmosis	Hydrocephalus, blindness, mental retardation
Varicella	Skin scarring, limb reduction defects, muscle atrophy, mental retardation
Syphilis	Abnormal teeth and bones, mental retardation
Cytomegalovirus	Growth and developmental retardation, microcephaly, hearing loss, ocular abnormalities
Herpes (primary)	Pregnancy loss, growth retardation, eye abnormalities
Herpes (active)	Vertical transmission at delivery
Chemicals	
Methylmercury	Cerebral atrophy, spasticity, mental retardation
Lead	Pregnancy loss, CNS damage
Polychlorobiphenyls (PCBs—ingested)	Low birth weight, skin discoloration
Maternal Disorders	
Insulin-dependent diabetes mellitus	Congenital heart defects, caudal deficiency, neural tube defects, limb defects, holoprosencephaly, pregnancy loss
Hypo/hyperthyroidism	Goiter, growth and developmental retardation
Phenylketonuria	Pregnancy loss, microcephaly, mental retardation, facial dysmorphism, congenital heart defects
Hypertension	Intrauterine growth retardation
Autoimmune disorders	Congenital heart block, pregnancy loss
Reproductive Toxins	
Cigarette smoking	Pregnancy loss, low birth weight
Hyperthermia	Neural tube defects
Chronic alcoholism	Growth and developmental retardation, microcephaly, craniofacial dysmorphism
Therapeutic radiation	Growth and developmental retardation, microcephaly

critical periods. **Figure 8-2** illustrates critical periods and body systems affected by teratogens across the course of prenatal life.

THE 3RD WEEK

A key feature of the third week is the organization of the embryonic disk into three layers: endoderm, mesoderm, and ectoderm. The **endoderm** is the germ layer from which the digestive system, many glands, and parts of the respiratory system are formed. The **mesoderm** is the germ layer that forms many muscles, the circulatory and excretory systems, and the dermis, skeleton, and other

supportive and connective tissues. The **ectoderm** is the primary embryonic cell layer from which the skin, the nervous system, and other structures will evolve. All of the organs and tissues of developing infants will emerge from these three layers of cells. By the end of the third week, an embryo will have the rudiments of important body structures that have emerged from one or more of these layers.

Differentiation of the embryonic disk into the three layers begins when cells from the layer that forms the floor of the amniotic cavity proliferate and migrate to form a line in the center of the embryonic disk called the *primitive streak*. As cells accumulate, the primitive streak will elongate, move inward (infold), and form three distinctive areas:

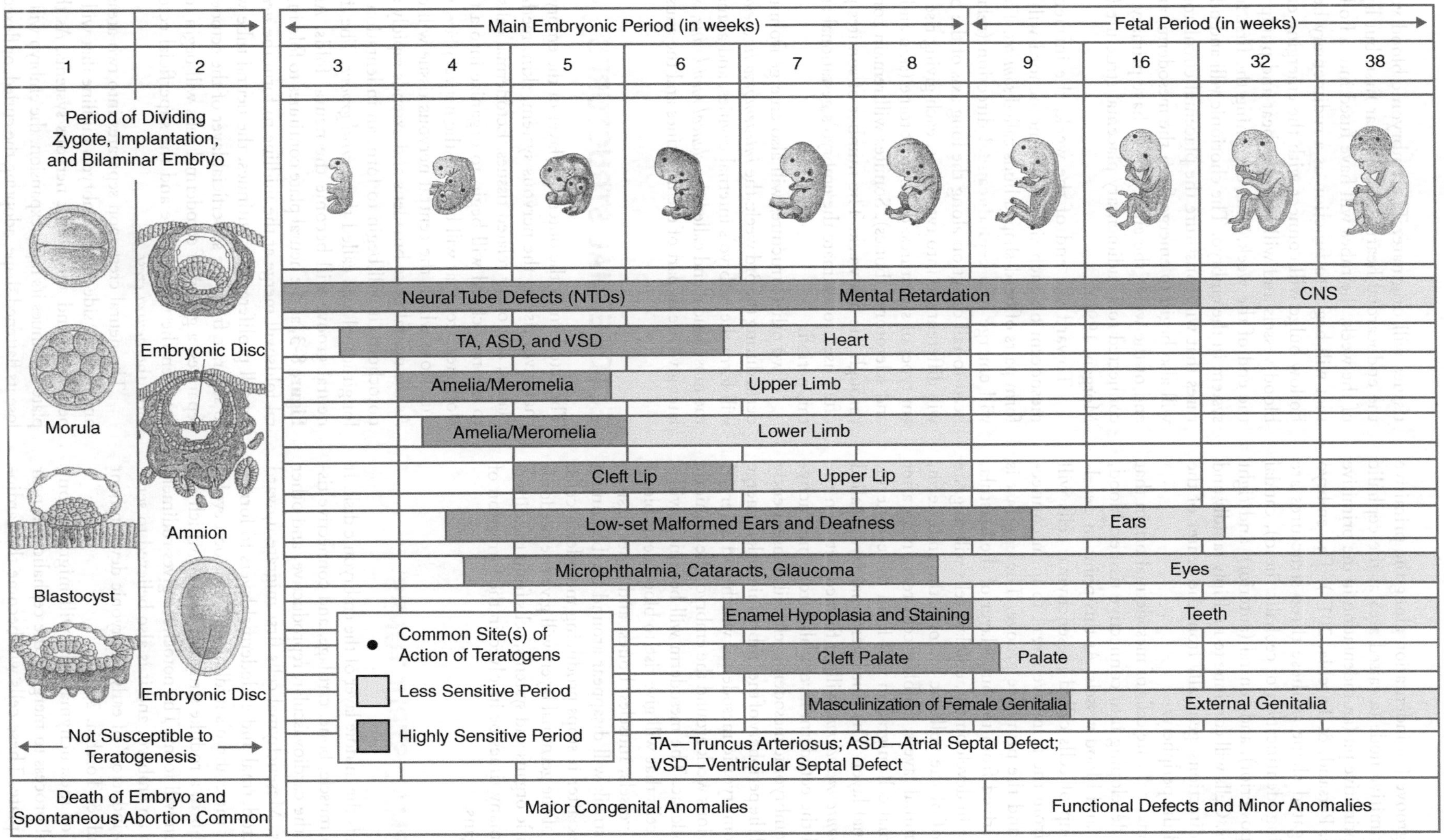

Blue denotes highly sensitive periods when major birth defects may be produced.

Figure 8-2 Summary of Critical Periods in Prenatal Development reprinted from The Developing Human: Clinically Oriented Embryology, 9th ed., K. L. Moore, et al, Critical Periods © 2013, with permission from Elsevier the primitive groove (an indentation along the primitive streak), the primitive node (a raised area at the cephalic end), and the primitive pit (an indentation in the primitive node) (Moore, Persaud, & Torchia, 2011). The embryo takes an elongated shape as these three structures are formed, allowing identification of cephalic (head), caudal (tail), dorsal (posterior), and ventral (anterior), and right and left surfaces. Cells will continue to multiply rapidly and migrate in all directions, generally from the center of the embryo toward the periphery.

Mesenchymal cells are cells of mesodermal origin that are capable of developing into connective tissues, blood, and lymphatic and blood vessels. At this point in development, a group of cells called mesenchymal cells will migrate away from the primitive streak to form connective tissue around the primitive groove. The epiblast is a tissue type derived from the outer layer of the blastula, and at this time in development, epiblast cells will migrate toward the roof of the yolk sac to form the endoderm, one of the germinal layers. Epiblast cells remaining after the mesenchymal cell migration will form the ectoderm, another germinal layer. The third germinal layer, called the *intraembryonic mesoderm,* will be formed between the endoderm and the ectoderm layers, also from mesenchymal cells. Intraembryonic mesoderm cells will subsequently migrate toward the periphery of the embryonic disk to merge with the extraembryonic mesoderm, which had emerged during the previous week around the embryo, the amniotic sac, and the yolk sac. The mesoderm will become a widespread layer of cells that will give rise to blood cells, blood and lymphatic vessels, muscles, bones, and other tissues. The primitive streak will disappear around the beginning of the 4th week after it stops producing mesoderm cells. Although each of the germinal layers will give rise predominantly to specific organs and systems, cells from the different layers will many times be involved in the formation of the various organs.

MESODERMAL STRUCTURES

The mesoderm is the middle layer of the embryonic disk. It will give rise to muscle, bone, cartilage, and connective tissues, as well as the cardiovascular, reproductive, and other internal organs. Mesenchymal cells first migrate upward between the ectodermal and endodermal layers to form a hollow chord at the embryo's midline that will soon evolve into the notochord, a rodlike structure around which the vertebral column will form. The notochord gives rudimentary stability to an embryo, and it is also believed to serve as "the primary inductor" of early embryonic development (Moore, Persaud, & Torchia, 2011).

A portion of mesenchymal cells will migrate along the notochordal process to merge at the cephalic end near the prechordal plate. These cells will become the cardiogenic mesoderm from which the heart and other vascular

tissues will originate. The embryonic blood vessels and the endocardial heart tubes appear first, but by the end of the week, the tubes will have fused into a hollow bulge that will begin to function as a rudimentary heart. This hollow bulge will connect with the emerging embryonic blood vessels and will begin to beat and pump blood by the end of the week, thus becoming the first functional system in the embryo. The chorionic villi and other structures that will constitute the placental circulatory system will also begin to emerge from the mesoderm, and by the end of the week, the embryo will have primary stem villi connected to a rudimentary placental structure (Sawin & Morgan, 1996).

Toward the end of the week, the intraembryonic mesoderm on each side of the notochord will begin to form pairs of bead-shaped buds called *somites.* The somites will emerge in a cephalocaudal direction (relating to a head-to-tail direction along the long axis of the body) and will differentiate into two types, each giving rise to different types of structures: dermomyotome (skin and muscles) and sclerotome (bones). Somites will remain conspicuous through the 5th week. The number of somites present is often used to estimate the embryo's gestational age during this period.

Two other structures will also emerge from the mesoderm during the 3rd week: the *intraembryonic coelom,* which will form the embryo's internal cavities, and a small area at the most caudal end called the *cloacal membrane,* which will later give rise to part of the intestines and the anus.

ECTODERMAL STRUCTURES

The ectoderm is the outermost layer of the embryonic disk that gives rise to the nervous system, skin, teeth, various glands, and other related tissues. Ectodermal cells adjacent to the notochord will begin to organize into a thickened elongated area that will become the neural plate, the structure from which the central nervous tissue will originate. As the neural plate broadens and extends rapidly along the notochord, it will begin to form an indentation along its longitudinal axis called the *neural groove.* The lips of the neural groove will become the neural folds. As seen in **Figure 8-3**, as the neural plate continues to fold in, the neural folds will merge at the midline to form the *neural tube.* As cell proliferation continues, the neural tube will begin to separate from the superficial layer of the ectoderm. As it separates, a group of ectodermal cells will begin to migrate between the neural tube and the superficial ectoderm to form the *neural crest.*

The neural crest soon separates into two areas of cells, one on each side of the embryo's midline that will form the peripheral and autonomic nervous systems. As the neural plate continues its rapid expansion, the embryo will gradually lose its flattened shape, adopting the curled, or flexed, posture it will maintain until birth. This process begins during the

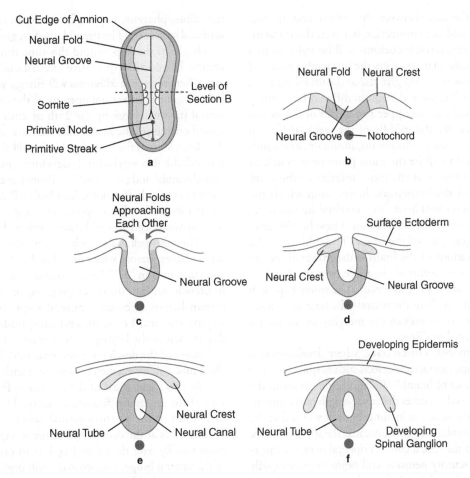

Figure 8-3 Stages of Formation (Infolding) of Neural Tube

3rd week and continues through the 4th week. It is called the *cephalocaudal folding of the embryo*. The outermost cells of the ectoderm will begin to differentiate into epidermal cells while nervous system development continues.

ENDODERMAL STRUCTURES

The endoderm will give rise to most of the digestive, urinary, and respiratory structures (Graham & Morgan, 2002). As cephalocaudal folding progresses, two pockets will appear in the endoderm, one at the cephalic end and one at the caudal end. These pockets represent the areas where the foregut and the hindgut will develop. Toward the end of the 3rd week and the beginning of the 4th week, the primordial gut tube will be formed from the portion of the yolk sac that remains inside the embryo, as the endoderm and the endoderm-lined yolk sac folds in. By around day 19 or 20, the embryo will also begin to fold lengthwise. This process is called *lateral folding of the embryo*. Lateral folding is the result of expansion of the paraxial mesoderm and the emerging somites.

By the end of the 3rd week, the embryo will have a distinguishable human resemblance. Although it will still be mostly flat, it is beginning to curl. It will have clearly identifiable cephalic, caudal, dorsal, and ventral surfaces. Several structures will be evident, including the bulge of the developing heart and inner organs; the oropharyngeal membrane at the cephalic end; the neural plate extending along the dorsal region; the somites at the middorsal section; and the cloacal membrane and plate at the caudal end. The embryo will have 4 to 12 somites by the end of this period. It will remain connected to the yolk sac through the yolk stalk (Moore, Persaud, & Torchia, 2011).

THE 4TH WEEK

The first part of the 4th week marks the beginning of the organogenesis phase, during which all of the embryo's organs and the internal cavities will be formed. The embryo will become strongly curved by the end of the 4th week as a result of its cephalocaudal folding; the cephalic fold will be deeper than the caudal fold as a result of the cephalic-to-caudal developmental progression. The embryo's ventral surface will close during the 4th week from the combination of lateral and cephalocaudal folding. As the embryo continues to fold ventrally, the space between the embryo and the yolk sac will decrease, and the connection between the intraembryonic and extraembryonic coeloms will be reduced to a small duct. The stalk that connects the intraembryonic and extraembryonic structures will give rise to the umbilical cord.

Brain tissue will grow and begin to differentiate rapidly during the 4th week, as the upper two-thirds of the neural tube wall enlarges. By the middle of the week, the brain will consist of three vesicles: forebrain, midbrain, and hindbrain. The forebrain will be the most prominent vesicle at this stage. The forebrain is the most anterior of the three primary regions of the embryonic brain, from which the cerebral hemispheres will arise. The cerebral hemispheres are the two halves of the brain cerebrum. These hemispheres make up the largest part of the brain. The middle of the three primary divisions of the brain is the midbrain of the embryo. The most posterior of the three primary divisions of the embryo's brain is the hindbrain. The spinal cord will begin to form as the walls of the neural tube become thicker and begin to close as a result of the merging of the lateral folds along the dorsal midline.

This is an extremely critical stage, where developmental alterations may cause neural tube defects such as spina bifida or anencephaly (absence of brain).[4] When it begins to form, the developing spinal cord occupies the entire length of the emerging spine, but by the time the infant is born, it will end at the level of the upper lumbar vertebras, because the spine will have grown longer than the spinal cord. Peripheral nerves, consisting of motor and sensory neurons, will begin to grow rapidly toward the end of the 4th week from the ventro-lateral sides of the developing spinal cord and from occipital neural crest cells. The ventral motor neurons will appear first. These are the neurons that activate muscle cells. Motor neuron development is followed by the appearance of dorsal sensory neurons. Dorsal sensory neurons are nerve cells that conduct impulses from a sense organ to the central nervous system. The axons of the motor fibers will grow fast, seeking out and migrating toward specific muscles. Sensory fibers will grow more slowly. The emerging nerves will migrate toward and into the limbs as the limbs are developing. It is believed that chemical markers at the target organ attract and direct nerve axons to establish correct connections (Sperry, 1963, as cited in Bruer, 2001). Axons that connect with the incorrect structure will not become functional and will eventually degenerate.

The cephalic end of the embryo will begin to resemble a human head as the forebrain grows and the oropharyngeal membranes and heart tube migrate ventrally. At this stage three pharyngeal arches will emerge from the oropharyngeal membrane on the ventral surface of the embryo immediately below the forebrain. These arches will give rise to the maxilla,

mandible, pharynx, larynx, face, mouth, tongue, and other orofacial structures. The thyroid, the first gland to emerge, will also begin to develop around this time from the pharyngeal arches. The otic pits (primitive internal ears) and a thickened area where the eyes and retinas will emerge will appear around the 26th day. The ventral opening at the cephalic end of the neural tube will close by the 25th or 26th day, whereas the caudal opening of the neural tube will close approximately two days later, around the 28th day. Limbs will also begin to appear around the 4th week. Limb development will progress in cephalocaudal and **proximodistal** (from the center, or midline, moving outward) directions. Arm buds will appear around day 26, but leg buds will not appear until approximately the 28th day; proximal segments will emerge before distal segments.

The 4th week is also an important developmental period for cardiorespiratory structures. The heart tube will elongate and curve into an "S." The cardiovascular system will continue to branch out into the developing organs and the lymphatic system begins to emerge. Several respiratory structures—larynx, trachea, bronchii, and lung buds—will begin to differentiate as the laryngotracheal groove emerges at the ventral aspect of the developing pharynx. Initially the laryngotracheal tube will have a direct connection with the pharynx.

At this stage, most of the gut hangs from the posterior wall of the emerging peritoneal cavity. The first sign of the formation of the gastrointestinal system is the emergence of liver buds at the caudal end of the foregut. The liver will grow rapidly over the following days to occupy a large area of the ventral bulge. The stomach will begin to form shortly after as a small dilatation at the lower end of the foregut.

By the end of the 4th week, the embryo will be somewhat cylindrical and about 4 mm long, will have well-defined body cavities and a tail at its caudal end, and will have approximately 26 to 28 pairs of somites (Moore, Persaud, & Torchia, 2011). Other cells will continue to differentiate into the various organ systems, but the cardiovascular system is the only system that will be considerably functional by the end of the 4th week.

The most common congenital anomalies associated with this developmental period are epigastric hernias (abdominal organs growing into the amniotic cavity, outside the abdominal wall) and spina bifida (defect in the center of the spinal column). Epigastric hernias will result from failure of the ventral fusion of the lateral folds, whereas spina bifida is caused by failure of the dorsal fusion of the neuropores and lateral folds. Tracheoesophageal fistulas may also occur if the trachea and the pharynx fail to separate adequately (Moore, Persaud, & Torchia, 2011).

THE 5TH AND 6TH WEEKS

These two weeks are characterized by major differentiation and growth of many organs and structures. By the 5th week, the placental circulation system will be functional, carrying

---

[4] The incidence of *neural tube defects (NTD)* has decreased significantly since preconceptional and periconceptional folic acid supplementation has been in use. Conversely, exposure to folic acid antagonists increases the NTD risk (Hernandez-Diaz, Werler, Walker, & Mitchell, 2001).

oxygen and nutrients from the mother to the fetus through the umbilical cord (Graham & Morgan, 2002). The head will experience the greatest growth during this period because of the cephalocaudal progression of development. By the 5th week, the brain will have divided into five vesicles; the cerebral hemispheres will form from the most cephalic vesicle of the forebrain and will gradually cover other brain structures. Brain waves can be recorded as early as the beginning of the 6th week (Hamlin, 1964). Cranial nerves will also begin to emerge between the 5th and the 6th weeks. The cranial nerves are composed of 12 pairs of nerves that emerge from brain tissue.

Primitive eyes covered by eyelids will appear between the 5th and the 6th weeks, as well as auricular hillocks and primitive external ear canals (Moore, Persaud, & Torchia, 2011). The mouth area will also be clearly identifiable by the 5th week. An enlarged area of the frontonasal processes of the pharyngeal arches will become the nasal placodes from which the nose will later emerge. By the 6th week, the nasal placodes from each side will merge at the midline, creating the primordial lower lip. The palate will also begin to form between the internal surfaces of the developing maxilla as the nasal prominences merge, but its development will not be complete until the 12th week. The nasal pits will deepen to form the nasal sac and nostrils.

During the 5th week, the upper limbs will look like paddles, with digital rays appearing distally on the hand plates. By the end of the 6th week, the upper limbs will have a complete cartilaginous skeleton and rudimentary elbow joints. Foot plates will begin to emerge by the 6th week, but will become more prominent by the 7th week. The 5th through the 8th week is the most sensitive period in the development of the limbs. Exposure to teratogens during this period will affect the limbs or part of the limbs that will be developing at the time of exposure. Upper limbs and proximal segments of the limbs will be affected earlier, whereas lower limbs and distal segments will be affected during the 7th and 8th weeks. Intermediate segments of a limb may be affected less frequently, resulting in absence or reduction of one or more bones. The drug thalidomide is a classic example of a teratogen that selectively affects the development of the limbs, especially if administered in the window of 24 to 42 postconceptional days (Hepper, 2003).

Critical developmental changes in many other body organs and systems will occur during the 5th and 6th weeks. Emergence of the heart septum—a membranous structure between the two heart atria or between the two heart ventricles—initiates the division of the heart into atrial and ventricular chambers. All four chambers of the heart will be formed by the 7th week. Development of the respiratory system will include branching of the lung buds into two bronchial buds, as well as appearance of a rudimentary pleural cavity and a primordial diaphragm. The developing lungs and heart will descend into the thorax

region by the end of the 6th week. The cardiovascular system will be functioning fairly well by this stage, but the respiratory system will not become functional until much later, because most of its development will occur toward the end of the fetal period.

The developing stomach bulge will expand during the 5th and 6th weeks and rotate clockwise until it assumes its mature position around the 8th week. During the 6th week, the intestines are elongating much faster than the abdominal cavity is enlarging, forcing a loop of the intestines to herniate into the umbilical cord. The intestines remain herniated until the 10th week, when they spontaneously begin to rotate into the abdominal cavity when space becomes available.

The most common congenital anomalies likely to occur around the 5th and 6th weeks include cleft lip and cleft palate. Lip and palate defects occur when the placodes and related structures fail to fuse at midline. Cleft palate defects may also occur at later stages, because the palate continues developing into the 12th week. Other abnormalities in the development of the pharyngeal arches include U-shaped cleft palate, retrognathia (retracted jaw), micrognathia (small jaw), and nasal airway abnormalities. Disturbed neural crest development may result in esophageal atresias as well as abnormalities of the heart and the great vessels (Otten et al., 2000). Other common developmental anomalies that may occur during this period include cardiac septal defects, limb anomalies, and abnormalities associated with persistent herniation or malrotation of the intestines.

THE 7TH AND 8TH WEEKS

One of the most important developments toward the end of the 7th week is the formation of cartilage and the beginning of *ossification* in the developing upper body. **Ossification** is the formation of bone or the conversion of fibrous tissue or of cartilage into bone. Craniofacial bones will emerge from neural crest cells that had migrated earlier into the pharyngeal arches. The vertebras and ribs will emerge from sclerotome somites. Most flat and long bones will emerge from mesenchymal cells that had organized earlier into sheaths of connective tissue or into cartilage formations.

Ossification begins with mesenchymal cells differentiating into osteoblasts (bone-forming cells) and osteoid tissue. Bones will primarily form from calcium phosphate accumulating in the osteoid tissue between the osteoblasts or, in the case of the long bones, in primary ossification centers of the cartilage formations. The clavicles and upper limbs will calcify first. Ossification of the vertebras and the lower limbs will occur later, during and after the 8th week. The trunk and limbs will elongate as their pre-bone structures calcify. The embryo will adopt a less curved appearance as bones begin to form around the spine. Bones will continue to ossify throughout the entire fetal period as well as postnatally.

Wrist joints will appear around the 7th week as limb development continues to progress proximodistally. Notches will form between the digital rays of the hand plates, initiating the development of the fingers. By the end of the 7th week, the embryo will have hands with wrists and webbed fingers as well as fan-shaped feet with emerging toes. The webs between the fingers and the toes will have disappeared within a week. At that point, all joints of the body will resemble the adult form, and the limbs—including hands and feet—will have their adult appearance.

By the 7th week, the embryo's heart will have primitive aorta, carotid, subclavian, and pulmonary arteries. The primordial pharynx will have elongated and established connections with the mouth and the esophagus. The cloaca will separate into two tubes: urogenital (giving rise to urogenital structures) and anorectal (giving rise to the rectum and anal canal). A layer of cloacal membrane ectoderm at the end of the developing anal canal will perforate to form the anal opening. Nonfunctional kidneys will have moved to their permanent location by the 8th week.

By the end of the embryonic period, the embryo will be approximately 5 cm long and will have a well-defined large head (approximately one-half the embryo's crown-to-rump length) and a smooth neck. Facial characteristics present will include low-set ears with distinguishable auricula, widely separated eyes, eyelid folds above and below the eye, forward-facing nostrils, and a complete upper lip. The embryo will have all of its rudimentary organs, well-formed limbs, and arteries, veins, nerves, cartilage, and muscles growing into the various body parts and systems, providing nutrition and functional support to the emerging structures. It will have three circulatory systems: umbilical or placental, embryonic, and vitelline. The umbilical or placental system will disappear at birth; the vitelline system will become part of the portal (liver) system; and the embryonic system will mature into the infant's cardiovascular system. Each circulatory system will have its own network of arteries and veins.

DEVELOPMENT OF BODY STRUCTURE IN THE FETAL PERIOD

The end of the 8th week and the beginning of the 9th week signal one of the most important milestones in prenatal development. It is that particular moment when the developing embryo begins to look clearly human and is considered a fetus. It is the point beyond which arguments about the beginning of human life decrease (Richardson & Reiss, 1999). It is also the moment beyond which exposure to teratogens will not necessarily cause widespread or lethal damage, because all of the organs and body systems have already been formed. Short-duration exposure to teratogens may cause placental functional deficits and fetal growth

restriction more than birth defects (Graham & Morgan, 2002). Any birth defect caused by mild to moderately harmful teratogens after this period will likely be localized to a specific part of the body; large or prolonged exposure or highly harmful teratogens may cause fetal death.

The fetal period is one of rapid fetal and placental growth as cell proliferation and hypertrophy or hyperplasia continues (England, 1996; Moore, Persaud, & Torchia, 2011). Between 9 weeks postconception and term age, the fetus will grow from about 5 cm to 36 cm (crown-to-rump length) and will increase in weight from about 8 g to between 3400 and 3600 g (Moore, Persaud, & Torchia, 2011).[5] From the 10th through the 20th week, the fetus will grow primarily in length, but after the 20th week weight gain will predominate, whereas the rate of length growth will begin to decline. Organ and tissue differentiation will continue, particularly during the first 4 to 8 weeks of the fetal period. Bones will continue to ossify and remodel throughout the entire fetal period (Moore, Persaud, & Torchia, 2011). The rate of growth of the head will decrease as the rate of growth of the extremities increases, beginning to give the fetus a more proportional appearance.

Although fetal development is most often obstetrically monitored by trimesters counting from the last menstrual period, the developmental milestones that occur during this period are best described in blocks of 4 to 5 weeks, counting from the moment of conception (Sawin & Morgan, 1996). The following sections highlight the most important developmental changes in the fetus from the 9th week through term age.

THE 9TH THROUGH 12TH WEEKS

During the period of the 9th through the 12th week, the fetus will continue to grow, body parts will become more detailed, and various body processes and systems will become functional. Crown-to-rump length will double between the 8th and the 12th weeks. After the 9th or 10th week, fetal growth and development may be monitored using ultrasound imaging, making it possible to identify a number of structural and functional anomalies in the fetus or the placenta. A well-formed cartilaginous skeleton (**chondroskeleton**) may be identified at the lowest portion of the skull, the spine, rib cage, scapulas, and extremities by the 10th to 11th weeks (Jirasek, 2001). Cartilaginous ribs may be visible under the skin. Ribs will grow first toward the ventral midline, fusing with the costal cartilages toward the end of this period. By the 12th week, the primary ossification centers will have appeared in the skull and all long bones. The head will continue to grow somewhat faster than the rest of the body, therefore remaining disproportionately

---

[5] There is some variability in the embryonic and fetal measurements reported in the literature. The measurements reported by Moore, Persaud, and Torchia (2011) are used in this chapter because of the credibility of the source.

large by the 12th week. The upper limbs will approximate their proportional full-term length in relation to the rest of the body, but the lower limbs will remain proportionally shorter by the end of the 12th week.

By the 9th week, the hands and feet will be well developed. Between the 9th and the 12th weeks, fingernails will begin to form (toenails will emerge later). The eyelid folds will fuse and will remain fused until the end of the 24th week. The ability to swallow will emerge, enabling the fetus to ingest amniotic fluid for nourishment and lung development. The kidneys will develop lobes and connecting tubules and begin to function. Fetuses will begin to produce urine around the 9th week; by the 12th week, they will be urinating into the abdominal fluid. External genital organs, particularly the penis, will be well defined by the 12th week, thus making it possible to distinguish the sex of the fetus through ultrasound.

During this time, there is continued vascularization. **Vascularization** is the growth of blood vessels into a tissue or organ with the result that the oxygen and nutrient supply is improved. Fetal-placental circulation will improve because of the continued development of vascularization. The placenta will also begin to remove waste products urinated by the fetus into the amniotic fluid.

THE 13TH THROUGH 16TH WEEKS

Fetal growth will be very active during the period of the 13th through the 16th week. The rate of growth of the head will have slowed down considerably in relation to the caudal structures and lower limbs. By the 16th week, the entire body will be more proportional, and the legs will approximate their full-term proportional length. Ossification will also be very active during this period, enabling the identification of many bones through ultrasound by the 16th week (Sawin & Morgan, 1996). Blood vessels will be superficial and clearly visible under the thin skin (England, 1996). By the 13th week, blood will begin to reach the lung epithelium as a result of ongoing capillary proliferation (Sawin & Morgan, 1996).

THE 17TH THROUGH 20TH WEEKS

Fetal changes occurring during the period of the 17th through the 20th week are not as remarkable as those of previous stages. The rate of growth of the fetus will have decreased markedly. By the end of the 20th week, all body structures will have approximated or reached their final position, and size proportions and will resemble their full-term appearance. The skin of the fetus will be covered with fine hair called *lanugo*, and a layer of a greasy paste called *vernix caseosa*. The vernix caseosa will protect the fetus from injury to the skin (Moore, Persaud, & Torchia, 2011). Another important development during this period is the emergence of adipose tissue and heat-producing brown fat (Moore, Persaud, & Torchia, 2011). Brown-fat accumulation will enable the fetus to maintain body heat toward the end of the fetal period (England, 1996). Accelerated lung maturation is still another important development of this period, preparing the fetus for survival. By the end of the 17th week, all elements of the lungs will be present, although nonfunctional.

Fetuses suspected of or at high risk for having congenital heart disease may be diagnosed as early as 18 to 20 weeks postconception, when the heart is no bigger than a thumbnail, with a specialized diagnostic procedure called *fetal echocardiography* (Schonberg, 2012). Infants with congenital heart disease often have other congenital or genetic anomalies or malformations (Schonberg, 2012). These infants often undergo chromosomal and high-resolution ultrasound diagnostic studies in utero to identify other potential anomalies and to establish an early intervention plan to address the presenting conditions. *Magnetic resonance imaging (MRI)* may be used after the 20th week to diagnose fetal anomalies with greater precision when diagnosis through ultrasound is uncertain (Schonberg, 2012). Examples of conditions that may be diagnosed with MRI include a variety of brain abnormalities and amount of lung tissue present in fetuses whose lung development is compromised, such as those with diaphragmatic hernias (Schonberg, 2012).

Another diagnostic procedure that can be effectively used to identify abnormalities in the developing embryo as early as 7 weeks postconception is *transabdominal embryofetoscopy*. Although this type of study increases the risk of spontaneous abortion, the use of thin-gauge needles has decreased this risk considerably (Quintero, Abuhamad, Hobbins, & Mahoney, 1993). Furthermore, the benefits of early diagnosis often offset the slightly higher miscarriage risk the procedure may carry.

THE 21ST THROUGH 25TH WEEKS

Several key milestones occur during the period of the 21st through the 25th week, the most important one being the enhanced probability of survival for infants born prematurely after the 23rd week who are provided with intensive life support. Survival before 21 weeks postconception and of infants weighing less than 500 g is rare. One of the factors improving survival after 22 weeks is the accelerated weight gain, during which the fetuses nearly double their weight. Enhanced lung development and the beginning of the production of *surfactant* (a substance that promotes alveolar functioning) around the 22nd week will further enhance the fetus's chances of survival (Sawin & Morgan, 1996); however, infants will continue to have a high mortality rate by the 26th week because of respiratory and central nervous system immaturity. Moreover, many infants who survive premature birth at such early ages will develop secondary disabilities.

By the 21st week, the eyes will be completely developed and primitive rapid eye movements may be observed. By the end of the 25th week, the fetus will have eyebrows and open eyelids with eyelashes. Taste buds will have emerged on the tongue and mouth. The skin will continue to appear thin, wrinkled, and reddish. The volume of amniotic fluid will increase as the kidneys develop and the fetus's ability to urinate into the amniotic cavity improves. Decreased production of urine by obstruction of the urinary tract or other factors will diminish the amount of amniotic fluid that accumulates, resulting in a condition called **oligohydramnios** (Graham & Morgan, 2002). Oligohydramnios occurs most frequently during the third trimester and may have other causes, such as placental insufficiency (Moore, Persaud, & Torchia, 2011).

Oligohydramnios may cause a number of fetal abnormalities, the main ones being pulmonary hypoplasia (underdevelopment) and compression of the umbilical cord, which may cause serious damage to the fetus, including death (Moore, Persaud, & Torchia, 2011). The fetus's ability to swallow amniotic fluid will also be improving during this time. Any problem that interferes with the fetus's ability to swallow will cause a condition called **polyhydramnios**, manifested by excessive accumulation of amniotic fluid. Both of these conditions will affect the fetus's development toward the end of the pregnancy.

THE 26TH THROUGH 29TH WEEKS

The period of the 26th through the 29th week is characterized by increased weight gain, fat accumulation, and accelerated maturation of the respiratory and central nervous systems. The fetus will gain about 700 g (roughly 1½ lb) of weight and by the end of the 29th week, will weigh approximately 1700 g (over 3½ lb). Infants born before the 28th week will probably weigh under 1500 g and therefore will be classified as **very low birth weight infants (VLBW)**. These infants have a higher risk of neonatal complications (Sawin & Morgan, 1996).

Pulmonary maturity will accelerate by the 28th to the 29th week. Neural regulation of respiration will be well established, and the lungs will be sufficiently developed to breathe air, should the infant be born prematurely. **Fetal viability** exists when a fetus is sufficiently developed to live outside the uterus. Fetal viability at this stage will be much improved, and risk for disability will be lower, but prematurely born infants will still require temperature support because of limited subcutaneous fat and immature *thermal regulation*. Thermal regulation refers to the fetus's ability to maintain body temperature outside the womb environment. Because this is a transitional phase for the respiratory system, respiratory problems associated with minor delays in maturation in infants born prematurely around this period are not uncommon. The risk for other neonatal complications, particularly serious ones, will be low after

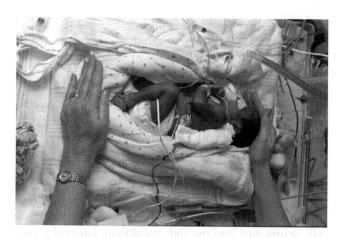

Figure 8-4   Premature Infant Care

the 28th week. As illustrated in **Figure 8-4**, the external support for immature body systems in premature infants is provided in a specialized medical environment that is very different from the uterus.

By the 29th week, the fetus will have all of the external characteristics of full-term infants, including full-term body proportions, open eyes, a head full of hair, fingernails and toenails, and less wrinkled skin because of increased subcutaneous fat. The fetus will still be covered with lanugo and a thick coat of vernix caseosa, but the skin will appear thicker and less reddish than during the previous period. All of the neonatal reflexes will be present, although not fully developed.

THE 30TH THROUGH 34TH WEEKS

Weight gain will continue at an accelerated pace, and by the 34th week, the fetus will have reached another important weight-related milestone: that is, the 2500 g (5½ lb) mark, when an early-born fetus will no longer be considered premature by weight. Infants born between the 30th and the 32nd weeks will likely require transitional temperature support because thermal regulation may not be completely developed, but the probability of surviving without problems will be high. Thermal regulation will be better established by the end of the 32nd week of gestation; thus, most infants born after this point will need only minimal transitional temperature support, if any, and will survive without complications. In contrast, 50 to 65 percent of infants born before 34 weeks postconception or weighing under 1800 g will have respiratory difficulties and frequent respiratory pauses called *apneic episodes* (Gomella, 1999). If prolonged or very frequent, such apneic episodes may compromise the infant's well-being. The incidence of apnea, however, has declined since the 1990s, with the introduction of preventive neonatal therapies such as caffeine and surfactant administration. Infants who have difficulty coming out of an apneic episode may require stimulation (for example, tactile, auditory, vestibular). Periodic breathing is another common respiratory pattern of premature infants born before 34 weeks of gestation. Periodic breathing usually causes no problems unless pauses are frequent and prolonged. The maturity of the fetus at 34 weeks is comparable to that of a full-term neonate. The fetus will look like a smaller full-term infant, with a head full of hair, pinkish and smooth skin, and a plumpish appearance resulting from increased subcutaneous fat accumulation toward the end of the period.

THE 35TH THROUGH 38TH WEEKS (FULL-TERM)

The fetus will gain approximately 900 g (approximately 2 lb) during the period of the 35th through the 38th weeks. At the time of birth, average weight will be about 3.4 kg (7½ pounds). Fat will accumulate at a rate of 14 g per day in the final weeks of the pregnancy (Moore, Persaud, & Torchia, 2011), providing the infant with much improved insulation and less need of temperature support. Chemical thermoregulation will be improved. The fetus will be prepared to sustain feeding, elimination, and respiration once separated from the placenta. The onset of labor is heralded by multiple factors, including multiple fetal and maternal hormone signals (Mendelson, 2009). It is important the infant be born close to the 40-week gestation mark, as prolonged time in the uterus postterm can be harmful to a fetus.

PRENATAL DEVELOPMENT OF BODY FUNCTION

Perhaps the most important rationale for the study of prenatal development is the fact that not only structure, but also functions or behavior develop in the months in utero. Improving ability to look inside the uterine environment without disturbing or harming the fetus through ultrasound and other radiographic methods have allowed a much better understanding of the normal development of these functions.

MENTAL FUNCTIONS

Of course, studies of mental functions in fetuses are extremely limited and must largely be inferred from observation. However, beginning in the 1940s, an increased interest in prenatal experience as a foundation for postnatal behavior was begun. The study of fetal behavior has been enhanced by ultrasound imaging (Yigiter & Kavak, 2006). Yigiter & Kavak (2006) reported a definition of fetal behavior that is any observable action (or reaction) to an external stimulus. These authors expressed the goal that integrity of the nervous system prenatally could be assessed by an examination of preterm infant behavior. In fact, an assessment

of preterm infant behavior, known as the Kurjak Antenatal Neurodevelopmental Test (KANET), has been developed and has been successfully reported to predict abnormal neurologic outcome from prenatal behavior observation (Abo-Yaqoub, Kurjak, Mohammed, Shadad & Abel-Maaboud, 2012). The KANET is a test named for its principal author and that observes fetal behavior, largely motor in nature, resulting in a score that is hoped to be a valid reflection of brain function (Kurjak, Stanojevic, Prodojevic, Lausin, & Salihagic-Kadic, 2012).

As is true in neonates, one insight into brain function is the regulation of level of arousal. Since the 1980s, four fetal behavioral states have been identified as precursors to the six behavioral states observed postpartum in term neonates. A **behavioral state** is a period of coordinated activity, which in the fetus is punctuated by periods of rest. As mentioned, postnatal behavioral states are considered to be among the most important aspects of behavior in newborn infants. Behavioral state may be defined as the infants' level of arousal mediating responsivity to environmental inputs. The presence of behavioral states in the fetus once again represents the continuity between prenatal and postnatal life. Fetal behavioral State 1F is quiescence, in which there are no fetal eye movements and occasional startles are seen. State 2F is characterized by frequent movements, with associated heart rate changes. State 3F is characterized by eye movements without gross body movements, and State 4F is continuous movement, with eye movement and an unstable and rapid heart rate (Hepper, 2003).

Infants born beyond 35 weeks will respond in similar ways to full-term newborns in most respects. Behavioral states will be well defined, with clearly identifiable sleep and wake states ranging from deep sleep to crying, and smooth transitions between states. Infants born after 34 weeks will be able to escalate to a full cry when upset, but healthy infants born before states have been established will tend to cry less frequently and less intensely when they reach term age than healthy full-term newborns will. Although full-term infants will be able to cry when hungry or in discomfort, infants born prematurely may need close monitoring because they may have difficulty demanding care or expressing their needs through crying or fussing. Quiet alertness will be much improved as infants approach term age. By 36 weeks, most newborn infants will be able to sustain attention for a sufficiently prolonged period to engage in social interaction with a caregiver or to focus on a non-human stimulus for brief periods. The ability to socially interact will make full-term infants active participants in family and society life.

SENSORY FUNCTIONS AND PAIN

Once again, sensory functions must be interpreted from observable physiologic or movement responses in a fetus, rather than from reported subjective experience of the sensation. There are some sensory experiences, such as vision, which are very limited in the uterine environment. The fetus probably has the greatest exposure to sound, touch, and movement. Sound has been studied more than any other sensation, probably because it is an easy stimulus to administer. Studies have shown the fetus clearly responds to sound with a change in movement as early as 24 weeks gestation and with a change in heart rate as early as 28 weeks gestation (Hepper, 2003). Background sounds present in the fetal environment include sounds of placental flow, the mother's heart rate, and digestive sounds. In management of pain in preterm infants, Ludington-Hoe & Hosseini (2005) reported using skin-to-skin contact, commonly known as "kangaroo care" prior to the infant having a heel stick procedure and found this reduced the infant's negative behavioral and physiologic responses significantly as compared to a control condition. Skin-to-skin contact involves laying the infant on the mother's chest, so the infant is exposed not only to the mother's skin, but also to sounds such as the mother's respiration and heart rate, which are familiar and comforting.

Touch is experienced by fetuses from contact with their own body parts, as well as with the constraints of the uterine wall. Research done in the 1940s demonstrated the fetus is capable of response to a tactile stimulus by 8 weeks gestation, making touch the first sensation to show functional activation (Hepper, 2003). Pain experience of the fetus is unknown from a subjective perspective, but a wealth of study on preterm infants substantiates responsiveness to pain including crying, facial grimacing, physiologic change, and elevated cortisol (Luddington-Hoe & Hosseini, 2005).

Movement is another sensory experience to which fetuses are exposed extensively in the prenatal environment. Fetuses are moving actively from about the 8th gestational week. In addition, a fetus is being moved along with the mother. The vestibular system of the inner ear is presumably well developed from this stimulation, and the fetus (premature infant) shows some ability to right itself with respect to gravity from about the 25th week of gestation (Hepper, 2003).

CARDIOVASCULAR, HEMATOLOGICAL, IMMUNOLOGICAL, AND RESPIRATORY SYSTEMS

The heart is the first major organ to develop and begin function in the embryo, with primitive circulation established by the 21st day of life, or by the beginning of the 4th embryonic week. The heart, which develops from cardiogenic mesoderm underneath the prochordal plate, is connected to a reverse fetal circulatory system in which oxygenated blood from the placenta is carried *toward* the heart by the venous system (Moore, Persaud, & Torchia,

2011). The blood entering the heart largely bypasses the lungs in a right to left shunt, exiting in the arterial system and becoming progressively deoxygenated as it is carried away from the heart. Eventually, the deoxygenated blood is carried back to the placenta via the umbilical arteries. Within a few seconds after birth, infants must begin to breathe on their own and must shift from fetal circulation to adult circulation, with oxygenation beginning to occur in the lungs. Crying immediately after birth facilitates lung expansion and the beginning of respiration. The shift from fetal to adult circulation will require closure of the ductus arteriosus and the foramen ovale, two openings that create the anatomic basis for the right to left shunt, enabling circulating blood to bypass the lungs. The *ductus arteriosus* is the passageway that exists between the pulmonary trunk and the aorta that normally closes within the first few hours after birth. Once adult circulation is established, most infants will demonstrate physiologic stability, including thermoregulatory and cardiorespiratory responses. These changes are discussed in greater detail in the following chapter, with fetal circulation illustrated in **Figure 9-1**.

After 36 weeks of gestation, respiratory difficulties are rare. Respiration rates become more regular and slower as the fetus approaches term age, but infants born with very low birth weights will usually have higher respiration rates when they reach term age than will full-term newborns. Such newborns will, in most cases, spontaneously adopt normal respiratory patterns, having practiced the paradoxical pattern of respiration for months in utero (Hepper, 2003). Both heart rate and respiratory rate of prematurely born infants also tend to be higher at term age than for full-term newborns.

NEUROMUSCULOSKELETAL AND MOVEMENT-RELATED FUNCTIONS

Intrauterine fetal body movements have been studied extensively as an indicator of fetal maturation and well-being. Two seminal papers in the 1980s by De Vries, Visser, and Prechtl (1982, 1985) provided elaborate descriptions and characterization of fetal movement. The authors list over 20 characteristic movement patterns of the fetus, such as startles, stretches, hiccups, paradoxical breathing, twitches, and head movements. It is interesting to note the authors include ventroflexion of the head as an observable movement in utero; however, postnatally, it will take several months before that behavior emerges in the context of gravity. This is yet another illustration of the diverse behavioral repertoire that is developing before birth.

One clear trend with increasing maturation is increasing periodicity to fetal movement. Periods of relative rest alternated with periods of activity are characteristic as a fetus approaches term. In fact, the incidence and duration of movement bursts will remain stable, but they will be more spaced apart (Ten Hof et al., 2002). Although the decrease in body movements has been traditionally attributed to intrauterine crowding or greater quiescence, recent evidence suggests that motor activity decreases because of developmental maturation (that is, greater stability and motor control), rather than either increase in quiet states or space restriction (Ten Hof et al., 2002). A similar decrease in motor activity is observed in infants born prematurely as they approach term age.

CONTEMPORARY MEDICAL ISSUES REGARDING PRENATAL DEVELOPMENT

Of course, in the twenty-first century, with the extraordinary technology available to study intrauterine behavior, it is also necessary to discuss medical and scientific issues surrounding the beginning of human life. Meyer (2008) argues when human life begins is *not* obvious as a positivistic fact and suggests tolerance for a variety of opinions. Kurjak, Carrera, McCullough, and Charvenak (2007) elaborated on the problem. These authors argue that at least three questions are involved. The first question is when human *biologic* life begins, which is a matter of science. The second is when health care professionals become obligated to protect human life, which these authors argue is a philosophical and ethical question, subject to greater controversy than the first. Finally, the question exists about how health care professionals should respond to disagreements about when human life begins, which they argue is the subject of ethics. This approach illuminates the complexity of the questions involved, and it is clear the matter will continue to be debated politically and legislatively. Rehabilitation professionals should remain informed about these issues as part of their understanding of prenatal development.

One issue that provokes such a controversy is that of human stem cell research. Stem cells are cells that are largely undifferentiated and retain the ability to develop into several different types of cells. The human stem cells in question are the pluripotent cells of the embryonic blastocyst. These cells can be maintained in culture for years in a suspended undifferentiated state. When they are ready to be used, scientists attempt to force them to differentiate into desired cells for whatever therapeutic intervention is being investigated (Hibaoui & Feki, 2012). This, of course, is also controversial as these cell lineages are from germinal phase embryos obtained for in vitro fertilization. Current U.S. policy limits human stem cell research to those stem cell lines in existence prior to 2001. A Stem Cell Research Enhancement Act to loosen restrictions, passed in Congress in 2005 and 2007, was vetoed by the president in both instances (Moller, 2008). The National Institutes of Health (NIH) approved the first clinical trial using embryonic stem cells in treatment for spinal cord injury (Hibaoui & Feki, 2012). Although the use of embryonic stem cells remains mired in controversy, other sources of stem cells have been developed. For example, stem cells have been obtained from amniotic fluid and umbilical cord blood (Meyer, 2008). Most recently, of great promise, scientists have been able to take human epithelial cells and revert them to a pluripotent state by introducing four genes. These cells, called induced pluripotent stem cells (iPS) are believed to have the pluripotency of human embryonic stem cells, without incurring ethical and moral challenges (Moller, 2008). Furthermore, the possibility of rejection due to immune challenge is also eliminated by iPS, which are derived from a person's own body cells. The production of iPS has led to another line of investigation, that is, whether other cells from an individual can be reprogrammed to replace cells that have been implicated in disease, such as cancer cells (Hibaoui & Feki, 2012). There is no doubt that, looking into the future of medicine and health care, the lessons learned from human genetics and embryology will play a key role in therapy for a variety of health conditions.

SUMMARY

Prenatal development is a fascinating and complex process. This chapter summarizes some relevant aspects for people working in rehabilitation, including the effect of teratogens on development during critical periods and the potential therapeutic use of pluripotent cells in the treatment of conditions such as spinal cord injury and other neurologic diseases. Perhaps of most importance, therapists should appreciate the enormity of change in body structures and function in prenatal life, which prepares humans to be actively participating members of the postnatal environment by the time of birth.

Understanding prenatal development is essential for physical and occupational therapists working with young children. In addition, as medical advances push the boundaries of our understanding, issues such as when life begins and the use of stem cells will continue to be important social issues that may impact personal lives as well as professional practice.

CASE 1

Jeanine

Jeanine is a 36-year-old woman who is pregnant for the third time—this time with twins. She didn't start trying to get pregnant until she was 34 years old, and she has had two miscarriages since then. She is thrilled that she is past the 20-week point in this pregnancy. Overall, she has felt fairly good—hardly any morning sickness, although in the first trimester, she was a little tired. She did everything she could do to protect this pregnancy: ate well, didn't smoke or drink, and got plenty of rest. At her 22-week doctor visit, the doctor said she had oligohydramnios evident on ultrasound. The fetuses were showing signs of distress in ultrasound heart rate monitoring. Jeanine was sent home with a form to monitor fetal movement and told to call her doctor to check in. However, before she could do that, she started to have labor contractions. She came to the hospital, and they bought some time in stopping the contractions with medication; however, about 10 days later, Jeanine delivered 24-week gestation twins: Robbie and Rachel.

The twins were in critical condition for the first few weeks as their lungs were so underdeveloped. They were given artificial surfactant. The twins' size was appropriate for gestational age, which the doctors said was a good sign. When Jeanine first saw her babies, two days after they were born, she cried. They didn't look real to her. They were so small they could fit in the palm of her husband's hand. While they were on the ventilator, they looked very floppy and sick. The nurses attempted to keep them in a flexed position through use of blanket rolls. They couldn't cry because of the ventilator, but they did have spontaneous movements and facial grimaces.

As the weeks progressed, Robbie and Rachel seemed to have a will to live. However, they continued to face struggles. Because of the long time on the ventilator, they both developed bronchopulmonary dysplasia. Like most premature infants, each had a patent ductus arteriosus and a heart murmur, which the cardiologist monitored. They were not very physically attractive babies because they lacked body fat, and their heads were molded somewhat and elongated in the anterior-posterior direction (flattened). Everyone noticed how Robbie liked to be swaddled. It decreased his fussiness and improved his respiratory status. However, no matter what the nursery staff did, Rachel seemed irritable. One day, after the babies were off the ventilators, the nursery staff decided to lay them in the same isolette for a trial. Rachel scooted close to Robbie, who placed his body in contact with hers. Rachel had improved physiologic status due to diminished stress. It was as if the babies were used to being in contact in utero, and when they could reestablish that familiarity from the womb, it made them much calmer.

This case study illustrates what happens when a fetus becomes a baby too soon, when all the body systems are still at a fetal level of maturation, but the environment is very intense and includes everything from gravity to lights and stimulation. For infants as young as Robbie and Rachel, nurseries often implement a minimal-stimulation protocol to minimize the time the babies are touched or handled. Likewise, where possible, attempts are made to avoid extremely bright lights and loud sounds. Every attempt is made to position the babies in flexion, as they would be in utero but are too weak to assume at birth. The long-term effects of such extreme prematurity are constantly studied, and the fact that these babies are kept alive at all is a miracle. Most babies born prematurely do surprisingly well by school age, depending, of course, on how early and how little they were initially. Therapists work to provide an environment that minimizes the trauma to these infants, who by all rights should still be in utero.

Continues

Case 1   *Continued*

Guiding Questions

Some questions to consider:

1. Take the sections of the chapter regarding the development of structures and functions in utero from 22 weeks of gestation to term birth. These twins had to develop those behaviors in the extra-uterine environment. What are the key differences, and how might they have a long-term impact on developmental outcome?
2. Consider environment as a contextual factor. What are the differences between intra- and extra-uterine environments? How can therapists try to minimize the stress of extreme prematurity by environmental modification?

CASE 2

Emmett

My name is Emmett. I'm 22 years old, and I have a disability called arthrogryposis, which affects my joints and general movement. I've had many operations, of which some have been a great success and some have been a waste of time. The operations started before my first birthday, and with every operation there were new braces and casts, and lots of time with the physical and occupational therapist.

They say that this all started about 5 weeks after my mom became pregnant with me. No one knows why but the joint spaces in my arms and legs did not develop as they were supposed to. Because my limbs did not move right, the skin, muscles, and tendons also did not develop right. The surgeries were intended to make my limbs bend in the right place, so I could have ordinary experiences like wearing shoes or being able to reach my mouth. In spite of all the surgeries, I am now confined to a wheelchair. My legs will not hold me up, and I cannot move my ankles or feet.

Although I use a lot of devices to do everyday things, I still need a personal attendant to help me get ready every morning. I am attending college and hope to become an accountant. I am on the slow track rather than the fast track because I was not that great of a student earlier in my life. I never fit in, and I found that people often did not expect much of me. I did not expect much of myself either! The truth is that although my arms and legs do not work for me, there is nothing wrong with my brain. I like math and I like being in my own apartment. Since I have been in college, I have made friends and can go out to movies and restaurants with them. We have fun going to places that are not wheelchair accessible sometimes, because that makes everyone uncomfortable!

They tell me that my condition was random, that there is a strong chance that any child I have would develop typically. It is hard to think about. I wonder whether any woman will ever love me in that way. I also wonder what I would do if an ultrasound told me that my unborn child had the same condition. I have a good life. My life has not been like other people's lives though. I think I would be a good father . . . but I would rather any child of mine had a more ordinary path.

Continues

Case 2 *Continued*

Guiding Questions

Some questions to consider:

1. Using the text and tables presented in the chapter, describe the critical stages in development of the musculoskeletal system, and identify when arthrogryposis might develop.
2. What is the relationship between the closed and cramped environment of the uterus and the positional deformity seen in children with arthrogryposis at birth?

Speaking of
Genetics and Biology

ANNE CRONIN, PhD, OTR/L
PEDIATRIC OCCUPATIONAL THERAPIST

As aspiring therapists and health care providers, you may wonder why you need to learn the biology of what goes on before a person is born, and certainly before a person is your patient. One reason why a basic understanding of prenatal development is needed for contemporary practice is that the rapid improvement in medical technology allows infants to survive at increasingly early times in their gestation, and these children born too soon need therapy support. Another compelling reason is that such knowledge is a tool for understanding and organizing the exponential increases in understanding human genetics. In clinical settings, you will meet both children and adults who have been labeled as having a "genetic disorder" that is rare, newly identified, or has no clinical documentation of its functional impact. For example, birth defects common to the early weeks of gestation, during the formative period for the neural tube, are anencephaly, cephalocele, and the Chiari malformations associated with hydrocephalus. These are profound disorders with a pervasive influence on functional performance.

Additionally, disorders may be specific to an embryologic cell layer, and this is valuable knowledge for therapists to have. Cystic fibrosis is a genetic disorder of the endoderm germ layer. Although cystic fibrosis is primarily perceived as a respiratory disorder, the endoderm is actually the cell layer from which the digestive system, many glands, and parts of the respiratory system are formed. Reflecting this, children with the disease typically have digestive as well as respiratory problems. Arthrogryposis multiplex congenital is a disorder of mesodermal development that results in insufficient and atypical development of the muscles, skin, skeleton, and connective tissues.

Although it may be difficult for clinicians to know and remember all of the possible genetic conditions and their functional manifestations, an understanding of prenatal development provides an invaluable tool for clinical reasoning as you address the needs of your clients.

REFERENCES

Abo-Yaqoub, S., Kurjak, A., Mohammed, A. B., Shadad, A., & Abel-Maaboud, M. (2012). The role of 4-D ultrasonography in prenatal assessment of fetal neurobehaviour and prediction of neurological outcome. *Journal of Maternal, Fetal, and Neonatal Medicine, 25*(3), 231–236.

Bruer, J. T. (2001). A critical and sensitive period primer. In D. B. Bailey, J. T. Bruer, F. J. Symons, & J. W. Lichtman (Eds.), *Critical thinking about critical periods* (pp. 3–26). Baltimore: Brookes.

De Vries, J. P., Visser, G. H., & Prechtl, H. R. (1982). The emergence of fetal behavior. 1. Qualitative aspects. *Early Human Development, 7,* 301–322.

De Vries, J. P., Visser, G. H., & Prechtl, H. R. (1985). The emergence of fetal behavior. 2. Quantitative aspects. *Early Human Development, 12,* 99–120.

England, M. A. (Ed.) (1996). *Life before birth* (2nd ed.). London: Mosby-Wolfe.

Gomella, T. L., Cunningham, M. D., Eyal, F. G., & Zenk, E. (1999) *Neonatology: Management, procedures, on-call problems, diseases and drugs (a Lang clinical manual).* Stamford, CT: Appleton & Lange.

Graham, E. M., & Morgan, M. A. (2002). Growth before birth. In M. Batshaw (Ed.), *Children with disabilities* (pp. 53–70). Baltimore: Brookes.

Hadlock, F. P. (1994). Fetal growth. In M. R. Harrison, M. S. Golbus, & R. A. Filly (Eds.), *Ultrasonography in obstetrics and gynecology* (3rd ed.). Philadelphia: W. B. Saunders.

Hamlin, H. (1964). Life or death by EEG. *Journal of the American Medical Association* (October 12, 1964), 190, 112–114.

Hepper, P. (2003). Prenatal psychological and behavioral development. In J. Valsiner & K. Connolly (Eds.), *Handbook of developmental psychology* (pp. 48–71). London, England: Sage Publications.

Hernandez-Diaz, S., Werler, M. M., Walker, A. M., & Mitchell, A. A. (2001). Neural tube defects in relation to use of folic acid antagonists during pregnancy. *American Journal of Epidemiology, 153,* 961–968.

Hibaoui, Y., & Feki, A. (2012). Human pluripotent stem cells: Applications and challenges in neurological diseases. *Frontiers of Physiology, 3,* 267. E pub ahead of print. doi:10.3389/fphys.2012.00267.

Jirasek, J. E. (2001). *An atlas of the human embryo and fetus—A photographic review of human prenatal development.* New York: Parthenon Publishing Group.

Kanavakis, E., & Traeger-Synodinos, J. (2002). Preimplantation genetic diagnosis in clinical practice. *Journal of Medical Genetics, 39,* 6–11.

Kim, R., & Clark, A. T. (2014) Hatching human blastocyst. *Molecular Reproduction and Development, 81*(3), 283. E pub ahead of print. doi:10.1002/mrd22313

Kurjak, A., Carrera, J. M., McCullough, L. B., & Charvenak, A. (2007) Scientific and religious controversies about the beginning of human life: The relevance of the ethical concept of the fetus as a patient. *Journal of Perinatal Medicine 35*(5), 376–383.

Kurjak, A., Stanojevic, M., Prodojevic, M., Lausin, I., & Salihagic-Kadic, A (2012). Neurobehavior in fetal life. *Seminars in Fetal & Neonatal Medicine, 17*(6), 319–323. E pub ahead of print. doi:10.1016/j.siny.2012.06.005

Ludington-Hoe, S. M., & Hosseini, R. (2005). Skin to skin contact analgesia for preterm infant heel stick. *AACN Clinical Issues, 16*(3), 373–387.

Mendelson, C. R. (2009). Mini-review: Fetal-maternal hormone signaling in pregnancy and labor. *Molecular Endocrinology 23*(7), 947–954.

Meyer, J. R. (2008). Finding ethically acceptable solutions for therapeutic human stem cell research *Ethics & Medicine: An International Journal of Bioethics 24*(1), 1–13.

Moller, M. (2008). Human embryonic stem cell research, justice and the problem of unequal biological access. *Philosophy Ethics Humanity Medicine.* E pub. doi:10.1186/1747-5341-3-22

Moore, K. L., Persaud, T. V. N., & Torchia, M. G. (2011). *The developing human: Clinically oriented embryology* (9th ed.). Philadelphia, PA: Elsevier.

Nishimura, H., Tanimura, T., Semba, R., & Uwabe, C. (1974). Normal development of early human embryos: Observations of 90 specimens at Carnegie Stages 7 to 13. *Teratology, 10,* 1–5.

Nussbaum, R. L., McInnes, R. R., & Willard, H. F. (Eds.) (2007). *Thompson and Thompson genetics in medicine* (7th ed.). Philadelphia: W. B. Saunders.

O'Rahilly, R., & Muller, F. (Eds.) (1987). *Developmental stages in human embryos.* Washington, DC: Carnegie Institution of Washington, Publication 637.

Otten, C., Migliazza, L., Xia, H., Rodriguez, J. I., Diez-Pardo, J. A., & Tovar, J. A. (2000). Neural crest–derived defects in experimental esophageal atresia. *Pediatric Research, 47,* 178.

Pearson, H. (2002). Developmental biology: Your destiny from day one. *Nature, 418,* 14–15.

Polifka, J. E., & Friedman, J. M. (2002). Medical genetics: 1. Clinical teratology in the age of genomics. *CMAJ-JAMC, 167,* 265–273.

Quintero, R. A., Abuhamad, A., Hobbins, J. C., & Mahoney, M. J. (1993). Transabdominal thin-gauge embryofetoscopy: A technique for early prenatal diagnosis and its use in the diagnosis of a case of Meckel-Gruber syndrome. *American Journal of Obstetrics and Gynecology, 168,* 1552–1557.

Richardson, M. K., & Reiss, M. J. (1999). What does the human embryo look like, and does it matter? *The Lancet, 354,* 246–248.

Sawin, S. W., & Morgan, M. A. (1996). Dating of pregnancy by trimesters: A review and reappraisal. *Obstetrical and Gynecological Survey, 51,* 261–264.

Schonberg, R. L. (2012) Birth defects and prenatal diagnosis. In M. Batshaw, N. Roizen, & G. Lotrecchiano (Eds.), *Children with disabilities* (pp. 347–361). Baltimore, MD: Brookes.

Stanojevic, M., Kurjak, A., Salihagic-Kadic, A., Vasili, O., Miskovic, B., Shadded, A., Ahmentr, B., & Tomasovic, S. (2011). Neurobehavioral continuity from fetus to neonate. *Journal of Perinatal Medicine, 39*(2), 171–177.

Ten Hof, J., Nijhuis, I. J. M., Mulder, E. J. H., Nijhuis, J. G., Narayan, H., Taylor, D. J., Westers, P., & Visser, G. H. A. (2002). Longitudinal study of fetal body movements: Nomograms, intrafetal consistency, and relationship with episodes of heart rate patterns A and B. *Pediatric Research, 52,* 568–575.

University of New South Wales. (2012). *Carnegie Stages.* Retrieved from http://php.med.unsw.edu.au/embryology/index.php?title=Carnegie_Stages

Virtual Human Embryo Project (VHE). (2014). Retrieved from http://www.ehd.org/virtual-human-embryo

Yigiter, A. B., & Kavak, Z. M. (2006). Normal standards of fetal behavior assessed by four-dimensional sonography. *Journal of Maternal Fetal Neonatal Medicine, 19*(11), 707–721.

CHAPTER 9

The Newborn

MaryBeth Mandich, PT, PhD,
Professor and Chairperson,
Division of Physical Therapy,
West Virginia University,
Morgantown, West Virginia

Objectives

Upon completion of this chapter, readers should be able to:

- Describe the developmental tasks of neonates, including physiologic and behavioral dimensions;

- Discuss the impact of the birth of a baby on the family;

- Describe the characteristics of premature at-risk newborns and contrast these with those of term neonates; and

- Describe the challenges a birth of a premature newborn places on the family.

Key Terms

anticipatory grief

asymmetrical tonic neck reflex (ATNR)

attractor well

biologic risk

bronchopulmonary dysplasia (BPD)

cerebral palsy

developmentally appropriate care

ductus arteriosus

efficacy

engrossment

entrainment

environmental risk

epigenetics

foramen ovale

gag reflex

gastroesophageal reflux (GER)

hypoxic ischemic
  encephalopathy (HIE)

interactive behaviors

intrauterine growth retardation (IUGR)

intraventricular hemorrhage (IVH)

jaundice

kangaroo care

kernicterus

labyrinthine righting reactions

meconium

minimal-stimulation protocol

Moro reflex

myelination

neonatal abstinence syndrome (NAS)

neonatal intensive care unit (NICU)

neonatal neck-righting reaction

neonatal period

neurogenesis

neuromotor behavior

oral motor reflexes

palmar grasp reflex

patent ductus arteriosus (PDA)

periventricular leukomalacia (PVL)

persistent fetal circulation

persistent pulmonary hypertension

phasic bite reflex

physiologic immaturity

placing reactions

plantar grasp reflex

postural support reaction

preterm infant

primitive stepping

pulmonary hypertension

reflex

respiratory distress syndrome (RDS)

retinopathy of prematurity

rooting reflex

small for gestational age (SGA)

societal-level risk factors

suckling

suck-swallow reflex

synaptogenesis

term infant

tonic labyrinthine reflex

INTRODUCTION

The birth of an infant is an irrevocable and life-altering event. Based on increasing knowledge of the competencies and behaviors of the human fetus, we know that birth represents not the beginning of human behaviors but rather a continuation of behaviors already emerging in utero. However, the challenge for newborns is adaptation to an immensely altered environment that includes gravity and the exposure to air, sound, light, and other stimuli. Babies must take over the functions of respiration and nutrition previously supplied by the placenta. Many body functions and some aspects of body structures, as outlined in the ICF framework, are forced to adapt to these environmental modifications in the first hours and days of life.

For a family, the birth of an infant is an enormous adaptive challenge. The ICF model addresses functions of individuals, but also makes links to the influence of attitudes, supports, and relationships in the environment. Environmental issues are very dynamic during the newborn period. Although many parents approach childbirth with the professed belief that nothing will change after the baby is born, this attitude rarely persists beyond the first few days of parenthood.

These developmental life tasks are challenging in the normative term-birth experience. However, because of the medical ability to save infants who are increasingly younger and sicker, more infants are facing the challenges of prematurity and at-risk birth. Since the early 1970s, the impact of preterm, at-risk birth on infants and their families has been extensively studied. A large number of professionals are involved in supporting these infants and their families in making transitions as easily as possible. It is important for professionals to understand, therefore, both the challenges facing term and at-risk newborns.

THE TERM INFANT

A full-term birth is the birth of a baby 37 weeks or more in gestational age, with the newborn called a **term infant**. A **preterm infant** (also called premature infant) is an infant born at less than 37 weeks gestation. Preterm infants are at greater risk for short- and long-term complications, including disabilities and impediments in growth and mental development. Newborn infants, whether term or preterm, must in the space of an instant take a first breath and begin to adapt to an environment that is extremely different from the aquatic environment of the womb, in which gravity is eliminated, physiologic support is largely provided, and all sorts of environmental stimuli are filtered through amniotic fluid. For the most part, term infants make this transition quite effectively over the first few hours and days of life. The first 4 weeks after birth are known as the **neonatal period**, and babies are commonly referred to as *neonates*. The transitions of the neonatal period encompass all domains of function.

BODY STRUCTURE AND FUNCTION

As discussed in Chapter 8, body structures are formed prenatally. In fact, body structure development, or *morphogenesis*, is most rapid in the embryonic period. Beginning with the fetal period of development, and continuing into postnatal life, structural maturation is driven by functional demands. A number of physiologic systems must respond to the demands of birth. One of the most immediate needs of newborn infants is to acquire oxygen. In utero, the lungs are not necessary to provide oxygen to a fetus, because the majority of oxygenation occurs through the placental circulation. Therefore, the fetal circulatory system bypasses the lungs for the most part as illustrated in **Figure 9-1**. This bypass is called the *right-to-left shunting of blood*, meaning that the blood passes from the right side of the heart directly to the left without passing into the pulmonary circulation. This right-to-left shunting of blood occurs through two major valves. The first, the **foramen ovale**, is an opening between the two atrial chambers of the heart. The second, the **ductus arteriosus**, is the passageway that exists between the pulmonary trunk and the aorta (Lindsay, 1996).

Normally, the ductus arteriosus closes within the first few hours after birth and the foramen ovale within the first two weeks. Occasionally, these pathways do not close off normally, resulting in a persistent postnatal shunting of blood and an associated failure of the pulmonary vascular beds to open and permit sufficient perfusion of the lungs. This condition is known as **persistent fetal circulation** and the associated condition of **persistent pulmonary hypertension**. As the name implies, pulmonary hypertension is high vasomotor tone in the pulmonary vasculature, which helps to keep the fetal circulation away from the lungs and moving through the ductus and foramen ovale. In a normal term birth, these vascular beds should open postpartum, allowing blood flow into the lungs for oxygenation. Failure to do so is considered persistent fetal circulation, which is most commonly seen in slightly preterm infants, 34 to 38 weeks old. It is a medical emergency and must be treated aggressively for the infants to survive. Failure of the ductus arteriosus to close is known as **patent ductus arteriosus (PDA)** and is a condition often seen in premature infants. In most cases, the ductus closes with maturation (Shepherd, Hanshaw, & Lane, 1999).

Another system that experiences dramatic change postpartum is the liver and its ability to make red blood cells (hemopoetic activity). Because of this change, most newborns experience an increase in bilirubin levels in the blood from the breakdown of red blood cells at 24 to 72 hours after birth. This increase in bilirubin causes the infants' skin to have a yellowish cast, known as **jaundice**. Normally, the bilirubin level increase is benign and never approaches levels that would cross the blood-brain barrier. However, bilirubin levels are routinely monitored postpartum, and if the levels increase to a certain point, intervention is warranted.

The most conservative interventions involve placing the infants in direct sunlight. The more aggressive intervention involves placing the infants under phototherapy lights in the blue spectrum or on phototherapy crib pads. The phototherapy light helps metabolize the bilirubin. Excessive bilirubin levels lead to a condition called **kernicterus**. When the bilirubin levels reach the point where the blood-brain barrier is crossed, certain parts of the brain are particularly susceptible. In particular, the basal ganglia, buried deep in the cerebral hemisphere, are susceptible in kernicterus, and before the current era of management, damage to this area resulted in children who had a type of cerebral palsy known as *choreoathetoid* (Long & Toscano, 2002). **Cerebral palsy** is the most common congenital (present from birth) disorder of childhood. It affects muscle tone and coordinated movement, and can result in problems with eating, bladder and bowel control, breathing, and learning. Although the choreoathetoid type of cerebral palsy has become rare in the Western world due to advances in prenatal and perinatal care, it is still occasionally seen, particularly as a sequelae of extreme prematurity.

Of course, the issue of nourishment is another challenge for neonates. Within the first few hours of life, infants normally take their first feeding. Even immediately postpartum, infants will often, if laid upon their mother's chest, attach to a breast and begin to suck. The mother produces a nutritive substance called *colostrum* for the first 48 to 72 hours after birth. This substance is viscous, clear, and full of antibodies that are passed from mother to infant. Normally, if the mother is breast-feeding, her milk comes in after the first few days. Breast-feeding has been known to have many positive effects on newborns and infants in the first year of life. First, and most important, breast-feeding protects newborns from infections and therefore reduces infant mortality. Breast-feeding has also been shown in some studies to have long-term impact on factors such as serum cholesterol, obesity, and even intellectual development (WHO, 2012). A recent study showed that social engagement, including breast-feeding, lowered newborn cortisol levels in the first six hours of life. Cortisol is a hormone secreted when infants are stressed (Elverson, Wilson, Herzog, & French, 2012), and high cortisol levels are associated with poorer health outcomes throughout life.

The process of elimination, or voiding, also undergoes change in the first few days postnatally. Initially infants void a thick, tarry substance known as **meconium**. This substance is normally voided in utero as well but is absorbed

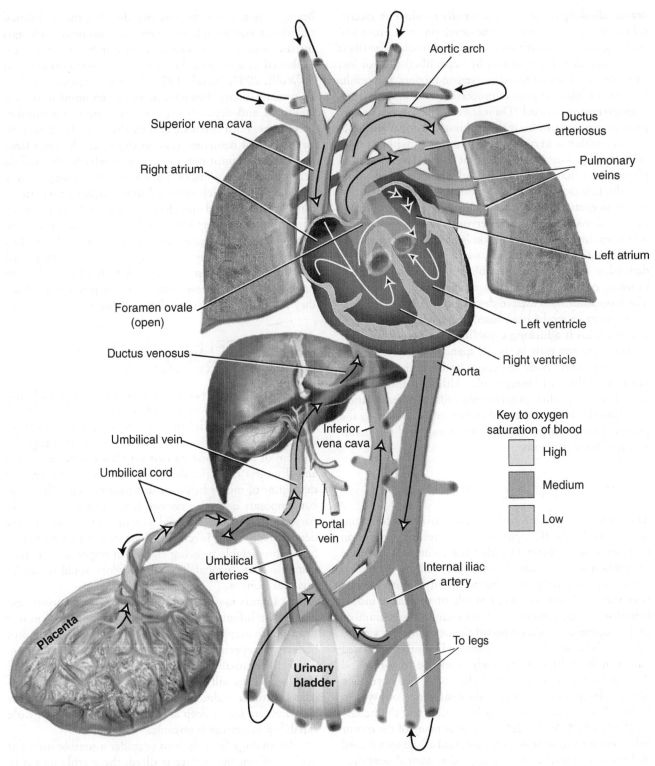

Figure 9-1   Fetal Circulation before Birth

in the amniotic fluid. Meconium staining of the amniotic fluid is one sign of fetal distress, and it is possible for infants to swallow the meconium during labor and birth. This is called *meconium aspiration,* and it is a condition that can result in asphyxia and brain damage if not recognized and treated (Shepherd, Hanshaw, & Lane, 1999).

The newborn central nervous system has largely completed cellular differentiation by the fifth gestational month. **Neurogenesis** is the term applied to the differentiation of new nerve cells. Subsequent development of the nervous system is a function of other processes. For example, *myelin* is the fatty substance that covers and protects nerves, allowing nerve fibers to rapidly conduct an electrical potential. **Myelination** is the developmental process of building a myelin sheath on the nerves to insulate the fibers and ensure that messages sent by nerve fibers are not lost en route. Myelination speeds nerve conduction, and results in more efficient cognitive processing and more refined sensory-motor control (Dubois et al., 2014). A related process, **synaptogenesis**, is the building of specialized junctions at which a nerve cell communicates with a target cell. Myelination and synaptogenesis are developmental phenomena that continue through the preschool years, and the functional impact of these processes will be discussed in greater length in later chapters. Further development and maturation of the nervous system is dependent on the environment. Myelination is particularly dependent on adequate infant nutrition, whereas synaptogenesis is dependent on nerve fibers establishing useful connections or losing connections that are not functionally meaningful. The term *plasticity* is used to describe the ability of the nervous system to model itself based on activity over synaptic circuits. This is a lifelong capability, but the capacity for change is greatest early in the life span.

In summary, body structures and functions in newborns are inherently inseparable. Although the prenatal period is a time when programmed cellular differentiation underlies the establishment of body form, exposure to the postnatal environment activates functions that direct maturation of body structure.

MOVEMENT FUNCTIONS

The study of **neuromotor behavior**, or movement functions as classified by the ICF, provides an interesting application of motor control theory in a historical context. Work done on anencephalic infants (infants born without a cerebral cortex) in the early part of the twentieth century showed that these infants displayed much of the same motor behavior as term neonates. For this reason, a large number of developmental studies reflected the maturationist view of neonatal behavior. This view, espoused by such renowned names in the field of infant study as Myrtle McGraw and Arnold Gesell, states that the behavior of newborns is a direct reflection of the parts of the central nervous system (CNS) that are functionally capable of directing this behavior (Goldfield & Wolff, 2002). Because many of the motor behaviors seen in neonates are processed at the spinal cord and brain stem levels, it was thought that normal newborns were largely subcortical creatures. It was not until the neurobehavioral studies of the latter part of the twentieth century revealed the immense variability and function of the neonates' behavioral repertoire that the view of neonates as functioning at subcortical levels was rejected.

Likewise, for motor behavior, the maturationist view held that motor behavior developed hierarchically in conjunction with the progressive maturation of the higher brain centers. Over the past two decades, the traditional reflexive, hierarchical frame of reference has been challenged by the premise that neonatal motor behavior is best explained by a systems theory of motor control (Goldfield & Wolff, 2002; Horak, 1991; Thelen & Spencer, 1998). In systems theory, behavior at any given point in time is emergent and depends on the interaction of a number of systems, both intrinsic and extrinsic to the organism. In the case of neonates, systems theory challenges a large number of assumptions about motor behavior (Goldfield & Wolff, 2002). Work by Thelen and Heriza suggests that the manner in which neonatal motor behavior has traditionally been studied and characterized is valid only for the environmental constraints in which the behavior occurs. For example, neonates are clearly capable of kicking when supine and performing a stepping pattern when supported in an upright position. Thelen and Fisher found that the only difference in these patterns is the posture in which they are produced (Heriza, 1991; Thelen & Fisher, 1982).

MOTOR REFLEX FUNCTIONS: NEONATAL REFLEXES

The neonatal reflex was traditionally considered the building block of neonatal motor behavior (Goldfield & Wolff, 2002). A **reflex** is defined as a stereotypic obligatory response to a given stimulus. Newer theorists challenge the concept of reflexes, stating that very few normal behaviors actually meet the strict definition of reflex. A conceptual descriptor of motor behavior in neonates that reflects the contemporary notion of systems is the term **attractor well**. An attractor well is a preferred pattern of movement. A very deep attractor well is reflected by a motor pattern that is highly predictable in being elicited in response to a given stimulus. Many neonatal motor behaviors would fall under this classification.

As infants mature and motor behavior repertoire expands, the infants experiment with a number of motor strategies to accomplish functional movement. The motor behavioral repertoire becomes less predictable and more variable. Eventually, through processes of maturation and learning, babies will develop preferred strategies to accomplish functional tasks. The preferred strategies are attractor wells that are not as deep as those of early life, where little variability in strategy is possible.

An analogy for this is to consider a marble on a flat surface. When the surface is tilted, the marble moves in any direction in response to the tilt. If the surface is topographically changed to have peaks and valleys (wells), the marble will move toward the well, but in different circumstances, it can vary its path. However, if the attractor well is very deep, the marble will nearly always find that well, irrespective of the stimuli around it (Shumway-Cook & Woollacott, 2012). These very deep attractor wells typify the motor behavior of newborns. However, the old terminology of *reflexes* is commonly used in the literature and in the clinical environment. Therefore, the so-called *neonatal reflexes* are described separately as follows in the ensuing discussion. Keep in mind that current research is challenging the stereotypic and obligatory nature of the normal patterns of movement, going so far as to say that these aforementioned characteristics are signs of abnormality. Rather, these patterns previously thought of as reflexes are highly preferred strategies that are not obligatory in that they can be altered under various circumstances, such as internal and external environmental characteristics (Goldfield & Wolff, 2002).

One final concept is extremely important in understanding the role of these neuromotor patterns that have traditionally been called reflexes. That is, many of the patterns seen in term newborns must be *integrated* to permit more complex and mature neuromotor patterns to develop. Integration means that the reflexive pattern is no longer a highly predictable or preferred pattern. Maturation of the nervous system in combination with environmental experience and practice promotes the development of more variable patterns of neuromotor behavior that underlie functional accomplishments (Eliot, 1999). It is very important to understand, though, that while integration means the reflex is no longer a dominant feature of infant behavior that is easily visible, the pattern itself has not been erased from memory. In fact, the pattern of the neonatal reflexes can be brought out in stressful situations as well as when the nervous system sustains damage. The reemergence of these patterns following neurologic damage such as stroke or head injury presents a challenge to therapists in positioning and handling clients. Therefore, it is important to learn the typical stimulus-response characteristics of these patterns, not only to understand normal infant development but also to understand how to intervene in a therapeutic situation. These so-called infant reflexes are described in the following text and photos, and are summarized in **Table 9-1**.

Oral Motor Reflexes

Among the earliest reflex behaviors observed are the reflexes associated with eating and swallowing. **Oral motor reflexes** are those reflexes specific to the muscle actions of the mouth and oral area. Several oral motor reflexes are present in healthy newborns. See **Table 9-1** for a summary of reflex activity in neonates.

Suck-Swallow Reflex

Of all the neonatal motor behaviors, the most basic is the one associated with the intake of nourishment, or the **suck-swallow reflex**. First appearing around the 28th week of gestation, this pattern is well established by birth. The stimulus to elicit this pattern is downward pressure on the tongue, and the response is a rhythmical sucking

movement. The early oral motor behavior of the neonate is differentiated from the more mature patterns developed by the end of the first early infancy, or the first three postnatal months. Neonates tend to respond with a total forward and down movement of lips, tongue, and jaw followed by a backward and upward retraction. Thus, neonates are actually pressing the nipple or teat to the hard palate and using a process of positive pressure, or expression, to obtain milk. The amount of negative pressure or suction that neonates can generate is limited because of weakness of the lip, tongue, and cheek musculature. This neonatal pattern of movement is called **suckling**. Over the first few months of life, infants begin to develop the ability to disassociate lip, tongue, and jaw movement and create negative pressure, or suction, in the intra-oral cavity. When this occurs, the pattern more resembles a mature pattern and is known as *sucking*. The normal suckling pattern of neonates is highly rhythmical and is characterized by a burst of several sucks followed by a pause. The rhythmicity of this pattern is important, and dysfunction in developing this pattern is often a problem for premature infants in making the transition to oral feeding. Typically, the suck-swallow pattern is linked, with a burst of sucks followed by a swallow (Goldfield & Wolff, 2002).

Phasic Bite Reflex

Neonates have a **phasic bite reflex**. This reflex is elicited by pressure on the gums, with a normative response being an up-and-down motion of the jaw that often accompanies the feeding behavior. A sustained bite in response to touch in or near the mouth, which infants are unable to release, is a *tonic bite reflex,* and is never normal. This type of abnormal pattern may be indicative of CNS damage, as in perinatal asphyxia (Kedesky & Budd, 1998).

Gag Reflex

The **gag reflex** develops later in utero than the primary feeding reflexes, not making its appearance until the 34th week of gestation. The gag reflex is elicited by touch of the posterior half to third of the tongue or the soft palate/uvula region. The normal response is a gagging pattern. The gag reflex plays an important role in feeding development in preterm infants. Because of its relatively late appearance, it is one factor associated with the standard caregiving practice of avoiding oral feeding in preterm infants until they have reached approximately the 34th gestational week (Kedesky & Budd, 1998).

Rooting Reflex

Another neonatal behavior associated with feeding is the familiar **rooting reflex** (see **Figure 9-2**). The rooting reflex

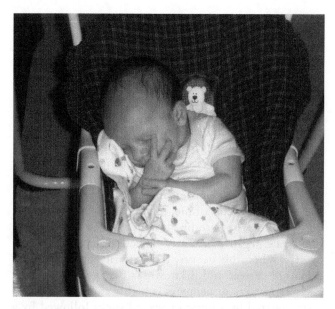

Figure 9-2   Rooting Reflex as Infant Gets Hand to Mouth

is elicited by perioral touch. The stimulus is to stroke on either side of an infant's cheek. A normal response is to turn toward the stimulus. If the upper lip is stroked, the infant extends the head. If the lower lip is stroked, mouth opening occurs. This reflex is the vestige of early patterns allowing newborns of other species born with their eyes closed to seek out the maternal teat (Hepper, 2002; Kedesky & Budd, 1998).

Tonic Labyrinthine Reflex

Tonic postural reflexes are activated by head and neck movements and influence the distribution of muscle tone throughout the body. The **tonic labyrinthine reflex** plays a role in mediating the strong early patterns of flexion seen in newborns (see **Figures 9-3** and **9-4**). The sensory trigger for this reflex is head position. When infants are prone, systemic flexion is facilitated; and when infants are supine,

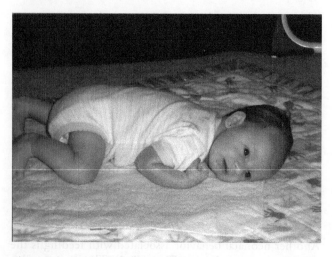

Figure 9-3   Resting Posture in Prone—Position Dominated by Flexion

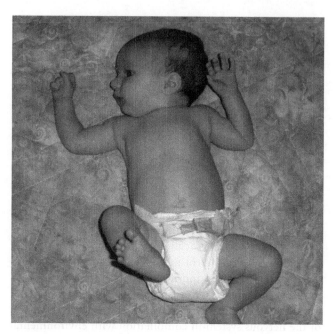

Figure 9-4   Resting Posture in Supine—Still Flexed but More Inclination toward Extension

systemic extension is facilitated. Thus, the effect of the tonic labyrinthine reflexes is to pull infants into the supporting surface; therapists describe this as being pulled *into gravity* (Hepper, 2002).

Labyrinthine Righting Reactions

From the moment infants enter a gravity environment, the tonic labyrinthine reflexes are in competition with the development of antigravity behaviors. An antigravity behavior is an active movement upward, away from the supporting surface. In newborns, antigravity behaviors are mediated by the **labyrinthine righting reactions**. The righting reactions as a group are a number of upper brain stem–mediated responses that either align the body with respect to gravity or the support surface, or rotate the body parts into alignment with each other, thereby permitting the individual to change positions, as in rolling. The labyrinthine righting reaction is the first to appear. The stimulus for this reflex, as in the tonic labyrinthine reflex, is position of the head or body in space. However, in this case, the response is an antigravity response, allowing an infant to lift up into extension when prone, or lift into flexion from the supine position. At birth, the labyrinthine righting reactions are barely evident but can be seen when infants are held in prone suspension and can lift their head into alignment with the body. Alternatively, parents see evidence of labyrinthine righting when they lay their newborn facedown and the baby slightly lifts and turns his or her head to the side. Often, the amount of head righting evident is variable in accordance with the arousal level of the infant. Infants who are

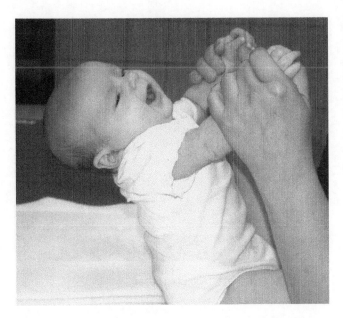

Figure 9-5   Head Lag in Pull-to-Sit Maneuver

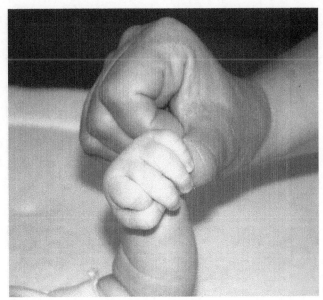

Figure 9-6   Palmar Grasp

agitated or crying may lift their head up farther. Another test of early labyrinthine righting is to pull a newborn to a sitting position. Normally the head lags back into extension for most of the pull to sit; however, as the infant approaches the supported sitting position, there are brief attempts to bob the head erect (see **Figure 9-5**).

Over the first 6 months of life, the labyrinthine righting reaction totally subsumes the tonic labyrinthine reactions such that by 6 months, infants can fully extend in prone and will lift the head to help in the pull-to-sit maneuver.

Neonatal Neck Righting

The first of the rotary righting reactions to develop is the **neonatal neck-righting reaction**, which is also present at birth. This is an immature example of the rotary righting reactions. The task accomplished by rotary righting reactions is to allow the infant to transfer from one postural set to another (that is, prone to supine). The neonatal neck-righting reaction is immature in that when the infant's head is turned passively, the body follows "like a log," rotating in a nonsegmental fashion. Because of the lack of antigravity control at birth, combined with immature rotary righting reactions, the neonatal neck righting is not sufficient to complete a roll from supine to prone position. Rather, it will allow the infant to roll from back to side and vice versa. The truly mature rolling pattern is not seen until approximately 4 months of age.

Grasp Reflexes

The grasp reflexes are highly predictable in newborns. Most obvious is the **palmar grasp reflex** (see **Figure 9-6**). This pattern occurs in response to pressure

in the palm, usually by an examiner placing a finger in the infant's palm. The response is that the infant's fingers curl around the examiner's finger, appearing to grasp. The **plantar grasp reflex** is similar, but the stimulus is a pressure across the metatarsal heads just under the toes (see **Figure 9-7**). The response is grasping of the toes (Hepper, 2002). This pattern is seen later as infants try to stand. The plantar grasp reflex represents a very primitive attempt at balance.

Placing Reactions

The **placing reactions** are also present in both hands and feet. The stimulus to these reactions is to stroke the back

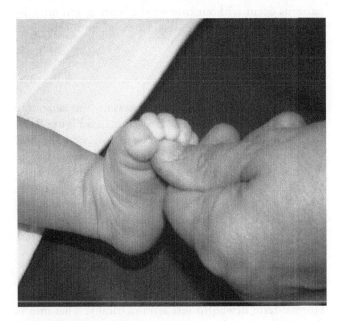

Figure 9-7   Plantar Grasp

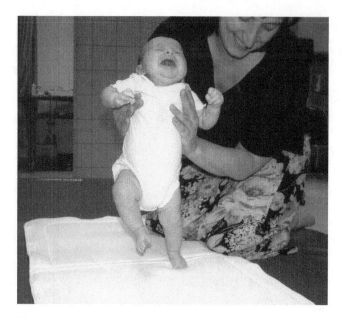

Figure 9-8   Primitive Stepping Pattern

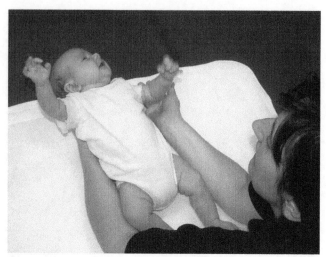

Figure 9-9   Moro Reflex (Abduction Phase)

of the hand or top of the foot as against a tabletop. Infants will lift the limb in flexion, and then extend the limb as if to place it on the table.

Standing Reactions

Two key patterns are seen in standing. One is the **postural support reaction**. When infants are held in vertical suspension and the feet are placed on the surface, the positive support reaction mediates extension through the lower limbs. If an infant is subsequently tipped slightly forward, she will spontaneously and reciprocally flex one leg and extend the other in alternating patterns. This is called **primitive stepping** (see **Figure 9-8**). Both of these patterns occur without true weight bearing and must be integrated to permit true weight bearing and walking to occur (Hepper, 2002).

Moro Reflex

A key pattern used in all neonatal assessment to determine neurologic integrity is the **Moro reflex** (see **Figure 9-9**). In the Moro reflex, the infant's head is dropped backward, stimulating the vestibular system of the inner ear. The response to the stimulus is abduction of the arms, followed by adduction of the arms across the chest (Hepper, 2002). The Moro is also a very predictable aspect of normal newborn behavior. Total absence of this reflex is a sign of neurologic problems. Asymmetry of the Moro may indicate a problem such as a brachial plexus palsy or stroke.

Asymmetrical Tonic Neck Reflex

Normal-term newborns rest asymmetrically. That means their head is turned to one side or the other, virtually never

remaining in the midline. Beginning at birth and peaking over the first 2 months of life, a typical postural set is mediated by the **asymmetrical tonic neck reflex (ATNR)** (see **Figure 9-10**). The stimulus for the ATNR is turning the head to one side. The response is very typical. The upper and lower limbs on the side toward which the infant is looking (that is, the face side) extend. The upper and lower limbs facing the back of the head (the skull side) flex. This creates a postural set symbolic of the en guarde position in fencing, so the pattern is sometimes referred to as the *fencing position* (Hepper, 2002). The ATNR is believed to play a role in establishing linkages between the dominant hand and the eyes, because it tends to be stronger to the right in most infants. An obligatory ATNR or persistence of the ATNR beyond 4 to 5 months of age is an unfavorable neurologic sign. The ATNR must be integrated to permit more mature behaviors, such as hands to midline and hands to mouth to emerge.

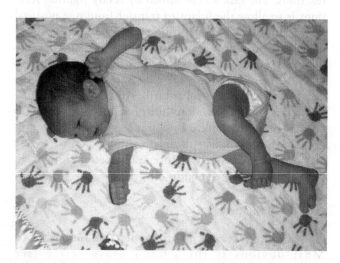

Figure 9-10   ATNR Pattern in the Supine Position

TABLE 9-1 Summary of Reflex Activity in Neonate

I. The primitive gravity-dependent influences of the tonic labyrinthine reflexes compete with the very early development of the labyrinthine righting reaction.

Tonic Labyrinthine Reflex (Prone, Supine)

Onset	Prenatal
Integration	6 months
Position	1. Prone 2. Supine
Procedure	Observe the child's tone and posture in prone and supine positions. Child in prone, lift head; evaluate presence of flexor tone. Child in supine, pull-to-sit, noting presence of extensor tone.
Response	Prone, flexor tone dominates; child will not lift head. Supine, extensor tone dominates; child will not flex in pull-to-sit.
Significance	Persistence will preclude ability to roll and to develop antigravity behaviors.

Labyrinthine Righting Reaction

Onset	Birth to 2 months
Integration	Persists through life
Position	Hold child vertically under the arms, tilting child in space.
Procedure	Tilt child's body in all directions.
Response	Head orients to vertical position and is steady, maintained in proper orientation to environment.
Significance	Persistence will prohibit antigravity behaviors; this is the starting point for the Landau reflex.

II. The hands are predominantly flexed; grasping (finger and toe flexion) is dominant.

Palmar Grasp Reflex

Onset	Birth to 2 months
Integration	4 to 11 months
Position	Place child supine with head in midline and hands free.
Procedure	Place index finger into the infant's hands with pressure over the metacarpal heads.
Response	Fingers will flex around the examiner's.
Significance	Cannot utilize volitional reach and grasp until integrated.

Plantar Grasp Reflex

Onset	Prenatal
Integration	9 months
Position	Place child supine with head in midline and legs relaxed.
Procedure	Place firm pressure against volar aspect of foot, directly below toes.
Response	Plantar flexion of toes occurs.
Significance	Indicates an immature attempt to maintain stability; should disappear in standing, coinciding with mature postural equilibrium.

III. The newborn is born with certain reflexes ensuring survival.

Rooting Reaction

Onset	Prenatal
Integration	3 months

Continues

TABLE 9-1   Summary of Reflex Activity in Neonate   *(continued)*

Position	Place child supine with head in midline.
Procedure	Using your finger, stroke the perioral skin at the corner of the mouth, moving laterally toward the cheek, upper lip, and lower lip.
Response	Infant turns head toward stimulus; if to lower lip, mouth tends to open.
Significance	Is rarely absent when infant is not satiated; absence may indicate CNS depression.

Suck-Swallow Reflex

Onset	Prenatal
Integration	2 to 5 months
Position	Place child supine with head in midline.
Procedure	Place finger or nipple into the infant's mouth.
Response	Rhythmic suckling movements occur; lips, tongue, and jaw move synchronously, first down and forward, then up and back.
Significance	Rarely suppressed in nonsatiated infant; absence may indicate CNS depression.

IV. The infant's motor abilities in postural control and mobility are composed of some of the following additional characteristic patterns.

Traction Response

Onset	Prenatal
Integration	2 to 5 months
Position	Place child supine with head in midline.
Procedure	Grasp child's wrists and pull toward sitting position.
Response	Flexion of shoulders, elbows, wrist, and fingers occurs.
Significance	Persistence will inhibit voluntary use of arms.

Moro Reflex

Onset	Prenatal
Integration	5 to 6 months
Position	Place child supine with head in midline.
Procedure	Support infant's head and shoulders with hands and allow head to drop back 20 to 30 degrees with respect to trunk, stretching neck muscles.
Response	Abduction of the upper extremities with extension of the elbows, wrists, and fingers occurs, followed by subsequent adduction of the arms at the shoulders and flexion at the elbows.
Significance	Is part of any standard neurologic assessment of newborns; although frequently the adduction component is variable, total absence of this reflex is usually indicative of neurologic abnormality.

Galant's Response (Incurvation of the Trunk)

Onset	Prenatal
Integration	By end of third postnatal month
Position	Place infant prone (in horizontal suspension) over your hand.
Procedure	Stroke with pressure along a paravertebral line.
Response	Trunk curves with shortening on the stimulated side.
Significance	May be useful in early evaluation of children with spina bifida to determine where trunk muscles are innervated.

Continues

TABLE 9-1 Summary of Reflex Activity in Neonate *(continued)*

Neonatal Neck Righting

Onset	Prenatal
Integration	Second trimester as mature neck righting develops
Position	Place child supine with head in midline.
Procedure	Lift and turn child's head to side.
Response	Child's body follows "like a log," that is, nonsegmentally.
Significance	Often persists in the presence of spasticity; will prohibit normal de-rotative rolling.

Asymmetric Tonic Neck Reflex (ATNR)

Onset	Birth to 2 months
Integration	4 to 6 months
Position	Place child supine.
Procedure	Have child turn head to one side.
Response	Extension of the arm and leg to which the face is turned occurs, along with flexion of the opposite limbs, producing an apparent "en guarde" fencing posture.
Significance	In normal development probably is responsible for early linkages between eyes and hands. Is not uncommonly apparent in the motor behavior of adults and children with CNS damage; when present and obligatory, prevents symmetrical behaviors, hand to mouth, and may contribute to the development of scoliosis.

Placing Reactions (Arms and Legs)

Onset	Arms = birth; legs = prenatal
Integration	By end of third postnatal month
Position	Hold child upright, in vertical suspension.
Procedure	Brush the dorsum of child's hand or foot against tabletop.
Response	The limb lifts in flexion, then is followed by extension as if to place it on the table.
Significance	Seen in CNS damage.

V. Movement patterns of the lower extremities are strongly reciprocal and reflect the spinal cord organization of the agonist/antagonist relationships between flexors and extensors. Central pattern generators (clusters of neurons which fire in alternate sequence) may be involved.

Flexor Withdrawal

Onset	Prenatal
Integration	By end of third postnatal month
Position	Place child supine with head in midline and legs relaxed.
Procedure	Apply noxious stimulus, such as pinprick, to sole of foot.
Response	Stimulated leg reacts with flexion at hip, knee, and ankle, withdrawing the extremity.
Significance	A withdrawal to a painful stimulus persists throughout life; however, it becomes localized to just a jerk of the ankle; the reflex is correctly named for the total withdrawal of the limb and is integrated in early life.

Crossed Extension

Onset	Prenatal
Integration	By end of third postnatal month
Position	Place child supine with head in midline.

Continues

TABLE 9-1	Summary of Reflex Activity in Neonate *(continued)*

Procedure	Hold one leg straight; apply firm pressure or noxious stimulus to sole of foot.
Response	Flexion, adduction, and then extension of the opposite leg.
Significance	Represents spinal cord neural networks that will lay the foundation for reciprocal pattern of locomotion.

Neonatal Positive Supporting

Onset	Prenatal
Integration	By end of third postnatal month
Position	Support infant in vertical suspension with your hands under arms and around trunk.
Procedure	Allow feet to make contact with support surface.
Response	Co-contraction of lower extremity muscles occurs, with limb support of minimal body weight.
Significance	Indicates normal muscle tone; if persists, may be associated with high muscle tone, as in spastic diplegia.

Spontaneous Stepping

Onset	Near birth
Integration	By end of third postnatal month
Position	Support child as in vertical suspension as described previously, but lean infant's body weight forward.
Procedure	Hold infant upright in vertical suspension, touching feet to support surface. Lean infant slightly forward to elicit stepping.
Response	Alternating stepping movements occur.
Significance	May persist, as in spastic diplegia.

CONTROL OF VOLUNTARY MOVEMENT IN THE NEONATAL PERIOD

The reflexive patterns of behavior just described dominate newborns' motor behavior. Functionally at birth, newborns' motor behavior is fairly limited and gravity dependent. This means that newborns are unable to work against gravity and move upward against gravity. In prone position, newborns are able to lift the head and turn it from side to side. Flexion is noted in upper and lower limbs. In supine, the head is typically turned to the side. Reciprocal kicking is noted. Infants will direct hand to mouth with varying degrees of success. In pull-to-sit, there is total head lag, but when infants are held supported in sitting, the head will bob erect into a neutral position. In supported standing, there is some acceptance of weight, but the standing pattern is immature and the weight is largely supported.

It is easy to see that if neuromotor behavior alone is considered, it could be assumed that an infant's nervous system is extremely immature. It used to be thought that the higher cortical centers were not active in newborn infants, because many of the reflexive patterns as described previously are present in anencephalic infants. However, studies of other aspects of newborn infant behavior do not support that assumption.

MENTAL FUNCTION AND BEHAVIORAL STATE

One of the most important aspects of behavior in newborn infants is the concept of behavioral state. *Behavioral state* may be defined as the infants' level of arousal mediating the responsivity to environmental inputs. The notion of behavioral state can be studied at two levels. The first level is physiologic and includes such data as analyzing the brain activity of the infants. The second is behavioral, analyzing the infants' behavioral response to stimulation (Wilhelm, 1993).

Physiologic studies of infant behavioral state utilize data such as the study of brain wave activity through electroencephalograms (EEGs). Basically, there is an attempt to identify clusters of brain activity that are differentiated from other clusters and that correlate with level of arousal. From these studies, it has been found that the first signs of behavioral state organization are not seen until infants reach 32 weeks gestational age. Between 32 weeks and term, there is increasing organization of characteristic cycles such that by term, three identifiable states are seen. These loosely correspond to wakefulness, rapid eye movement (REM) sleep, and non–rapid eye movement (NREM) sleep (Freudigman & Thoman, 1994). Other states are termed transitional.

Behavioral state as measured from the infants' behaviors such as responsivity to stimuli has become the benchmark for all assessment of term infant behavior. First classified for evaluative purposes by neurologist Heinz Prechtl in 1974, six behavioral states have been identified. The concept of behavioral state was further defined and incorporated into the Neonatal Behavior Assessment Scale (BNBAS) (Brazelton & Nugent, 1995). Since the widespread incorporation of behavioral state into that assessment, common definitions for the behavioral states are as follows, always indicated by the Roman numerals preceding them:

- *Behavioral State I* is deep sleep, corresponding to NREM sleep. There is no eye movement, there are no spontaneous startles, and infants are difficult to rouse.

- *Behavioral State II* is active, or REM, sleep. In this state, startles are elicited. Infants may make spontaneous movements but will settle down quickly.

- *Behavioral State III,* in which infants are in transition from sleep to wakefulness. One eye may be open, or both eyes may partially open. Infants appear to rouse but then seem drawn back into sleep.

- *Behavioral State IV* is extremely significant because of its importance in establishing social relationships and early learning. This state is called *quiet alert* and is the optimum behavioral state for evaluation (see **Figure 9-11**). In this state, infants do not have a great deal of extraneous body movement. They are visually attentive and will fixate on a stimulus.

- *Behavioral State V* is active alert. Infants maintain eyes open, but extraneous body movements interfere with sustained attention.

- *Behavioral State VI* is crying. Infants are aroused but are crying and therefore do not engage in interaction.

Infants' behavioral state determines their responsiveness to different stimuli; therefore, it is extremely important that assessments be done as close to Behavioral State IV as possible. Infants may appear abnormally unresponsive during an exam if the entire exam is carried out in nonoptimal behavior states (Brazelton & Nugent, 1995).

SENSORY FUNCTIONS

As the preceding discussion implies, the behavioral assessment of state is largely dependent on the infants' response to sensory stimulation. Term newborns have all senses functioning, although some are relied upon more than others. The sense of smell is highly developed in term newborns. Studies have shown that as early as the first week of life, infants can distinguish breast milk from their mother soaked on a breast pad from that of another women (Schaal et al., 1980). Likewise, the sense of taste appears to develop fairly early. Studies have shown that infants display preferences for different tastes. In a study by Mendella and Beauchamp (1996), when vanilla was added to either breast milk or formula, infants sucked longer and consumed more milk. These authors concluded their study by suggesting that one additional benefit of breast-feeding was that infants are exposed to a rich experience of foods that may help familiarize them with dietary habits of a given culture.

The sense of touch is very well developed in newborn infants. The somatosensory cortex, which processes touch information, is the most mature of the sensory cortical areas at birth (Lundy-Ekman, 2012). Klaus, Kennell, Plumb, and Zuehlke (1970) described the immediate postpartum behavior of infant-mother dyads. They reported that mothers typically initiated a period of massage of their newborns, beginning on the extremities and ending with palmar contact on the trunk. Bystrova et al. (2009) reported that mother-infant relationship was affected as long as a year after birth by skin-to-skin contact and early suckling, or both. The authors concluded, as have many others, that the first postnatal hours are important to the formation of the mother-infant bond. The importance of touch to the mother-infant relationship was first proposed in the classic Harlow study, which showed that infant monkeys would prefer a cloth-covered surrogate to a wire-covered surrogate that dispensed food (Harlow, 1958). The prominent infancy researcher Tiffany Field has studied the effects of massage on premature infants and found that massage can enhance weight gain and improve sociobehavioral responses. Massage has also been shown to positively affect the performance of neonates on habituation items of the Brazelton Neonatal Behavioral Assessment Scales (NBAS) (Scafidi, Field, & Schanberg, 1993). Many studies have shown that physiologic indices of stress in infants may be

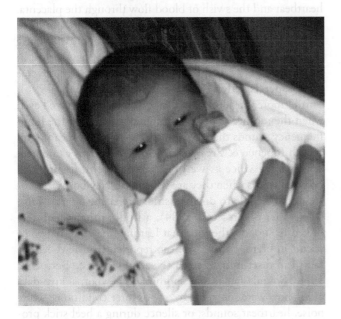

Figure 9-11 Newborn in Behavior State IV

impacted by tactile stimulation. Feldman, Rosenthal, and Eidelman (2014) reported preterm infants who received maternal touch through a caregiving protocol known as "kangaroo care" demonstrated effects in multiple systems up to 10 years of age. In summary, the tactile system is fairly well functioning in term newborns at birth, and provision of sensory input over that system appears to enhance the well-being of sick or distressed infants.

Related to the sense of touch is the vestibular/proprioceptive sensory modality. This modality mediates the responsivity to position and movement. Of all sensory experiences, perhaps none is as practiced at birth as this, for infants have been moving in an aquatic environment for some months. Once exposed to the extrauterine environment of gravity, the infants' motor responses are primarily the source of inferences about the functioning of this system. For example, the Moro and labyrinthine reactions occur in response to vestibular inputs. The classic work of Korner and Thoman (1970) showed that the infants' level of arousal was affected by positioning, with the upright position promoting a more alert state. Rocking, which has long been a way to quiet fretful infants, is also a vestibular mediated sensory experience.

The two sensory systems that have received the most attention in infant research are those of vision and hearing. With respect to vision, prior to the mid-twentieth century it was believed that for all intents and purposes, newborn infants were blind, because of the inability to form meaningful perceptions (Lamb & Campos, 1982). Fantz reported breakthrough studies on visual perception in infants in the 1960s. These classic studies showed that newborn infants had clear visual preferences. For example, infants preferred black-and-white patterned stimuli to gray, and a facial stimulus to a neutral stimulus (Fantz, 1961; Fantz, 1963). Subsequently, it was suggested that it was the high contrast inherent in the face pattern, not the face itself that was appealing to newborns (Lamb & Campos, 1982). However, more recent work continues to contribute to the premise that there is something about the human face that has intrinsic appeal to newborns. Walton, Bower, and Bower (1992) reported that by 1 to 2 days of age, infants seem to recognize images of their mother's face as compared with the face of a stranger by changes in the infant's sucking response. These same authors have reported that infants seem to be able to discriminate the mother's face and recognize it through a variety of rotations and transformations (Walton, Armstrong, & Bower, 1997). Slater et al. (1998) have reported that early in the first week of life, infants seem to look longer at faces judged to be attractive by adults.

It is also pertinent to understand some of the limits of an infant's vision. For example, it is known that visual acuity at birth is not the same as that of normal adults, that is, 20/20. Because of difficulties in accurately determining visual acuity in newborns, there is a range of estimated acuity somewhere between 20/300 to 20/800 (Cohen, DeLoache, & Strauss, 1979). Another way to view the research on visual acuity in newborns is that they see best

objects that are about 8 to 12 inches from their face, about the distance of the mother's face when cradling the infant in a traditional *en face* feeding position.

Another area of research on infant vision that has received recent attention is the ability of infants to perceive color. For some period of time, studies on color preference were confounded by brightness, a problem that was resolved in more recent studies that control the brightness variable (Cohen, DeLoache, & Strauss, 1979). It is fairly well established, however, that infants react to colors as early as 4 months of age. This research, like the studies on visual acuity, is difficult to determine definitively in newborns. One general summary statement about newborn color preference can be made. It is clear that, in combination with the previous findings about infants preferring stimuli of high contrast, the traditional pastel colors of the newborn nursery have little appeal to newborns. Adams, Courage, and Mercer (1994) studied newborns and reported that they could clearly discriminate the red color only from a nonchromatic patch of consistent luminescence. As a result of this consensus, a number of toys for infants made up of black, white, and red have been marketed.

A summary of neonatal visual abilities is as follows. First, neonates clearly have the ability to see, process, and react to visual stimuli, although this ability is not fully mature at birth. Neonates prefer high contrast in visual stimuli and seem to prefer the human face. They are able to discriminate the maternal face within the first week of life. To optimally stimulate infants, the object should be held relatively close (8 to 12 inches) from the infant's face. Finally, neonatal color vision is very limited. It seems to first be evident in the red portion of the spectrum.

In addition to vision, the hearing capabilities of newborn infants have been studied extensively. Unlike vision, the auditory system has been extensively stimulated in utero, with the most common sounds being those of the mother's heartbeat and the swish of blood flow through the placenta. However, as reported earlier, the fetus clearly responds to auditory stimuli in the external environment, including the mother's voice. Studies have shown that newborns can distinguish between their mother's and a stranger's voice (DeCasper & Fifer, 1980; Spence & Freeman, 1996). Furthermore, the ability to distinguish voices occurred even when the mother's voice was filtered, taking out the high-frequency sounds that assist in the detection of meaningful speech (Spence & Freeman, 1996). Newborns can detect a whispered voice as well but are unable to distinguish between voices when they are whispered. Newborns did not appear to be able to distinguish or prefer the father's voice (DeCasper & Prescott, 1984), a finding that was interpreted to support the idea that learning the maternal voice occurs in utero. It has also been reported that newborn infants can discriminate pitch (Nazzi, Floccia, & Bertocini, 1998). Sounds can also be soothing to newborns. Five-day-old infants were subjected to one of three conditions: white noise, heartbeat sounds, or silence during a heel-stick procedure. It was found that infants in both of the stimulus conditions (white noise and heartbeat) showed less reactive response to the invasive procedure (Kawakami, Kurihara, Shimizu, & Yanaihara, 1996).

Integration across several senses also appears to occur in newborns. Meltzoff and Borton (1979) demonstrated that infants who experienced tactile exploration of a certain shape of pacifier displayed a visual preference for that pacifier later. There is also evidence that newborns can imitate behaviors that are already within their behavioral repertoire. In the classic work on neonatal imitation done by Meltzoff and Moore (1977), infants were shown to imitate common movements such as tongue thrusting and mouth opening. Infants have also been shown to imitate facial expressions in a study by Kaitz, Meschulach-Sarfaty, and Auerbach (1988). Morrongiello, Fenwick, and Chance (1998) have shown that infants as young as 2 days could seemingly learn audiovisual pairings and reacted when the expected pairings did not occur.

As evidenced by the preceding studies, normal newborns actually show a quite sophisticated behavioral repertoire in terms of responding to various aspects of the environment. From the time of birth, human newborns are processing and reacting to information from the environment.

ACTIVITY AND PARTICIPATION

Not only do newborn infants enter a new physical environment at birth, making necessary structural and functional adaptations, neonates are now able to begin participating in a social environment. All active behaviors directed at gaining the attention of others are called **interactive behaviors**. Abilities such as imitation of behaviors are part of such interactions. The newborns' interactive abilities also play a key role in the development of social attachments, as to the parents. Immediately postpartum, the mother and infant undergo characteristic behaviors that seem to have the rhythmicity associated with all social interactions. For example, when two adults are speaking to one another, the speaker will not only verbalize but also make facial gestures and body movements. The listener will not speak but shows engagement in the exchange through various body movements and facial gestures. When the speaker is finished, the person who listened will typically engage in a verbal response, and the roles of the interaction are reversed. At birth, a rudimentary variation of this social exchange appears to be present (see **Figure 9-12**). This linked behavioral exchange has been called **entrainment**.

The famous developmental psychologist John Bowlby proposed in the 1950s that infants have innate social capabilities (Karen, 1994). Condon and Sander (1974) described the entrainment of infants' movements with their mother's voice with infants only a few hours old. In their classic study, these authors observed films of infants during

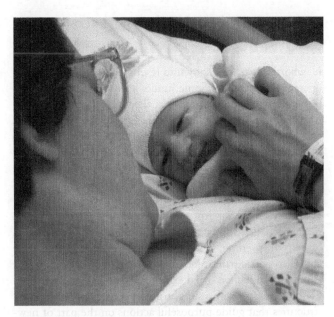

Figure 9-12   Newborn and Postpartum Mother in Entrainment

the presentation of taped speech. They found that there was a relationship between distinct limb movements and speech. Klaus and Kennell suggest (1982) that the responses or signals put forth by infants during entrainment are important elements in the formation of attachment. Brazelton (1963) says that these early communications with the infants help the parents begin to see their newborns as individuals and to adjust their own behaviors to the infants' signals. This premise of the importance of early social interaction with neonates is challenged by the often necessary separations that occur during a preterm or at-risk birth, which will be discussed later.

COMMUNICATION

Communication is a complex phenomenon, which develops rapidly over the early postnatal years. The examples of interactive behavior described previously imply that newborns have a beginning ability to communicate. As discussed in Chapter 5, communication includes both receptive and expressive dimensions. Gervain, Berent, and Werker (2012) used optical imaging to record brain activation in newborns exposed to spoken language. They reported the neural foundations of language acquisition to be present at birth. May and colleagues (2011) used near-infrared spectroscopy to study brain activation patterns in newborns exposed to native language, unfamiliar language, or nonlanguage sounds. These authors found differential brain activation patterns in response to the unfamiliar language, indicating infants discriminated and responded to these language sounds. It appears newborns are able to perform some of the functions of receptive language; however, expressive functions remain limited to pre-intentional and then intentional nonverbal forms of behavior.

LEARNING AND APPLYING KNOWLEDGE

Newborns have been shown to respond to both classical and operant conditioning. Some studies have suggested that newborns can remember stories that they heard read aloud prenatally (DeCasper & Fifer, 1980). Farroni, Menon, Rigato, and Johnson (2007) reported newborns between the second to fourth days of life did not discriminate or prefer fearful versus neutral faces, but preferred happy faces to neutral. These authors interpreted these results to reflect perceptual learning, postulating that newborns have experience with happy faces, but not fearful facial expressions. Trevarthen (2011) summarized an extensive body of research in the cognitive capabilities of newborns, emphasizing that newborns have a remarkable ability to participate intersubjectively to attract and engage adults in productive social exchanges that facilitate learning. He presented evidence supporting activation of higher brain structures that guide purposeful actions on the part of newborns to support learning from the earliest days of life. From the perspective of the developing nervous system, all of these behaviors support the presence of a basic form of cognition.

ENVIRONMENTAL AND FAMILY ISSUES

The birth of a child is a significant life event. Svejda and colleagues (1982) suggest that one of the tasks of the first 4 weeks of life is the establishment of *biorhythmicity*. Anyone who has brought a newborn home from the hospital knows how completely the normal rhythms of life are disrupted for the first weeks. This, in combination with the normal hormonal fluctuations of the postpartum mother, usually creates some element of stress. In fact, the birth of a child has sometimes been referred to as a "life crisis." Subsequently, authors have used less dramatic labels for the so-called transition to home, but there is no one who would suggest that there is not some element of stress in the situation. Rarely are the parents getting enough sleep, as the aforementioned biorhythms are in the process of being established. Postpartum mothers experience tremendous swings in hormones, which usually allow them to function through the transition but in some cases may result in more severe disturbances, such as *postpartum depression*. Fathers, on the other hand, must adjust as well. They may feel the additional financial burdens of a new baby. A heightened sense of family responsibility may be felt. In addition, first-time fathers worry about factors such as the well-being of their wife and new baby, how well they will make the transition to fatherhood, and how their relationship with their wife will change over time (McNall, 1976).

Cowan, Cowan, Coie, and Coie (1978) suggested that irrespective of parental philosophy about gender roles, more traditional roles tend to emerge in the early postpartum weeks, with mothers spending more time with their infants in

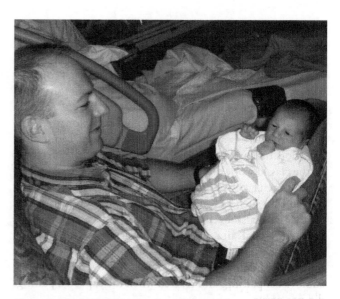

Figure 9-13   New Father Engrossed with Son

caregiving. However, Parke and Lamb both pioneered research on fathers and reported that fathers are capable of establishing attachments to their infants at around the same time as the mothers (Lamb, Frodi, Hwang, Frodi, & Steinberg, 1982). Furthermore, studies by Parke (1979) have shown that fathers are capable of responding to their infant's cues, interpreting infant signals, and feeding their infants effectively (see **Figure 9-13**). The term **engrossment** has been used to describe the sense of absorption, preoccupation, and interest that fathers have in their newborn (Greenberg & Morris, 1974).

In families where there are other children at home (that is, the mother is multiparous), the postpartum adjustment of necessity must include the siblings (see **Figure 9-14**). Trause and Irvin (1982) summarize the research on sibling adjustment. For the most part, becoming a sibling is seen to be traumatic.

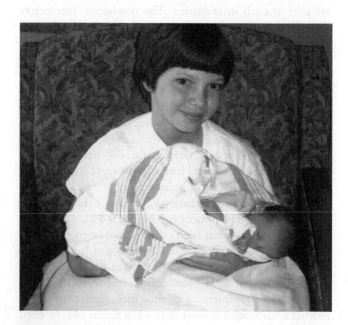

Figure 9-14   New Big Sister

A study by Legg, Sherick, and Wadland (1974) reported that most of the new siblings reported feeling negative emotions such as jealousy. There appears to be an age effect in that the younger the child, the more significant the problems.

Trause and colleagues (1977, 1981) were responsible for the early documentation of the return of dependence behaviors in new siblings under the age of 3. Despite this often challenging transition, in by far the majority of cases the family adaptation to the newborn occurs successfully, and the infant is integrated into the rhythms of family life.

GENDER AND CULTURAL ISSUES

Culture and gender issues are difficult to isolate specifically to the neonatal period. Most studies examine more than the neonatal period. With respect to gender, the preceding discussion identified some of the effects of parental gender on typical patterns of interaction with a newborn. What about the gender of the infant? Gender issues illustrate cultural practices. In some cultures the birth of a male infant is much more highly prized than the birth of a female infant. In Western cultures, traditional parents (defined as the father as the primary breadwinner and the mother as primary caregiver) tend to interact more with sons than with daughters. However, in one interesting study, Lamb and colleagues (1982) reported that in nontraditional Swedish families, parents tended to interact more with daughters. The authors speculated that parents in nontraditional families possibly overcompensated for their perception that girls were traditionally given less attention than boys.

Cultural practices affect not only the birth process but the immediate postpartum period as well. Infants are shown to respond preferentially when the mother has ingested culturally typical food. This may be a way of acclimating infants to normative food preferences for a given culture. There are also cultural differences in caregiving of neonates. In some cultures, leaving infants to cry for longer periods of time is valued to develop independence. In other cultures, such as American, infants are quickly picked up and soothed, rocked, and subjected to calming voices in speech and song. Japanese infants are said to have a more quiet temperament. Finally, contact with the parents is very different between cultures. In some cultures, infants are almost never physically separated from the mother, being carried on cradleboards and pouches. In Eastern cultures, it is not uncommon for infants to sleep with the parents, not only immediately after birth but also for some time thereafter.

THE AT-RISK INFANT

Processes of neonatal development and the transition to extrauterine life are complicated in the normal circumstances surrounding birth. However, a number of infants fall into the category of "at risk," which even further complicates this early period. Risk is traditionally thought of as arising from either biologic or environmental factors. **Biologic risk** is related to factors in the infant or the mother that are known to have potentially adverse consequences for the infant (Shonkoff & Phillips, 2000). Such risk factors include genetic problems, disease or disability in the mother or infant, maternal age, maternal smoking or drug use in pregnancy, **intrauterine growth retardation (IUGR)**, and prematurity. The label IUGR is a term applied to infants who fail to reach obstetrical growth norms while in utero. The related term, **small for gestational age (SGA)**, refers to infants born at less than the 10th percentile for weight based on gestational age (Shepherd, Hanshaw, & Lane, 1999). In most cases, infants who are labeled as IUGR would also be SGA, but it is possible that infants can have intrauterine growth retardation that is not as serious as to cause them to fall below the 10th percentile and therefore be in the SGA category. **Environmental risk** is related to factors in the infants' environment that may have a potentially adverse effect on the infants, such as low socioeconomic status (SES), inadequate parental caregiving, neglect or abuse, poor nutrition, and so on (Shonkoff & Phillips, 2000).

Unfortunately for infants, biologic and environmental risk factors often correlate. For example, there are definite biologic risks for an infant of a teenage mother who smokes during the pregnancy; however, environmental risks such as poor nutrition, low SES, and inadequate parental caregiving are not uncommonly associated with this scenario. Thus, biologic and environmental risk factors often combine and escalate the effects of each other to the detriment of the infants. *Protective factors,* as described in Chapter 2, are factors that help to ameliorate risk, according to the life course theory and health development model. They may be either environmental (family support) or constitutional (physical attractiveness) (Shonkoff & Phillips, 2000). Protective factors are measurable attributes associated with positive outcomes, especially in the presence of adversity or high risk levels (Gest & Davidson, 2011).

Prematurity and associated sequelae will be dealt with at length in subsequent paragraphs. A brief review of some of the other risk factors is as follows. Obviously, **societal-level risk factors** such as teenage pregnancy and maternal drug and alcohol abuse are often discussed. The risk factor in a teenage pregnancy is first and foremost biologic. The immature physical development of the mother may affect the pregnancy, resulting in an infant that is born too small or too early. Likewise, a teen mother may not have adequate nutrition, both before and during the pregnancy. Few teenagers are conscious of eating a healthy diet, not only for them, but to sustain another life. Once the infant is born to a teenage mother, the baby is frequently brought home to the maternal home. Grandparents are often extended caregivers in the family system. The father may not be part of the family. If the father does try to assume a paternal role, he is frequently struggling to support the family financially. For teenage parents, who have their own developmental tasks to conquer, mastery of the superimposed task of parenting is often difficult to impossible.

SUBSTANCE ABUSE

By far the majority of research on risk has been done on the issue of substance abuse by a mother during pregnancy. The two general categories of substance abuse are alcohol and drugs. The effects of prenatal exposure to alcohol are well known and may be classified by effect. The first, and most serious, is *fetal alcohol syndrome (FAS)*. This syndrome is associated with characteristic physical features, microcephaly (small head), and often mental retardation. The second is called *fetal alcohol effects syndrome (FAES)*. In this case, the alcohol abuse by the mother was not as severe in either amount or duration as in the preceding case. Nevertheless, the infants may have softer neurologic signs, such as learning and attention problems or lowered IQ (Pierog, Chadavasu, & Wexler, 1977). The amount of alcohol required to produce these syndromes is surprisingly small, as little as 2 to 3 ounces a day (Moore, 2003).

Prenatal drug use has also been shown to affect developing fetuses, as manifested in the behavior of the newborns. One drug extensively studied in the 1980s and 1990s was cocaine. Studies have clearly demonstrated short-term effects of maternal use of cocaine. *Cocaine-exposed infants* often show behavioral irritability, difficulty in quieting, and poor feeding (Phillips, Sharma, Premachandra, Vaughn, & Reyes-Lee, 1996). Whether or not there are long-term effects on infants of maternal cocaine abuse are less clear, but the preponderance of evidence suggests that most effects are in the neonatal period, and that long-term effects, if any, are subtle. Furthermore, long-term effects of maternal cocaine abuse are difficult to separate from other socioeconomic variables. Other drugs that have been studied include street drugs such as heroin. Infants born to mothers who are addicted to heroin typically must go through drug withdrawal and display associated symptoms such as rapid breathing and irritability (Householder, Hatcher, Burns, & Chasnoff, 1982).

Since the year 2000, use of prescription opioids (painkillers) for nonmedical purposes has increased significantly, including in pregnant women, thereby presenting a new substance to add to the list of potentially harmful agents in newborns. **Neonatal abstinence syndrome (NAS)** is a term used to describe postpartum behavioral and physiologic effects on neonates of exposure to drugs in utero. Infants born with NAS are subjected to higher levels of mortality and morbidity. Recent studies indicate more than a doubling of cases of NAS associated with nonmedical use of prescription painkillers in pregnancy (Creanga et al., 2012).

SMALL FOR GESTATIONAL AGE

The term *small for gestational age (SGA)* is used to describe infants born at less than the 10th percentile for weight. When infants are born with low birth weight (less than 2500 g), and are also SGA, the term *intrauterine growth*

retardation (IUGR) is used to describe the outcome. The consequences of IUGR have primarily been shown to relate to attentional and activity disorders; however, the outcome appears to interact with the support in the postnatal environment. In other words, environmental risk appears to bring out the tendencies for attentional disorders in infants who are IUGR, but a supportive environment may help minimize the consequences (Robson & Cline, 1998). IUGR reflects poor fetal nutrition during pregnancy. One common cause of IUGR is maternal smoking, which deprives the fetus of oxygenation.

HIV EXPOSURE

Over the past two decades, the incidence of infants infected with human immunodeficiency virus (HIV) has increased dramatically, creating an international health crisis, particularly in some parts of the world, such as sub-Saharan Africa. The mechanism of transmission of the disease is believed to be from mother to infant through the placental circulation. Alternatively, fetal contact with the mother's blood and body fluids through vaginal delivery is another means of transmission. Infants who contract the HIV virus from the mother are considered HIV-exposed and have a high probability of developing full-blown pediatric acquired immunodeficiency syndrome (AIDS) in the first 2 years of life; however, identification in the neonatal period is not common because the presence of maternal antibodies may block identification (Rainville, 1999). In the United States, incidence rates of infants born with HIV by transmission from the mother have steadily declined since its peak in 1992. However, there remains significant racial disparity in the data. In 2009, incidence of perinatally acquired HIV infection per 100,000 was 9.9 in African American babies, declining from a rate of 15.2 in 2007. Rates for white Americans declined in the same period from 0.8 to 0.1, and for Hispanics from 2.1 to 1.7 (per 100,000). "Opt-out" prenatal testing for HIV is strongly recommended by the Centers for Disease Control and Prevention (CDC) to further reduce these numbers (CDC, 2012). This has been attributed to better identification of mothers who are HIV-positive, improved antiretroviral drug treatment of mothers, drug prophylaxis in infants, and improved labor and delivery practice. However, HIV exposure in infancy remains a serious international public health issue (Fowler, Gale, Lampe, Etina, & Owor, 2010).

PRETERM INFANTS

The definition of *term infant* and *preterm infant* is a direct estimate of the duration of the pregnancy, dated from the mother's last menstrual period. This is called *gestational age. Gestational age* is the common terminology associated with dating the age of preterm infants. Infants are defined as preterm if born before the 37th week of gestation. A term pregnancy is considered 38 to 42 weeks gestation. The week discrepancy (37 to 38 weeks) is attributed to various classification systems. Prematurity must be considered in conjunction with birth weight. A birth weight less than 2500 grams is considered *low birth weight (LBW)*. Therefore, many premature infants are also low birth weight. Infants weighing less than 1500 grams at birth are considered to be *very low birth weight (VLBW)*, and infants weighing less than 1000 grams are considered to be *extremely low birth weight (ELBW)* (Shepherd, Hanshaw, & Lane, 1999). Although the landscape is an ever-changing one, recent reports suggest that acceptable limits of viability (50 percent chance of survival without significant neurodevelopment impairment) are at the 23rd to 24th week of gestation, with birth weight above 400 grams. Although there are reports of infant survival at 22 weeks gestation, these reports are likely linked to fewer deaths in the delivery room, and statistical evidence for long-term survival of these infants is not positive (Zayek et al., 2011).

CHARACTERISTICS OF PRETERM INFANTS

Preterm infants differ from term infants in many important ways. First, there is the obvious **physiologic immaturity**. The most important body system in considering physiologic immaturity is the lungs. The development of the lungs in the last postnatal trimester in utero is in large part what enables the successful transition to extrauterine life at term birth. Conversely, when infants are born too soon, the immaturity in the lungs creates a condition known as **respiratory distress syndrome (RDS)**. Nearly all preterm infants have this condition, which is attributable to a lack of surfactant. A major improvement in care of preterm infants in the 1990s was the development and routine administration of an artificial surfactant, which helps to promote maturation of the lungs. Still, one of the more common adverse outcomes of prematurity is the development of a chronic lung condition known as **bronchopulmonary dysplasia (BPD)**. BPD is a progressive scarring of the lungs creating an emphysematous-like function. The etiology of BPD is multifactorial, but probably related to prolonged ventilation of immature lungs; therefore, infants who do not wean well from the ventilator are considered to be at risk for this condition (Long & Toscano, 2002).

Other aspects of physiologic immaturity include the cardiac system. As stated earlier, the circulatory system in utero is one that involved a right-to-left shunt of blood, bypassing the lungs, which are not needed in the fetus because it receives all oxygenation through the placenta. Patent ductus arteriousus (a prolonged opening of the ductus) is not uncommon. This condition usually resolves itself with maturation but occasionally requires surgical intervention.

Another condition exists when the shunting of the blood persists beyond the perinatal period. This is known as persistent fetal circulation (discussed earlier in this chapter), and is treated by aggressive oxygenation through special ventilators or through extracorporeal membrane oxygenation (ECMO). Because persistent fetal circulation is associated with diminished blood flow through the lungs, the vascular resistance in the lung capillary beds stays extremely high, creating a condition known as pulmonary hypertension.

The gastric system is also immature in preterm infants. In particular, the sphincter that holds food in the stomach is often underdeveloped and weak. Thus, after infants finish feeding, the stomach contents can reflux into the esophagus, creating a heartburn-like condition known as **gastroesophageal reflux (GER)** (Long & Toscano, 2002). This condition is extremely common in premature infants and can produce behaviors such as incoordination in swallowing, feeding aversion, and arching. Because therapists often work with feeding problems in the nursery, these behaviors are important to identify. Treatment for GER ranges from very modest interventions to very aggressive. Typically, the first intervention attempted when GER is suspected is thickening of the feeds. Also, keeping the infant in a semi-upright position, by elevating the bed or placing the infant in a sling on a reflux board, is helpful. Antacid medications are also routinely prescribed. Finally, there is a surgery called a *Nissen procedure* that can be done to tighten the sphincter.

The musculoskeletal system of preterm infants is noticeably different from that of term infants, as can be seen by just walking into a room where infants are lying in their isolettes. Preterm infants are predominantly hypotonic prior to approximately 34 weeks gestational age. The development of muscle tone progresses from lower extremities to upper, in a caudalcephalic direction. Claudine Amiel-Tison characterized the development of preterm infants across three dimensions: passive tone, active tone, and reflex tone. Passive tone primarily defined the resting postures and resistance to passive movement of preterm infants. *Active tone* described normal righting reactions in horizontal and vertical suspension, and *reflex tone* described the postnatal evolvement of reflexes (Amiel-Tison, 1968). The tests of passive muscle tone are still in common use today and reflect the development of muscle tone. The skeletal system of preterm infants is very malleable. This is especially important because, if careful positioning is not done, preterm infants can develop an elongated skull in the sagittal plane. This condition is sometimes referred to as *craniofacial molding*. Likewise, tightness in the shoulder girdle and external rotation of the hip can persist for some time after hospital discharge.

The nervous system of preterm infants is also immature and can be susceptible to insult. One type of insult that is not uncommon results from a lack of oxygen due to asphyxia and is known as **hypoxic ischemic encephalopathy (HIE)**. Fragile blood vessels near the ventricles of the brain can rupture, causing **intraventricular hemorrhage (IVH)**. Another adverse outcome for the vulnerable nervous system is **periventricular leukomalacia (PVL)**, characterized by necrosis and cavitation of the white matter of the brain. PVL may develop following a vascular insult such as IVH or in isolation, presumably due to some insult to the neural tissue (Long & Toscano, 2002).

The neurologic immaturity of normal preterm infants can manifest itself in several ways. Preterm infants are more tremulous than term infants, and *clonus,* a reflex that is a rhythmic alternation of muscular contraction and relaxation in response to quick stretch, is commonly seen. Specifically, behavioral states as a reflection of neurologic maturity are different in preterm versus term infants. Infants less than 36 weeks gestational age do not have clear sleep or behavioral state patterns when compared with term infants, although emergence of these patterns begins as early as 26 weeks gestation. Rapid eye movements become synchronized to EEG patterns around 30 to 31 weeks gestation (Scher, 2008). Therefore, the maturation of these patterns, as typically happening in utero, is an important feature of cortical maturation. In fact, characteristics of preterm infant EEG activity have been used to predict developmental outcome in preterm infants (Scoppa et al., 2012). Developmentalists such as Heidelise Als have built upon the work of T. Berry Brazelton, expanding the concepts of the Brazelton assessment to attempt to describe the interactive maturity of premature infants. Als described five developmental subsystems that are undergoing maturation through the synergy of a number of differing external and internal factors. These subsystems are autonomic (physiologic functioning), motor, state organization, attention or interaction, and regulatory. Als went on to describe the behaviors of infants that signal engagement or disengagement across the various subsystems (Als, 1986).

Finally, the visual system of preterm infants is fragile and susceptible to compromise. One common problem associated with prematurity is **retinopathy of prematurity (ROP)**, caused by ischemia, or lack of blood flow to the eyes. It can result in visual impairment and blindness (Mechoulam & Pierce, 2003). ROP is related to excessive oxygen levels that can lead to abnormal patterns of retinal vascularization and destruction of vascular endothelial cells (Claxton & Fruttiger, 2003). Currently, common treatments for ROP include laser surgery to remove the abnormal vascularization and promote normal vascular growth.

CHARACTERISTICS OF PRETERM INFANT ENVIRONMENT

Preterm infants are cared for in a very special environment known as the **neonatal intensive care unit (NICU)**. NICUs are typically considered Level III nurseries, meaning that they have the ability to resuscitate infants. The birth of a premature infant is a medical crisis, due to the immaturity in physiologic systems discussed previously. In fact, the term *golden hour* has been borrowed from care of trauma patients, where it refers to organization and implementation of standard clinical care protocols. In the birth of premature infants, the term refers to implementation of practices that improve the adaptation of the infants in the delivery room, thereby increasing potential for improved long-term outcomes (Bissinger & Annabale, 2010). The intensive care in an NICU really refers to intensive nursing care. The nurse-to-infant ratio in a typical NICU is very low. Typically, after the infants "graduate" from intensive care, they move on to a step-down unit (NSDU, or neonatal step-down unit), where the nurse-to-infant ratio is higher.

The necessities of medical caregiving in these nurseries create a very abnormal environment for preterm infants, who normatively should be in a totally flexed position in a dark, aquatic environment. This environment provides multisensory stimulation. The lighting in an NICU is high, and in many cases there is no diurnal cycling of the lights as would occur in a normal environment. The high light has been suggested to affect the developing retina (Glass, 1990). In addition, studies have shown that infants react physiologically to the lighting in the environment. Gordon-Shogan and Schumann (1993) found, in a study using infants as their own controls, that rapid increases in lighting were associated with a decrease in oxygen saturation. Many investigators have reported that when light-dark cycles are implemented, preterm infants tend to improve in physiologic and behavioral parameters (Young, 1996).

Noise is also an issue in the NICU. The noise in the nursery is largely caused by medical equipment. Isolettes do not protect infants from these noise levels, which have been likened to that of light traffic or machinery; however, noise levels in the nursery can peak at levels consistent with a busy airport. As in the case with light, the noise levels in the nursery have been shown to adversely affect both behavioral and physiologic parameters (Young, 1996).

Finally, patterns of caregiving involving somatosensory stimulation are unique in the NICU. Not surprisingly, preterm infants are more likely to be touched for medical procedures (such as drawing blood, adjusting lines and leads) or physiologic caregiving (diaper change, positioning, turning) than in a social context (rocking, rubbing, skin-to-skin contact). Like other forms of stimulation, the typical handling of these infants can produce physiologic distress, including oxygen desaturation, apnea, decreased heart rate (bradycardia), and increased respiratory rate.

Developmentally Appropriate Care

The compilation of evidence regarding the nature of the NICU environment has resulted in decades of research on **developmentally appropriate care**. Developmentally appropriate care does not have a single definition, but includes some of the features included in the following discussion. Developmentally appropriate care seeks to minimize the iatrogenic effects of prematurity by increasing sensitivity of caregivers to infant cues (Samra, McGrath, Wehbe, & Clapper, 2012). Heidelise Als, mentioned previously, has numerous publications describing various aspects of developmental care, She has been a key figure in the description, implementation and assessment of developmental care. For example, one key publication (Als et al., 2004) demonstrated that developmentally appropriate care can alter both structure and function of the brain of preterm infants. One key aspect of developmental care is careful attention to infant stress related to handling directed at medical caregiving as opposed to comfort. One strategy to address this problem is the implementation of **minimal-stimulation protocols**. In these protocols, caregivers attempt to cluster caregiving procedures such that the infants have the ability to settle into quiet behavioral states and rest between disturbances (Young, 1996). Some studies have shown that by careful handling of preterm infants, including attention to positional support and infant behavioral cues, the amount of time in fretful behavioral states, with its associated physiologic costs, is reduced (Becker, Brazy, & Grunwalk, 1997). Another popular area of research, as mentioned earlier, is the effect of providing supplemental tactile stimulation such as massage on preterm infants (Field, Scafidi, & Schanberg, 1987; Scafidi et al., 1993). Another form of intervention in the NICU designed to promote more normative patterns of sensory and social stimulation is the concept of **kangaroo care**, where an infant is laid inside the parent's clothes in skin-to-skin contact. This procedure, conceptualized in Sweden, has been suggested to promote a thermal homeostasis for infants without having to introduce abnormal stimulation through machines. Other advantages of kangaroo care are the skin contact and the social bonding with the parents (Bosque, 1995). As mentioned earlier, longitudinal studies following preterm infants up to 10 years of age have now documented long-term benefits associated with kangaroo care (Feldman et al., 2014).

Some of the most recent studies of developmental care focus on the emerging science of epigenetics. *Epigenesis* describes the development of an organism as it moves from a relatively unstructured state to a more ordered and differentiated state over the course of developmental time. **Epigenetics** is the study of heritable changes in gene expression or cellular phenotype caused by mechanisms other than changes in the underlying DNA sequence. Preliminary results from this emerging field of research suggest that maternal handling and positive sensory experiences in early life modify gene transcription, particularly in the production of hormones and enzymes that positively affect the developing brain (Samra et al., 2012). Further study is also warranted on epigenetic adaptations by infants that may enhance short-term survival, but have long-term negative consequences on the nervous system (Gudsnuk & Champagne, 2011).

In summary, developmentally appropriate care has a foundation in biological processes and has been shown to be the best practice in caring for preterm infants. Provision of developmentally appropriate care is typically overseen in a transdisciplinary fashion by a number of professionals, including occupational and physical therapists, as well as nurses or developmental psychologists.

SOCIAL EFFECTS OF PRETERM BIRTH

In the 1970s, due to the work of a number of researchers, including Klaus and Kennell (1982), the importance of parental contact with infants in the immediate postnatal period was conclusively demonstrated. These studies have significantly changed labor and delivery room practices as well as hospital care by promoting the need of infant and parents to have time together in the immediate postpartum period. However, these findings beg the question of the situation that is typical in preterm birth. In preterm births, the infants are typically resuscitated if necessary, shown to the mother, and whisked away to the NICU. The NICU is frequently in a different hospital, and the infants are transported by ambulance or helicopter, leaving the postpartum woman behind. Even in the relatively optimal situation where the NICU is in the delivery hospital, the medical needs of the infants result in maternal-infant separation almost immediately.

Parent-neonate separation is a prevalent problem associated with preterm births. The short-term consequences of this separation are well documented. Parents of preterm infants report a wide range of psychological responses. One of these typical responses, **anticipatory grief**, occurs when parents are afraid that the infant will not survive, so engage consciously or subconsciously in protective behaviors. Examples of such behaviors might be choosing not to take advantage of visiting with their baby, delaying the naming of the infant, and not wanting to talk about the baby (Sweeney, Gutierrez, & Beachy, 2012)

Another response that is widely reported is a sense of lack of efficacy. **Efficacy** is the personal sense that you are competent and effective in your life roles. The mother of a preterm infant is seeking to reinforce her efficacy as a caregiver. Efficacy is reinforced when she is able to take care of her infant, including feeding, as well as to calm her infant when crying. Infants with irregular biorhythms or difficult temperaments, or who are poor feeders, do not promote these feelings of efficacy in their mothers, and this can lead to additional stress. Because these infants have so many medical needs that are attended to by professionals, the parents may feel detached and that they cannot take care of their baby. They report feeling as if the baby belongs to someone else. The separation that parents of a preterm experience is physical as well as geographical. By physical separation, we mean that the medical caregiving equipment prevents the parents from holding, touching, and talking to a baby as would otherwise be done. Despite these short-term consequences, many parents of preterm infants do ultimately attach to their infant and place the NICU experience in perspective.

Professionals working with families in this vulnerable situation can help minimize the stress on infants and families. Nurseries that provide a welcoming atmosphere to families, allowing them to stay at their infant's bedside, promote attachment. Professionals should be careful to instruct the parents in how to care for their infants and support parents in their early attempts at caregiving. Culp, Culp, and Harman (1989) showed that parents who observed their preterm infant's performance on developmental assessment showed less anxiety and improved confidence in their ability to deal with their infant's cues. It has been shown that coping behaviors of parents of preterm infants can be enhanced by providing them with information and emotional support (Cusson & Lee, 1994). There are many ways that professionals interacting with preterm babies and their parents can promote positive interactions. These include helping parents to recognize their infant's cues, helping them with support groups after discharge, and teaching parents about play and caregiving strategies (Holloway, 1997).

SUMMARY

Much of the focus on newborns centers on the maturation of body structures and body functions. The ability to participate as a family member emerges as infants develop control over their physiologic functions. The life tasks associated with the neonatal period for both newborns and the family are quite dramatic and cross all domains of behavior. It is remarkable that in most cases, the challenges of birth and the neonatal period are successfully met with relatively little difficulty. There are, however, situations of both biologic and environmental risk that can negatively affect this life transition. Professionals working with neonates to promote positive outcomes for all concerned often focus on individuals in the infants' environment to foster the development of healthy and supportive relationships.

Speaking of
Practice in the NICU

MARYBETH MANDICH, PT, PhD,
PEDIATRIC PHYSICAL THERAPIST

My first experience working with these special babies came when I was in graduate school. I walked into the neonatal intensive care unit (NICU) and was totally overwhelmed. The first baby I saw was large by today's standards—probably around 2000 g. But the baby looked so small to me! I remember picking up the baby to test head control and all the alarms went off. I nearly dropped the baby, and I thought I had done something really terrible.

Since that time, I have had a fascination with the world of these tiny babies born too soon. They should be in a flexed position, in a dark, aqueous environment, listening to their mother's heartbeat and muted voice. Instead, these babies are placed in the intensive care environment of lights, sounds, pinpricks, and monitors. I have always wondered what the world seems like to them and, also, what effects it has on them both immediately and long-term. It seems incomprehensible to me that this aberrant environment could not have some sort of impact on the baby.

One of the studies we did a few years ago really emphasized what I mean. As a therapist, I am interested in making life better for these infants, helping them to function in the environment. We did a study of infant swaddling and found that, as a result of something as simple as swaddling, the babies had a more positive behavior state for a greater proportion of the time. Likewise, it reduced their incidence of apnea and bradycardia. Something so simple, which caregivers have done for infants the world over, actually appears to have medical benefit. I listened to Dr. Kennell many years ago (of the Klaus and Kennell theory of maternal-infant bonding). He was discussing the positive effects on labor and delivery of having a woman, called a *duenna*, there to support the mother. The effects were remarkable. He later commented that if these effects had been a drug, everyone would want to know where to get it. But because it was a human intervention, people were hesitant to believe the results.

I think the same applies to the NICU. The simplest intervention can make life better for these babies. For that reason, I cannot stop searching for those tiny things that we can do to help these precious little ones.

CASE 1

Elise

Elise is a 36-year-old woman. She waited to get pregnant and then sustained two miscarriages before having a baby, Joshua, who was born at 26 weeks gestation. The time in the neonatal intensive care unit was very difficult. Elise stayed away from her husband in the Ronald McDonald House of the teaching hospital where Joshua was born. That caused some family stress because her husband, John, wanted to be there and got frustrated at Elise's "hormonal" and emotional reports. Joshua had respiratory distress syndrome, and bronchopulmonary dysplasia developed. He was put on medicine for reflux. He had a small intraventricular hemorrhage (Grade II) on the right.

Elise was very frustrated by the fact that she couldn't hold Joshua. When she was finally allowed to try to feed him by mouth, two months after he was born, he displayed arching and fussy behavior, and she felt as if she couldn't take care of her own baby.

Eventually, Joshua's problems resolved, and he was discharged from the nursery, but he had to receive oxygen and be on a breathing monitor. The first few weeks at home, Joshua seemed to have no development of rhythmic patterns of sleeping and waking. He cried a good bit, and his voice sounded pathetic and raspy. When Joshua went back for his clinic visit two weeks after discharge, he hadn't gained any weight.

Joshua was discharged when he was approximately 40 weeks gestational age, but by that time he was chronologically 3½ months old. Elise wondered if Joshua was delayed because he didn't do anything that a 3-month-old baby would do. The pediatrician suggested a referral to an early intervention program to give Elise some support.

The therapist associated with early intervention did a developmental assessment when Josh was 1 month adjusted age and found that his behavior was approximately that of a newborn. He seemed tired and listless and had a very significant head lag. The therapist suggested some positioning strategies and showed Elise how to swaddle Joshua. Some sensory techniques were attempted to try to calm him. The therapist showed Elise how attentive Joshua was to her face and voice when he was in a quiet behavioral state.

Over the next 6 months, Joshua was weaned off oxygen. He began to display the motor behaviors of his adjusted age. The therapist continued to come to the home and give suggestions about activities to do with Joshua. Overall, however, John, Elise, and Joshua are now doing much better and enjoying each other very much.

Guiding Questions

Some questions to consider:

1. What aspects of Joshua's early life differed from that of a typical term infant? How could developmentally appropriate care improve his transition to home?
2. What is the importance of touch in early life? How could you use that knowledge to help Joshua's mother in care?
3. Joshua's parents had a difficult time with the NICU experience and the separation from their baby. What are typical aspects of postpartum behavior in parent-infant interaction, and how did those differ in Joshua's case?

CASE 2

Kayla

Kayla was born at 24 3/7 weeks gestation with a birth weight of 570 g (1 lb, 4 oz) to a 30-year-old mother who had good prenatal care. She was born vaginal breech delivery with Apgar scores of 4 at 1 minute and 7 at 5 minutes. In the NICU, Kayla was placed on a high-frequency oscillating ventilator (HFOV) for 21 days until she was weaned from respiratory support at 56 days of life. Since birth, Kayla has had severe bronchopulmonary dysplasia and has been fed using a nasogastric tube.

Kayla was referred for OT and PT services at 32 weeks postconceptual age for developmentally supportive positioning, feeding support as she weans off the tube, and to assist Kayla's caregivers in identifying and responding to Kayla's cues. When assessed, Kayla was restless and became irritable with hands-on care. She demonstrated increased extensor posturing of her head, trunk, and extremities. Sensitivity to sound and light were also noted. Kayla had very low tolerance to handling and position changes during care. Kayla was unable to utilize any self-calming behaviors and was difficult to calm with external supports. She did respond to flexed positioning and firm touch when provided for long enough for her to relax into the position.

Kayla's mother visits her every day, but is fearful about handling Kayla. When Kayla is stressed, she has increased heart rate and oxygen desaturation. In addition, Kayla is gaining weight poorly because she has difficulty sleeping. Her mother worries about the warnings of the monitors on Kayla and does not know how to calm her. Kayla does not accept a pacifier at this time. To be ready for discharge, Kayla (now 3½ lb) needs to weigh 5 lb, and Mom needs to feel comfortable with her care.

Guiding Questions

Some questions to consider:

1. What can therapists who are working with Kayla do to improve her mother's confidence in handling her baby?
2. As Kayla matures, what are some aspects of developmental care that might be helpful?
3. What should Kayla be able to do from a motor perspective as she approaches term gestational age? What can be done to ensure her motor development is not impacted by NICU care?
4. What reflexes should Kayla demonstrate and when?

REFERENCES

Adams, R. J., Courage, M. L., & Mercer, M. E. (1994). Systematic measurement of human neonatal color vision. *Vision Research, 34,* 1691–1701.

Als, H. (1986). A synactive model of neonatal behavioral organization: Framework for the assessment of neurobehavioral development in the premature infant and for support of infants and parents in the neonatal intensive care environment. In J. K. Sweeney (Ed.), *The high-risk neonate: Developmental therapy perspectives* (pp. 3–53). New York: Haworth Press.

Als, H., Duffy, F. H., McAnulty, G. B., Rivkin, M. J., Vajapeyem, S., Mulkem, R. V., Warfield, S. K., Huppi, P. S., Butler, S. C., Conneman,

N., Fischer, C., & Eichenwalk, A. C. (2004) Early experience alters brain structure and function. *Pediatrics, 113*(4), 846–857.

Amiel-Tison, C. (1968). Neurological evaluation of the maturity of newborn infants. *Archives of Disease in Childhood, 43,* 89–93.

Becker, P. T., Brazy, J. E., & Grunwalk, P. C. (1997). Behavioral state organization of very low birth weight infants: Effects of developmental handling during caregiving. *Infant Behavior & Development, 20,* 503–514.

Bissinger, R. L., & Annabale, D. J. (2010) Thermoregulation in very low-birth weight infants during the golden hour: Results and implications. *Advances in Neonatal Care, 10*(6), 351.

Bosque, E. M. (1995). Physiologic measures of kangaroo versus incubator care in a tertiary-level nursery. *Journal of Obstetrical, Gynecological and Neonatal Nursing, 24,* 219–226.

Brazelton, T. B. (1963). The early mother-infant adjustment. *Pediatrics, 32,* 931–938.

Brazelton, T., & Nugent, J. K. (1995). Neonatal Behavioral Assessment Scale. *Clinics in Developmental Medicine (No. 137)* (3rd ed.). Philadelphia: J. B. Lippincott.

Bystrova, K., Ivanova, V., Edhborg, M., Matthiesen, A. S., Ransjo-Arvidson, A. B., Mukhamedrakhimov, R., Uvinas-Mobert, R., & Widstrom, A. M. (2009). Early contact versus separation: Effects on mother–infant interaction one year later. *Birth, 36*(2), 97–109.

Centers for Disease Control (CDC). (2012). *HIV among pregnant women, infants, and children in the United States.* Retrieved from http://www.cdc.gov/hiv/pdf/risk_WIC.pdf

Claxton, S., & Fruttiger, M. (2003). Role of arteries in oxygen induced vaso-obliteration. *Experimental Eye Research, 77*(3), 305–311.

Cohen, L. B., DeLoache, J. S., & Strauss, M. S. (1979). Infant visual perception. In J. Osofsky (Ed.), *Handbook of infant development* (pp. 393–438). New York: John Wiley & Sons.

Condon, W. S., & Sander, L. (1974). Neonate movement is synchronized with adult speech: Interactional participation and language acquisition. *Science, 183,* 99–101.

Cowan, C., Cowan, P., Coie, C., & Coie, J. D. (1978). Becoming a family: The impact of a first child's birth on the couple's relationship. In W. Miller & L. Newman (Eds.), *The first child and family formation.* Chapel Hill: University of North Carolina Press.

Creanga, A., Sabel, J., Wasserman, C., Shapiro-Mendoza, C., Taylor, R., Barfield, W., Cawthon, L., & Paulozzi, L. (2012). Maternal drug use and its effect on neonates: A population-based study in Washington state. *Obstetrics & Gynecology, 119*(5), 924–933.

Culp, R., Culp, A. M., & Harmon, R. J. (1989). A tool for educating parents about their premature infants. *Birth, 16,* 23–26.

Cusson, R. M., & Lee, A. L. (1994). Parental interventions and the development of the preterm infant. *Journal of Obstetric Gynecologic & Neonatal Nursing, 23,* 60–68.

DeCasper, A. J., & Fifer, W. P. (1980). Of human bonding: Newborns prefer their mothers' voices. *Science, 208,* 1174–1176.

DeCasper, A. J., & Prescott, P. (1984). Human newborns' perception of male voices: Preference, discrimination and reinforcing value. *Developmental Psychology, 17,* 481–491.

Dubois, J., Dehaene-Lambertz, G., Kulikova, S., Poupon, C., Huppi, P. S., & Hertz-Pannier, L. (2014). The early development of brain white matter: A review of imaging studies in fetuses, newborns and infants. *Neuroscience, 276,* 48–71.

Eliot, L. (1999). *What's going on in there? How the brain and mind develop in the first five years of life.* New York: Bantam Books.

Elverson, C. A., Wilson, M. E., Herzog, M. A., & French, J. A. (2012). Social regulation of the stress response in the transitional newborn. *Journal of Pediatric Nursing, 27*(3), 214–224.

Fantz, R. L. (1961). The origins of form perception. *Scientific American, 204,* 66–72.

Fantz, R. L. (1963). Pattern vision in newborn infants. *Science, 140,* 296–297.

Farroni, T., Menon, E., Rigato, S., & Johnson, M. (2007). The perception of facial expressions in newborns. *European Journal of Developmental Psychology, 4,* 2–13.

Feldman, R., Rosenthal, Z., & Eidelman, A (2014). Maternal-preterm skin-to-skin contact enhances child physiologic organization and cognitive control across the first 10 years of life. *Biological Psychiatry, 75*(1), 56–64.

Field, T. M., Scafidi, F., & Schanberg, S. (1987). Massage of preterm newborns to improve growth and development. *Pediatric Nursing, 13,* 385–387.

Fowler, M., Gable, A., Lampe, M., Etina, M., & Owor, M. (2010). Perinatal HIV and its prevention: Progress toward an HIV-free generation. *Clinics in Perinatology, 37*(4), 699–719.

Freudigman, K., & Thoman E. (1994). Ultradian and diurnal cyclicity in the sleep states of newborn infants during the first two postnatal days. *Early Human Development, 38*(2), 67–80.

Gervain, J., Berent, I., & Werker, J. (2012). Binding at birth: The newborn brain detects identity relationships and sequential position in speech. *Journal of Cognitive Neuroscience, 24*(4), 564–574.

Gest, S. D., & Davidson, A. J. (2011). A developmental perspective on risk, resilience, and prevention. In M. K. Underwood & L. H. Rosen (Eds.), *Social development: Relationships in infancy, childhood, and adolescence* (pp. 427–454). New York: The Guilford Press.

Glass, P. (1990). Light and the developing retina. *Documenta Opthalmologica, 74,* 195–203.

Goldfield, E. F., & Wolff, P. H. (2002). Motor development in infancy. In A. Slater & M. Lewis (Eds.), *Introduction to infant development* (pp. 61–82). Oxford: Oxford University Press.

Gordon-Shogan, M., & Schumann, L. L. (1993). The effect of environmental lighting on the oxygen saturation of pre-term infants in the NICU. *Neonatal Network, 12,* 7–13.

Greenberg, M., & Morris, D. (1974). Engrossment. The newborn's impact upon the father. *American Journal of Orthopsychiatry, 44,* 520–531.

Gudsnuk, K., & Champagne, F. (2011). Epigenetic effects of early developmental experiences. *Clinics in Perinatology, 38*(4), 703–717.

Harlow, H. F. (1958). The nature of love. *American Psychologist, 13,* 673–685.

Hepper, P. G. (2002). Prenatal development. In A. Slater & M. Lewis (Eds.), *Introduction to infant development* (pp. 39–60). Oxford, England: Oxford University Press.

Heriza, C. (1991). Motor development: Traditional and contemporary theories. In *Contemporary management of motor control problems* (pp. 99–126). Alexandria, VA: American Physical Therapy Association.

Holloway, E. (1997). Parent and occupational therapist collaboration in the neonatal intensive care unit. *American Journal of Occupational Therapy, 48,* 535–538.

Horak, F. B. (1991). Assumptions underlying motor control for neurologic rehabilitation. In *Contemporary management of motor control problems* (pp. 11–27). Alexandria, VA: American Physical Therapy Association.

Householder, J., Hatcher, R., Burns, W., & Chasnoff, I. (1982). Infants born to narcotic-addicted mothers. *Psychological Bulletin, 92,* 453–468.

Kaitz, M., Meschulach-Sarfaty, O., & Auerbach, J. (1988). A re-examination of newborns' ability to imitate facial expressions. *Developmental Psychology, 24,* 3–7.

Karen, R. (1994). Astonishing attunements: The unseen emotional life of babies. In *Becoming attached: Unfolding the mystery of the infant-mother bond and its impact on later life* (pp. 347–359). New York: Time-Warner Books.

Kawakami, K., Kurihara, H., Shimizu, Y., & Yanaihara, T. (1996). The effects of sounds on newborn infants under stress. *Infant Behavior and Development, 19,* 375–379.

Kedesky, J. H., & Budd, K. S. (1998). Assessment of environmental factors in feeding. In *Childhood feeding disorders* (pp. 79–114). Baltimore: Brookes.

Klaus, M. H., & Kennell, J. H. (1982). *Parent-infant bonding.* St. Louis: C.V. Mosby.

Klaus, M. H., Kennell, J. H., Plumb, N., & Zuehlke, S. (1970). Human maternal behavior at first contact with her young. *Pediatrics, 46,* 187–192.

Korner, A., & Thoman, E. (1970). Visual alertness in neonates as evoked by maternal care. *Journal of Experimental Child Psychology, 10,* 67–78.

Lamb, M. E., & Campos, J. J. (1982). Sensory and perceptual development. In *Development in infancy: An Introduction* (pp. 57–91). New York: Random House.

Lamb, M. E., Frodi, A. M., Hwang, C. P., Frodi, M., & Steinberg, J. (1982). Effect of gender and caretaking role on parent-infant interaction. In R. Emde & R. Harmon (Eds.), *The Development of attachment and affiliative systems* (pp. 109–118). New York: Plenum Press.

Legg, C., Sherick, I., & Wadland, W. (1974). Reaction of pre-school children to the birth of a sibling. *Child Psychology & Human Development, 5,* 3–39.

Lindsay, D. (1996). *Functional human anatomy* (pp. 447–448). St. Louis: Mosby.

Long, T., & Toscano, T. (2002). *Handbook of pediatric physical therapy* (2nd ed.). Philadelphia: Lippincott Williams & Wilkins.

Lundy-Ekman, L. (2012). *Neuroscience: Fundamentals for rehabilitation* (4th ed.). Philadelphia: W. B. Saunders.

May, L., Byers-Heinlein, K., Gervain, J., & Werker, J. F. (2011) Language and the newborn brain: Does prenatal language experience shape the neonate neural response to speech? *Frontiers in Psychology, 2,* 222.

McNall, L. K. (1976). Concerns of expectant fathers. In L. K. McNall & J. T. Galeender (Eds.), *Current practice in obstetrics and gynecology.* St. Louis: C.V. Mosby.

Mechoulam, H., & Pierce, E. A. (2003). Retinopathy of prematurity: Molecular pathology and therapeutic strategies. *American Journal of Pharmacogenomics, 3*(4), 261–277.

Meltzoff, A. N., & Borton, R. W. (1979). Intermodal matching by human neonates. *Nature, 282,* 403–404.

Meltzoff, A. N., & Moore, M. K. (1977). Imitation of facial and manual gestures by human neonates. *Science, 198,* 75–78.

Mendella, J., & Beauchamp, G. K. (1996). The human infant's response to vanilla flavors in mother's milk and formula. *Infant Behavior & Development, 19,* 13–19.

Moore, K. (2003). Human birth defects. In K. Moore, T. Persaud, & W. Schmitt (Eds.), *The developing human* (7th ed.; pp. 167–201). Philadelphia: W. B. Saunders.

Morrongiello, B., Fenwick, K., & Chance, G. (1998). Crossmodal learning in newborn infants: Inferences about properties of audiovisual events. *Infant Behavior & Development, 21,* 543–554.

Nazzi, T., Floccia, C., & Bertocini, J. (1998). Discrimination of pitch contours by neonates. *Infant Behavior & Development, 21,* 779–784.

Parke, R. M. (1979). Perspectives on father-infant interaction. In J. Osofsky (Ed.), *Handbook of infant development* (pp. 549–590). New York: John Wiley & Sons.

Phillips, R. B., Sharma, R., Premachandra, B. P., Vaughn, A., & Reyes-Lee, M. (1996). Intrauterine exposure to cocaine: Effect on neurobehavior of neonates. *Infant Behavior & Development, 19,* 71–81.

Pierog, S., Chandavasu, O., & Wexter, I. (1977). Withdrawal symptoms in infants with fetal alcohol syndrome. *Journal of Pediatrics, 90,* 630–633.

Rainville, E. B. (1999). Prenatal and perinatal risk factors. In S. M. Porr & E. B. Rainville (Eds.), *Pediatric therapy: A systems approach* (pp. 22–60). Philadelphia: F. A. Davis.

Robson, A., & Cline, B. (1998). Developmental consequences of intrauterine growth retardation. *Infant Behavior & Development, 21,* 3331–3344.

Samra, H., McGrath, J., Wehbe, M., & Clapper, J. (2012). Epigenetics and family-centered developmental care for the preterm infant. *Advances in Neonatal Care, 12*(55, Supplement 1), S2–S9.

Scafidi, F. A., Field, T. M., & Schanberg, S. M. (1993). Factors that predict which preterm infants benefit most from massage therapy. *Developmental & Behavioral Pediatrics, 14,* 176–180.

Schaal, B., Montaganer, H., Hertling, E., Bolzoni, D., Moyse, A., & Quichon, R. (1980). Les stimulations olfactives dans les relations entre l'enfant et la mere. *Reproduction, Nutrition, Development, 20,* 843–858.

Scher, M. S. (2008). Ontogeny of EEG-sleep from neonatal through infancy periods. *Sleep Medicine, 9*(6), 615–636.

Scoppa, A., Casani, A., Cocca, F., Colettsa, C., DeLuca, M. G., DiManso, G., Grappone, L., Pozzi, N., & Orfe, L. (2012). aEEG in Preterm infants. *Journal of Maternal, Fetal, and Neonatal Medicine, 25*(Supplement 4), 139–140.

Shepherd, J. T., Hanshaw, J. K., & Lane, S. J. (1999). Working in the neonatal intensive care unit. In S. M. Porr & E. B. Rainville (Eds.), *Pediatric therapy: a systems approach* (pp. 313–378). Philadelphia: F. A. Davis.

Shonkoff, J. P., & Phillips, D. P. (2000). *From neurons to neighborhoods: The science of early childhood development.* Washington, DC: National Academy Press.

Shumway-Cook, A., & Woollacott, M. (2012). *Motor control: Translating research into clinical practice* (4th ed.). Philadelphia: Lippincott, Williams & Wilkins.

Slater, A., VonderSchulenburg, C., Brown, E., Badinock, M., Butterworth, G., Parsons, S., & Samuels, C. (1998). Newborn infants prefer attractive faces. *Infant Behavior & Development, 21,* 345–354.

Spence, M., & Freeman, M. (1996). Newborn infants prefer the maternal low-pass filtered voice, but not the maternal whispered voice. *Infant Behavior & Development, 19,* 199–212.

Svejda, M. J., Pannabecker, B. J., & Emde, R. N. (1982). Parent-to-infant attachment: A critique of the early "bonding" model. In R. Emde & R. Harmon (Eds.), *The development of attachment and affiliative systems* (pp. 88–93). New York: Plenum Press.

Sweeney, J. K., Gutierrez, T., & Beachy, J. (2012) Neonate and parents: Neurobehavioral perspectives in the NICU and follow-up. In D. Umphred, T. Rolando, M. Lazaro, & G. Burton (Eds.), *Neurological rehabilitation* (6th ed.; pp. 271–316). St. Louis: Mosby.

Thelen, E., & Fisher, D. M. (1982). Newborn stepping: An explanation for a "disappearing" reflex. *Developmental Psychology, 18,* 760–775.

Thelen, E., & Spencer, J. P. (1998). Postural control during reaching in young infants: A dynamic systems approach. *Neuroscience and Biobehavioral Reviews, 22*(4), 507–514.

Trause, M. A., & Irvin, N. A. (1982). Care of the sibling. In M. Klaus & J. Kennell (Eds.), *Parent-infant bonding* (pp. 110–130). St. Louis: C. V. Mosby.

Trause, M. A., Boslett, M., Voos, D., Rudd, C., Kennell, J. H., & Klaus, M. H. (1977). A birth in the hospital: The effect on the sibling. Abstract #70 in *Pediatric Research, 11,* 383.

Trause, M. A., Voos, D., Rudd, C., Klaus, M., Kennell, J., & Boslett, M. (1981). Separation for childbirth, the effect on the sibling. *Child Psychology & Human Development, 12,* 32–39.

Trevarthen, C. (2011). What is it like to be a person who knows nothing? Defining the active intersubjective mind of a newborn human being. *Infant and Child Development, 20,* 119–135.

Walton, G. E., Armstrong, E. K., & Bower, T. G. R. (1997). Faces as forms in the world of the newborn. *Infant Behavior & Development, 21,* 537–543.

Walton, G. E., Bower, M. J., & Bower, T. G. (1992). Recognition of familiar faces by newborns. *Infant Behavior & Development, 15,* 265–269.

Wilhelm, I. (1993). Neurobehavioral assessment of the high-risk neonate. In I. Wilhelm (Ed.), *Physical therapy assessment in early infancy* (pp. 35–70). New York: Churchill Livingstone.

World Health Organization (WHO). (2012). *10 facts on breastfeeding.* Retrieved from www.who.int/features/factfiles/breastfeeding/en/index.html

Young, J. (1996). *Developmental care of the premature baby.* London: Bailliere Tindall.

Zayek, M., Trimm, R., Hamm, C., Peevy, K., Benjamin, J., & Eyal, F. (2011). The limits of viability: A single regional unit's experience. *Archives of Pediatric and Adolescent Medicine, 65,* 126–133.

CHAPTER 10

Infancy

MaryBeth Mandich, PT, PhD,
Professor and Chairperson,
Division of Physical Therapy,
West Virginia University,
Morgantown, West Virginia

Objectives

Upon completion of this chapter, readers should be able to:

- Describe the developmental tasks of infants across all domains of performance;

- Name the major behavioral milestones of each period of infancy;

- Describe the characteristic reflexes and reactions associated with each period of infancy, and discuss how these relate to motor behavior;

- Discuss the interaction between domains of performance, such as the relationship between object permanence and stranger anxiety;

- Identify why a thorough knowledge of developmental sequence is important for therapists;

- Identify and discuss the social roles of infants, including a thorough definition and discussion of the concept of attachment and its implications; and

- Define developmental delay, and discuss its significance.

Key Terms

abnormal development
affordance
astasia
avoiding reaction
balance
body-on-body righting reaction (BOB)
body-on-head righting reaction
   (BOH)
cruising
developmental delay
equilibrium reactions
hypotonia
inferior pincer grasp

lateral grasp
locomotor pattern
lordosis
mature rotary neck righting
optical righting reaction
palmar grasp
plagiocephaly
postural control
postural equilibrium
postural set
posture
prehension
protective reactions

radial digital grasp
raking
righting
stereotypy
stranger anxiety
superior pincer grasp
symmetrical tonic neck reflex
   (STNR)
synaptic pruning
toddling
torticollis
transfer pattern
transient developmental delay

INTRODUCTION

The term *infancy* is used here to describe the period of life from birth through 12 months of age. It is a time of rapid physical growth as well as rapid developmental maturation. Newborns are largely dependent, although able to exert more control over the environment than once was thought. However, by the end of infancy, children show significant environmental mastery across multiple domains of behavior. The near total gravity dependency and limited mobility of newborns are replaced at 1 year by an ability to move from place to place and manipulate objects in the environment. The limited communication skills of newborns are replaced at 1 year of age by the purposeful use of language as a communication skill. Finally, by 1 year of age, infants have adopted a clear social participation role, with characteristic temperament and a style of interaction with both family and others.

The processes that underlie this change in the first year of life are both intrinsic and extrinsic. Normally developing infants will experience maturation and growth in all body systems. However, it is the incredibly rapid maturation of the central nervous system (CNS) that is especially important in the first year of life. This CNS maturation supports much behavioral change over the first year (Eliot, 1999). Despite the important role played by innate functions, the effect of the environment is not to be underestimated (Scarr, 1992). The role of environment in infancy is evident in many ways. First, cross-cultural study of different caregiving practices demonstrates their impact on infant development (deVries, 1999; Shonkoff & Phillips, 2000). Second, studies of infants who have had negative

environmental experiences through deprivation, abuse, or overstimulation confirm the fact that such experiences negatively impact developmental acquisition of behavior (Chang & Merzenich, 2003; Teicher et al., 2003). Finally, many studies, both animal and human, confirm the interaction effect of environmental experiences and neural maturation (Eliot, 1999; Johnston, Nishimura, Harum, Pekar, & Blue, 2001).

The first year of life is a remarkable and fascinating time in the human life span. Professionals working with children who are developing normally or who have special needs derive great satisfaction from the opportunity to have an impact on the human potential represented by the infancy period.

BODY STRUCTURE AND FUNCTION: CHANGE OVER THE FIRST YEAR

In the first year of life, growth continues at a very rapid rate. The average male infants grow 6.75 inches (17.2 cm), and the average females grow 3.25 inches (7.1 cm). These measurements represent an increase in length of approximately 50 percent (Payne & Isaacs, 2012). Recent data indicate that average term infants in the United States weigh 7.5 pounds, which is a slight decrease since 1990 (Donahue, Kleinman, Gillman, & Oken, 2010). Infants tend to lose some of their birth weight in the first postnatal days and return to birth weight by the end of the second week. By 5 to 6 months, birth weight has doubled, indicating a rate of growth of approximately an ounce a day. In the second half of infancy, weight gain slows down to about ½ ounce a day. By the end of the first year, typically, birth weight has tripled (Payne & Isaacs, 2012). A newborn's head is a greater proportion of the body than at 1 year. A newborn's heart rate ranges from 120 to 140 beats per minute but slows over the first year to approximately 80 to 100 beats per minute. Blood pressure in infants is also lower than in adults. Normative blood pressure at birth is around 80/55, and the systolic pressure increases gradually so that at 1 year, normal blood pressure is approximately 95 to 100/55 (Choukair, 2000).

THE FIRST YEAR OF LIFE: AN OVERVIEW

The first year of life is commonly subdivided into periods of 2 to 3 months. These periods are defined by characteristic accomplishments. In this text, development during the first 12 months is organized into four time frames, each consisting of 3 months. These periods of 3 months are defined as early infancy (birth to 3 months), middle infancy (4 to 6 months), late infancy (7 to 9 months), and

infancy transition (10 to 12 months). Within each period, accomplishments are categorized and discussed according to domains typically associated with developmental assessment. These domains are gross motor, fine motor/adaptive behavior, person-social behavior, and cognitive language. A summary of development over the first year across these periods may be found in **Table 10-1** (Long & Toscano, 2002; Schulman, 2010).

For clarity, some important terms will be introduced prior to the discussion of infant development. The process of bringing the body parts into alignment is known as **righting** (VanSant, 1995). The process of reestablishing the center of mass over the base of support once displaced is known as **postural equilibrium**. **Posture** is the alignment of the body at any given point in time, including both biomechanical and neuromotor elements. **Postural control** is the ability to maintain the body in a position by keeping the center of gravity over the base of support or returning it over the base of support following displacement, for the dual purposes of orientation and stability (Payne & Isaacs, 2012; Shumway-Cook & Woollacott, 2012). There are two classifications of postural control—static and dynamic. *Static postural control* is the ability to sustain or hold a quiet position, whereas *dynamic postural control* is the ability to maintain alignment of body parts during movement. **Balance** is another

TABLE 10-1	Summary of Development during first Year of Life			
EARLY INFANCY: Birth through 3 Months				
Gross Motor	**Fine Motor**	**Oral-Motor**	**Cognitive-Language**	**Personal-Social**
Present: ATNR; tonic labyrinthine; labyrinthine righting Behavior: • Lifts head in prone (NB) • Lifts head 45 degrees (1–2 mo.) • Lifts head 90 degrees (2–3 mo.) • Increasing extension at rest • Predominantly asymmetrical (NB) • Total head lag in pull-to-sit (NB), which decreases (1–3)	Present: ATNR; palmar grasp reflex; upper extremity traction Behavior: • Hands closed most of the time with spontaneous opening (NB) • Hands swipe at mouth (NB) • Inserts hand in mouth and sucks (1) • Hands open (1–3) • Grasps object placed in palm briefly	Present: Suck-swallow reflex; phasic bite reflex; rooting Behavior: • Suckling pattern • Bottle/breast-fed • Vigorous suck • Coordinates suck, swallow, and respiration	Behavior: • Cries • Coos • Vocalizes when not crying • Chuckles	Behavior: • Cries to communicate • Calms to human face and voice • Visual tracking not across midline (NB) Across midline 180 degrees (3 mo.) • First smile (2–3 mo.)

Continues

TABLE 10-1   Summary of Development during first Year of Life   *(continued)*

MIDDLE INFANCY: 4–6 Months

Gross Motor	Fine Motor	Oral-Motor	Cognitive-Language	Personal-Social
Integrated: All primitive reflexes ATNR, TLR, palmar grasp, stepping, supporting Appears: Body-on-body righting Rotary neck righting Protective extension down and forward Prone equilibrium STNR Behavior: • Rolls prone to supine, supine to prone (4–6) • Full prone extension (6) • Lifts head and helps in pull-to-sit (5) • Midline behavior: hands and feet to mouth • Sits propped (5–6) • Supported standing with weight bearing	Integrated: Palmar grasp Behavior: • Hands are closed at rest less of the time • Hands to midline in play (4) • Grasps object placed in palm (4) • Predominantly ulnar palmar grasp (5–6) • Reaches (5–6) • Rakes (5–6)	Integrated: Rooting reaction Phasic bite reflex Behavior: • First spoon feeding: Upper lip not active (4) • Disassociation of lips, tongue, jaw begins with true sucking (4) • Voluntary suck: increased negative pressure in oral cavity (4) • Upper lip activates in removing food from spoon	Behavior: • Secondary circular reactions—infant acts on environment to prolong interesting experiences • Disyllabic utterances • Increase in sounds produced • Babbling begins (5–6)	Behavior: • Early play • Infant shows delight • Laughs and chuckles

LATE INFANCY: 7–9 Months

Gross Motor	Fine Motor	Oral-Motor	Cognitive-Language	Personal-Social
Integrated: STNR Appears: Protective extension; side (7–8); backward (9–10); sitting equilibrium (7–8) Behavior: • Sits erect independently (7–8) • Commando crawls (7–8) • Assumes sitting (8–9) • Pushes to hands and knees (8–9) • Rocks in hands and knees (8–9) • Quadruped may begin (9)	Behavior: • Radial palmar grasp (7) • Lateral pincer grasp (8–9) • Voluntary release	Behavior: • Eats well from spoon (7) • Early solids, uses munching pattern (7–9)	Behavior: • Babbles clear vowel-consonant sounds • Secondary circular reactions (4–8) change to coordination of secondary reactions (8–9) • Aware of ability to manipulate environment • Object permanence develops	Behavior: • Shows anger and fear • Will protest if caregiver leaves • Demonstrates early signs of caregiver attachment • Becomes an "emotional being"

Continues

TABLE 10-1 Summary of Development during first Year of Life *(continued)*

TRANSITIONAL INFANCY: 10–12 Months

Gross Motor	Fine Motor	Oral-Motor	Cognitive-Language	Personal-Social
Appears: Equilibrium quadruped (9–10); Standing (11–12) Behavior: <ul><li>Assumes and maintains quadruped (10)</li><li>Creeps on hands and knees (10–11)</li><li>Pulls to stand (10–11)</li><li>Cruises at furniture (10–11)</li><li>Walks with two hands held, then one hand held</li><li>Walks independently</li></ul>	Behavior: <ul><li>Inferior pincer grasp (10–11)</li><li>Pincer pad-to-pad grasp (11–12)</li><li>Superior pincer tip-to-tip grasp (12)</li></ul>	Behavior: <ul><li>Eats solids with tongue lateralization</li><li>Appearance of diagonal and rotary jaw movement</li></ul>	Behavior: <ul><li>First true word (11–12)</li><li>Babbles more sounds</li><li>Object permanence more secure</li><li>More sophisticated means-end relationships</li></ul>	Behavior: <ul><li>Shows an attachment style</li><li>Stranger anxiety</li></ul>

word for postural stability, which is when the body is maintained in equilibrium at rest (static equilibrium) or during movement (dynamic equilibrium) (Shumway-Cook & Woollacott, 2012). Finally, **postural set** is the alignment of body parts at any given point in time.

Prehension is the use of the hands for grasping, holding, and manipulation of objects. To accomplish a prehensile task, several components are necessary. These include the ability to approach the object in space, known as *reach;* the ability to position and close the hand around the object, known as *grasp;* the ability to move the object while it is held, known as *manipulation;* and the ability to release the object when desired (Duff, 1995). These different components of fine motor control mature variably over the first year, with grasp being one of the earliest functions, beginning as a reflex and progressing to increasing volition.

EARLY INFANCY: BIRTH TO 3 MONTHS—AN OVERVIEW

The first 3 months of life are a transition period for infants (and their family). The changes that occur over the first 3 months are cumulative but not dramatic. Infants are laying the groundwork for the remarkable achievements of the ensuing months. In motor development, there is increasing postural extension and increasing ability in antigravity control, especially of the head and arms. The arms develop and begin to explore space. Early communication progresses

from crying to gurgling and cooing. Infants get to know Mom and Dad and begin to clearly express preferences. Their cognitive development is mostly manifested through attention, visual fixation and following, and habituation to familiar stimuli.

Gross Motor Development

As previously discussed, newborns' movements are heavily influenced by the deep attractor wells of behavior otherwise known as *reflexes*. Antigravity behavior in prone is limited at birth to lifting and turning the head from side to side (see **Figure 10-1A**). Over these first months, this ability improves significantly, so that by 4 months of age, the head can be lifted up to 90 degrees, and infants are able to look around (see **Figure 10-1B**). Concurrent with this improved head control in prone, the infants' arms begin to prop, so that by 4 months, their elbows are tucked under their body, and relatively soon after they are able to use their increasing antigravity control as a base on which to shift their weight to one side, which is a preparatory pattern toward rolling from prone to supine (see **Figure 10-1C**). These abilities coincide with the diminishing influence of the tonic labyrinthine pattern in prone and the increasing labyrinthine righting abilities.

In supine, newborns are once again gravity-dependent. Grasping their forearms and pulling them to a sitting position while assessing the righting of their head usually tests the amount of antigravity control they

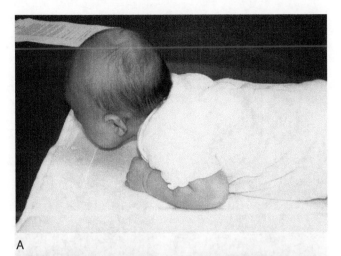

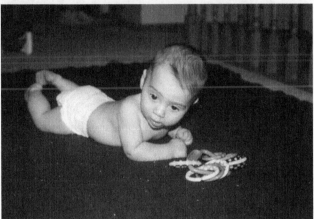

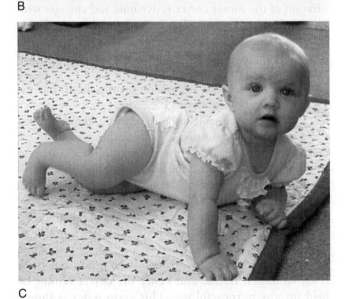

Figure 10-1 Maturation of Prone Behavior: A. 1–2 months; B. 3–4 months; C. 4–5 months

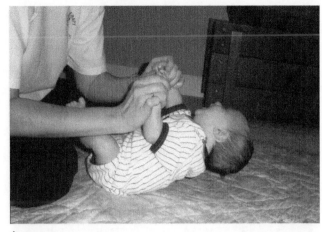

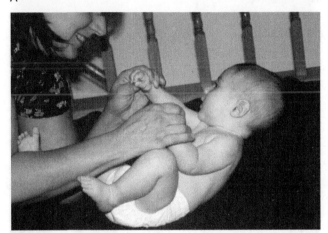

Figure 10-2 Decrease in Head Lag in Pull-to-Sit: A. Newborn; B. 5 months

(**Figure 10-2B**). Once newborns are sitting, their head will fall forward on their chest, but brief periods of righting are seen; however, by the end of early infancy, sitting with head stable and upright is seen (see **Figure 10-3A** through C).

In the upright position, when a baby is held in vertical suspension, righting against gravity likewise develops over the first 3 months of life. At birth, the influence of the supporting reaction produces a successive extension of the lower limbs without true weight-bearing support. When held in supported standing, the newborn also displays a rhythmic alternating stepping movement (see **Figure 10-4**). These stepping patterns are similar in kinematic characteristics to the patterns of supine kicking, and it has been proposed that early kicking and stepping are similar patterns differing only in postural set in which they occur (Thelen & Fisher, 1982). Using Thelen's terminology, patterns such as kicking and stepping have been referred to as stereotypies. A **stereotypy** is an intrinsic nonpurposeful movement pattern that repeats itself. It appears to be intrinsic and therefore does not depend on sensory feedback to be elicited (Payne & Isaacs, 2012).

have from the supine position. At birth, in the pull-to-sit, there is nearly complete head lag (see **Figure 10-2A**), but by 4 months of age, infants show minimal head lag

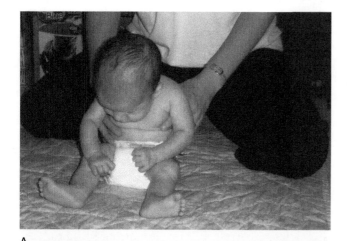

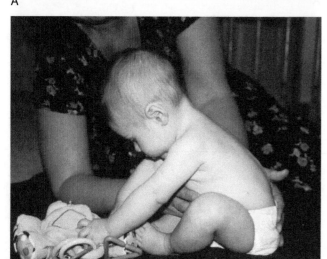

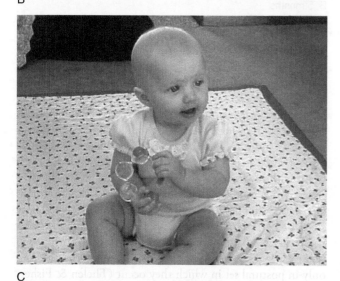

Figure 10-3 Maturation of Sitting Behavior: A. Newborn (supported); B. Increasing extension at 4–5 months; C. Sits erect at 6–8 months

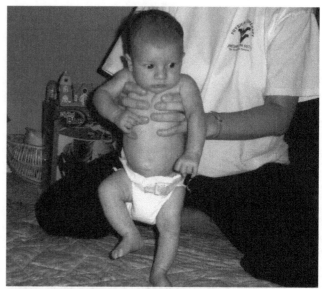

Figure 10-4 Reflexive Stepping Behavior in Newborn

Fine Motor Development

Many factors influence the development of fine motor skills during infancy. For the development of fine motor control, three things are needed: (1) the capacity for motor control of the fingers; (2) somatosensory feedback to the motor system; and (3) translation of somatosensory information onto a motor planning guiding appropriate hand configurations (Henderson & Pehoski, 2006). The functional organization of the motor cortex is dynamic and changes with hand use and experience. This is important because during infancy there is increasing motor activity in the hand, including opposition of the thumb and the movement of grasp distally to the fingertips.

At birth the hands are predominantly fisted, but the pattern is never obligatory in the normal case. An infant's hands will open spontaneously. In addition, the infant will swipe at the mouth, sometimes inserting the entire fist in the oral cavity. Typically, it takes a few months for an infant to truly engage in thumb-sucking behavior, although occasionally this is seen perinatally. Throughout the first 3 months, infants increasingly keep their hands open, so that by 4 months of age, their hands are open most of the time.

In newborns, grasp is reflexive and nonfunctional. Newborns' fingers will close around an object when pressure is applied across the metatarsal heads, but there is no volitional release and hence the object cannot be held for any purposeful use. This grasp reflex is shown in **Figure 10-5**. It gradually diminishes over the first few postnatal months.

Likewise, at birth there is no purposeful reaching pattern, although there is believed to be a kind of reaching called *visually triggered reaching*. This means that early in life infants are able to see a target and will attempt to approach the target with their arms (Shumway-Cook &

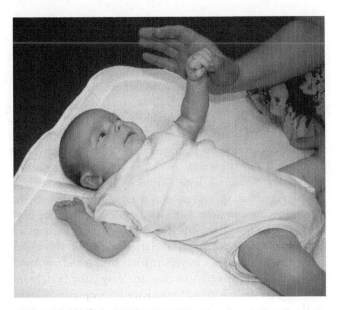

Figure 10-5 Reflexive Grasp in Newborn

Oral-Motor Development

Neonates demonstrate the suckling pattern, as described in Chapter 9. The suckling pattern exemplifies the developmental principle of general to specific in that there is little disassociation of lips, tongue, and jaw in this pattern. Likewise, neonates show the reflexive behaviors described previously of phasic bite, suck-swallow, and gag. Most infants are bottle- or breast-fed through the first months. Even if cereal is introduced in this period for medical reasons or reasons of convenience, it is often mixed with formula in the bottle. Young infants are not efficient spoon-feeders. The major occurrence in oral-motor behavior between birth and 3 months is the increasing volitional aspects of the suck-swallow pattern. There is better lip closure, and infants will demonstrate mouth opening and anticipatory behaviors as the bottle approaches their mouth (Koontz-Lowman & Lane, 1999). Concurrent with these changes, there is an increase in negative pressure in the oral cavity, which is the beginning of the transition to a mature suck pattern.

Cognitive and Language Development

The production of sound is related to oral-motor development in that the muscle control developed early in feeding also underlies the production and differentiation of sounds. In Chapter 5, there was much discussion of early communication behaviors. At birth, an infant's communication is pre-intentional and is predominated by crying. During crying, the mouth is open and the tongue is observed to shape and cup, much as it does in feeding. With increasing control of lips, tongue, and jaw through the first few months, infants begin to vocalize. The earliest vocalizations, occurring around 1 to 2 months of age, are cooing and gurgling sounds usually used to indicate pleasure during feeding. By the end of the early infancy period, infants are typically using open-mouth, monosyllabic utterances (Long & Toscano, 2002). Intentional communication also begins at this time.

Cognitive development in the first year of life is difficult to assess and is largely judged indirectly through observation of behaviors. From a Piagetian perspective, the first 3 months of life comprise the reflexive stage and primary circular reactions. In the *reflexive* stage of the first month, infants respond to the world based on prewired responses to stimulation, as in the sucking reflex when an object is placed in the mouth. However, as infants enter the stage of *primary circular reactions,* the hallmark of repeating interesting actions occurs. This may start very simply, as infants might begin to repeat actions such as sucking or looking at hands to maintain an interesting phenomenon.

Historically, it was initially thought that infants had very little cognitive capability—in fact, the tradition was to view infants as functioning at a subcortical level of the

Woollacott, 2012). Newborns have semidirected swipes, usually at the mouth, as described previously. By 3 months of age, they have more directed swipes, batting at objects placed above the head in preparation for true reach; however, the hands are largely open as the arm is extended, making grabbing of the object impossible. Thelen describes these waving motions of the arms as an example of a stereotypy involving upper extremities (Payne & Isaacs, 2012). Near the end of early infancy, infants begin to be able to sustain grasp on an object placed in the hand.

Henderson and Pehoski (2006) note that "the hand is both a motor and a sensing organ and there is a tight interplay between these two functions" (p. 7). The first motor actions of the hands and eyes are guided by an infant's interest in acquiring perceptual and sensory information. This is important to note, because children with sensory impairments (such as blindness) have atypical patterns of hand skill development simply because of the differences in their sensory experiences. The development of fine motor skills does have some predictable maturational aspects, but is also highly variable based on the environmental conditions within which the child is maturing. Cultural child-rearing practices influence many of the learning conditions in infancy. How much time a baby is held, the space afforded the infant for explorations, the sensory qualities of the environment available to the infant, and the social rewards for particular activity patterns will all influence early hand use (Henderson & Pehoski, 2006).

Similar to the development of grasp, the first pattern of object release is a reflexive behavior. An **avoiding reaction** is a reflexive behavior involving finger extension as an infant withdraws and abducts the fingers in response to touch on the hand (Henderson & Pehoski, 2006). This reflexive pattern serves as an automatic mechanism to facilitate finger extension, often resulting in an involuntary, or automatic, release.

nervous system, primarily due to observation and interpretation of motor behavior. However, research done beginning in the mid-twentieth century has changed this view significantly. During the fetal period, between 100 and 200 billion nerve cells or neurons are formed (Feldman, 1999).

As mentioned in preceding chapters, the first 2 years of life are critical for brain development. During that period, myelin is being laid down. In addition, neurons establish elaborate synaptic connections with each other. The first 2 postnatal years are thought of as a time of synaptic sculpturing, with synaptogenesis occurring while other synapses and neurons are disappearing or becoming dormant (synaptic pruning). **Synaptic pruning** is the process of preserving the most-used neurons, synapses, and dendrites while gradually eliminating synaptic connections that are not used. This combined result of synaptogenesis and synaptic pruning is heavily related to environmental experience in both human and animal studies (Eliot, 1999). Therefore, provision of a nurturing and supportive environment for infants is extremely important in determining their ability to maximize their innate potential. At the end of this chapter, the effects of environment on early development will be discussed in some detail.

In light of new knowledge about the nervous system, as well as newer, more sophisticated studies of infant development using experimental paradigms such as habituation and physiologic monitoring, much more information is available about what infants "know." In early infancy, visual acuity and visual tracking improve. By 4 months of age, infants are able to visually track across midline consistently. They continue to prefer patterns with high contrast, such as black and white, but by the end of the period, there is indication that they can make distinctions between lights of different wavelength and begin to perceive color in groupings similar to those of adults (Teller & Bornstein, 1987). Using a checkerboard with various numbers of squares, a number of researchers have demonstrated that infants prefer patterns of increasing complexity with increasing age (McCluskey, 1981). In general, it is also thought that over the first few months, infants begin to respond less with a defensive reaction to a novel stimulus— such as a light, unexpected touch—and more with an approach, or orienting, response (Resiman, 1987).

Personal-Social Development

At birth newborns will show emotions, especially distress due to physical discomfort. Over the first 3 months, they will begin to show increasing periods of positive affect, including turning toward a pleasurable stimulus (Sroufe, 1996). By the end of the period, they are clearly showing social pleasure by smiling. Infants are able to differentiate between their mother and a stranger within the first weeks of life (Masi & Scott, 1983). Infants in the first few months are capable of imitating activities that are already in their

behavioral repertoire, such as opening the mouth or sticking out the tongue.

Temperament and interaction style are relatively stable aspects of infant behavior. Infants have been classified as *externalizers,* who have a great deal of facial expression and low physiologic reactivity, and *internalizers,* who have a relatively flat affect but are highly physiologically reactive (Field, 1990). Chess and Thomas (1996) have developed a classification of three main temperament types: easy, difficult, and slow to warm up. An *easy* baby shows curiosity in novel situations, high rythmicity in behaviors such as sleeping and eating, and moderate emotional intensity. In contrast, a *difficult* baby will have moods that are more negative and be less adaptable in general. A *slow-to-warm-up* baby shows less activity and is relatively calm; however, this baby would approach a novel situation with withdrawal and shows more negative affect than the easy baby (Feldman, 1999). The sensitivity and reactivity to people and events in the environment that constitute temperament have been shown to be relatively stable over time and hence are probably heavily attributable to innate processes (Field, 1990).

MIDDLE INFANCY: 4 TO 6 MONTHS— AN OVERVIEW

The period of 4 to 6 months of age is one of major change in motor behavior. In gross motor behavior, infants learn to master antigravity control in both prone and supine positions. The first independent sitting occurs, as does the first transfer of postural set from prone to supine and supine to prone. Infants develop functional use of the hands, and are able to reach and grasp an object with a characteristic palmar grasp. Near the end of the period, infants may be beginning to transfer objects from hand to hand. In language, a greater variety of sounds is produced, including disyllabic utterances. Infants begin babbling during this period. Cognitive development is seen in activity on the environment, especially activity designed to prolong interesting phenomena. These are the secondary circular reactions. By 6 months, infants are developing object permanence. In personal-social development, they express joy and delight and engage in early play activities, such as peekaboo (see **Table 10-1**).

Gross Motor Development

In the middle infancy period, there is a significant change in gross motor ability, both in terms of posture and in terms of mobility. Because motor behavior rapidly grows more sophisticated, it is worthwhile to discuss some terminology that will be helpful in describing further motor development. Motor behavior is generally the result of muscle contraction. Exclusive of smooth and cardiac muscle, which will not be discussed here, motor behavior usually produces two functional consequences: holding or moving. Postural patterns control the alignment of the center of mass over the base of support and the relative alignment of body parts. Mobility patterns perform one of two functions.

The first type of mobility pattern is a **transfer pattern**. A transfer pattern permits people to transfer or translate from one postural set to another, as in going from lying down to sitting up or from prone to supine. A **locomotor pattern** moves, or translates, the entire body through space, as in crawling or walking. At birth, an infant's motor repertoire is very limited. Postural control is reflected only in very brief periods of righting the head in the postural sets of prone and sitting. Also, at birth there are no mobility patterns of either the transfer or locomotor types. Infants are very dependent on a caregiver for these functions. We have seen how over the first 3 months of life, infants' postural control develops in various postural sets so that by the beginning of the 4th month, they are able to prop up in prone on elbows, lifting the head and maintaining control. In supported sitting, they are able to maintain the head in a stable position, and in pull-to-sit, their head no longer lags. There is increasing symmetry in the supine posture as well. By the beginning of the 4th month, they can bring hands to midline and keep the head in midline to explore them. However, through the end of this period, they are still dependent in transfer and locomotor patterns.

In the 4th through the 6th month, infants make dramatic gains in motor ability across all the dimensions described. In this period, all the early dominant patterns of posture and movement, characterized by deep attractor wells, such as the tonic labyrinthine, asymmetrical tonic neck, grasp, stepping, and grasp reflexes, have been integrated. As this occurs with maturation of neuromotor and musculoskeletal systems, more functional motor behavior is permitted. Some characteristic patterns develop that underlie these new abilities, many of which appear at 4 to 6 months of age.

A series of righting reactions mediated by the CNS appear fully in the period of 4 to 6 months. The purpose of these righting reactions as a group is first of all to orient the head (and body) in space and the body parts with respect to each other and, second, to rotate the body parts into alignment with each other. The first, labyrinthine righting, has been defined as movement of the head into alignment with gravity in response to position in space, as detected by the vestibular system of the inner ear. Labyrinthine righting appears at birth in the limited abilities of infants in antigravity control, but it is fully mature by the 6th month. A related reaction, **optical righting reaction**, serves the orientation function of postural control, by positioning the head in response to the visual environment. The **body-on-head righting reaction (BOH)** rotates the head into alignment with the body or the surface on which the body is lying. These righting reactions all serve a postural function, whereas the other two righting reactions are known as *rotary righting reactions,* which serve a mobility function. The early

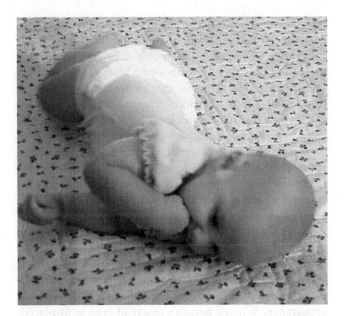

Figure 10-6   Rotary Righting Reaction

neonatal neck righting reaction is replaced by **mature rotary neck righting** in this period. The stimulus for rotary neck righting is rotation of the head and neck, in which the body de-rotates back into alignment. The **body-on-body righting reaction (BOB)** is similar, but in this case a rotary stimulus is applied along the long axis of a limb segment, and the body de-rotates into alignment. **Figure 10-6** illustrates body-on-body righting as rotation among body parts.

As a group, these righting reactions are present in the period of 4 to 6 months and reflect changes in neural maturation. Traditional thinking was that the emergence of these reactions was a determinant factor in the coincident emergence of postural control. However, contemporary thought in the systems model identifies changes in the neuromuscular response patterns as only one of several reasons for changes in behavior underlying milestone acquisition. Other factors to be considered include changes in the musculoskeletal system, maturation of sensory systems, and development of organizational strategies to process sensory input and development of internal representations to map these inputs. There is sound preliminary evidence that the emergence of milestones as traditionally reported is related to the postural set assumed in testing—in other words, that postural set interacts with the motor skill, and that when infants are put in different postural sets, the skill that may be observed is different. Simply put, infants may be able to demonstrate reaching easier in supported sitting than in supine. Furthermore, there is evidence that some of the postural reactions can respond to training (Shumway-Cook & Woollacott, 2012). Taking all current information into account, it appears that the development of the postural reactions, such as righting, plays a role in the acquisition of motor milestones; however, the role represents just one component of a complex system and is not as determinant as was once believed.

There are two other sets of postural reactions that contribute to balance. The first are the **protective reactions**. Protective reactions are also known as *parachute reactions*, indicating that these reactions provide a safety response for children. The stimulus that elicits these reactions is consistent—a displacement of center of mass such that the body cannot recenter over the base of support. In this case, the arms come out in extension to catch or protect the proximal body parts. The parachute reactions develop in a prescribed sequence, the first one being in response to downward displacement at approximately 5 months of age, followed by the anterior protective extension response at about 6 months of age (Shumway-Cook & Woollacott, 2012; VanSant, 1995).

The final set of postural reactions, which serve the function of balance, are the **equilibrium reactions**. These reactions, unlike the protective reactions, come into play in an attempt to reestablish the center of mass over the base of support in displacement. They have a very characteristic appearance. When a person's center of mass is displaced, the trunk responds by curving sideways against the direction of the displacement. Meanwhile, the limbs on the side that the displacement occurs are increasing their tone for weight bearing. The opposite arm and leg abduct. These equilibrium reactions also develop sequentially, with the prone reaction the first to appear at approximately 5 to 6 months of age (Shumway-Cook & Woollacott, 2012).

In terms of motor behavior, then, an infant's behavior is no longer dominated by primitive patterns with deep attractor wells. The righting reactions have all developed, as well as protective extension forward and down and the earliest equilibrium reaction. One observable change is increasing antigravity postural control. From 4 months, when infants are able to prop on elbows, the infants begin to lift up even higher in prone, propping on hands by 4 to 5 months of age (**Figure 10-1C**). By 6 months of age, when held in horizontal (prone) suspension, infants perform total antigravity extension, traveling through the hips. This pattern is known as the *Landau reaction* (see **Figure 10-7**), which is at least in part a combination of the postural righting reactions (Shumway-Cook & Woollacott, 2012). This mastery of total antigravity

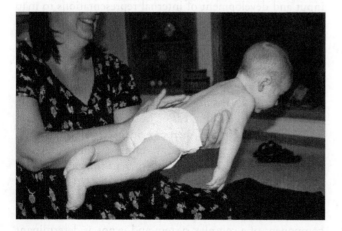

Figure 10-7 Landau Reaction at Approximately 5 to 6 Months

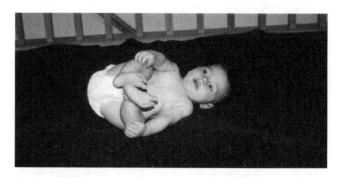

Figure 10-8 Hands-to-Feet Behavior at 4 to 5 Months

control is considered critical in some therapies, and is also known as the *pivot prone pattern* or *prone extension pattern.*

Infants' antigravity control in supine also changes dramatically from 4 to 6 months. By 4 months, infants can keep the head in midline and engage hands, but by 5 months or so, they can also bring feet to midline and will often play with hands and feet to mouth (see **Figure 10-8**).

This ability reflects increasing antigravity or flexor postural control in supine. Likewise, when infants are pulled to sitting beginning at about 5 months, they actually anticipate that movement and lift their head in an attempt to help (see **Figure 10-2B**). Antigravity control also manifests itself in sitting. An infant's spine, initially rounded in supported sitting during early infancy, now begins to show extension. At 4 months, the extension of neck and cervical spine is evident, but by 6 months, the extensor posture has traveled into the thoracic and lumbar spines, showing the normal curves in the cervical and lumbar spine (see **Figure 10-3B**). The first independent sitting typically occurs around 5 months of age. This sitting uses the arms for support, with the infant's legs positioned crossed and turned out in a style known as ring sitting. One final "reflex" of postural tone appears in this period. This is the **symmetrical tonic neck reflex** (STNR). Like its ATNR counterpart, the stimulus for the STNR is position of the head as detected by joint receptors in the neck. However, in this case, the head is flexed or extended. The response is for the arms to follow the postural attitude of the head and the legs to do the opposite. For example, when the neck is flexed, the arms flex and the legs extend. When the neck is extended, the arms extend and the legs flex. As shown in **Figure 10-9**, it is easy to see how the posture of the latter position relates to the earliest independent sitting (head extended, arms extended, legs flexed).

In standing, infants perform an interesting transition during 4 to 6 months. Recall that the earliest standing is heavily reflexive, with infants requiring a great deal of extrinsic support and bearing little true body weight. In the transition to upright control and true weight bearing, infants early in this period display **astasia**, which means "without stance." In this pattern, infants draw up legs and feet when attempts are made to place them in supported standing (VanSant, 1995). Parents will often interpret this pattern as an infant wishing to play a "jumping" game. During middle infancy,

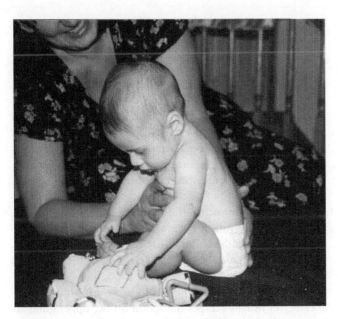

Figure 10-9   *Sitting Propped in Symmetrical Tonic Neck Reflex Position*

astasia disappears, and there is true weight bearing with an increasingly erect stance (VanSant, 1995).

With respect to mobility patterns of transfer, infants in middle infancy develop the first ability to change from one postural set to another with rolling. Rolling occurs in prone when an infant, who has been experimenting increasingly with postural control in prone on elbows by shifting weight, actually shifts weight enough to accomplish a complete transition, combined with the increasing rotation of body segments.

Traditional milestones for American infants give the first roll as occurring from prone to supine at 4 to 5 months and subsequently supine to prone at 5 to 6 months (see **Figure 10-10**). Cultural practice may influence this

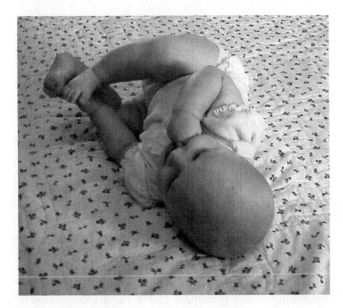

Figure 10-10   Rolling

sequence, however, as American babies are now spending more time in supine due to the "Safe to Sleep" public health initiative (formerly known as the Back to Sleep campaign), the sequence of acquisition of rolling milestones has become less clear (Dewey, Fleming, & Golding, 1998). This initiative was aimed at reducing the incidence of *sudden infant death syndrome (SIDS)*, because major epidemiologic studies show that countries where people have always placed infants in supine to sleep have a lower incidence of SIDS than do countries where infants are placed prone.

Davis, Moon, Sachs, and Ottolini (1998) reported on a prospective study of 351 infants who slept in either prone or supine positions. This study found that earlier attainment of motor milestones was associated with prone sleeping, including rolling prone to supine, sitting propped, creeping, crawling, and pulling-to-stand. However, they found no significant difference according to sleep position in the age of walking.

In summary, there is variability in attainment of early postural and mobility milestones that is affected by sleep position, but that this age of attainment does not adversely affect developmental outcome. In any case, by 6 months of age, infants are rolling freely from prone to supine and back. Locomotor patterns that move the body through space have yet to develop; however, a precursor pattern often appears during this period. This pattern is a prone or abdominal pivot in which an infant raises up on hands, and turns in a circle, bending the arms and legs on one side of the body.

Fine Motor Development

There is also remarkable change in the function of the arms and hands in the period of middle infancy. After an extended period of using the hands to explore the sensory qualities of their environment, infants become interested in mastering objects for functional purposes. As infants learn that they can have an effect on the environment, they become motivated to intentionally grasp and hold objects. At the start of this period, around 4 months of age, when an object is placed in a child's hand, he or she will use an *ulnar palmar grasp to* hold the object. This is based initially on the palmar grasp reflex described in Chapter 9, which is involuntary. By the time infants are 5 months old, they use a voluntary palmar grasp pattern. A **palmar grasp** (also called a *primitive squeeze grasp*) is characterized by a pronated hand and flexion of all fingers to hold an object against the palm without use of the thumb. With this grasp pattern, the wrist is usually flexed, which occurs because the hand is often extended beyond the object, which is approached laterally, with all fingers closing around the object to the palm (Shumway-Cook & Woollacott, 2012). By 6 months, infants are grasping with a similar palmar grasp, but with wrist neutral. As they continue to use the palmar grasp pattern, it begins to move away from the ulnar side of the hand and infants use both tactile and visual information to begin to plan movements and to prepare the hand for grasp by opening and shaping the hand prior to grasp.

Also, around 6 months of age, infants learn to control grasp and use grasp to move things into either their visual field, or their mouth. In addition, sometime around 5 to 6 months, infants begin to show the pattern of **raking**, in which a small object such as cereal or a raisin is approached with open hands and fingers, which cover the object like a rake, then attempt to sweep the object into the palm by closure of fingers. By the end of the period, some investigators indicate that infants can perform a primitive transfer of a cube from one hand to another. This is an early indicator of release, because one hand can release the object as the other grasps it (Duff, 1995). By 6 months, infants are usually able to hold a bottle with both hands as well.

Reaching also becomes much more functional at this time, with the appearance of visually guided reaching. Whereas *visually triggered reaching* is important in the initiation of reach by prospectively seeing an object and initiating reaching, *visually guided reaching* is feedback dependent. Visually guided reaching requires the coordination of proprioceptive information from the hands with the visual inputs (see **Figure 10-11**). Visually guided reaching develops in the second period, concurrent with improved postural and upper extremity control (Shumway-Cook & Woollacott, 2012). This means that by 6 months of age, infants are able to reach and obtain an object such as a cube that is offered.

In this time period, infants also begin a transition from the reflexive avoiding reaction to the development of a purposeful reach. Although infants are unable to control the pattern, by 6 months, they will release objects accidently, often when the object contacts another resisting surface such as during bimanual play. During this period, infants practice finger extension in play and exploratory activities seen in patting and touching movements.

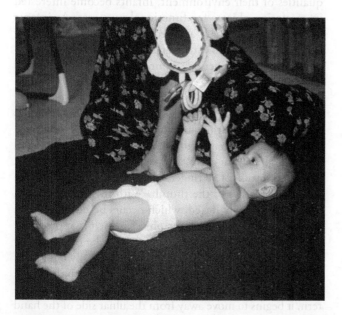

Figure 10-11 Reaching (for Toy)

Oral-Motor Development

The oral-motor pattern used for sucking from the bottle is changing in middle infancy. Because lips, tongue, and jaw no longer move as a complete unit, or are disassociated, the jaw is able to stabilize for the nipple, with the lips forming a tight seal. This generates increased negative pressure in the oral cavity, and the pattern becomes true sucking as opposed to the suckling pattern of early life, which depends largely on positive pressure or expression. Likewise, the sucking pattern comes under voluntary control around 4 months of age.

Around 4 months, the first spoon-feeding is also offered, usually infant cereal. Infants approach the first spoon-feeding with an immature repertoire of movement, stroking the tongue forward and back out of the mouth in an attempt to manage the bolus of food. The upper lip is initially not active in scraping the food off the spoon; rather, a caregiver usually scrapes the spoon off the upper gums to remove the bolus. Using this rather inefficient pattern, a great deal of food is often lost onto the chin. By the end of this period, 6 months of age, the upper lip becomes active to sweep food off the spoon, and spoon-feeding becomes more efficient. By this time, an infant's diet includes stage-one baby foods, which are of consistently pureed texture. Infants will also demonstrate food preferences at this time.

The first teeth often appear at around 6 months (Kedesdy & Budd, 1998). In part depending on this acquisition, solid food may be offered to infants. If this is done, infants are able to bring food to the mouth and perform an early munching pattern, using an up-and-down jaw motion. Likewise, it is highly variable whether infants have been presented a cup this young, but if they have, an attempt to suckle liquid from the cup with ensuing liquid loss is usually the result.

Cognitive-Language Development

The sounds that are emitted in this period of middle infancy have a much greater variety and typically begin to be bisyllabic rather than monosyllabic babbling. Initially, infants babble the sounds heard in all languages, but they begin to refine their babbling to the speech sound of their own language by 6 to 7 months. Sound becomes a form of secondary circular reaction, which is the Piagetian period encompassing 4 to 6 months. In secondary circular reactions, infants volitionally repeat activities that produce interesting results. Unlike primary circular reactions, which are primarily focused on infants, secondary circular reactions are focused largely on the environment, as infants learn that things can be controlled. For example, during this stage, infants begin to notice that the sounds they make influence what happens in the environment; therefore, they repeat interesting sounds (Feldman, 1999). Infants also engage in outright laughter during social exchanges.

The cognitive acquisitions of 4- to 6-month infants also include repetitive actions on objects in the environment. Infants may squeeze, pat, or shake an object to produce interesting sounds. Near 6 months, infants begin to experiment with the object permanence concept. *Object permanence* is the realization that objects continue to exist once they are outside the direct visual field. By 6 months, infants are able to obtain a partially hidden object and may begin to experiment with object permanence by purposefully dropping something and watching to see what happens.

Personal-Social Development

In the 4- to 6-month period, infants, as already stated, will express delight, laughter, and joy during social exchange (see **Figure 10-12**). There is early play across affective, vocal, and motor dimensions (Sroufe, 1996). The reciprocal exchange in interactions, which was rudimentary in the early months, is now fully developed. During this period, games like pattycake and peekaboo usually begin. Although an infant's role is mostly of delighted observer at this early stage, these are important aspects of early play. In addition, in this period, infants show a clear preference for parents or caregivers, although when a caregiver leaves, an infant is easily distracted and consoled (Lamb & Campos, 1982).

LATE INFANCY: 7 TO 9 MONTHS: AN OVERVIEW

In late infancy, infants are able to manipulate objects with hands while in a stable sitting position. They also develop the first mobility pattern, allowing translation from place to place. Grasp becomes refined enough to pick up small objects, and they are able to hold two objects at once, as well as transferring objects from hand to hand. Infants display clear babbling sounds, typically including "Mama" or "Dada," or both, but the sounds are not yet discretely applied to the appropriate person. Infants can begin to use tools to manipulate, and object permanence is a key cognitive construct that is developing in this period. Concomitant with the development of object permanence, infants begin to show increasing distress when a caregiver leaves or when a stranger appears. Infants are now emotional beings.

Gross Motor Development

The period of late infancy is one in which infants make great strides in transfer and locomotor ability, establishing security in postural sets that are progressively up against gravity. At the beginning of this period, infants are able to perform the abdominal-pivot locomotor pattern but are not able to crawl from one place to another. Around 7 months of age, they develop the ability to crawl with their belly on the floor. This belly-down type of locomotion is known as *belly crawling* or *commando crawling* (named after the type of locomotor pattern soldiers use). This is the first true locomotor pattern.

In terms of postural set, infants at the beginning of this period were already sitting, but arms were used as props or supports. Around 7 to 8 months of age, they develop the ability to sit upright without using hands for support (see **Figure 10-3C**). This subsequently allows the hands to be free for manipulation when sitting. The development of sitting erect coincides with the appearance of the sideways protective reactions, and the sitting equilibrium reactions develop shortly thereafter. Infants will be able to sit erect for a while before posterior protective extension reactions develop, usually around the 9th month (see **Figure 10-13**).

As is evident in **Figure 10-14**, the maturation of sitting balance allows infants to lean forward and return to upright without balance loss. Note also that they are able to sit erect before they are able to assume the sitting position.

The transfer from lying to sitting positions usually occurs around the 8th month, and is heavily rotary in nature

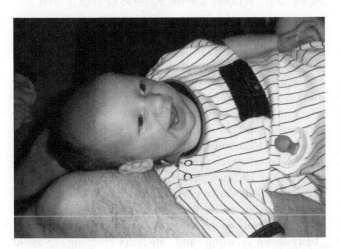

Figure 10-12 Infant is social participant and expresses pleasure.

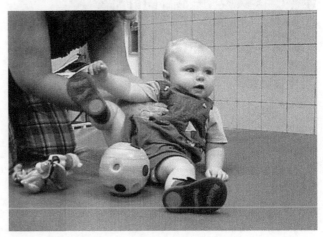

Figure 10-13 Protective Extension Side/Back

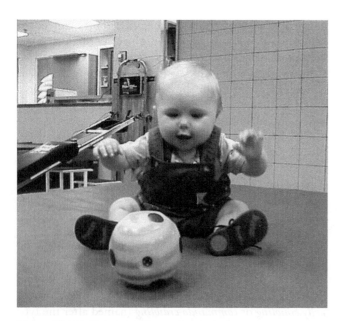

Figure 10-14   Sitting equilibrium permits leaning forward.

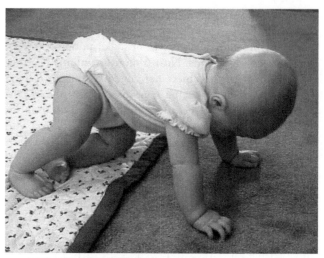

Figure 10-16   An infant experiments with assumption of all-fours position.

(see **Figure 10-15**). An infant's limited abdominal muscle strength, in addition to body shape, precludes symmetric sit-up patterns at this early age.

In prone, while the early locomotor pattern of crawling is being perfected, infants are also progressively pushing up against gravity. They push up on hands and attempt to flex the hips and knees under the body. Initially, this is a crude attempt, and they often fall forward onto their arms; however, gradually they are able to coordinate the demands of the quadruped position (see **Figure 10-16**). These demands include a stable horizontal trunk with flexion at hips, knees, and shoulders, but with extension of elbows and wrists. Often, as infants seek stability in the all-fours, or quadruped, position, it will appear as if they are rocking forward and backward (see **Figure 10-17**). This quadruped rocking

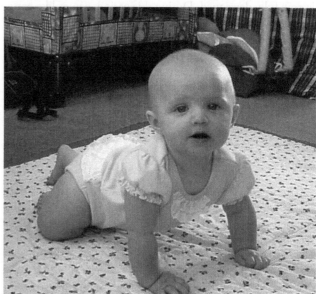

Figure 10-17   An infant who has mastered all-fours position.

is practice of graded eccentric and concentric closed kinetic chain muscle activity, which is representative of the sort of activity demanded of the lower limb for gait. The ability to perform a locomotor pattern in quadruped develops usually around 9 to 10 months.

The terminology that is associated with these early locomotor patterns is unfortunate. To the lay public, the quadruped locomotor pattern is often referred to as crawling; however, developmentalists use the term *creeping* to describe the all-fours pattern, and *crawling* is reserved for the earlier belly-down pattern (Payne & Isaacs, 2012). A simple convention for individuals working with children to use is simply to describe the pattern more fully, as in "belly-down crawling" and "all-fours creeping" to avoid confusion.

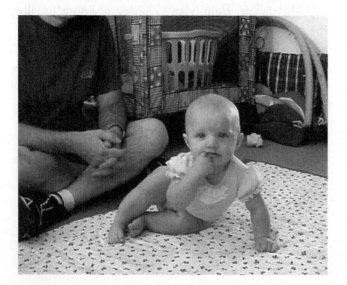

Figure 10-15   Rotary Pattern Used to Get to Sitting Position

Fine Motor Development

The fine motor development of late infancy is especially significant with respect to prehensile function of the hands. During this period, two important phenomena occur: One is disassociation of thumb and fingers, with increasing activity of the thumb, and the second is a progressive movement radially of grasp functions. By 7 months of age, an infant's palmar grasp has usually transitioned to the radial side of the hand, with the force of the grasp occurring more on the radial than the ulnar side. By about 8 months, infants are able to refine the raking pattern of 6-month-olds and can grasp a small object such as a raisin with the pad of the thumb to the side of the index finger. This may be thought of as a **lateral grasp** (also called a *scissors grasp*).

During this time period, the action of the thumb begins to differentiate from the actions of the fingers. The earliest grasp pattern in which the thumb is active is usually the radial digital grasp. The **radial digital grasp** pattern is when an object is held distally (in the fingers rather than the palm) and children grasp an object with the thumb, index, and middle fingers. The activation of the thumb independently of the fingers is a significant feature of infant hand development. It has been said that 40 to 70 percent of normal hand function is provided by the opposition of the thumb (Duff, 1995).

Another key element of hand function in this period is release. Voluntary release occurs in the 7- to 9-month period, and infants will begin to enjoy games that involve placing objects in containers and then dumping them out to start the game over again (Duff, 1995). The disassociation of the fingers allows infants to isolate the index finger, and during this period they will poke at a small object of interest (Koontz-Lowman & Lane, 1999). This isolation of the index finger is also used for pointing, which can serve as a form of communication. The combined effect of these developments in fine motor function is the ability to play and manipulate toys (see **Figure 10-18**).

Oral-Motor Development

In the period of late infancy, solid foods are introduced. Infants are quite effective in eating from a spoon, and their upper lip is active. The activity of the upper lip in general produces a stronger seal on the bottle. Overall, there is increasing disassociation and control of lips, tongue, and jaw. Infants mouth almost every object that is presented, in part in an effort to decrease discomfort associated with teething. Cup drinking is still inefficient, although there is less liquid loss. As mentioned previously, the first solid food is presented in this period. Infants can hold a soft cracker or teething biscuit and bring it to their mouth, holding their jaw closed over a soft solid until they bite off a piece. Chewing is nonrotary, and jaw movement is an up-and-down movement known as *munching*. This munching pattern is in part a reflection of the fact that the tongue is not yet actively lateralizing, or moving food from side to

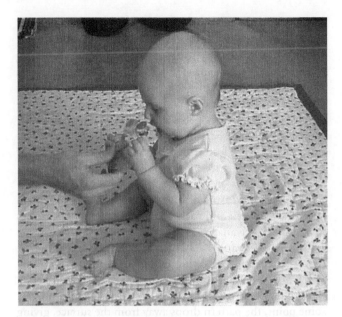

Figure 10-18 Proximal gross motor and advancing fine motor control allow infants to play with toys.

side in the mouth. If food is placed in the mouth laterally, however, infants are able to lateralize the tongue, and some rotary-diagonal jaw movement appears (Koontz-Lowman & Lane, 1999).

Cognitive-Language Development

In late infancy, language development has progressed to clear babbling of sounds of the spoken language. In English, "Ma-ma" or "Da-da," or both, are usually heard, although often not yet applied specifically as names of the parents. As mentioned earlier, the first sounds represent primary circular reactions, in which infants will repeat an interesting sound just to hear it again. Babbling in part represents secondary circular reactions. Infants continue to experiment with interesting sounds, and begin to use the sounds to control the environment. This raises an interesting question regarding language development. It takes nearly a year for the first true word to be uttered. What takes infants so long to attain this milestone? There are two potential sources of complexity in language development that impact the length of time it takes to acquire words. The first is the *phonology*, or the complexity of the sound production. It has been estimated that more than 70 muscles and eight to ten body parts must be directed under neural control to utter a one-syllable word (Acredolo, Goodwyn, Horobin, & Emmons, 1999). The second source of complexity is the *cognitive structure development* that underlies the purposeful use of patterns of sound as language. During this time, infants pass from secondary circular reactions into a coordination of secondary schema.

This phase of coordination of secondary circular reactions is marked by several key factors. Beginning at about

8 months, with the onset of this stage, infants begin purposeful manipulation. As part of this stage, infants will push one toy out of the way to reach another toy that is lying underneath it (Feldman, 1999). Object permanence begins to develop in earnest in this period. For example, an infant will search for a toy that is hidden while he is watching. The development of object permanence also has large implications for personal-social milestones, including demonstration of negative affect around strangers. These two major changes—searching for hidden objects and becoming upset around strangers—represent a large behavioral shift that indicates an increasing ability on the part of an infant to coordinate present and past events using memory processes (Sameroff & Cavanagh, 1979).

A 7- to 9-month-old infant also is developing in sensory-perceptual areas. For example, in the classic "visual cliff" experiment, infants were allowed to crawl over a Plexiglass surface with a checkered pattern underneath. At some point, the pattern drops away from the surface, giving the illusion of a "cliff." Infants as young as 6 to 7 months would not crawl over the cliff (Gibson & Walk, 1960). Further studies have shown that the development of depth perception is related to the cortical developments that support binocular vision (Eliot, 1999). One of the related concepts arising from the visual cliff paradigm is the concept of **affordance**. An affordance is an interaction between the person and the environment that determines possibilities for action. For example, in the visual cliff experiments, infants could use touch of the surface as an affordance to decide whether or not to continue crawling. If encountering a puddle when walking, an adult would examine the affordances in the situation and determine whether to walk around it or jump over it. Affordances are perceived, and therefore the ability to recognize them is an indicator of perceptual processing (Cole, Chan, Vereijken, & Adolph, 2013). Early intervention providers may use affordances in the form of toys or positioning equipment to encourage acquisition of developmental behaviors.

Personal-Social Development

The concept of object permanence is a major cognitive foundation for the development of attachment and for reactivity to strangers, which begins in this period of late infancy. Before this time, infants demonstrate an "out of sight, out of mind" worldview with respect to parents or other caregivers leaving. This worldview begins to change at about 7 months of age, and infants begin to protest the departure of specific people, especially parents. At this time they are initially unwilling to be consoled by substitutes, a behavior that has been called *separation protest* (Lamb & Campos, 1982).

Another factor that influences personal-social development in late infancy is the increasing mobility of infants. Before 7 months, infants would be unable to attempt to sustain contact by any means other than crying. However, in this period, they have some form of prone locomotion, so it is possible to try to follow a parent or caregiver upon leaving. This behavior of trying to maintain or prolong contact with a caregiver will emerge fully in the next phase.

During this period, infants will become more fully engaged as social beings. They will interact with other infants by attempting to touch them and by increasing vocalizations. They will also purposefully initiate interactions with a caregiver, explore the caregiver by touching his or her face, and attempt to manipulate interactions (Sroufe, 1996).

By 9 months, infants are "emotional beings" (Sroufe, 1996). This term reflects the fact that infants now have become sensitive to the meaning of events. Infants from 7 to 9 months will begin to demonstrate the emotion of anger. For example, anger may be expressed when an expected consequence does not occur. Fear, as mentioned previously, also begins to appear in this period, particularly when a stranger is introduced. The fact that infants show distress to specific stimuli, will use affect as a motivation, and will seek help for maintaining an interesting game or experience all support the idea of this major developmental milestone of becoming an emotional being occurring in this phase.

INFANCY TRANSITION: 10 TO 12 MONTHS—AN OVERVIEW

At the beginning of the transition period from the 10th to the 12th month, proficiency in quadruped mobility is developing. By the end of this period, at 12 months, infants typically take the first steps. It will take some time before gait and postural mechanisms mature to adultlike patterns. Grasp is secure, and infants can pick up even the smallest object. They are independent with finger-feeding and drink from a cup. In this period, the first true purposeful object-release pattern emerges. The first word is also said sometime in this period. They also display clear maternal or caregiver attachment behaviors at this time, and stranger anxiety is a typical phenomenon.

Gross Motor Development

The infancy transition period represents the culmination of an extremely rapid progression of gross motor milestone acquisition. At the beginning of infancy transition, infants have successfully pushed into the all-fours, or quadruped, position and rocks. As they gain stability in this position, the ability to sustain quadruped emerges, followed shortly by the locomotor pattern of hands-and-knees creeping. Not all children progress through this period. One study reported that 82 percent of normal infants used creeping on all fours as their pre-walking locomotor pattern. Other patterns identified included *shuffling* in a sitting position, rolling, and belly-crawling. About 7 percent of infants did not demonstrate any pattern before they initiated walking.

Some of the infants who did not use the all-fours locomotor pattern showed a transient hypotonia, especially those in the belly-crawling, sitting, and shuffling classifications. **Hypotonia** is a condition of diminished state of muscle tension and diminished resistance of muscles to passive stretching. These hypotonic infants walked later than the infants who performed quadruped creeping or who skipped the phase entirely (Robson, 1984).

From these and similar data, it may be concluded that it is not necessary to pass through the quadruped creeping phase to develop standing and walking. However, failure to do so, especially if using the alternative patterns, may be associated with delayed onset of walking. Furthermore, some children who have impaired motor control may show a preference to avoid the quadruped creeping pattern; despite that fact, the pattern has elements that might prove to be of therapeutic benefit. For example, children who would benefit from this pattern in particular are children with Down syndrome, who need to develop the rotary movement and graded control, and children with hemiplegia, who need to develop bilateral weight bearing.

Shortly after children begin to creep, they will get to a piece of furniture and initiate a pull-to-stand. They should ideally pass through the half-kneel position to reach standing. Infants will often explore this ability to pull-to-stand when waking up in the middle of the night. As shown in **Figure 10-19**, they will pull up at crib or playpen rails.

Interestingly, infants will be able to pull-to-stand before being able to lower, and will often cry the first few times this occurs. It will not take infants long to figure out how to get down, but until they do, parents may be distressed to find that an infant who was formerly sleeping through the

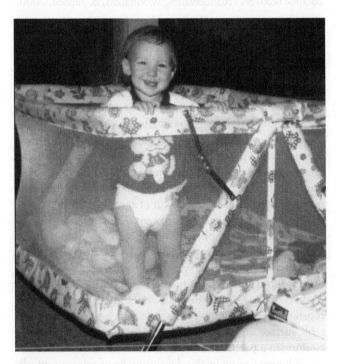

Figure 10-19 An infant demonstrates the result of pull-to-stand and readiness to cruise.

night now awakes and pulls-to-stand, crying for a parent to come to the rescue once successfully standing.

After pulling-to-stand, infants will typically move sideways around furniture. This pattern is called cruising. **Cruising** is a locomotor pattern that uses an abduction, lateral shift mobility pattern with extrinsic postural support. Gradually, infants typically free one hand from the support surface and move between pieces of furniture, such as a coffee table and the couch. Meanwhile, parents are typically "walking" with infants by this time, holding first two hands and then one hand to provide support. A 10- to 12-month-old will be demonstrating true weight bearing through the legs but does not yet have the postural control for independent gait.

Sometime around the first birthday, infants take the first independent steps. Bipedal gait is the definitive locomotor pattern for humans. Early infant gait does not have the smoothly coordinated, effortless appearance of mature gait. In fact, early gait is so distinctive that it even has a unique name applied, **toddling,** and these early walkers are called by the associated name, *toddlers.* Several features characterize toddling, or immature gait. The upper extremities are held up and out from the body in abduction. There are several reasons given for this pattern of the arms. It has been suggested that this is a "readiness" pattern for the infants to catch themselves should they fall. It has also been suggested that this pattern represents the effort to maintain an upright trunk in extension when postural control is still immature. The lower trunk is in extension, with lumbar lordosis. **Lordosis** is the inward curvature of a portion of the lumbar and cervical vertebral column. Associated with this lordosis is protuberance of the infant's belly. This pattern is associated with the relatively inactive abdominal musculature at the end of the first year. The lower limbs are abducted in a wide base of support. This increased base of support is a common compensation for immature balance reactions (see **Figure 10-20**).

As an infant takes early steps, the cadence is often rapid, because there is inadequate control for sustained unilateral stance. Hence, the appearance is almost as if the infant is falling from one leg and catching with the other (see **Figure 10-21**). It will take approximately another two years of practice before the infant's postural and mobility patterns in gait resemble those of the adult (Sutherland, Olshen, Cooper, & Woo, 1980).

Normal adults have a series of so-called strategies they use to sustain postural control. These include an *ankle strategy,* in which the ankle musculature contracts in response to a backward or forward displacement. This strategy helps move the center of mass over the base of support and comprises the typical postural sway seen in quiet stance. The ankle strategy is used when the displacement is small and the standing support surface is firm. A second strategy is the *hip strategy,* which is used when the standing support surface is soft or is smaller than the base of support provided by the feet. The hip strategy is also used in larger or faster displacements. The *stepping strategy* allows people to step

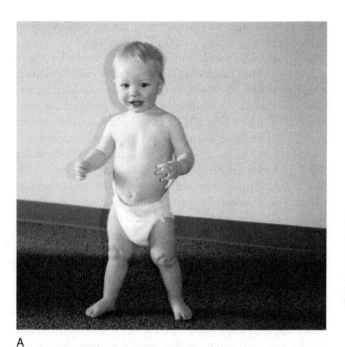 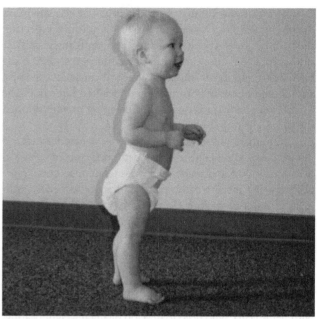

A   B

Figure 10-20   Front and Side Views of a Typical Infant in Standing Posture at 1 Year

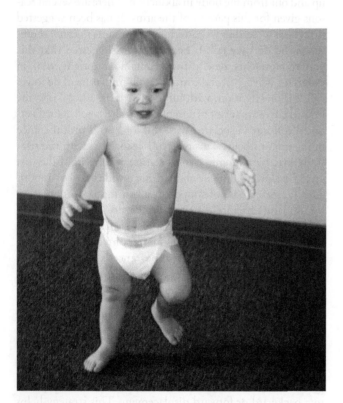

Figure 10-21   Walking at 1 Year

and reestablish the base of support. This is used when the disturbances are large, so that the base of support cannot be recovered. These three strategies are an example of *muscle synergies,* defined as the functional coupling of groups of muscles that operate together as a unit (Shumway-Cook & Woollacott, 2012).

It has been found that after three to six months of walking experience, toddlers demonstrate the hip strategy; however, the amount of abdominal muscle activation in this strategy is less than that of adults until 7 to 10 years of age (Woollacott et al., 1998). Likewise, it has been found that it takes one to three months of walking experience before toddlers are able to successfully use a stepping strategy for balance recovery (Roncesvalles, Woollacott, & Jensen, 2000).

Fine Motor Development

At about 10 months, typically developing infants can further oppose the thumb so that it approximates the volar surface of the index finger. This is known as an **inferior pincer grasp**. Control moves through the phase distally, first to the pad of the index finger. The pad-to-pad opposition of thumb and index finger is considered a pincer grasp. The most discrete and controlled grasp is between the tip of the thumb and the tip of the index finger, such as one might use a needle in sewing. This **superior pincer grasp** appears around 1 year of age (Duff, 1995).

Starting in this developmental period, there is an increased interest in objects and an increase in object play. Purposeful release of grasped objects first occurs when infants hold an object at midline with both hands, and then pull the object out of one hand into the other. This is a forced, or resisted, release. Near the same time, infants explore other resisted release patterns such as releasing an object against a table surface, or opening the hand by dragging it down the clothing of a parent or other innocent bystander.

The next stage in the development of release typically involves flinging an object, combining elbow, wrist, and finger extension in a synergistic, ballistic movement. New developmental activities that emerge with this skill include dropping food and toys in play. With increasing reach, grasp-and-release abilities, which are supported by developments in other domains, including cognitive, infants begin to demonstrate adaptive skills. *Adaptive skills* may be considered those skills that permit infants to perform self-care. Usually by 1 year of age, infants begin to take off clothing, often starting with their socks. They will hold out their arms to assist with dressing. Fine motor skills, including grasp-and-release patterns, will continue to refine throughout early childhood.

Oral-Motor Development

Infants from 10 to 12 months develop proficiency with eating solid foods, feeding themselves with their fingers. The chewing pattern is more mature, with a mix of up-down and rotary/diagonal components. Infants at this time are able to drink independently from a "sippy" cup. Although infants at 12 months are quite proficient with removing food from a spoon or fork, parents are still often hesitant to allow them to try to self-feed using utensils. Infants still cannot efficiently scoop the food onto a spoon and, if presented a spoon already filled, will pronate and wave it around just as often as getting it to the mouth. In the case of using a fork, it is easier for infants to get the food on the fork by spearing it; however, most parents are concerned that infants will jab themselves with the tines. Often, however, infants in this period will begin to show a desire for independence with some of these activities.

Cognitive-Language Development

In this transition period, the first word usually emerges. Typically, by 12 months, infants specifically apply "Mama" and "Dada" to the appropriate people and may have one or more additional words. Often, these early words are names for pets, siblings, or other family members. This phase encompasses the cognitive phase of coordination of secondary circular reactions begun in the previous phase. Infants' ability to manipulate using tools continues to be refined. They will spend long periods playing games such as putting blocks in a plastic milk bottle and dumping them out. Object permanence continues to become more secure. Infants routinely search for hidden objects; however, they can still be fooled. For example, if someone hides a toy under one cup with an infant watching but subsequently moves the object, he often continues to focus on finding the object in the first hiding place (Feldman, 1999).

Personal-Social Development

In this transition phase, attachment behaviors are clearly developed. A child's emotional, cognitive, and physical maturity enable her to use the mother as a "secure base" from which to explore the world (Sroufe, 1996). Children at 10 to 12 months will fall into one of the three classifications of attachment behavior: securely attached, avoidant, or insecurely attached. *Securely attached infants* will seek to maintain proximity with a caregiver (in this case, let's say it is the mother) and will react with negative emotion when she leaves. When the mother returns, the infants will go immediately to her. When the mother is present, these infants will leave her to explore the room, referencing back to her visually or approaching her at intervals, as if to make sure she is still there. *Avoidant infants* do not seek proximity to the mother, and when she returns, they tend to ignore her. *Ambivalent infants* will seek contact with the mother and become distressed when she leaves, but when she returns, these infants may display anger at her and resist comforting.

A recently added category of attachment is *disorganized-disoriented*. In this category, infants will show inconsistent behavior that is often self-contradictory. These infants may be the least securely attached (Feldman, 1999).

Also in this stage, infants will show true **stranger anxiety,** which has been developing over the past several months. This is differentiated from the *stranger protest* in that stranger anxiety has an anticipatory quality to it. An infant may react negatively to strangers, as in a clinic room, before the stranger has actually approached the infant and while the parent is still present.

VARIATIONS IN DEVELOPMENT

This chapter has presented an overview of the sequence of acquisition of key behaviors in the first year of life. It is important to remember that the exact time of milestone acquisition is highly variable and less important than the sequence itself. Traditionally, individuals who want to assess the performance of infants in the first year of life use the developmental sequence of milestone acquisition. The infants' capabilities are compared against the normative sequence, and a judgment is made of whether or not their performance falls in the range of normal variability. Failure to fall within the normative range of milestone acquisition is labeled as developmental delay. **Developmental delay** is less a diagnosis than a descriptor. In other words, a description of developmental delay says only that a child is slow in acquiring milestones; it does not imply a specific etiology of delay. For example, developmental delay may be due to a known condition such as Down syndrome, or it may be identified in a former premature infant with risk factors but no known specific cause for delay.

Developmental delay may be global or focal. In some cases, delays in all areas of development are noted, as in the case of a child with Down syndrome. Conversely, the delay may be restricted to only some areas, such as motor or language development. The determination of the areas of deficit helps in determining etiology. Thus, if an infant's delay is restricted to language, it would be imperative to determine if the child has a hearing impairment. If the delay seems to be most significant in the motor areas, a problem such as cerebral palsy may be the reason. Cerebral palsy, by definition, is not a diagnosis. Rather, it is a description of clinical sequelae resulting from a defect of lesion of the brain in early life that manifests in primarily neuromotor systems with secondary impact on musculoskeletal and other systems (Wilson-Howie, 1999).

Developmental delay may be distinguished from abnormal development. Developmental delay is primarily a quantitative concept—that is, it refers to how many of the normative milestones an infant has acquired—whereas abnormal development refers less to the quantitative than the qualitative aspects of development. **Abnormal development** is a pattern or sequence of behavior acquisition that differs from typical patterns in quality and form and includes aspects that are not seen in the typical sequence. For example, an infant who had a mild stroke might be at the slow end of normal ranges in timing of milestone acquisition, but the qualitative aspects of movement make the parents worry that something is wrong. An infant with a diagnosis of mental or psychiatric impairment might show an abnormal quality of attachment behavior.

Of course, abnormal development and developmental delay often coexist, as in the case of an infant with cerebral palsy. These infants will show stereotypic patterns of posture and movement that look abnormal, and they are bound by these patterns so that acquisition of milestones does not occur on time. It is also important to remember that not all developmental conditions can be diagnosed immediately in infancy. For example, a child with cerebral palsy may acquire early milestones within the normative range but fall off later in the first year.

Finally, there is a **transient developmental delay**. In this case, an infant fails to acquire early milestones but catches up later in the first year. Transient delay is often seen in infants who had a difficult perinatal course, and it seems that the brain as well as other body systems take some time to recover. Transient delay is not equivalent to the observation that premature infants tend to develop according to their gestational rather than chronologic age. Therefore, when assessing the developmental milestones of premature infants, the convention is to adjust the infants' age for prematurity. Subtracting the number of weeks an infant was premature from the infant's chronologic age obtains the adjusted age. Thus, an infant who was born 8 months ago is that chronologic age. However, suppose that infant was a 28-week-gestation premature infant. Because a term pregnancy is dated at 40 weeks, that infant is 12 weeks, or 3 months premature. Therefore, the adjusted age and associated normative milestones would be at the 5-month level. Adjustment for prematurity is traditionally done in developmental assessment until the infant has reached 2 years of age. Therapists and other professionals who work with infants need to know the normative patterns and sequences of development in the first year to correctly identify problems and design appropriate interventions.

CONTEXTUAL FACTORS: EFFECTS OF CULTURE AND ENVIRONMENT

Motor development, which has a predictable sequence with a largely innate component, may be thought of as relatively "privileged." This means a wide range of caregiving practice can be tolerated without a negative effect on the developmental outcome (Eliot, 1999). This is an important factor in cases where infants may have to be casted or have other kinds of constraints for a few weeks or months in the first year. Otherwise, normally developing children should not demonstrate significant delays as a result of this intervention. This is not to infer that motor development is completely unaffected by environmental experience. Relatively small changes in cultural and caregiving practices can produce small variations in timing and sequence of milestone acquisition. Cross-cultural studies of development have also shown that caregiving practices can affect the pattern of development (Cintas, 1988); however, in most cases, the ultimate outcome of walking around 1 year of life is unchanged.

The "Safe to Sleep" program, as described previously, represented an instituted change in national caregiving practice. This change slightly affected the pattern but not the outcome of developmental milestone acquisition (Davis et al., 1998). Although this change in caregiving practice did not significantly affect motor development, an interesting side effect of this program has emerged. Because infants in the first 3 months of life spend much more time in supine than previously, and because the posture of these infants is predominantly asymmetrical, the developing musculoskeletal system is subjected to these positional forces. In particular, the skull with its open fontanelle tends to mold according to the pressure of the support surface. As an infant rests in supine with the head turned to one side or the other, the sternocleidomastoid muscle that turns the head can become asymmetrically tight. The result of this is a large number of infants who are diagnosed with *positional plagiocephaly* and *torticollis* (Cummings, 2011). **Plagiocephaly** is a term used to describe flattening of one side of the skull with contralateral skull bulging in the frontal area. **Torticollis** is congenital damage to the sternocleidomastoid muscle in the neck that results in a shortening or excessive contraction of the muscle, resulting in both limited range of motion in both rotation and lateral neck bending. This limits head turning to the opposite side, creating a vicious cycle. Congenital torticollis has become such a high incidence referral to physical therapy that clinical practice guidelines have been published to help therapists provide evidence-based interventions (Kaplan, Coulter, & Fetters, 2013).

There are several treatments for positional plagiocephaly. Prevention is the most optimal intervention, which is done by educating parents to have infants in prone ("tummy time") 15 minutes at least three times a day. Physical therapy can be used to stretch the tight neck muscles and encourage positional symmetry. Finally, a molding helmet can be used to shape the skull. Studies have shown that parent education and physical therapy work best if done before 4 months of age, and helmets work best if implemented at 5 to 6 months of age (Cummings, 2011; Kluba, Kraut, Reinert, & Krimmel, 2011). **Figure 10-22** is an illustration of the skull deformation that occurs in positional plagiocephaly.

Furthermore, all of the findings discussed here do not imply motor development is never adversely affected by caregiving practice. In studies of infants who were raised in extremely deprived environments, such as orphanages in third world countries, motor development may be seriously affected. The reason for the problems of these infants may be multifactorial, and include nutrition.

Psychosocial development is definitively affected by the emotional environment of infants. The quality of the attachment developed in the first year of life forms the basis for the types of relationships infants form later in life (Feldman, 1999). Securely attached infants are believed to have learned how to regulate emotional arousal and how to depend on others for assistance when needed (Sroufe, 1996). Rodriguez and Tucker (2011) reported attachment of a mother to her parents was a factor in determining whether or not the mother would turn into an abuser herself. These authors disputed as overly simplistic the notion that children who were abused are more likely to become abusive parents. This notion, which was accepted through the latter part of the twentieth century, had its roots in Bandura's social learning theory. More recently, however, there have been attempts to determine why some children who were abused do not become

abusive parents. Rodriguez and Tucker's (2011) study found that if a mother had a perceived positive attachment relationship to any adult figure, she was more likely to break the cycle of abuse, despite being at risk, than a mother who had a history of poor attachment. Music (2009) reviewed literature on the effects of child neglect across the spectrum. He cited literature on reactive attachment disorder (RAD), which is a clinical diagnosis applied to children who are completely apathetic and withdrawn in social situations to the point of being antisocial. This diagnosis was first applied to children who were subjected to extreme neglect in institutional settings. However, Music also reviewed the effects of less extreme neglect, saying these children tend to lack empathy and be avoidant. Finally, Music applied the neurobiological premise of "experience expectancy" to explain some of the characteristics seen in these children. Experience expectancy means the nervous system is prepared to receive inputs, such as social exchange, touch, and comforting in early infancy. Failure to receive these inputs may result in permanent alterations in social behavior (Music, 2009).

In the examples of motor development and psychosocial development discussed previously, the need for a supportive environment is identified. This raises the question of the effect of poverty on child development. Given the national and international economic hardships since 2007, an increasing number of children are growing up in poverty. Isaacs (2011) reported increases in child poverty from 18 percent in 2007 to 22 percent in 2010, with large variations by state. Over the same time period, the number of poor children increased by 3 million to a total number of 16 million in 2010. Brooks-Gunn and Duncan (1997) summarized reports on effects of poverty on children. The authors reported that, in addition to increased risk of mortality and childhood illness such as asthma, there are effects of poverty on factors such as cognitive development and school achievement. The authors reported the effects of poverty were greater in early childhood and greater for long-term rather than short-term poverty. Low family income was found to have greater negative impact on cognitive- and achievement-related outcomes than emotional outcomes, although children in poverty were more likely to have emotional and behavioral problems than their more affluent peers.

As mentioned throughout earlier portions of this text, the developing brain is highly plastic, due to the rapid synaptogenesis and the extensive myelination that occurs in the first 2 years of life. The current standard of intervention is based on the fact that the earlier a problem is identified, the greater the likelihood that intervention will have a positive effect, because of maximizing the neural resources available to children due to plasticity. A recent study showed a significant difference in language development for children from low socioeconomic status (SES) families when exposed to early cognitive enrichment (Cates et al., 2012). The premise that early environmental enrichment can help children overcome biologic and environmental challenges is the basis for the Individuals with Disabilities Education Act, Part C, Early Intervention. This act is discussed extensively in Chapter 21 of this text.

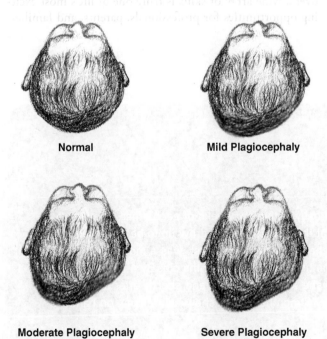

Normal

Mild Plagiocephaly

Moderate Plagiocephaly

Severe Plagiocephaly

Figure 10-22   Positional Plagiocephaly

THE FOUNDATION OF INFANCY

In Chapters 1 and 2, there was extensive discussion of both the ICF and life course theory, including the Health Care Development Model. The USHHS concept paper about the life course model has as a core tenet the notion that early experience influences later health. In addition, the model talks about critical or sensitive periods and the importance of environment to health (USHHS, 2010). Arguably, the first postnatal year of life is a critical foundation for later health.

Therapists and developmental specialists providing early intervention should always remember the importance of the first year. Ultimately, the goal of early intervention is to promote positive development in this critical period. The outcome of "health" as defined in the ICF is full participation in life (WHO, 2001). For infants in the first year, participation typically emerges in the context of family. That is why best practice in early intervention is often home based. Therapists and others must be familiar with normal development, as well as with risk and protective factors to promote a normal developmental outcome. For infants over the first year, this means going from being dependent in mobility and control to having rudimentary environmental mastery in terms of locomotion and use of the hand. This is necessary for exploration of the environment, which promotes cognitive development. Infants as social beings should feel attachment and should have a nurturing care provider. The infants' environmental control is beginning to expand to the use of symbols in the form of language by the end of the year. The task of early intervention specialists is often challenged by environmental contextual issues such as poverty, lack of stable living arrangements, parental substance abuse, and other factors. Through education of parents about how to promote normal development, it is hoped that infants can overcome biologic and environmental risk factors and have mastered the normal developmental accomplishments of the first year to provide a platform for future life course development.

SUMMARY

The first year of life rivals only the fetal period in its rapidity of developmental change, and from the aspect of behavior, it is the most dynamic period of change across the human life span. In gross motor development, infants progress from being relatively dependent on external support for something as simple as head control to being able to walk independently. In fine motor development, they progress from a nonfunctional reflexive grasp to being able to pick up the smallest of objects. In oral motor development, the first year marks progress from a total diet of liquid taken by bottle or breast to a slightly modified mature diet, including drinking liquids from a cup and finger-feeding diced solids.

Communication and language skills progress in the first year from being limited to nature and extent of crying to one or more single words, including identification of parents by name. Finally, in personal-social development, as infants become toddlers, they have typically developed attachment to one or several primary caregivers and are active participants in social relationships. To watch infants progress from relatively dependent newborns to curious, active toddlers who exert mastery over a wide array of skills is truly one of life's most exciting opportunities for professionals, parents, and families.

CASE 1

Meghan and Amy

Sheila and Terri are good friends, and they each had a baby within six weeks of each other. They were very excited to be pregnant together and were sure that their babies would grow up to be "best friends." They both had baby girls. However, Sheila's baby, Meghan, who was born first, was a model baby from the start. Meghan was sleeping through the night by the time she was 2 months old. By 4 months, she was rolling over and beginning to sit up. By 6 months, she was sitting well, and shortly after that, she started to turn into a semi–hand-and-knees position. By 8 months of age, she was creeping on hands

Continues

Case 1   *Continued*

and knees, and by 10 months of age she was walking. Meghan had a vocabulary of four words at 1 year and was a very social child.

On the other hand, Terri's little girl, Amy, was a very difficult child. She was irregular in all her patterns and clearly had a difficult temperament. For the first two months, Amy cried nearly all night long, and Terri and her husband were up trying to quiet her until the early hours of the morning, not getting very much sleep themselves. Amy hated to be on her stomach, and the only position where she was semi-happy was in her infant swing, where she spent a lot of time those first months. At 6 months of age, Amy was rolling from her back to her stomach, but not stomach to back. She was barely sitting propped. By 8 months of age, Amy would sit and play with toys briefly, but nothing interested her for long. Amy did not start pulling-to-stand until she was close to 1 year of age. She was saying only "Ma-ma" and "Da-da" at 1 year of age.

Sheila and Terri and their spouses were having dinner one night. After they got home, Terri's husband commented that he was worried because Amy seemed "slow." He wondered why Amy wasn't walking yet. Terri burst into tears and said she felt like she was a failure as a mother.

This case study illustrates the individual variability in infants. Meghan, who was an infant with an easy temperament, was developing at an accelerated rate. Amy, on the other hand, had a difficult temperament and was a more demanding child. She was less open to new experiences and more demanding of caregiver attention. But both children were developing normally. It would be important to make sure that Terri and her husband could appreciate Amy's uniqueness and recognize that Meghan's relative acceleration will make very little difference over time.

Guiding Questions

Some questions to consider:

1. A developmental axiom is that "development is variable in form but predictable in consequence." Apply this axiom to the case of these two infants.
2. Amy does not like to be in the prone position. What are the developmental milestones that arise out of the prone position and the antigravity control encouraged in that position? What potential structural problem could Amy have developed if she has an extreme aversion to the prone position?
3. What are some environmental affordances that could be used to encourage Amy to develop upright locomotor skills such as cruising and walking?

CASE 2

Manuel

Julie and Tim have been unable to have children. They are very excited when they find out they have been approved to adopt a child from an orphanage in a South American country. They gather their resources and fly to pick up their new son, Manuel. There is no medical history available. Manuel is about 10 months old when they adopt him.

Continues

Case 2 *Continued*

They bring Manuel back to the United States. He is a very quiet baby. He lies quietly and rarely cries. Manuel is barely sitting forward propped. He has a head lag in pull-to-sit. Manuel refuses to eat anything, taking only the bottle. He occasionally makes babbling sounds, but he has very little affect. He does not get upset, no matter who is holding him. Manuel will reach and grasp toys but drops them after a brief period of exploration.

Julie and Tim are very worried. Although they already love little Manuel, they were assured that the baby they were adopting was "normal" and did not have any kind of neurologic problem. The pediatrician has an MRI done, and there is no brain damage. Julie and Tim ask about a referral to early intervention. When the early intervention team visits Julie and Tim, they conclude that there are definite delays; however, without knowing Manuel's medical history (whether he was term or preterm), it is difficult to determine the severity of the delays. The early intervention team encourages Julie and Tim to provide a rich, supportive environment for Manuel. They explain brain plasticity and suggest that there is a good chance that Manuel will respond to their activity suggestions.

By 18 months of age, Manuel seems like a different child. He is clearly attached to Julie and Tim and speaks four to six words. He is walking well and eating solids. Although they continue to work especially on Manuel's language development, they are thrilled with their little boy and feel they have seen firsthand the effect of environment on development.

Guiding Questions

Some questions to consider:

1. Review the developmental sequence discussed in the chapter. To the knowledge of the parents, Manuel is 10 months old when he is adopted. What should a 10-month-old be doing across all domains of development?
2. Explain why Manuel seems like a different child at 18 months of age. What impact does environment have on his emerging behavior? Relate this to the term *neuroplasticity*.
3. Why does early intervention play an important role in this case? Describe activities the early intervention team probably recommended for Manuel, based on his initial level of function.

Speaking of
The Parent-Infant Bond

SUSAN LYNCH, MD, NEONATOLOGIST, DIRECTOR OF WEST
VIRGINIA UNIVERSITY, NEONATAL FOLLOW-UP CLINIC

As a pediatric resident, you tend to view your work in terms of illness and acute care. Your concerns are focused around how to identify and treat sickness in children. You learn how to recognize an ear infection, and how to select the correct antibiotic to treat that infection. Neonatologists like myself complete a fellowship in which we are faced with the responsibility of learning a huge body of science, and the sometimes overwhelming task of incorporating this knowledge into day-to-day care of premature and sick infants. Again, the focus is on sickness. You learn to

Continues

Speaking of *Continued*

make acute, even emergent decisions. You put an immense effort into becoming the best you can be at taking care of babies—once again, however, focusing primarily on the well baby–sick baby continuum.

As years go by and I develop more perspective, I realize that as daunting and as rewarding as taking care of sick infants is, the real meaning of what I do is reflected in families. Every year, I never cease to be amazed by the strength of the parental bond, the ability of mothers and fathers to selflessly love and care for their infants. I believe these abilities sometimes surprise even parents themselves.

Often, after particularly poignant interactions with parents, I find myself quietly reflecting on this attribute. For example, it is not uncommon for me to see a mother, sitting at the bedside of her critically ill infant day after day, laying her head down and sleeping on the corner of the bed to get some rest. Recently, I had to deliver some bad news to a father about his infant's condition, and he responded by saying, "We were told that we could never have children due to my wife's illness. Our son is a gift from God and we know he would not take away such a gift. We know he will be okay."

You can read about and study attachment and bonding. But until you have experiences such as those I have described, you cannot begin to appreciate the power of that relationship between parent and infant. Each family, unique in its beliefs and traditions, welcomes the infant and nurtures the infant, thereby creating a new relationship or bond. The strength of that bond in terms of love and dedication never ceases to amaze and inspire me.

REFERENCES

Acredolo, L. P., Goodwyn, S. W., Horobin, K. D., & Emmons, Y. D. (1999). The signs and sounds of early language development. In L. Balter & C. Tamis-LeMonda (Eds.), *Child psychology: A handbook of contemporary issues* (pp. 116–139). Philadelphia: Psychology Press.

Brooks-Gunn, J., & Duncan, G. (1997). The effects of poverty on children. *The future of children: Children and poverty, 7*(2), 55–71.

Cates, C. B., Dreyer, B. P., Berkule, S. B., White, L. J., Arevalo, J. A., & Mendelsohn, A. L. (2012). Infant communication and subsequent language development in children from low-income families: The role of early cognitive stimulation. *Journal of Developmental and Behavioral Pediatrics, 33*(7), 577–585.

Chang, E. F., & Merzenich, M. M. (2003). Environmental noise retards auditory cortical development. *Science, 300*(5618), 498–502.

Chess, S., & Thomas, A. (1996) *Temperament: Theory and practice (basic principles into practice).* New York: Brunner/Mazel.

Choukair, M. (2000). Blood chemistry/body fluids. In G. K. Siebert & R. Iannone (Eds.), *Harriet Lane handbook* (pp. 119–180). St. Louis: Mosby.

Cintas, H. M. (1988). Cross-cultural variation in infant motor development. *Physical & Occupational Therapy in Pediatrics, 8,* 1–20.

Cole, W. J., Chan, G. L., Vereijken, B., & Adolph, K. (2013). Perceiving affordances for different motor skills. *Experimental Brain Research, 225,* 309–319.

Cummings, C. (2011). Positional plagiocephaly. *Paediatrics & Child Health, 16*(8), 493–496.

Davis, B. E., Moon, R. Y., Sachs, H. C., & Ottolini, M. C. (1998) Effects of sleep position on infant motor development. *Pediatrics, 102*(5), 1135–1140.

DeVries, M. W. (1999). Babies, brains and culture: Optimizing neurodevelopment on the savanna. *Acta Paediatrica Supplement, 88*(429), 43–48.

Dewey, C., Fleming, P., & Golding, J. (1998). Does the supine sleeping position have any adverse effects on the child? II. Development in the first 18 months. ALSPAC study team. *Pediatrics, 101* (1), E5.

Donahue, S. M., Kleinman, K. P., Gillman, M. W., & Oken, E. (2010) Trends in birthweight and gestation length among singleton term births in the United States: 1990–2005. *Journal of Obstetrics & Gynecology, 11s*(2p1), 357–364.

Duff, S. V. (1995). Prehension. In D. Cech & T. Martin (Eds.), *Functional movement across the lifespan* (pp. 313–353). Philadelphia: W. B. Saunders.

Eliot, L. (1999). *What's going on in there? How the brain and mind develop in the first five years of life.* New York: Bantam Books.

Feldman, R. S. (Ed.) (1999). *Child development: A topical approach.* Upper Saddle River, NJ: Prentice Hall.

Field, T. (1990). *Infancy.* Cambridge, MA: Harvard University Press.

Gibson, E. J., & Walk, R. D. (1960). The "visual cliff." *Scientific American, 202,* 64–71.

Henderson, A., & Pehoski, C. (Eds.). (2006). *Hand function in the child: Foundation for remediation* (2nd ed.). St. Louis: Mosby.

Isaacs, J. (2011). *The recession's ongoing impact on America's children*. Retrieved from http://www.brookings.edu/research/papers/2011/12/20-children-wellbeing-isaacs

Johnston, M. V., Nishimura, A., Harum, K., Pekar, J., & Blue, M. E. (2001). Sculpting the developing brain. *Advances in Pediatrics, 48,* 1–38.

Kaplan, S. L., Coulter, C., & Fetters, L. (2013) Physical therapy management of congenital muscular torticollis: An evidence-based clinical practice guideline (from the Section on Pediatrics of the American Physical Therapy Association). *Pediatric Physical Therapy, 25*(4), 384–394.

Kedesdy, J. H., & Budd, K. S. (1998). Assessment of environmental factors in feeding. In *Childhood feeding disorders* (pp. 79–114). Baltimore: Brooks.

Kluba, S., Kraut, W., Reinert, S., & Krimmel, M. (2011). What is the optimal time to start helmet therapy in positional plagiocephaly? *Plastic and Reconstructive Surgery, 128*(2), 492–498.

Koontz-Lowman, D., & Lane, S. J. (1999). Children with feeding and nutritional problems. In S. Porr & E. B. Rainville (Eds.), *Pediatric therapy: A systems approach* (pp. 379–423). Philadelphia: F. A. Davis.

Lamb, M. E., & Campos, J. J. (1982). *Development in infancy.* New York: Mosby.

Long, T., & Toscano, T. (2002). *Handbook of pediatric physical therapy* (2nd ed.). Philadelphia: Lippincott, Williams & Wilkins.

Masi, W. S., & Scott, K. G. (1983). Preterm and full-term infants' visual responses to mothers' and strangers' faces. In T. Field and A. Sostek (Eds.), *Infants born at risk: Physiological, perceptual and cognitive processes* (pp. 173–179). New York: Grune & Stratton.

McCluskey, K. A. (1981). The infant as organizer: Future directions in perceptual development. In K. Bloom (Ed.), *Prospective issues in infancy research* (pp. 119–136). Hilldale, NJ: Lawrence Erlbaum Associates.

Music, G. (2009). Neglecting neglect: Some thoughts about children who have lacked good input, and are "undrawn" and "unenjoyed." *Journal of Child Psychotherapy, 35*(2), 142–156.

Payne, V. G., & Isaacs, L. D. (2012) *Human motor development: A lifespan approach.* New York: McGraw-Hill.

Resiman, J. E. (1987). Touch, motion and proprioception. In P. Salapatek and L. Cohen (Eds.), *Handbook of infant perception: From sensation to perception* (vol. I; pp. 265–303). Orlando, FL: Academic Press.

Robson, P. (1984). Prewalking locomotor movements and their use in predicting standing and walking. *Child Care, Health and Development, 10,* 317–330.

Rodriguez, C. M., & Tucker, M. (2011) Behind the cycle of violence, beyond abuse history: A brief report on the association of parental attachment to physical child abuse potential. *Violence and Victims, 26*(2), 246–256.

Roncesvalles, M. N. C., Woollacott, M. H., & Jensen, J. L. (2000). The development of compensatory stepping skills in children. *Journal of Motor Behavior, 32,* 110–111.

Scarr, S. (1992). Developmental theories for the 1990s: Development and individual differences. *Child Development, 63*(1), 1–19.

Schulman, L. (2010). Baby's first year: Developmental milestones, what's happening, month-by-month. Retrieved from http://www.ivillage.com/babys-first-year-developmental-milestones/6-a-127191?p=2

Shonkoff, J. P., & Phillips, D. P. (2000). *From neurons to neighborhoods: The science of early childhood development.* Washington, DC: National Academy Press.

Sameroff, A. J., & Cavanagh, P. J. (1979). Learning in infancy: A developmental perspective. In J. Osofsky (Ed.), *Handbook of infant development* (pp. 344–392). New York: John Wiley & Sons.

Shumway-Cook, A., & Woollacott, M. (2012). Motor control issues and theories. In *Motor control: Translating research into clinical practice* (4th ed., pp. 1–20). Baltimore: Lippincott, Williams and Wilkins.

Sroufe, L. A. (1996). *Emotional development: The organization of emotional life in the early years.* New York: Cambridge University Press.

Sutherland, D. H., Olshen, R., Cooper, L., & Woo, S. (1980). The development of mature gait. *Journal of Bone & Joint Surgery, 62A,* 336–353.

Teicher, M. H., Andersen, S. L., Polcari, A., Anderson, C. M., Navalta, C. P., & Kim, D. M. (2003). The neurobiological consequences of early stress and childhood mal-treatment. *Neuroscience and Biobehavioral Reviews, 27*(1–2), 33–44.

Teller, D., & Bornstein, M. (1987). Infant color vision and color perception. In P. Salapatek & L. Cohen (Eds.), *Handbook of infant perception: From sensation to perception* (vol. I; pp. 185–236). Orlando, FL: Academic Press.

Thelen, E., & Fisher, D. M. (1982). Newborn stepping: An explanation for a "disappearing reflex." *Developmental Psychology, 18,* 760–785.

U.S. Department of Health & Human Services Health Resources and Services Administration Maternal and Child Health Bureau (USHHS). (2010). Rethinking MCH: The life course model as an organizing framework. Bureau of Maternal & Child Health. Retrieved from http://mchb.hrsa.gov/lifecourse/rethinkingmchlifecourse.pdf

VanSant, A. (1995). Development of posture. In D. Cech & T. Martin (Eds.), *Functional movement development across the lifespan* (pp. 275–294). Philadelphia: W. B. Saunders.

Wilson-Howie, J. M. (1999). Cerebral palsy. In S. Campbell (Ed.), *Decision making in pediatric neurologic physical therapy* (pp. 23–83). New York: Churchill Livingstone.

Woollacott, M., Burtner, P., Jensen, J., Jasiewics, J., et al. (1998). Development of postural responses during standing in healthy children and in children with spastic diplegia. *Neuroscience and Biobehavioral Reviews, 22,* 583–589.

World Health Organization (WHO). (2001). *ICF: International classification of functioning, disability and health.* World Health Organization. Retrieved March 10, 2014 from http://www.who.int/classifications/icf/en/

CHAPTER 11

Family and Disability Issues through Infancy

Anne Cronin, PhD, OTR/L, FAOTA,
Associate Professor, Division of
Occupational Therapy, West Virginia
University, Morgantown, West Virginia

Objectives

Upon completion of this chapter, readers should be able to:

- Describe how the severity, the visibility, and the prognosis of the condition may impact the development of infants later in life;

- Discuss the impact of poverty on the family and on the family's ability to respond to an infant's health concerns;

- Define what makes a newborn infant high-risk and recommended high-risk infant follow-up care;

- Explain the potential impact of prolonged uncertainty on parental function;

- List some possible impacts of having an at-risk infant as a sibling;

- Compare and contrast family-centered care with trauma-informed pediatric care; and

- Explain the principles underlying ethical professional decision making and its application to the care of infants with serious and chronic illness.

Key Terms

associations

birth defects

cerebral palsy

children with special health care
   needs

chronic disease

chronic sorrow

congenital infections

early intervention

failure to thrive

family-centered care

health care ethics

high-risk infants

iatrogenic health problems

infant mortality rate

neural tube defects

orofacial clefts

palliative care

Part C of the Individuals with
   Disabilities Education Act

poster child

stigma

syndromes

technology-dependent children

trauma-informed pediatric care

uncertainty in illness theory

ventricular septal defect

CASE 1

Jaxon

Jaxon was born at 36 weeks gestation with a neural tube defect (myelomeningocele) and hydrocephalus. The level of his lesion is L-1. He is now 8 months old (7 months adjusted age) and is followed by the state birth to 3 program, receiving both PT and OT services. Jaxon lives with and is cared for by his grandmother. Jaxon's mother is 15 and is working to finish high school. Jaxon's father (also 15) visits often, but seems very overwhelmed and distressed during these visits. Since Jaxon's mother is usually in school when the early intervention therapists are in the house, she does not get involved in his "therapy" and does not seem to understand his condition. Jaxon's grandmother is worried about her daughter's detachment and wants her to be more active in the care of her son.

Jaxon is alert and sociable, interested in all the sounds and people around him. He loves to play peekaboo and enjoys lying on his back and playing with his play gym. He knows his name and is beginning to imitate babble. Jaxon's grandmother describes him as an easy, happy baby. He eats well, drinking from a bottle and taking pureed foods from a spoon. He is beginning to finger-feed breakfast cereal and other small soft bites of food.

Jaxon prefers to play on his back, and he will roll from prone to supine, but not from supine to prone. He is not sitting independently, but happily sits in a variety of supportive baby seats. He no longer has a head lag in pull-to-sit, but is unable to get into a sitting position without support.

Jaxon will reach for and hold his plastic teething rings. He has learned to drop his toys, and laughs as he does it, but cannot recover the toy on his own. When he loses his toys, he cries loudly. Most of the time his mother and grandmother either hang toys over him or attach them to his baby seat because they want him to be happy. Jaxon is able to control his eyes to look at distant objects and can follow people and pets with his eyes as they move around the room. He loves the television and will watch even adult shows (his grandmother's soap operas) happily without fussing.

Continues on page 244

INTRODUCTION

The birth of a baby is, in most cases, eagerly anticipated. Long before a baby's birth, many parents make elaborate plans for their child and their child's future. Even when development is typical and the family has strong environmental supports, the addition of an infant to a family is a life-changing event. Although the bulk of this textbook focuses on typical life span development, a significant proportion of people have at least some periods of their lives where they face atypical challenges. For this reason we will, in this text, occasionally reflect on alternate developmental trajectories. The developmental path that is the focus of this chapter is the challenges of illness, impairment, and child disability. In this chapter, this developmental path will be considered primarily from the point of view of the parents.

Even when birth and delivery proceed as expected, additional support may be needed to help facilitate the development of parenting confidence and competence (Fowler et al., 2012). The parents' fantasies about the ideal child impact their expectations of themselves as parents and of the demands they will experience in the care of their child (Hugger, 2009). When faced with an infant who does not reflect the fantasized ideal, parents face an intense period of emotional stress (Abery, 2006; Bingham, Correa, & Huber, 2012; Glidden, Billings, & Jobe, 2006; Hugger, 2009). For some families, the diagnosis of disability occurs before the child is born. Congenital disorders such as spina bifida and Down syndrome can often be diagnosed through medical technology before the birth of the child. Glidden, Billings, and Jobe (2006) found that when parents were aware of a child's disability prior to birth, they used coping strategies more effectively.

When a baby is born too early, the family must adjust not only to their immediate needs but also to a potentially changed life course. Maroney (n.d.) comments that "the birth of a premature infant is a journey few are aware of unless they are faced with the overwhelming experience. The joy of giving birth is often coupled with fear, guilt, loneliness, and anger. A helpless infant confronts every part of your belief system and challenges every aspect of your life." Infants who are born early or born with a medical problem may have a prolonged period of hospitalization after birth. Power and Franck (2008) report that while the infant is hospitalized, parents generally want to participate in their child's care, especially by participating in those activities of daily living associated with routine infant care. An additional role expected of the parents of hospitalized infants is the monitoring and coordination of services for their child (Jefferies, 2014). By participating in the care of their infant, parents are encouraged to develop a sense of efficacy in their parenting role, as discussed in Chapter 9.

After the initial shock and the immediate need for medical support, the parents may have a period of time where the development of their child is closely monitored

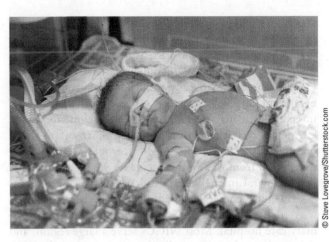

Figure 11-1 Babies born with health problems can be greatly helped by medical technologies, but these same technologies can make it hard for parents to build an attachment to their newborn.

and the child's developmental outcome is in question. Although many premature infants recover fully from their birth experience, some do not. It is at this point parents often have difficulty coming to terms with their child and begin a process of mourning as a parent accepts characteristics of the actual rather than the "ideal child" (Hugger, 2009). This mourning period may become extended over the lifetime of the child in cases of serious disability or illness. Olshansky (1962) first described **chronic sorrow** as a normal grief response that continues over time in a situation such as parenting a child with severe disabilities, which has no predictable end. Because the situation is ongoing, the sadness or sorrow is cyclic and recurrent. Chronic sorrow is also progressive and can intensify even years after the initial sense of loss, disappointment, or fear. Olshansky noted that when the diagnosis of a physical disability or cognitive impairment is given, parents realize their lives will never be the same again, nor will their lives unfold as imagined. Roos (2002) viewed chronic sorrow as "a living loss that cannot be removed" (p. xvii), and that is therefore cyclical, pervasive, and progressive. Persistent feelings of grief may limit a parent's ability to respond to their infant's cues. This is especially true in a highly medically intrusive environment such as a neonatal intensive care unit where an infant may have a variety of tubes and monitors attached, such as those on the infant pictured in **Figure 11-1**. Prolonged hospital care intrudes upon parental interactions and parent-infant bonding.

ATTACHMENT ISSUES

Attachment theory was described in Chapter 3 of this text. Its most important tenet is that an infant needs to develop a relationship with at least one primary caregiver for social and emotional development to occur normally. Infants become attached to individuals who are sensitive and responsive in social interactions with them, and who remain as consistent caregivers for some months during the period up to about 2 years of age. Parents who are sensitive and interactive with their child develop positive and supportive attachments. Parents who are unable to respond interactively, whether because of chronic sorrow or because of intrusive medical interventions, may develop insecure attachments (Shah, Clements, & Poehlmann, 2011). Newborn infants born prematurely or born with medical problems are quickly transferred from the mother's care to the specialized care of a neonatal intensive care unit (NICU). A NICU, as described in Chapter 9, provides highly specialized care and is a tertiary care center that is not a routine part of every primary care hospital. Most NICUs serve a large region, and sick newborns born in smaller hospitals are transferred to the NICU for care, even though the mother may remain in a smaller hospital. In rural communities, this may mean that the mother and child are separated, and the extended family may need to drive several hours to visit the NICU. This stress, in addition to the distress caused by the infant's health, can be overwhelming for families. A familiar national charity that attempts to help decrease this stress by providing housing for families near major children's health centers is the Ronald McDonald House Charities (2014).

Health care professionals working with infants both in hospital and community settings must understand the emotional challenges facing families as they deal not only with the complex medical care of their child, but also with chronic sorrow and less than optimal early attachment experiences. One focus in infant and family interventions is supporting attachment and helping to resolve grief associated with the birth of a "less than perfect" infant. Failure to address the emotional needs of infant-caregiver units can have enduring effects on infant outcome. Raine (2013) has reported high correlation between birth complications, maternal rejection, and high rates of violent crimes in longitudinal studies of infants who experienced both biologic and environmental risk. He also mentions the importance of appropriate early nutrition. This constellation of risk factors is very common in infants who begin life in a NICU, supporting the notion that a critical role of community-based care in high-risk infants is to support a positive family environment. Attachment has been reported as a critical factor in understanding resiliency, or the ability to achieve a desired outcome despite stressors as discussed in Chapter 2 (Gumley, Taylor, Schwannauer, & MacBeth, 2014).

Consider now the case of Jaxon, whose primary caregiver is his grandmother rather than his mother. Although there is no reason to be concerned that he is not nurtured by his grandmother, his mother's detachment may cause problems in the long run. Many grandparents value their caregiving roles because they feel that they are holding their family together (Force, Botsford, Pisano, & Holbert, 2000). Although the role may be valued over time, many grandparents who serve as primary caregivers report that they often felt isolated, overwhelmed, and depressed (Force et al., 2000).

Although it seems clear that it will benefit the whole extended family if Jaxon's mother finishes high school, her detachment may be a sign of depression or anxiety. Because Jaxon has a competent caregiver, his mother may fail to push herself to learn the caregiving skills needed to support her son's health. The physical and occupational therapists providing home care for Jaxon should plan their visits at times that both the mother and the grandmother are present. All educational efforts should be directed at both women, and Jaxon's mother should be given special "play" activities to help her learn how to interact positively with Jaxon and to have a distinct role that is not shared with Jaxon's grandmother. The case presents Jaxon's father as interested but without a clear role in his son's care. If possible, it would be ideal to also include Jaxon's father in activities that would help him to interact positively with his son.

HIGH-RISK INFANT CARE

Children with medical challenges, including those born prematurely, are likely to spend some time in a NICU and then be discharged to family care. Infants preparing to be discharged from the NICU that continue to have significant health problems or health conditions that leave them vulnerable to the development of additional health or developmental problems are considered **high-risk infants**. Infants who are high risk are also more at risk for insecure attachment at 12 months (Udry-Jørgensen et al., 2011). **Table 11-1** lists some factors that make an infant high risk.

Parents of high-risk infants may be dealing with psychological stress of their own. Placencia and

TABLE 11-1 Some Indicators of High-Risk Infant Status
Condition:
Birth weight of 1500 grams or less
Gestational age of less than 32 weeks
Intraventricular hemorrhage greater than Grade II
Congenital anomalies or intracranial abnormalities
Abnormal neurologic exam or seizures
Persistent pulmonary hypertension requiring nitric oxide
Infant of substance-abusing mother

Adapted from Purdy and Melwak, 2012. Reference Crediting: Purdy, I. & Melwak, M. (2012). Who is at risk? High-risk infant follow-up. *Newborn and Infant Nursing Reviews*, 12, 4, 221–226.

McCullough (2012) report that many mothers of high-risk infants experience symptoms of post-traumatic stress disorder (PTSD) associated with their child's birth and medical challenges. These authors noted the severity of the infant's medical complications is predictive of maternal PTSD symptoms. Mothers who have experienced this level of distress are likely to be guarded in their interactions with new health care providers who were not part of the early medical experiences of their child. In addition to the PTSD symptoms, mothers of medically fragile infants exposed to their child's long-term hospitalization are at risk for depression, especially immediately after their baby's discharge (Placencia & McCullough, 2012).

An essential role for occupational and physical therapists who work with newborns is preparing the family for the discharge of their child. Increasingly, infants are being discharged to home on oxygen, apnea monitors, high-calorie formulas, and nasogastric and gastrostomy feeding tubes. All of these devices require specialized care to maintain.

When an infant is identified as high risk, extensive discharge planning is needed so that the health of the baby is optimized. The first and most important discharge need is individualized parental education that includes hands-on practice with the management of any medical equipment that the infant will continue to need. In addition, the multidisciplinary team should develop a clear written discharge plan with the results of any diagnostic studies to be provided to the parents and to any health care personnel who will care for the child in the home community. In addition, the team must establish an individualized home care plan working with the parents to set up medication, feedings, and exercise schedules (Purdy & Melwak, 2012). Follow-up care and appointments must be coordinated. When Kuppala and colleagues (2012) reviewed current practices in high-risk infant follow-up care, a consistent finding was the need for a multidisciplinary team presence to support both the infants and the family. As mentioned previously, infants are being discharged from the high-risk nursery with increased demands placed on the family to provide supportive care.

One area of concern post-discharge is infant nutrition and growth. It has been documented that neurodevelopmental outcome later in childhood is related to the size of head circumference as an indicator of brain growth at 3 months of age (Neubauer, Greismaier, Pehhbock-Walser, Pupp-Peglow, & Kiechl-Kohlendorfer, 2013). Numerous additional studies support this correlation between adequate nutrition, brain development, and subsequent motor and cognitive neurodevelopmental outcome (Hay, 2008). Because infants discharged from the NICU may be sluggish feeders who may require supplementation of calories through nasogastric or other means of feeding, families are under enormous pressure to ensure the infant eats and thrives. **Failure to thrive (FTT)** is a diagnostic term describing insufficient weight gain or inappropriate weight loss. Therapists working in home-based early intervention programs should ask caregivers their perceptions of the feeding experience, and provide supportive suggestions to families to improve efficacy of infant feeding if problems are determined.

Some of these high-risk infants will be technology dependent when discharged from the hospital to home. The term **technology-dependent children** refers to children who cannot survive without medical technology such as mechanical ventilation or parenteral nutrition. These technology-dependent children are more medically unstable, and will require more frequent medical visits and hospital admissions in their follow-up care, placing greater care demands on parents and other family members (Toly, Musil, & Carl, 2012).

SIBLINGS OF MEDICALLY FRAGILE INFANTS

Bringing home an infant with complex medical needs will impact the entire family, and change family routines. One of the first changes to happen is that families focus and plan routines around the child with the intensive medical needs (Carnevale, Alexander, Davis, Rennick, & Troini, 2006). Heaton and colleagues (2005) interviewed siblings of technology-dependent children and found that most of the siblings had considerable household responsibilities (for example, cleaning, washing, and cooking), soon after their sibling came home. Some of these siblings went on to take on aspects of technical and nursing care. Many of the siblings provided supervision for other siblings, including their technology-dependent sibling. The experience of siblings will vary greatly both by the relative ages of the two children (siblings who are much older are likely to have more caregiving responsibilities), the other supports that a family has, and the degree and type of disability of a sibling with special needs. For this reason, few generalizations about the sibling experience can be made. There are additional challenges for all family members when a family member is medically fragile, and these challenges may result in emotional or behavioral impairments. Most studies of siblings have found that the majority report overall good mental health. There is evidence that a small proportion of siblings are at risk of emotional and behavioral problems associated with their experience of having a sibling with a disability (Giallo, Gavidia-Payne, Minett, & Kapoor, 2012).

FRAGMENTATION OF HEALTH CARE SERVICES

Once they leave the NICU, many at-risk infants and children with chronic conditions often receive the majority of their health care through specialty clinics. Specialty clinics offer many valuable services, but may lead to a fragmentation of care and poor case management between service providers. This can lead to misunderstandings and parental confusion about how to best meet a child's needs. In addition to their developmental challenges, children born prematurely are especially vulnerable to respiratory and viral illnesses, both of which are frequent causes for an infant's rehospitalization (Allen, Vessey, & Shapiro, 2009).

CHILD CARE ISSUES

Another challenge to coordinated care for children with special needs occurs when a primary caregiver is not a legal guardian of the child. This would be the case in the example of Jaxon in the beginning of this chapter. If Jaxon's mother is not involved in his daily care routines, she will not be able to give accurate histories when he attends appointments or when he has other medical problems. Jaxon's developmental sequence will not be typical because of his myelomeningocele. Clearly articulating his abilities and interests will help caregivers to better understand his needs. Jaxon will have unique medical concerns due to his condition as well. For example, it is common to monitor children with hydrocephalus closely to both determine the need for a shunt to reduce the pressure on his brain, and if he has a shunt, to adjust the shunt optimally. Jaxon's activity patterns will offer much insight into the need for shunt-related interventions. Ordinary parenting concerns such as sleeping and eating can become major stressors when paired with the demands of caring for a fragile or unstable infant.

Helping an infant get adequate sleep is another important parenting activity for all parents, but it is especially challenging for parents of preterm infants. These infants may need to have frequent nighttime feedings and may need special attention to positioning in their cribs. For these parents, the Safe to Sleep campaign (formerly known as the Back to Sleep campaign) is especially important. The back sleep position carries the lowest risk of a child experiencing sudden infant death syndrome. In addition there is evidence that babies who sleep on their backs are less likely to get fevers, stuffy noses, and ear infections. The back sleep position makes it easier for babies to look around the room and to move their arms and legs. When infants cannot sleep on their backs, due to medical of physical problems, special positioning strategies can be used to keep them safe and comfortable in side lying.

Another child care concern is that an infant may not be able to attend regular day care settings because of the likelihood of increased exposure to respiratory, gastrointestinal, and other infectious diseases. Many parents choose to stay at home with their infant rather than return to work because of the lack of an acceptable day care option. This choice is a complex one, because it also may mean that the family income is greatly reduced (with one parent not earning wages). It also may contribute to family isolation over time, because if the family does not have caregivers that they trust to manage their child, the family may be unable to engage in community activities and may not be able to get respite support during difficult times.

SOCIAL AND MEDICAL FACTORS RELATED TO DISABILITY IN INFANTS

The **infant mortality rate** is an estimate of the number of infant deaths for every 1000 live births. This is an important and often reported number because this statistic is often used as an indicator to measure the health and well-being of a nation. Data gathered in 2010 indicated an infant mortality rate in the United States of 6.05 per 1000 live births (CDC, 2012b). The five leading causes of infant mortality reported by the Centers for Disease Control (CDC), accounting for 57 percent of all infant deaths in the United States in 2013, are (1) serious birth defects; (2) preterm birth; (3) sudden infant death syndrome (SIDS); (4) maternal complications of pregnancy; and (5) injuries.

Birth defects (also called congenital abnormalities) are physical abnormalities that are present at birth. Birth defects are found in 2 to 3 percent of all newborn infants, and are not related to prematurity. *Major birth defects* are structural abnormalities that require medical and/or therapeutic intervention. *Minor birth defects* are abnormalities that do not cause serious health or social problems. When multiple birth defects occur together and have a similar cause, they are called **syndromes**. A syndrome mentioned earlier in this text is Down syndrome. Down syndrome is the most common chromosomal abnormality, affecting 11.8 babies per 1000 in the United States (CDC, 2012a). If two or more defects tend to appear together but do not share the same cause, they are called **associations**. The study of genetic associations is a new and growing field. Genetic association is not specifically causative of a condition but does affect susceptibility to common diseases and also influences the presentation of disease-related quantitative traits.

The infant mortality rate varies greatly by the race and ethnicity of the parents. For example, **Figure 11-2** shows that the infant mortality rate for non-Hispanic blacks is nearly twice the national average.

Looking briefly at the two top causes of infant mortality, congenital birth defects and preterm birth, the incidence of congenital birth defects has remained fairly stable, and does not vary significantly across race and ethnic groups (Allen, Vessey, & Shapiro, 2009). This is not the case for the second leading cause of infant mortality, preterm birth. The Centers for Disease Control and Prevention (CDC) estimated that 35 percent of all infant deaths in the United States in 2009 were related to preterm births (2013a). The incidence of preterm births varies greatly by both ethnic groups and by socioeconomic status, with lowest mortality seen mostly in Caucasian people of middle- and upper-income levels.

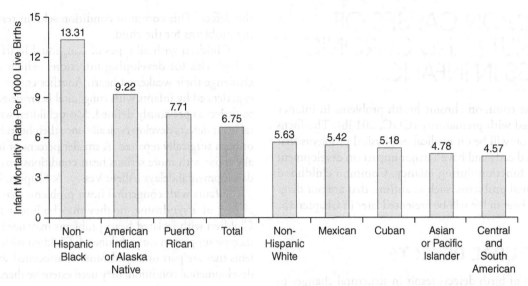

Figure 11-2 U.S. infant mortality rates vary greatly by race and ethnicity. Centers for Disease Control and Prevention and National Children's Health Service

The statistics show that for very preterm infants (less than 32 weeks of gestation), the infant mortality rates were 26 percent higher for non-Hispanic black and 14 percent lower for Central and South American infants than for non-Hispanic white infants, in a pattern very similar to the infant mortality rates shown in **Figure 11-2** (MacDorman & Mathews, 2011). Preterm birth is also a leading cause of long-term neurological disabilities in children (CDC, 2013b). When an infant is ill or disabled, the care of that infant requires extensive social, financial, and emotional reserves, as well as medical care. Families living at or near the poverty level may not be able to meet the infant's needs without external support. Many children lack the active support of two parents. The Children's Defense Fund (2010) reports that 38 percent of all children in the United States are being born to unmarried mothers. More surprising, 71 percent of non-Hispanic black children and 50 percent of Hispanic children in the United States are born to unmarried mothers. Children in single-parent homes are often also living at or near the poverty level. In these cases, even without the addition of illness or disability, these children may enter a cycle of chronic poverty. Parents with low financial resources, who would be marginally able to support typically developing children, may not be able to afford the costs associated with a child with a chronic illness.

The financial, employment, and child care pressures are very great in early adulthood, and especially in cases where the parents are very young or a parent also has a serious health condition, and caring for an infant with complex health needs may be beyond their ability. In many cases, grandparents are able to help support these young families, and sometimes actually assume the role of primary caregivers for their grandchildren as illustrated in **Figure 11-3**. The Children's Defense Fund (2010) reports that more than 2.7 million children in the United States live with grandparents who are

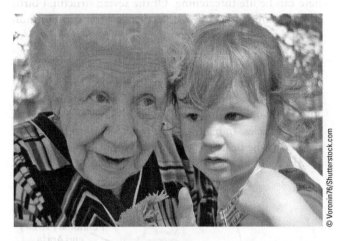

Figure 11-3 Increasingly, grandparents are involved as primary care providers to infants, especially infants with serious health problems.

responsible for them, and close to 20 percent of the grandparents raising their grandchildren live in poverty.

Children in poverty have a significantly higher incidence rate and severity level of disability. Women living in poverty may be less likely to seek prenatal care. Even when care is available at no cost to them, they must manage transportation to and from the medical visit, and must have the flexibility to leave their workplace to attend prenatal visits. Infants born too early and infants with serious illnesses require long hospitalizations, often in distant regional specialty care hospitals. In addition to the cost of medical care and medicines, these families must pay for lost time at work, as well as travel and lodging expenses. The impact of this can be dramatic. For example, Curtis and colleagues (2010) followed children born with serious health conditions, and it seemed that the economic and physical demands of caring for these children were associated with increases in the likelihood of both family overcrowding and homelessness.

COMMON CAUSES OF DISABILITY AND CHRONIC ILLNESS IN INFANCY

Many of the common chronic health problems in infancy are associated with prematurity (CDC, 2013b). The focus in this section will be on medical or physical problems that are diagnosed early and have a major impact on development and family function during infancy. Common childhood developmental problems, such as autism, that are not diagnosed until later in life will be presented later in Chapter 15.

STRUCTURAL DEFECTS

Many types of birth defects result in structural changes to the body. Some of these defects are very small and have no impact on function. Other defects, such as those presented here can be life threatening. Of the severe structural birth defects, congenital heart defects are the most common in the United States, affecting nearly one percent of—or about 40,000—births per year (CDC, 2011). Although there are many specific types of congenital heart defects, the most common type is ventricular septal defect (VSD) (CDC, 2011). A **ventricular septal defect**, as pictured in **Figure 11-4**, is an abnormal opening between the left and right ventricles. In many cases, a small VSD often closes on its own as the heart grows, usually within the first year of life. In more severe cases, surgery will be required to close

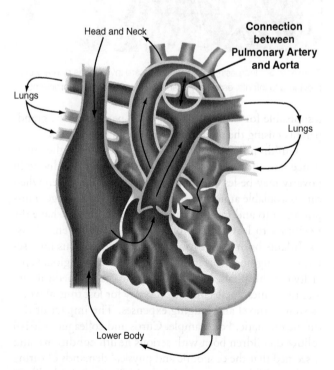

Figure 11-4 Ventricular septal defect is the most common congenital heart defect.

the defect. This common condition seldom results in lasting problems for the child.

Children with all types of congenital heart defects are at high risk for developing infections, which can further challenge their weakened heart. Another common problem experienced by infants with congenital heart defects is failure to thrive, as previously defined. Most children with congenital heart defects develop typically once their heart has matured or been surgically repaired. A smaller percent of infants, usually those with more serious heart conditions, may also show developmental delays (Allen, Vessey, & Shapiro, 2009).

Infants with congenital heart problems may have them as part of a syndrome, or they may be isolated problems. Children with isolated heart problems may need little to no therapy support in early childhood. Children with heart problems that are part of a syndrome, or associated with another developmental condition, may need extensive therapy support.

CLEFT LIP OR PALATE

Cleft lip or palate is the second most commonly occurring birth defect in the United States. Cleft lip and cleft palate are birth defects that occur when a baby's lip or mouth does not form properly. Together, these birth defects commonly are called **orofacial clefts**. As with congenital heart defects, orofacial clefts may comprise part of a syndrome or may be associated with another developmental condition. *Isolated orofacial clefts,* or clefts that occur with no other birth defects, make up about 70 percent of all orofacial clefts (CDC, 2012c).

Infants with a cleft lip with or without a cleft palate or a cleft palate alone often have problems with feeding, with ear infections, and sometimes with hearing loss. Although there are surgical corrections for these conditions, they usually cannot be initiated until an infant is at least 3 months old. For this reason, the first priority for the child's health is the establishment of adequate feeding. Cleft lip surgeries are the earliest to be done. Cleft palate surgeries are usually done at 9 to 18 months of age, and in severe cases, may require more than one surgical procedure to reconstruct the oral cavity (Allen, Vessey, & Shapiro, 2009). Infants with orofacial clefts may need speech therapy, but are not likely to be seen by occupational or physical therapy unless the cleft is part of a syndrome that includes other impairments.

NEURAL TUBE DEFECTS (NTD)

Neural tube defects (NTDs) are another one of the most common birth defects in the United States. An NTD is an opening in the spinal cord or brain that occurs very early in human development. When the neural tube does not close completely, an NTD develops. There are two main types of NTDs. *Open NTDs* occur when there is a herniation of nervous system tissue through the opening in the skull or vertebrae. There are several subtypes of open NTDs, the best known of which is myelomeningocele (also called spina bifida). With the open types of NTD, surgery is performed, sometimes in utero, to close the neural tube and prevent infection. This is the condition illustrated at the start of this chapter with the case of Jaxon.

The second type of NTD, *closed NTD*, is rare. The best known example of a closed NTD is tethered cord (NICHD, 2007). Referring to the discussion of neural tube development presented in Chapter 8, remember that the central nervous system closes to form a tube in the 4th week after conception. Subsequently, the spinal cord regresses relative to the developing vertebral column such that the spinal cord typically ends around the second lumbar vertebra. A long terminal ending, known as *filum terminale,* represents the end of the spinal cord as it courses through the lumbar canal and exits the dura in the sacral region. As the name implies, the tethered cord syndrome means the filum terminale is anchored, which produces a downward traction on the entire nervous system. Tethered cord syndrome may be associated with urologic problems, scoliosis, and progressive neurologic symptoms. One indication of tethered cord syndrome is the presence of stigmata such as sacral dimples or hair tufts (Hertzler, DePowell, Stevenson, & Mangano, 2010).

Open NTDs, or spina bifida aperta, can vary greatly in severity, with the treatment and functional limitation reflective of the specifics of each individual's condition. The functional limitations typically reflect the level of the lesion, whether in the brain or the spinal column and on how much nervous system tissue is involved. Initial treatment, sometimes done prenatally, is the surgical closure of the defect. Infants with NTDs may have any of the following associated problems: hydrocephalus, seizures, cognitive differences, musculoskeletal deformities, bowel and bladder problems, and latex allergies. Most children with NTDs require some supportive therapies in early childhood. For example, Jaxon, the case introducing this chapter, will need leg braces and intensive physical therapy in early childhood in order to learn to walk. As he matures, he may need adaptive devices to help him manage his self-care and school activities.

MUSCULOSKELETAL IMPAIRMENTS

Any condition that causes damage to the brain can potentially impact control of the muscular system. **Cerebral palsy (CP)** is an umbrella term used to describe a group of chronic conditions that first and foremost affect body movement and muscle coordination. CP is due to damage to the brain in early life and is therefore nonprogressive; however, functional abilities may improve, worsen, or remain the same over time (AACPDM, 2014). Cerebral palsy is an important condition for therapists to understand as it is the most common motor disability in childhood (CDC, 2013b). In neurological terms, cerebral palsy is not a single condition, but the manifested symptoms that are secondary to many kinds of cerebral damage. CP is vague as a diagnostic label, and includes several different subtypes and combinations of those subtypes.

The prevalence of CP was estimated as 3.1 per 1000 (8-year-old children) (Christensen et al., 2014). Children with cerebral palsy have difficulties in controlling muscles and movements as they grow and develop. The nature and extent of these difficulties may change as children grow. This is confusing to families, because the brain injury that caused the problem is nonprogressive. However, as children grow into adolescents and adults, they may seem to weaken because their limited muscle control may not be adequate to generate sufficient force to maintain upright postures, especially as needed for standing and walking. Depending on the precise area of the brain that is affected, there may be associated difficulties that become obvious during development (for example, in vision, hearing, learning, and behavior).

Abnormalities in muscle performance can be identified early in infancy. However, because of the plasticity of the nervous system, it is seldom possible to accurately predict the actual limitations children will experience later in life. Many children born prematurely are noted in early infancy to have hypotonia (lower than normal tension in the muscles). By the second year of life, the children may have developed typical muscle tension, may have developed an abnormal pattern of muscle activation (hypertonia or dystonia), or may continue to have low muscle tone. It is not unusual for a diagnosis not to be given until a child's motor development is nearly complete as doctors observe the child through the development stages of sitting, crawling, and walking. For this reason, studies that describe the incidence and types of cerebral palsy do not target infants; rather, they look at populations of school-aged children. The CDC (2013c) indicates that 77.4 percent of the children identified with CP at age 8 had spastic-type CP. Also at this age, about 58.2 percent of the children identified with CP could walk independently.

Children with cerebral palsy have limitations in motor control. This typically impacts functional limb use, but may also limit speech production. Speech, occupational, and physical therapists have an important role in supporting development in these infants and children, while providing support for the families. The early care for infants with cerebral palsy often involves a great deal of special equipment and special rules for the positions in which the child should eat, be bathed, sleep, and play. This can be overwhelming for families dealing with chronic sorrow and the physical demands of caring for a medically fragile infant.

DEFECTS CAUSED BY CONGENITAL INFECTIONS

A less publicized cause of chronic infant health problems is congenital infection. **Congenital infections** are infections contracted before or at birth from the mother. Most infections contracted by a mother during pregnancy do not affect the fetus, but some cross the placenta and cause harm. In these cases, the effect on the baby depends on the stage of pregnancy at which the infection occurs. In early pregnancy, the development of organs may be disrupted, and later in pregnancy, infections may result in a baby who is seriously ill at birth. Although less common in recent years due to widespread immunization, *maternal rubella* can lead to fetal heart abnormalities and impaired hearing and vision. The most common congenital infection today is *congenital cytomegalovirus (CMV) infection* (CDC, 2013c). This infection occurs widely in the population and has little impact on most people. In fact, the CDC reports that about 1 in 150 children is born with CMV infection, yet only about 1 of every 5 children of those born with CMV infection will develop permanent problems (such as hearing loss or developmental disabilities) due to the infection. Finally, as discussed in Chapter 9, global incidence of infant infection with the HIV virus continues to decline, but remains a focus of public health attention.

DEFECTS CAUSED BY GENETIC SYNDROMES

Genetics play a role in some birth defects. It is probable that genetic factors play a role in most of the structural birth defects described earlier. In genetic syndromes, the birth defect is programmed in the child's genetic structure. In general, genetic causes of birth defects fall into three general categories: chromosomal abnormalities, single-gene defects, and multifactorial influences. Prenatal environment can play a major role in the development of defects in all three categories, especially those linked to multifactorial causes. The influence of genetics on human development from a multifactorial perspective has been previously discussed in Chapter 2. Our discussion of genetic syndromes will be limited to the most common of the genetic syndromes that is typically followed by both physical and occupational therapy.

Down Syndrome

People who have Down syndrome suffer from moderate to severe cognitive impairment and a wide variety of birth defects that run together. In fact, there are more than 50 features of Down syndrome. But not every person with Down syndrome has all the same features or health problems. **Table 11-2** presents some of the most common of the defects that constitute Down syndrome.

Infants with Down syndrome often have difficulty coordinating the movements for eating and are slow to gain motor milestones in development. Although many adults with Down syndrome live semi-independent lives, as infants they

---

TABLE 11-2 Common Defects Associated with Down Syndrome

Category	Impairment
Body shape and size	• Short stature • Distended enlarged abdomen • A short, wide neck, sometimes with excess fat and skin • Shorter limbs and digits than would be expected for stature
Face shape and features	• Slanted eyes • A broad flattened nasal bridge • Small ears that may be set low on the head • Small irregularly shaped mouth and tongue; child's tongue may partly stick out
Physiologic or metabolic problems	• Congenital heart defects • Hypothyroidism • Gastrointestinal tract anomalies such as duodenal atresia and Hirschsprung's disease • Altered immune functions leading to high incidence of infections and other diseases • Hearing loss
Neurologic differences	• Hypotonia throughout the body with ligamentous laxity • Cognitive impairment • Seizure disorders • Sleep apnea

Down syndrome offers a clear example of a syndrome, a pattern of birth defects that occur together and have a similar cause.

benefit from intensive interdisciplinary intervention to help them reach their potential (Allen, Vessey, & Shapiro, 2009).

IATROGENIC HEALTH PROBLEMS

It was noted earlier that more preterm infants are surviving than ever before. Many of the problems that physical and occupational therapists address in infants who were born early fall into the category of iatrogenic problems. **Iatrogenic health problems** are medical or psychological problems that result from medical treatment. The aggressive ventilator support required to manage common respiratory problems in premature infants may result in chronic lung disease.

Bronchopulmonary dysplasia (BPD) is a serious lung condition that mostly affects premature infants who are born with serious respiratory distress syndrome (RDS) and need oxygen therapy to survive. If premature infants still require oxygen therapy by the time they reach their original due dates, they're diagnosed with BPD. This condition is considered iatrogenic because it is caused by the oxygen therapy; however, without the oxygen therapy, such infants would not survive. Infants with BPD may have associated health problems. Common associated health problems include upper airway anomalies, prolonged need for ventilator support, poor growth and nutrition, gastroesophageal reflux, cardiac conditions, seizures, and developmental delays (Allen, Vessey, & Shapiro, 2009). Many times children with BPD need a tracheostomy to help enhance their breathing during infancy. A tracheostomy, such as that pictured in **Figure 11-5**, can increase oxygen intake and reduce the effort needed to breath, but it may also limit oral eating and the development of oral communication.

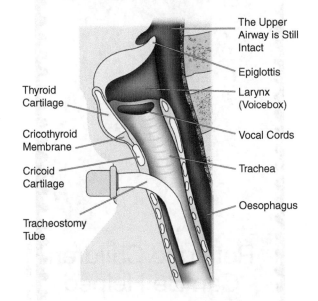

Figure 11-5 When infants need a tracheostomy tube to breathe, they may have difficulty gaining skills in eating, drinking, and oral communication.

CHRONIC AND DISABLING DISEASES IN INFANCY

A **chronic disease** is any disease or serious health condition that persists for three months or more. In infants, some diseases are considered chronic even though they have not persisted for three months. Any condition that an infant or child is diagnosed with that is expected to result in one or more of the following sequelae is considered chronic. Sequelae that define chronicity in children include a limitation of functions appropriate for the child's age, lasting disfigurement, dependency on medication or diet for the control of symptoms, dependency on medical technology, the need for more medical care or related services than is typical, and the need for special ongoing treatments at home (Stein & Silver, 2002).

Because not all chronic conditions in children need additional health, education, or social services, a secondary description was developed to identify children whose health condition qualifies them for supportive federal and state programs. The term *children with special health care needs* was used to describe this group of children. **Children with special health care needs** are legally defined as "those who have or are at increased risk for a chronic physical, development, behavioral, or emotional condition and who also require health and related services of a type or amount beyond that required by children generally" (McPherson et al., 1998). This legal definition focuses on the need for additional services rather than on a specific medical condition.

The overall incidence of most childhood conditions has been stable over the past 30 years. What has changed is the life expectancy of infants with these conditions. Advances in medicine including medications, improved diagnosis, and improved surgical techniques has led to a dramatic increase in the prevalence of infants, children, adolescents, and young adults requiring care for chronic conditions (Allen, Vessey, & Shapiro, 2009). Infants with chronic conditions are at risk for developmental delay or developmental disability. The presence of a serious health condition can limit a child's social contacts, physical environment, physical resources (such as respiration), and the ability to practice developmentally appropriate skills.

Palliative care is an area of health care that concentrates on reducing the severity of disease symptoms, and supports a positive quality of life in the presence of illness. This is ideally a multidisciplinary approach that supports both the patients and their family through addressing the physical, emotional, spiritual, and social concerns that arise with serious illness. A palliative care approach to occupational and physical therapy is often a central aspect in meeting the needs of chronically ill infants. In many instances, infants need a period of supportive therapy to help with developmental skill acquisition while the children physically grow enough for corrective surgery (as in the case of congenital heart conditions) or for a child's lungs to grow and mature (as in the case of BPD).

CHARACTERISTICS OF THE CONDITION

The greater the *severity* of an infant's health condition, the greater the likelihood the infant will face global developmental delays and the focus of infant care will be palliative. What is less obvious is that children at both ends of the illness severity spectrum are the ones at the greatest risk for developmental problems (Northam, 1997). Children with the most severe problems may be involved in lifesaving medical interventions, that support life, but that actually interfere with development. For example, children with BPD may have a tracheostomy to assist breathing and a gastroesophageal tube implanted to allow tube feeding so that they get enough nourishment to support health and lung growth. The "tubes" together with the cardiovascular limitation associated with the condition limit the development of motor, self-care, and communication skills. Children with intermediate levels of severity in their condition are the most likely to receive regular intervention for identified deficits, and the intervention is more likely to result in functional improvement than that seen with the more severely involved children.

At the other end of the spectrum, children with mild health or developmental conditions often adapt well, and their limitations are not always apparent. In these cases, both the parents and the child often deny the condition, and both may have unrealistic expectations about the child's potential function and performance. In many cases, this denial interferes with the identification of symptoms or developmental problems limiting ongoing medical management or therapeutic support for the condition. Often children with mild conditions may be overlooked, or may not actually qualify for services until they reach school age and begin to face challenges they are unable to adapt to. At this point, they may have emotional impairments in addition to the original disabling condition (Allen, Vessey, & Shapiro, 2009).

A second characteristic of the condition to consider is *visibility*. Visibility plays an important role in producing negative social reactions (Joachim & Acorn, 2000). When a condition is visible, such as Down syndrome or cerebral palsy, the child is at risk for stigmatization. A **stigma** is a social mark of disgrace associated with a particular circumstance, quality, or person. People in the social mainstream (those without stigma) often generalize from a particular disability to a variety of disabilities or imperfections. For example, it is a common complaint among wheelchair users that some people talk to people in a wheelchair as if they are mentally slow and hard of hearing. In this form of stigmatization, infants and children may be excluded from ordinary social interactions and may have low expectations set for them by the adults around them.

A second possible aspect of stigmatization is the belief that people who are disabled (and in our case, the parents of children with disabilities) are more virtuous than those who are not (Allen, Vessey, & Shapiro, 2009). A much maligned use of this sort of "virtuous" stigma is seen in the use of poster children in advertising and fundraising. A **poster child** is a child who has a disease and is pictured in posters to solicit funds for combating the disease. Charities have used poster children to raise money since the 1930s because it works. The stamp issued by the U.S. Postal Service in 1974 that is pictured in **Figure 11-6** shows an example of the use of a poster child to raise awareness and support fundraising.

Mike Erwin, a former Muscular Dystrophy Association poster child, comments that "When people see a child with leg braces and crutches, they feel sorry and drop a coin in the jar or call in the pledge. But once the fundraising drive is over, that image of the poor little poster child lingers. The general public absorbs the idea that people with muscular dystrophy, or polio—really all people with disabilities—are pitiable victims who want and need nothing more than a big charity to take care of them. Or, better, to cure them" (Erwin, n.d.).

The mixed message of what Erwin calls a "pity approach" [what another former poster child, Emily Rapp (2008), described as "feeling special and singled out") may impede the transition to adulthood and make independent living difficult. In addition, it has been argued that the poster child mentality seriously undermines the disability civil rights movement (which will be discussed in more detail in Chapter 19 of this text). The complaint of disability rights advocates is the implication that people with disabilities need pity and charity rather than accessible

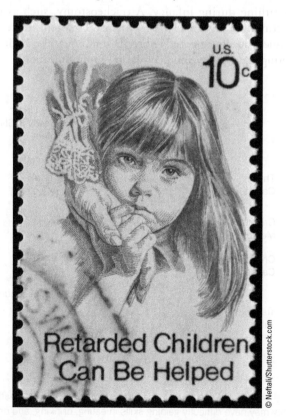

U.S. 10¢

Retarded Children Can Be Helped

© Neftali/Shutterstock.com

Figure 11-6   Although not a part of a specific fund-raising effort, this stamp uses pity to raise awareness for a cause.

TABLE 11-3   Dimensions of Stigma

Dimension	Definition of Dimension	Possible Parental Response
Concealability	The degree to which the condition can be hidden	Choosing concealing clothing.
		Limiting the infant's contact with people outside the family.
		Excessive focus on "normality," including resisting the use of assistive devices such as wheelchairs or splints.
Course of the Condition	The extent to which a condition changes over time, the *prognosis*	Denial of a negative trajectory, postponing or failing to seek intervention.
		Failure to use ordinary discipline, offering the child no limits on behavior because of the condition.
Strain	The effect of the condition's visibility and qualities on interpersonal relationships	Limiting the infant's contact with people outside the family, including limiting the family's participation in valued community activities.
		Choosing concealing clothing for "unsightly" medical appliances such as colostomy bags or tracheostomy tubes.
Aesthetic Qualities	The extent to which a condition affects a child's appearance	Choosing to emphasize a positive superficial feature, such as long pretty hair, sometimes to the point that it restricts therapeutic interventions such as positioning.
		Choosing cosmetic interventions rather than functional interventions.
Cause of Stigma	Whether the condition is congenital or acquired	Blaming one another for the condition, whether it might be prenatal parental behaviors (such as smoking during the pregnancy), or blaming others, such as the medical team if the infant's injury occurred after birth.
Peril	Dangers of being affiliated with a stigmatized child	Parent may choose to isolate the family, or just the child in question, limiting their exposure to the community.
		Parents may fail to seek appropriate care and developmental services for the child.

Adapted from (Allen, Vessey, & Shapiro, 2009). p. 23. Reference Creditng: Allen, P.J., Vessey, J.A., & Shapiro (2009). Primary Care of the Child with a Chronic Condition, 5th edition. St. Louis, MO: C.V. Mosby.

public transportation and housing, employment opportunities, and other civil rights that a democratic society should ensure for all its citizens (Erwin, n.d.).

Parents of infants with visible conditions must grapple with issues of stigma and pity at the same time they are learning to care for their child with special needs. Joachim and Acorn (2002) describe six dimensions of stigma as it is seen in chronic health conditions. Four of these dimensions, concealability, the course of the condition, strain, and aesthetic qualities, are particularly relevant to families dealing with infants with disabilities. **Table 11-3** presents these dimensions of stigma.

Physical and occupational therapists often develop extended personal relationships with the parents of the infants that they treat. For many families, the services of therapists and other health professionals are welcome as a support for the healthy development of their child. However, disability in infancy is especially difficult for families, and it is not uncommon that a family may welcome one type of therapy and not the other, or that they may welcome therapy but not the recommended therapeutic devices. Understanding

the family and the impact of disability on the family can be essential in meeting both the child and the family's needs.

FAMILIES, CULTURE, AND COPING WITH INFANT ILLNESS

There are many factors that impact the level of stress and amount of coping needed when parents learn that their child has a disability (Abery, 2006; Glidden, Billings, & Jobe, 2006; Gray, 2006). For most parents, it seems that the earlier the diagnosis, the better. As noted earlier in this chapter, parents who were aware of a child's disability due to prenatal testing were more effective in their coping than parents who had expected a typically developing child (Glidden, Billings, & Jobe, 2006). Although some conditions can be diagnosed before or at birth, many conditions are not evident until later in development. Parents often notice when their child is developing differently, or is slower to acquire skills than typical children. When they notice differences in their child, parents usually worry. Most and colleagues (2006) found that the older a child was at the time of diagnosis, the greater the level of stress the mother reported. Uncertainty about whether the child has a problem is a source of stress (Bingham, Correa, & Huber, 2012). When parents suspect a problem but there is no clear medical answer or diagnosis, they feel unsupported and do not have confidence in how to provide the needed care for their child.

This is important for health care professionals to understand. Developmental differences are often identified and therapy is initiated, even though the actual diagnosis is unclear. Many diagnoses used in early childhood are descriptive of the presenting problem, but offer parents little insight into the prognosis or long-term implications of the condition. Some of the common nonspecific diagnoses seen in infant and toddler intervention programs include developmental delay, pervasive developmental delay, and hypotonia. Other more specific and newer diagnostic labels, such as periventricular leukomalacia (PVL), offer much insight to neurologists, but provide little prognostic or functional information for therapists and parents. Although general labels like cerebral palsy have fallen out of favor since medical technologies allow diagnosis to be much more accurate, the parents of a child with PVL might be better served with the label of cerebral palsy (which is caused by many possible things including PVL), because they can search the Internet and find much more useful parent-focused information.

TRANSITION TO LIVING WITH A DIAGNOSIS

Santacroce (2003) noted that "uncertainty is the single greatest source of psychosocial stress for people affected by serious illness" (p. 45). Santacroce (2003) has applied a more general theory, the **uncertainty in illness theory (UIT)**, to the experience of parents with a chronically ill child. The UIT explains how uncertainty develops in patients with an acute illness and how patients deal with this uncertainty. Research on UIT has shown that uncertainty in illness decreases over time but returns with illness recurrence or exacerbation. The uncertainty is highest or most distressing while awaiting a diagnosis. After diagnosis, illness symptoms can lead to uncertainty when the symptoms change over time, or are unpredictable and inconsistent. Similarly, severe illness where the outcome is unknown has been reported to lead to uncertainty (Mischel, 2006).

A parent's transition to living with a diagnosis of a chronic health condition in their child begins with uncertainty, at the point when parents first become aware of their child's differences. The transition is a process that often continues throughout childhood, and involves the period during which all family members absorb the implications of the condition both for the child and for the family. In the first part of this transition, the *prediagnostic stage,* the family begins to explore resources and often seeks help through their pediatrician or primary health care provider. For some, this is a period of lay explanations ("he's just lazy") or symptom management, using things like extra rest and over-the-counter medications. When the conditions either do not resolve or worsen, the family often pursues more extensive testing. When this prediagnostic stage is prolonged, the parents' stress increases, and some parents lose confidence in their ability to care for their child (Allen, Vessey, & Shapiro, 2009).

The search for a medical diagnosis is the final part of the prediagnostic stage. This is a period of many appointments, many tests, and many long waits for results. As was stated earlier, a long prediagnostic stage can undermine the parents' confidence in caring for their child. Similarly a long medical prediagnostic period can erode the parents' confidence in the medical care providers. This is a period where stressed and frustrated parents may lash out at health care providers, institutions, and systems of care (Allen, Vessey, & Shapiro, 2009).

When a diagnosis is finally identified, parents often react with relief that the long period of uncertainty is over. The relief may soon be eclipsed by distress, especially when the diagnosis is of a terminal condition, and the parents must come to accept the likelihood that they will outlive their child. When it is a condition like autism that is not life threatening, yet which has no definitive cure, the family also faces many choices about which path to pursue in the care of their child. Santacroce (2003) notes that long-term uncertainty can interfere with a parent's ability to reliably monitor the child's health, to assign and enforce standards for behavior, and to promote the child's transition to self-management and eventually independent living. If the family had either a strongly negative, or a strongly positive response to the medical help they experienced in the prediagnostic stage, this experience is likely to influence their decision making about interventions at this stage.

After the child has a diagnosis and an immediate plan of action is developed, the next stage parents must face is living with the condition. In cases where the medical plan of action is clear, families develop confidence with the demands, and the impact of the condition on all family members becomes clearer. Parents of children with severe chronic conditions are often socially isolated by stigma and by caregiving burden. In this stage of living with the condition, some parents develop depressive symptoms or show evidence of post-traumatic stress disorder (Santacroce, 2003). The characteristics of the condition that cause the greatest family stress are conditions with sudden onset, conditions with instability or unpredictability in the course of the condition, conditions that are associated with functional limitations, and conditions that are highly visible (Allen, Vessey, & Shapiro, 2009).

CULTURE, BELIEFS, AND CHRONIC CONDITIONS

As discussed in Chapter 4, cultural identity and cultural beliefs can influence parenting and health decisions.

Understanding and respecting these influences is essential in providing care for infants and their families that must deal with serious illness and chronic health conditions. Cultural beliefs and values can be reflected in preferential treatment based on the infant's sex, beliefs about type and level of medical interventions that are acceptable, and beliefs about parenting responsibilities in the care of the infant.

Religious and spiritual beliefs are often central to family members' response to an infant's illness. Families may seek an explanation for the infant's difficulties in religious beliefs (for example, "I am being punished . . ."), or they may use their beliefs to find solace and strength ("God does not give me anything that I cannot handle."). Most hospitals have some sort of formalized Chaplin service to provide spiritual support to families. In rare instances, a family's religious or cultural beliefs may bring them into conflict with health care providers. In these cases, it is crucial to communicate clearly with both the family and the health care team interacting with the family. The main focus in such conflicts should be to preserve respectful relationships with the family and to ensure ongoing care for the child.

MAJOR LIFE AREAS

Disability has a pervasive impact on both infant development and the family. The ICF describes three major life areas, education, work and employment, and economic life. These major life areas have only a secondary relevance to infants. The area of education includes a category of informal education that might be loosely applied to infants. Informal education includes learning at home or in some other noninstitutional setting from parents or family members. Infants with serious health problems are often challenged to simply perform life-sustaining tasks such as eating, sleeping, and breathing. The demands of these tasks limit their opportunities to learn and practice skills that typically developing infants gain during the first year of life.

All three of the major life areas—education, work and employment, and economic life—are profoundly impacted for parents and caregivers of infants with serious illness or disabilities. Parents who were engaged in some stage of formal education prior to the birth of their child will almost always need to have a hiatus in their progress as they address the needs of their child. Some of these parents, especially those with lower socioeconomic resources who have little family support may not be able to return to the educational program at all. This will have a long-term impact on the financial and employment opportunities available to the parent.

Similarly, any existing work or employment situation will be challenged. Although family leave time for a newborn is commonly allowed, that allowed leave time rarely exceeds eight weeks. Many premature infants and those with serious birth defects spend more than eight weeks in the intensive care unit. Depending on individual circumstances, including the availability of spousal support,

flexibility within the workplace, the presence (and needs of) siblings, and the social support available to parents, some parents will lose their employment during this period of crisis. As with parents who were involved in educational programs, some of the parents may not be able to return to the workforce at all. The Children with Special Health Care Needs program provides health and medical supports for the child, so the cost of health care is less oppressive for families, but with the loss of employment or student status, many parents may lose their own health insurance coverage.

EARLY INTERVENTION AND SPECIAL EDUCATION SERVICE UNDER IDEA

Although we do not usually think of education in considering the needs of infants with chronic illness or disability, early intervention services for infants and toddlers with disabilities (birth through 3 years of age) have been a part of IDEA since 1986. This section of the law is commonly known as **Part C of the Individuals with Disabilities Education Act.** Through Part C evaluation, special services are to be provided to infants and toddlers at no cost to the parents. This program, in addition to the Children with Special Health Care Needs program, offers care for an infant once the baby has been discharged to the home. When the infant is medically stable and residing in the family home, supportive health services, including occupational and physical therapy, come to the child's home to provide family education, support, and therapy for the infant.

Early intervention, in this context, is the process of providing services, education, and support to young children who are deemed to have an established condition, those who are evaluated and deemed to have a diagnosed physical or mental condition (with a high probability of resulting in a developmental delay), an existing delay, or children who are identified as at risk of developing a problem that may impede their development. The purpose of Part C is to lessen the effects of the disability or delay. Services are designed to identify and meet children's needs in five developmental areas, including physical development, cognitive development, communication, social or emotional development, and adaptive development (Wright & Wright, 2012).

A central focus of Part C is family-centered care. **Family-centered care** assures the health and well-being of children and their families through a respectful family-professional partnership. It honors the strengths, cultures, traditions, and expertise that everyone brings to this relationship. Family-centered care is the standard of practice that results in high-quality services. Specifically, in family-centered care, service providers respect that each family is unique and that the family, not the health care provider, is the constant in the child's life. In the traditional medical model, the health care provider is considered the expert; in the model of family-catered care, the family members are identified as the experts on the child's abilities and needs. The family works together with service providers to make informed decisions about the services and support the child and family receives.

Although family-centered care is the ideal, it is best suited to interactions when an infant is not at high medical risk. There are instances such as traumas and medical emergencies in which the health care team must act quickly and decisively, and the family continues to need both support and information, although a true collaborative team model is not practical. In these cases, an adaptation of the family-centered care principles is applied. **Trauma-informed pediatric care** means incorporating an understanding of the impact of traumatic stress on ill or injured children and families while treating the medical aspects of trauma. In these cases, health care providers are expected to integrate an understanding of traumatic stress

into their routine interactions with children and families, in order to reduce the impact of difficult or frightening medical events, and to help children and families cope with emotional reactions to illness and injury (National Child Traumatic Stress Institute, 2011). **Figure 11-7** illustrates the foundation premises of both family-centered care and trauma-informed pediatric care side by side, with shared components shown as an overlap.

ETHICS AND CHILDREN WITH A CHRONIC CONDITION

Health care ethics are a set of moral principles, beliefs, and values that guide us in making choices about medical and health care. Our ethical responsibilities in a given situation depend in part on the nature of the decision and in part on the roles we play. For example, parents and their extended

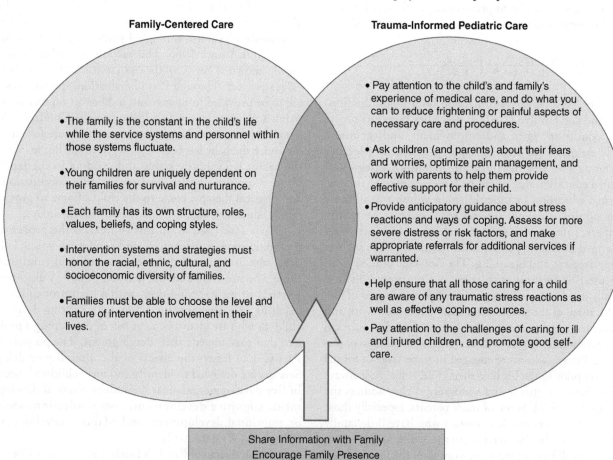

Family-Centered Care

- The family is the constant in the child's life while the service systems and personnel within those systems fluctuate.

- Young children are uniquely dependent on their families for survival and nurturance.

- Each family has its own structure, roles, values, beliefs, and coping styles.

- Intervention systems and strategies must honor the racial, ethnic, cultural, and socioeconomic diversity of families.

- Families must be able to choose the level and nature of intervention involvement in their lives.

Trauma-Informed Pediatric Care

- Pay attention to the child's and family's experience of medical care, and do what you can to reduce frightening or painful aspects of necessary care and procedures.

- Ask children (and parents) about their fears and worries, optimize pain management, and work with parents to help them provide effective support for their child.

- Provide anticipatory guidance about stress reactions and ways of coping. Assess for more severe distress or risk factors, and make appropriate referrals for additional services if warranted.

- Help ensure that all those caring for a child are aware of any traumatic stress reactions as well as effective coping resources.

- Pay attention to the challenges of caring for ill and injured children, and promote good self-care.

Share Information with Family
Encourage Family Presence
Develop Cultural Competence
Recognize Family Strengths and Needs
Listen for and Use the Family's Own Terms
Be Open to Other Healing Professionals and Customs
Show Respect By Working within the Family Structure

Figure 11-7 Although there are many important differences between family-centered care approaches and trauma-informed pediatric care, there are areas of overlap. In both cases, the best possible support of the child and the family is the goal.

TABLE 11-4	Basic Ethical Principles
Core Principle	**Definition**
Autonomy	To honor the patients (or family's) right to make their own decision; self-determination.
Beneficence	To help the patients advance their own good; to promote the welfare of people under your care.
Nonmaleficence	To do no harm, including no medical harm, cause unnecessary pain, or to try unproven or unneeded therapy.
Justice	To be fair and treat like cases alike; to offer consistent level of care based on need rather than based on a source of reimbursement.

families play different roles and owe different ethical obligations to each other than patients would to their physician. As health care providers, we must understand our own values and beliefs, and learn to detach ourselves at times to provide emotionally and culturally respectful care to a family. All health care professionals owe four main ethical principles to patients. These are presented in **Table 11-4**.

Culture and tradition influence both personal and professional ethics. Ethical health care decision making are complex when dealing with children, because adults make the decisions for children. An adult who chooses not to undergo heart surgery or to pursue cancer treatments is allowed to make that choice, and is supported with palliative care to the level desired. When a child has cancer or a heart condition that health care professionals have an effective treatment for, a parent who decides not to treat the condition presents an ethical challenge for health care providers. Beneficent decision making should include consideration of all treatment options that clearly benefit the infant or child and that the benefits clearly outweigh any associated burdens. Burdens that might be considered by physical and occupational therapists working with young children would include pain and emotional distress about immobilization or social isolation.

The term *nonmaleficence* relates to the health care providers' duty to prevent or remove harm. Harm could include medical harms, such as fractures or infections caused by a therapist's inattention to safe procedures. Another aspect of potential harm to a child is the introduction of experimental or alternative therapies to replace scientifically proven standard treatments. A parent, not a therapist, may choose to use an experimental or alternative treatment, and the health care provider can be important in helping the parent have as much information as possible in making the decision. Justice pertains to the provision of fair and equal treatment. This ethical principle requires that no particular criterion (for example, gender, wealth, religious beliefs, or parental lifestyle) should be a factor in deciding whether to offer or deny a service or intervention.

Each professional group has its own code of ethics that defines and describes the four principles presented earlier in terms relevant to that profession. Additionally, occupational and physical therapy practitioners typically collaborate with other hospital and early intervention service providers to promote a child's development and support family members and caregivers in optimizing a child's developmentally appropriate participation in home and community life. Some of the most challenging ethical considerations are those that occur in the hospital when infants or children are in an intensive care unit. All hospital-based health care providers should be aware that it is common for hospitals to have Institutional Ethics Committees that can serve as a valuable resource for both professionals and parents dealing with difficult ethical decisions.

SUMMARY

The ICF is an important view of human function that integrates the family into the performance factors that influence individual function (World Health Organization, 2001), and reflects a large body of research support about families and family development. Infants with chronic conditions are at a higher risk than other infants for negative developmental trajectories. The severity of the condition, the child's individual traits, family functioning, and the availability of social support networks all have an impact on child outcomes (Allen, Vessey, and Shapiro, 2009). Issues of socioeconomic status, culture, and ethics are environmental contextual factors that may be barriers or facilitators from the ICF frame of reference. These factors are especially relevant in the care of infants with serious illness and chronic disabilities as they affect family resources for both physical and emotional coping strategies. All families need support and education, and education provided needs to be culturally competent. Families will need, and be ready for, additional information at many points in their child's development. Physical and occupational therapists are well placed to partner with families and help provide needed support.

CASE 1

Jaxon . . . Continued

Initially, Jaxon's parents focused a great deal on "whether or not he would walk," but now, they are becoming concerned with his failure to develop even basic target skills like rolling and sitting. Jaxon is moving toward an age where typically developing infants can move around the house independently. His grandmother has not encouraged him to do a lot of moving around. The PT wants him to spend part of the day strapped into a low rolling seat that he can push across the floor by himself. He also needs to be put upright in a "stander" a couple of times a day. Consider the discussion in Chapter 6 of this text about embodied cognition. Jaxon's grandmother's decision may have a negative impact on both his physical and his cognitive development.

Guiding Questions

Some questions to consider:

1. Think about how to explain Jaxon's needs simply and clearly to both his mother and his grand-mother. You should do this in way that encourages them to do more without making them feel stressed or defensive.
2. On the Internet, look up a description of a "medical home." Define this and explain how it would be beneficial to Jaxon and his family.

CASE 2

Madison

Madison was born at 28 weeks gestation and was in the NICU for four months. She has a history of bronchopulmonary dysplasia, and now at 8 months of age chronologically (3½ months adjusted age), she is still on oxygen through CPAP, although only a eighth liter. Her mother just wants her to get off the oxygen, because she does not sleep well with a night nurse in the house. Madison is the third child in the family. She has two older brothers, Joey (3 years old) and Daniel (7 years old). She lives with both parents in a suburban area. Madison's father is an EMT, and her mother is a dietician. Currently, Madison's mother works only a few hours a week, because Madison's care is so specialized it takes much of her time.

Left alone, Madison will lie on her back and toss her head from side to side. She quiets when you pick her up, but she still has head lag in pull-to-sit. She had retinopathy of prematurity, and the ophthalmologist has prescribed eyeglasses for myopia and strabismus. Madison does not like her glasses, and because she is not moving around on her own, seldom wears them. She loves music and clearly recognizes the voices of the people in her family. She laughs and coos when someone holds her and "dances" with her to the music.

Madison kicks reciprocally and rolls from side to supine and is unable to hold her head up in prone, but when held upright, can keep her head in alignment with her body. Madison does not make eye

Continues

Case 2   *Continued*

contact, does not look at her hands or at toys, but will watch people (and the family cat) move about the room.

Madison is not yet reaching or using her hands much. Most of the time she holds her hands in a fist. She is happiest when held and carried by others. Whenever Madison is put down in prone, she screams loudly and inconsolably until someone "rescues" her. In supine she is quieter, but she is still fussy. Madison sleeps lightly, never more than three hours at a time.

Madison's mother says, "I guess I was lucky with the boys . . . Joey especially, he was such an easy baby." Madison's mother is clearly exhausted, and the early intervention team is concerned that she is getting disheartened and passive in her interactions with her daughter. She says she gets lonely at home with the two kids. Madison's father is supportive of his wife and of Madison, but works irregular hours and is not able to help much with child care.

Guiding Questions

Some questions to consider:

1. Although Daniel attends school most days, Madison's mother has the full-time care of two preschool children, one of whom is medically fragile. As the early intervention therapist, where should you focus your efforts in building a supportive home environment for Madison?
2. Madison's mother may benefit from some respite care. She cannot hire a regular babysitter because the caregiver needs to be able to respond to Madison's medical needs. Special respite services are not available in all communities. Look in your area. Is there a service that could help Madison's mother?
3. What sort of activities would you plan to engage Madison's brothers and make them feel included in her care?

Speaking of
Chronic Sorrow

SUSIE RITCHIE, RN, MPH, CPNP DEVELOPMENTAL
SPECIALIST AND PRIMARY CARE PROVIDER

During pregnancy, all parents anticipate the delivery of a perfect, healthy baby. Perhaps nothing is more devastating to mothers and fathers than learning their newborn has a condition that will prevent him or her from becoming a fully functioning independent adult.

For nearly 30 years, I have worked with infants and young children who have developmental concerns. Over that time, I have developed a great appreciation for the impact of the first few months, days, and hours after parents are given a diagnosis that will affect their child and their family for life.

During that time of initial diagnosis, when the loss of the "wished-for child" is acutely felt, mothers and fathers begin to grieve (Solnit & Stark, 1961). This grieving is part of a process of coming to terms with what that loss actually means for their child and their family. Some experience "chronic sorrow" that reflects a lifelong sadness (Olshansky, 1962).

I remember being asked to do a developmental assessment on a newborn with a rare genetic syndrome. When I entered the room, this lovely, articulate mother cried and told me, "The one thing I said to my husband during

Continues

Speaking of   *Continued*

this pregnancy was, 'I know that I can't handle a baby who isn't okay. I just won't be able to care for a child who is retarded or obviously deformed.' Now, here we are." Fortunately, like most, that mother did "handle" her daughter and did it beautifully. Now, 17 years later, this very bright young woman is about to enter college, despite her obvious physical obstacles. Although her parents rejoice in her accomplishments, they continue to grieve for the normal life experiences their child has been and will be denied because of her condition.

There is an excellent video produced by WinStar in 1999 entitled *For Love of Julian*. In this film, narrated by Susan Sarandon, mothers and fathers discuss that time when they learned that their child would not be like other children due to a developmental disability. The emotion displayed by these families, in many cases years after the birth of the infant, is extremely powerful. I would encourage anyone working with children who have special needs to watch such films, listen to parents, and observe family interactions closely. In doing this, we can all come to understand that "acceptance" of a devastating diagnosis may never be completely possible. Recognizing that "acceptance" is a process that lasts for many years, indeed throughout the life span of parents and their special child, hopefully allows professionals and families to grow together in positive and productive ways.

REFERENCES

Abery, B. H. (2006). Family adjustment and adaptation with children with Down syndrome. *Focus on Exceptional Children, 38*(6), 2–20.

Allen, P. J., Vessey, J. A., & Shapiro, N. (2009). *Primary care of the child with a chronic condition* (5th ed.). St. Louis, MO: C.V. Mosby.

American Academy for Cerebral Palsy and Developmental Medicine (AACPDM). (2014). Retrieved from http://www.aacpdm.org /patients/what-is-cerebral-palsy

Bingham, A., Correa, V., & Huber, J. (2012). Mothers' voices: Coping with their children's initial disability diagnosis. *Infant Mental Health Journal, 33*(4), 372–385.

Carnevale, F., Alexander, E., Davis, M., Rennick, J., & Troini, R. (2006). Daily living with distress and enrichment: The moral experience of families with ventilator-assisted children at home. *Pediatrics, 117*(1), e48–e60.

Centers for Disease Control and Prevention (CDC). (2011). Congenital heart defects: Data and statistics. Retrieved from http://www.cdc.gov/ncbddd/heartdefects/data.html

Centers for Disease Control and Prevention (CDC). (2012a). CDC features: Down syndrome cases at birth increased. Retrieved from http://www.cdc.gov/features/dsdownsyndrome/

Centers for Disease Control and Prevention (CDC). (2012b). *NCHS data brief: Recent declines in infant mortality in the United States, 2005–2011*. Retrieved from http://www.cdc.gov/nchs/data /databriefs/db120.htm

Centers for Disease Control and Prevention (CDC), (2012c). *Birth Defects: Cleft Lip and Cleft Palate*. Retrieved from http://www .cdc.gov/ncbddd/birthdefects/cleftlip.html

Centers for Disease Control and Prevention (CDC). (2013b). *Cerebral palsy: Data and statistics for cerebral palsy.* Retrieved from http://www.cdc.gov/ncbddd/cp/data.html

Centers for Disease Control and Prevention (CDC). (2013c). Cytomegalovirus (CMV) and congenital CMV infection. Retrieved from http://www.cdc.gov/cmv/trends-stats.html

Centers for Disease Control and Prevention (CDC). (2013a). *Reproductive health: Preterm birth*. Retrieved from http://www.cdc .gov/reproductivehealth/maternalinfanthealth/pretermbirth.htm

Children's Defense Fund. (2010). *State of America's children*. Retrieved from http://www.childrensdefense.org/child-research-data -publications/data/state-of-americas-children.pdf

Christensen, D., Kim, Doernberg, N., Maenner, M., Arneson, C., Durkin, M., & . . . Yeargin-Allsopp, M. (2014). Prevalence of cerebral palsy, co-occurring autism spectrum disorders, and motor functioning. Autism and Developmental Disabilities Monitoring Network, USA, 2008. *Developmental Medicine & Child Neurology, 56*(1), 59–65.

Curtis, M. A., Corman, H., Noonan, K., & Reichman, N. E. (2010). Effects of child health on housing in the urban U.S. *Social Science & Medicine, 71*(12), 2049–2056.

Erwin, M. (n.d.). *The kids are all right*. Retrieved from http:// thekidsareallright.org/index.html

Force, L. T., Botsford, A., Pisano, P. A., & Holbert, A. (2000). Grandparents raising children with and without a developmental disability: Preliminary comparisons. *Journal of Gerontological Social Work, 33*(4), 5–21.

Fowler, C., Rossiter, C., Maddox, J., Dignam, D., Briggs, C., Deguio, A., & Kookarkin, J. (2012). Parent satisfaction with early parenting residential services: A telephone interview study. *Contemporary Nurse: A Journal for the Australian Nursing Profession, 43*(1), 64–72.

Giallo, R., Gavidia-Payne, S., Minett, B., & Kapoor, A. (2012). Sibling voices: The self-reported mental health of siblings of children with a disability. *Clinical Psychologist, 16*(1), 36–43.

Glidden, L. M., Billings, F. J., & Jobe, B. M. (2006). Personality, coping style and well-being of parents rearing children with developmental disabilities. *Journal of Intellectual Disability Research, 50,* 949–962.

Gray, D. E. (2006). Coping over time: The parents of children with autism. *Journal of Intellectual Disability Research, 50,* 970–976.

Gumley, A. L., Taylor, H. E. F., Schwannauer, M., & MacBeth, A. (2014) A systematic review of attachment and psychosis: Measurement, construct validity and outcomes. *Acta Psychiatrica Scandinavica, 129*(4), 257–274.

Hay, W. W., Jr. (2008). Strategies for feeding the preterm infant. *Neonatology, 94*(4), 245–254.

Heaton, J., Noyes, J., Sloper, P., & Shah, R. (2005). Families' experiences of caring for technology-dependent children: a temporal perspective. *Health & Social Care in the Community, 13*(5), 441–450.

Hertzler, D. A., DePowell, J. J., Stevenson, C. B., & Mangano, D. O. (2010) Tethered cord syndrome: A review of the literature from embryology to adult presentation. *Neurosurgical Focus, 29*(1), E1–9.

Hugger, L. (2009). Mourning the loss of the idealized child. *Journal of Infant, Child & Adolescent Psychotherapy, 8*(2), 124–136.

Jefferies, A. L. (2014). Going home: Facilitating discharge of the preterm infant. *Paediatrics & Child Health (1205-7088), 19*(1), 31–36.

Joachim, G., & Acorn, S. (2000). Stigma of visible and invisible chronic conditions. *Journal of Advanced Nursing, 32*(1), 243–248.

Kuppala, V., Tabangin, M., Haberman, B., Steichen, J., & Yolton, K. (2012). Current state of high-risk infant follow-up care in the United States: Results of a national survey of academic follow-up programs. *Journal of Perinatology, 32*(4), 293–298.

MacDorman, M. F., Mathews, T. J. (2011). *Understanding racial and ethnic disparities in U.S. infant mortality rates.* NCHS data brief, no 74. Hyattsville, MD: National Center for Health Statistics.

McPherson, M., Arango, P., Fox, H., Lauver, C., McManus, M., et al. (1998). A new definition of children with special health care needs. *Pediatrics, 102,* 137–140.

Maroney, D. (n.d.). *Premature-Infant.com: Walking the road of hope and possibility with a premature infant.* Retrieved from http://www.premature-infant.com/index.html

Mischel, M. (2006). *What do we know about uncertainty in illness?* Japanese Society for Nursing Research. Retrieved from http://www.jsnr.jp/meeting/docs/31_02.pdf

Most, D. E., Fidler, D. J., Laforce-Booth, C. L., & Kelly, J. (2006). Stress trajectories in mothers of young children with Down syndrome. *Journal of Intellectual Disability Research, 50,* 501–514.

National Child Traumatic Stress Institute. (2011). *Healthcare toolbox: Trauma-informed pediatric care.* Retrieved from http://www .healthcaretoolbox.org/index.php/why-traumatic-stress-is -relevant-in-pediatric-health-care/tipc

National Institutes of Health/National Institute of Child Health and Human Development (NICHD). (2007). *Neural tube defects (NTDs): What are neural tube defects?* Retrieved from https://www.nichd.nih.gov/health/topics/ntds/conditioninfo/Pages /default.aspx

Neubauer, V. Greismaier, E., Pehhbock-Walser, N. Pupp-Peglow, U., & Kiechl-Kohlendorfer, U. (2013). Poor postnatal head growth in very preterm infants is associated with impaired neurodevelopment outcome. *Acta Paediatrica, 102*(9), 883–888.

Northam, E. A. (1997). Psychosocial impact of chronic illness in children. *Journal of Paediatrics and Child Health, 33*(5), 369–372.

Olshansky, S. (1962). Chronic sorrow: A response to having a mentally defective child. *Social Casework, 43,* 190–193.

Placencia, F., & McCullough, L. (2012). Biopsychosocial risks of parental care for high-risk neonates: Implications for evidence-based parental counseling. *Journal of Perinatology, 32*(5), 381–386.

Power, N., & Franck, L. (2008). Parent participation in the care of hospitalized children: A systematic review. *Journal of Advanced Nursing, 62*(6), 622–641.

Purdy, I., & Melwak, M. (2012). Who is at risk? High-risk infant follow-up. *Newborn and Infant Nursing Reviews, 12*(4), 221–226.

Raine, A. (2013). *The anatomy of violence* (pp. 182–273). New York: Pantheon Books.

Rapp, E. (2008). *Poster Child.* New York: Bloomsbury USA.

Ronald McDonald House Charities. (2014) Retrieved from http://www.rmhc.org/what-we-do

Roos, S. (2002). *Chronic sorrow: A living loss.* New York: Routledge.

Santacroce, S. (2003). Parental uncertainty and posttraumatic stress in serious childhood illness. *Journal of Nursing Scholarship, 35*(1), 45–51.

Shah, P. E., Clements, M., & Poehlmann, J. (2011). Maternal resolution of grief after preterm birth: Implications for infant attachment security. *Pediatrics, 127*(2), 284–292.

Solnit, A. J., & Stark, M. H. (1961). Mourning and the birth of a defective child. *The Psychoanalytic Study of the Child, 16,* 523–527.

Stein, R. E., & Silver, E. J. (2002). Comparing different definitions of chronic conditions in a national data set. *Ambulatory Pediatrics, 2*(1), 63–70.

Toly, V., Musil, C., & Carl, J. (2012). Families with children who are technology dependent: Normalization and family functioning. *Western Journal of Nursing Research, 34*(1), 52–71.

Udry-Jørgensen, L., Pierrehumbert, B., Borghini, A., Habersaat, S., Forcada-Guex, M., Ansermet, F., & Muller-Nix, C. (2011). Quality of attachment, perinatal risk, and mother-infant interaction in a high-risk premature sample. *Infant Mental Health Journal, 32*(3), 305–318.

World Health Organization. (2001). ICF: *International classification of functioning and disability.* Geneva, Switzerland: World Health Organization.

Wright, P., & Wright, P. (2012). *Wrightslaw: Early intervention (Part C of IDEA).* Retrieved from http://www.wrightslaw.com/info /ei.index.htm

CHAPTER 12

Development in the Preschool Years

Anne Cronin, PhD, OTR/L,
Associate Professor, Division of
Occupational Therapy, West Virginia
University, Morgantown, West Virginia

Objectives

Upon completion of this chapter, readers should be able to:

- Describe the motor and skeletal changes in the preschool years;

- Explain how language and perceptual development support the development of both fine motor and self-care skills;

- Describe the development of object use and its impact on the development of self-care and pre-academic skills;

- Identify the major power and precision grasp patterns and patterns of hand skill development in the preschool years;

- Describe school readiness, including physical and cognitive/behavioral task performance expectations;

- Differentiate typical characteristics of preschool play, and discuss the importance of play as a childhood occupation and in the development of functional skill; and

- Describe the contextual factors influencing preschool children and the influence of these factors on function and disability.

Key Terms

associative play

attunement play

Ayres Sensory Integration

bimanual coordination

body mass index (BMI)

calibration

constructive play

cooperative play

discriminative touch

dynamic postural stability

equilibrium reactions

executive attention

fine motor control

flow

games with rules

graphomotor skills

hand preference

haptic perception

in-hand manipulation

onlooker play

parallel play

perceptual motor skill

physical play

play with objects

postural stability

power grasp

pre-academic skills

precision grasp

pretense/sociodramatic play

school readiness

self-efficacy

sensory processing

solitary play

stability limits

static postural stability

static visual acuity

symbolic play

unoccupied play

visual discrimination

visual scanning

CASE 1

Trevor

Trevor was a quiet baby and was slow to develop motor control. Because of his delayed motor control, at 3 months of age, he began receiving early intervention physical and occupational therapy. At 1 year, he was diagnosed with cerebral palsy (spastic quadriplegia). Now 3 years old, Trevor has hypotonia (low resting tension in the muscles) in his postural muscle groups, but hypertonia (high resting tension) in his upper and lower extremities. He is dependent in all mobility and self-care functions.

At this time, Trevor (1) is rolling from prone to supine and supine to side, (2) is showing visual attention and reaching for objects, and (3) in supported sitting, brings his hands to midline and is able to sit briefly (about a minute) without support. He sits with a rounded back and falls backward with a hip extensor spasm from time to time. He does *not* have (1) protective extension, (2) hip stability in weight bearing, or (3) any locomotor pattern other than rolling. When supported in a standing device, he tends to be on his toes. Emerging skills include taking weight on his legs in a standing position and assuming an all-fours position.

Trevor is alert and interested in people and things around him. He reaches for toys but is unable to extend his arms fully and often misses his target. He has a raking palmar grasp pattern with his hands and often doesn't like the way things feel. Trevor needs support with positioning for feeding. He does not have adequate trunk control to sit independently.

Trevor is able to speak a few words, but they are difficult to understand. He has recently begun to attend the public special needs preschool. He attends the school five mornings a week and receives special education support as well as physical, occupational, and speech therapy to help optimize his development.

Continues on page 271

INTRODUCTION

In popular culture, infants transition from infancy to toddlerhood when they achieve the milestone of walking. This is an important transition, because the period of rapid neuromotor development slows and the developmental focus shifts from acquisition of motor control to acquisition of communication and social and behavioral control. As we will see, physiologic and motor control changes will continue at a rapid rate in the first 5 years of life, the preschool years. In the preschool years, the sudden expansion in communication and social skills will eclipse other areas in contributing to increased function. In Chapter 2, the concept of *sensitive periods* in development was introduced. In a sensitive period of development, neuronal connections are particularly susceptible to environmental input. There are several developmental sensitive periods in the preschool years. In infancy, the emphasis in development was in the areas of structure and function. In the preschool years, true interactive participation and activities occur. The personal and environmental contexts become increasingly apparent in their influence on the rate and types of skills acquired. Play, an activity that is intrinsically motivated and engaged in for pleasure, becomes more complex during this stage and is central to the process of preschool development. The Lego Foundation (2010) describes play as central to both the emotional well-being and mental health of children. Play in early childhood serves as a mirror on development and is an important human occupation throughout life. For this reason, this chapter will have an extensive discussion on play and the role of play in learning.

In the preschool years, many lasting health trajectories begin. Trends to sedentary lifestyles and obesity are one such trajectory that is increasingly seen in American preschoolers. At another level, many communities have early childhood swimming and "sports readiness" activity programs aimed at preschool children. Programs like these offer opportunities for play and learning in a social environment. The father and son pictured in **Figure 12-1** are engaged in a parent-child "learn to swim" program. These programs are tools to help develop a healthy lifestyle trajectory, rather than the unhealthy one mentioned earlier.

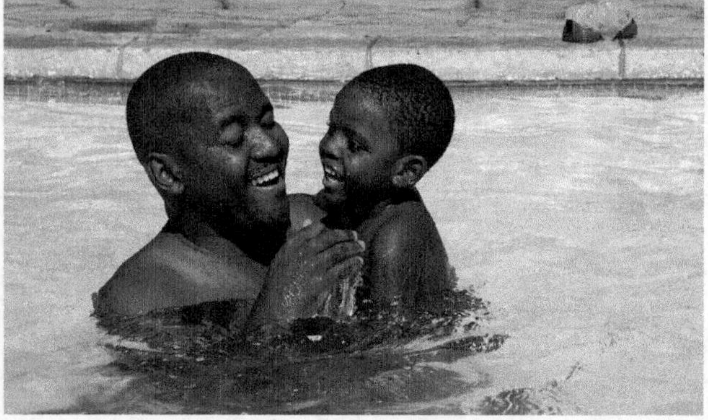

This is an important period of development to understand because it is in this period that some types of disability become apparent. Autism, cerebral palsy, muscular dystrophy, and many other disorders are first recognized, and families begin building relationships with therapists as their child leaves infancy and moves into the preschool years. The biggest group of childhood assessment tools, used by both occupational and physical therapists, focus on these developmental years because of the importance of this period to the long-range functional skill development of the child. This is also an impressionable period in social and emotional development. Persistent emotional distress, neglect, or the experience of trauma experienced during this period can have lasting impacts of personality development and mental health.

In the second through fourth developmental years, children acquire the basic skills needed to function within their social and cultural environment. These skills, called *developmental milestones,* usually appear in long lists of skills typical within a culture to a specific age group. In children 1 to 2 years of age, the cultural differences tend to reflect the family lifestyle and home routines. As the children gain language, they also assimilate cultural behaviors and values. The rate and pattern of specific skill development in areas of self-care and adaptive function may vary widely based on the early childhood environmental contexts. For this reason, developmental assessment should be based on the cultural mores within which children live. When children begin to use a fork, or chopsticks, or even a computer mouse, vary greatly by the children's exposure to and opportunity to practice the skills in question. In this chapter, developmental milestones will be considered generally, but the focus will be on the development of functional skills. Milestones are useful for screening children but do not give physical and occupational therapists adequate information to determine whether a delay is based on neuromotor, cognitive, or environmental causes.

© Daleen Loest/Shutterstock.com

Figure 12-1   Father and son engage together in physical play. Through this playful exchange, the father is also able to support the development of a healthy lifestyle.

BODY STRUCTURES AND FUNCTIONS

The changes in the body that we will focus on the most in this chapter are in brain and nervous system development. The preschool years are also a period of rapid physical growth and increased control of both body functions and movements. This is typically a period in which children love to explore their growing sensorimotor skills through active play. Children who are unable to engage in activity for health or other reasons may be slower to gain skills than their more active peers. Because of the high level of neural plasticity, there is an emphasis on early intervention and early identification of developmental differences.

This period affords the most productive time for therapists to make lasting changes in motor function.

BRAIN AND NERVOUS SYSTEM DEVELOPMENT

The brain's plasticity is at its postnatal highest in infancy and during the preschool years (Belsky & de Haan, 2011; James, 2010). From infancy to age 6, the brain grows to about 90 percent its adult size, and important developmental processes occur in terms of sensory development, fine motor, affective, and cognitive functions during this period (Moon et al., 2011).

Brain imaging studies show that for most children between 3 and 6 years, there is increased left hemisphere activity, which may be reflective of the dramatic rate of language development during this period. Increased myelination, synaptic development in the prefrontal cortex, occur extensively early in the preschool years. Around age 4, synaptic pruning in areas of the brain not being used begins and extends throughout childhood. These brain changes result in an improvement in the speed of information processing as well as improved attention, reasoning, and cognitive control. As first presented in Chapter 9, myelination speeds nerve conduction, and results in more efficient cognitive processing and more refined motor control (Moon et al., 2011). Infants, as we will recall from Chapter 10, move their hands in gross grasp patterns that begin as reflexes and mature to active voluntary grasps. During this period of development, infants lack the ability to isolate the movement of one finger from the movements of all fingers on that hand. This is because their nerves are insufficiently myelinated, and there is "overflow" of the nervous impulse to surrounding areas.

As preschool children act on their environment, learn, and develop skills, the neuronal pathways that they use most are strengthened. In typically developing children, the synapses that are most important to survival and optimal function will flourish, and useless connections will be removed. When children have some developmental challenge, such as a hearing loss that can result in overdependence on the visual system, pruning will occur in a pattern reflecting their needs and experiences. In some cases, this is adaptive, but in others the children may need additional stimulation to maintain and develop connections that they will need to function well later in life. Synaptic pruning results in *use-dependent brain organization*. This means that brain functions you use often are strengthened, and brain functions you seldom use may become less available (Henderson & Pehoski, 2006).

In the case of Trevor presented at the start of this chapter, it is clear that there are many activities that typically developing preschool children will engage in that Trevor cannot manage. Trevor is dependent on others for mobility, feeding, and social exchanges. This dependency may lead to a pattern of synaptic pruning that further exaggerates his disability. The focus on early childhood interventions for children like Trevor is to help them engage in a broad range of developmental activities and support the development of cognitive functions.

Another area where there is significant brain development is in the fibers linking the cerebellum to the cerebral cortex (Deoni, Dean, O'Muircheartaigh, Dirks, & Jerskey, 2012). This change contributes to the dramatic gains in motor coordination seen during the preschool years. The cerebellum is involved with both motor and cognitive development, and has a prominent role in processing temporal information. The cerebellum is believed to be involved with processing novel cognitive and motor tasks and in the acquisition of new cognitive and motor skills throughout life (Davis, Pitchford, Jaspan, McArthur, & Walker, 2010). The refinement of motor calibration and flow, discussed later in this chapter, occur because of increased cerebellar influence on cognitive and motor skills.

As noted earlier, there is much neural activity in the left hemisphere of the cortex during the preschool years. During this time, the left hemisphere develops more rapidly than the right, beginning the process of hemispheric *lateralization*. As the hemispheres lateralize, they specialize in function. This results not only in a hemisphere that is superior at processing language, but also in the development of hand dominance and sensory integration.

Although the process of brain lateralization begins in the preschool years, it is central to the development of academic skills. For this reason, further discussion of brain lateralization can be found in Chapter 13 on middle childhood.

PHYSICAL DEVELOPMENT

After age 1, a baby's growth in length slows considerably, and by 2 years, growth in height usually continues at a fairly steady rate of approximately 2 to 3 inches (6 cm) per year until adolescence. The best tool to determine whether a child's growth is adequate is the body mass index. The **body mass index** (BMI) is a calculation that uses height and weight to estimate how much body fat someone has. This tool does not rely on averages, but rather is a measure of the physiological state of the individual. Throughout these early years as the brain and central nervous system continue to grow, both nutrition and activity patterns impact this growth (Belsky & de Haan, 2011).

In the preschool years, children gain muscle bulk, coordination, and strength. Walking becomes smoother and more effortless, and children gain skill in running, jumping, and climbing. The rate and sequence of skill acquisition vary with the children's environment and social situation. Developmental screening tests list milestones like "pedals a tricycle," which assumes exposure and practice with tricycles or bicycles with training wheels. Health care professionals need to understand the qualitative changes in movement during this period to isolate motor skill delay from culture and environmental influences.

Another component of motor skills is the necessary physical energy to sustain performance of tasks. Typically developing preschool children are characteristically very energetic and prefer active play. Although they have high energy and activity levels, they may have limited endurance to sustain time-consuming tasks without problems of physical fatigue. Children who have been ill or have some types of impairments may lack the energy or endurance to practice motor skill, and may be slower to develop motor milestones.

Through the process of motor learning, preschool children engage in complex volitional motor behaviors that the individuals choose to use to meet a desired goal. Although volitional behaviors are present in term infants, they are very limited because infants do not yet have the postural control, perception, or mental functions needed to support complex actions. In the preschool years, children's

volitional behaviors grow in both complexity and in intent. **Table 12-1** provides some specific examples illustrating the increasing sophistication of motor skills through age 5.

COMMUNICATION FUNCTIONS

The whole of the preschool years are a sensitive period for language learning. Expressive and receptive vocabulary is expanding, and the semantic and syntactic structure of their language is becoming more complex. A more in-depth overview of the process of language development is presented in Chapter 5 of this text. This chapter will summarize these changes and

TABLE 12-1	Development of Motor Control	
Age	**Gross Motor**	**Fine Motor**
2 to 2½ Years	Walks up the stairs using reciprocal movements independently, although may still need help with going down stairs Able to walk backward Stands on toes Stands on one foot for a few seconds	Demonstrates a functional grasp and wrist control with using a spoon, some spillage Able to unbutton large buttons on clothing Able to turn the pages of a book one at a time Begins to create things with clay and modeling clay
2½ to 3 Years	Walks on a line with one foot in front of the other Walks on tiptoes Stays on one foot for two to three hops Pedals a tricycle	Able to manipulate small beads and pegs Able to hold an object with one hand while using the other hand to perform an action Scribbles spontaneously Turns over container to pour out contents
3 to 3½ Years	Stands on one foot for up to 5 seconds Balances on a balance beam Walks up and down the steps well, alternating feet Jumps with both feet	Able to hold up fingers to tell age Able to use enough force to roll modeling clay into worms or snakes Holds crayon or marker with the thumb, index, and middle fingers Dresses him or herself with help
3½ to 4 Years	Able to hop forward three or more times Rhythmically marches to music Moves forward and backward with agility Broad jumps forward up to 24 inches	Successfully manages small buttons Holds a drinking glass in one hand Draws a person with two to four body parts Able to use a one-button computer mouse
4 to 4½ Years	Able to climb up a ladder to the slide and slide down Can stand on one foot for up to 10 seconds Able to hop on one foot five times	Able to screw and unscrew nuts and bolts Able to touch each finger to the tip of the thumb Uses table utensils skillfully
4½ to 5 Years	Beginning to learn to pump the swing Running is controlled; can start, stop, and turn while remaining balanced Walks on tiptoe Gallops and skips	Able to manipulate squeeze bottles Hand preference is established Laces (but cannot tie) shoes Able to dial a telephone

emphasize how language development mirrors the development of cognitive abilities. In this age group, a lack of exposure to language results in a persistent, lifelong lack of language skills (Kuhl, Conboy, Padden, Nelson, & Pruitt, 2005).

By 3 years, most children have acquired nearly 1,000 words, and they can produce three-word sentences. During this time period, children can often be observed talking to themselves. This "private speech" reflects the beginning of thoughtful control of behavior. Through talking to themselves, children can try out ideas and experiment with possibilities. By the end of the preschool period, this private speech is largely internalized (Feldman, 2011). Between four and five the child's ability and desire to communicate expand rapidly. By four years the typical child can use connected sentences, tell experiences or simple events in sequence, reproduce short verses, rhymes, songs from memory and use sentences of at least five words. By five years the child can use words precisely and can use plurals and tense correctly. The five year old has also developed pragmatic language skills and can express him- or herself in a varied tone of voice and inflection. Between the ages of four and five the child becomes an effective communicator and can carry on extended conversations, can give information, convey ideas and ask thoughtful questions.

The case of Trevor illustrates the problem when preschool children are unable to express themselves using language. At school, Trevor's speech therapist has introduced some augmentative communication devices that speak for him. This paired with specialized seating and electronic switches the occupational therapist provided have made a big difference in his alertness and motivation in all areas. Trevor now can communicate using noun-verb combinations and can appropriately choose between several preprogrammed phrases in social interactions. Now that he can express himself, Trevor has been more cooperative and has developed improved compliance with his physical therapist and is beginning to walk in the classroom using a walker. As he gains confidence and skill with the AAC device and the walker, Trevor will be able to use these devices both at home and in the community, greatly expanding his sensorimotor experience and environmental contexts.

During the preschool period, language becomes the primary mechanism for making needs, feelings, and thoughts known to others, so this skill will be especially important for Trevor. By 5 years of age, children's vocabulary typically consists of about 5,000 to 8,000 words, and they speak in grammatically complex sentences. Communication and language are central to all of the developmental tasks of the preschool years. New skills are taught, usually with verbal instructions, games include story lines and dialog, and all types of social interactions require communication. Because of the close relationship between language and cognition, delays in the development of language can impact all areas of development.

Children who have difficulty gaining language skills will have difficulty engaging in learning activities and participation in activities in their homes and communities. Language delays in the preschool years often appear to adults in the child's world as a frustration with learning and play activities that involve talking to others, listening, or following directions. Children with language delays often seem inattentive to others and not interested in classroom activities. It is not uncommon for children with language delays to have negative behavioral outbursts, caused by their frustration with the inability to communicate. The discussion in Chapter 5 about alternative and augmentative communication strategies (AAC) introduced the idea of teaching sign language to prelinguistic children. Offering an alternative communication strategy for young children with delayed language development results in improved behavior and improved engagement in learning activities (Pizer, Walters, & Meier, 2007). One of the most common causes of language impairment in young children is autism. Because language development is so important in the preschool years, it is important to recognize language delays early and refer children with early warning signs for expert assessment. **Table 12-2** lists the some "red flags" for language development that all health care providers should be aware of.

AAC strategies, as described in Chapter 5, are often a routine part of the early childhood supports offered to children with autism spectrum disorders (Ganz et al., 2012). These AAC strategies are typically developed by a speech language pathologist, but should be understood and supported by the occupational and physical therapists working with the children.

SENSORY CHARACTERISTICS

Advances in neuroscience have shown the importance of the sensory systems and sensory feedback in all areas of learning and development (Smith, 2006). For example, in the preschool years, children assimilate and integrate information from visual, tactile, and proprioceptive senses as they learn to dynamically control their balance. Through sensory and social learning, preschool children develop a body image. *Body image* is a people's sense of their own physical appearance and physical abilities, usually in relation to others within their social environment. By 1 year of age, most infants recognize themselves when they look in the mirror. This early recognition of self expands through the preschool years so that by age 5, most young children have a strong sense of their bodies in terms of cultural values like beauty and strength (Burgess & Broome, 2012; Monteiro Gaspar, Amaral, Oliveira, & Borges, 2011). The development of body image is reliant on a child's ability to see and process visual sensory information. Strickling (2010) notes that "the blind child has an unusual dependence on a sighted person to mediate and help integrate his environment. This notion of dependence must be considered as a major factor in the blind child's development. The blind child has diminished control over his environment and can only control his inner world. As he withdraws into this world, he diminishes the need for social interaction. He may not understand that there is a complex world outside of himself, that he is separate from it,

TABLE 12-2 Red Flags for Language Development

- No back-and-forth sharing of sounds, smiles, or other facial expressions by 9 months or thereafter.

- No babbling by 12 months.

- No back-and-forth gestures, such as pointing, showing, reaching, or waving by 12 months.

- Does not turn to the person speaking when his/her name is called by 12 months.

- No words by 16 months.

- Does not use pointing or other "showing" gestures to draw attention to something of interest by 16 months.

- No simple pretend play, like feeding a doll or stuffed animal, and attracting your attention by looking up at you by 18 months.

- No two-word meaningful phrases (without imitating or repeating) by 24 months.

- Any loss of speech or babbling or social skills at any age.

Adapted from Greenspan, Prizant, & Wetherby, 2004. Reference Creditng: Greenspan, S., Prizant, B. & Wetherby, A. (2004). Hallmark Developmental Milestones. Retrieved from https://www.firstsigns.org/healthydev/milestones.htm

that he can both act on it and be the recipient of action." This example helps illustrate how the sensory-perceptual aspects of early childhood experiences broadly influence development. Adults who lose sensory functions later in life will not experience the pervasive change in learning and skill acquisition that is common in preschool children with sensory impairments.

Early in the preschool years, toddlers move and actively explore their environment. From this active exploration, there is a rapid growth in sensory perception. The children receive rich visual, somatosensory, auditory, and olfactory experiences that become paired with motor actions and learning. Through sensorimotor exploration, children begin to explore new motor actions. During this process of sensorimotor activity, the expansion of cerebellum function described earlier supports the development of increasingly sophisticated movements. The resulting controlled, volitional motor act that responds in a dynamic way to sensory perceptions is called a **perceptual motor skill.** Many of the traditional items on developmental screening tests for this age test specific perceptual motor skills like walking along a line, throwing a ball to a target, and climbing playground equipment. Children with deficits in sensory function or in sensory perception may be able to sit, stand, run, and jump but be unable to manage these complex perceptual motor skills.

A specific type of perceptual motor skill, *visual perceptual skill,* is an important developmental focus in the preschool years. Visual perceptual skills include recognizing colors, matching shapes and sizes, and understanding the spatial relationships between objects (over, under, through, beside . . .). Children with visual impairments must develop learning strategies to accommodate their limited or absent vision. These children have a unique developmental sequence and should not be assessed on standards developed for visually intact children. Additionally, these children have

a qualitatively different experience of their environmental contexts. Vinter and colleagues (2013) found support for the construct of embodied cognition when they studied blind children describing familiar objects. These researchers reported that that the blind children used descriptions that "evoked the tactile and auditory characteristics of objects significantly more often than the sighted children" (Vinter, Fernandes, Orlandi, & Morgan, 2013, p. 861).

Sensory Integration

The term **sensory processing** refers to a complex set of neurobiologic functions that enable the brain to understand what is going on both inside the body and in all of the environmental contexts in which individuals engage. This neurobiologic function has been the focus of interest and research in both occupational and physical therapy. **Ayres Sensory Integration** is a theory and treatment approach developed on an understanding of this process, and is used to guide clinical reasoning and intervention decisions. A. Jean Ayres introduced the theory as a frame of reference for therapy interventions in the late 1950s. Since then, many other researchers have contributed to development of this theory (Lane & Bundy, 2012), which describes the senses (auditory, vestibular, proprioceptive, tactile, and visual) as contributing to learning and to the development of important functional skills discussed in this chapter, including regulation of activity level and attention span, eye-hand coordination, visual perception, and many metacognitive functions.

Ayres Sensory Integration theory is a theory of brain-behavior relationships that allow us to interact and respond in purposeful ways dependent upon adequate organization of sensory information. Stimuli must be integrated and matched with past experience for accurate information to register, and for the generation of a meaningful response.

This is a powerful information-processing network that allows for input from one sensory system to facilitate or inhibit the entire system. This sensory integration process is innate, and it provides an innate drive to seek out new sensory experiences. The innate motivation to move and play that pervades early childhood is believed to be a normal, healthy outcome of sensory integration, which enhances the quality of all developmental processes (Lane & Bundy, 2012).

Children with significant difficulties processing specific sensory modalities may be described as having *sensory processing disorders*. These children often have difficulty acquiring the skills needed to perform well in both school and social environments. Sensory processing disorders typically occur as a result of innate developmental differences, but they also may occur when young children have had an extremely restricted early childhood experience. For example, young children who are immunosuppressed will need to be restricted in their play activities and their social contacts (Allen, Vessey, and Shapiro, 2009). This restriction will keep them from having typical sensorimotor experiences and may result in poor sensory processing.

Visual Skills

From infancy, vision is the sensory system that most motivates children to explore the world. Children can see and want to explore things well before they are independently mobile. This is one of the reasons for the popularity of infant walkers. The demanding pre-walker now has the ability to move in space and follow up on those enticing visual cues. With the increased understanding of embedded cognition and the links between active movement and learning, the importance of self-directed movement even in young children cannot be overestimated (Smith, 2006). Trevor's learning and understanding of both spatial and temporal aspects within the environment may be compromised if he does not develop a capacity for independent mobility. The use of a walker, as introduced by his physical therapist, can greatly enhance his overall functions, not simply his mobility.

Vision provides typical preschoolers with as much as 80 percent of all their learning (Braddick & Atkinson, 2013). Through vision, toddlers learn to imitate and experiment. Vision is also instrumental to the development of hand skills discussed later in this chapter. For the purpose of this discussion, the term *visual skills* will be used to describe the ability of individuals to use extraocular muscles to direct the eye. The primary eye movements used in vision are visual pursuits (also called *tracking*) and visual scanning (also called *saccadic eye movements*). Visual pursuits are slow, smooth movements, typically used as the gaze follows a moving object. **Visual scanning** involves short, rapid changes of fixation from one point in the visual field to another. Visual scanning is used when searching for something and in reading.

The eye is still immature at birth, and visual skills gradually develop throughout the first 5 years of life (Payne &

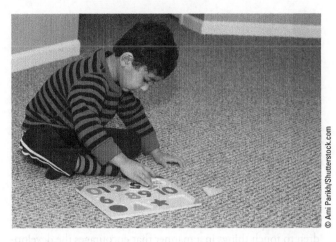

Figure 12-2   Completing puzzles requires both static visual acuity and eye-hand coordination.

Isaacs, 2012). Infants have efficient **static visual acuity**; this refers to the ability to discern details when both the person and the target are static. Static visual acuity is useful for reaching and grasping objects, the basic hand skills required in infancy and early in the preschool years. This skill is much used in preschool play activities, as illustrated in **Figure 12-2**. Static visual acuity is the ability tested in standard eye exams. It is important that visual problems are identified early, because failure to correct this type of problem can hinder the development of eye-hand coordination. As eye-hand coordination emerges, children experiment with hand movements and begin to develop fine hand and eye control.

Visual perception is a "mental function involved in discriminating shape, size, colour, and other ocular stimuli" (World Health Organization, 2001). Children first learn to recognize objects based on their general appearance. In early childhood, vision and touch experiences are usually paired, and through this pairing and the use-dependent nature of brain organization, the brain dynamically binds together visual and touch information (Henderson & Pehoski, 2006). Through this pairing, when you see something familiar you already know how it will feel. Similarly, when you feel something familiar, you already know how it will look.

This early ability is **visual discrimination**, and it includes the ability to distinguish specific features of an object like shape, size, and color. The visual discrimination of forms precedes children's ability to copy those forms in drawing tasks. As preschool children begin to experiment with crayons, they first make random marks, then can trace and imitate lines they see someone draw for them. After this, the children can copy simple lines and pictures, and finally they can draw the lines and shapes from memory.

By the age of 4, most children can follow simple instructions and copy patterns for art projects and early writing. This fact illustrates how closely visual and hand skill development are linked. Visually impaired children will be much slower to develop these hand skills, as their perceptions must be based on other discriminative cues, like touch perception.

Touch Skills

The sense of touch has many different functions in development. The type of touch that warns us of pain or danger is a very diffuse network that causes a protective alerting response. This type of touch is what causes one to startle when tickled from behind with a piece of grass. Light, moving touch is a trigger for this type of protective withdrawal response. Firm touch, as infants enjoy in swaddling, is a quieting or calming touch. Both of these early touch responses persist throughout life. As infants gain touch experience, they can begin to identify things as distinct from the more general protective and calming types of touch. This is accomplished by a neurologically newer (more complex) ability to discriminate types of touch. For children to touch things in a manner that encourages the development of perception and memory, their early protective reaction needs to be overridden by discriminative touch perceptions. **Discriminative touch** functions are those aspects of touch that we think about consciously, like how hard, smooth, or curved an object is. Discriminative touch is the type of touch that allows preschool children to learn to use their hands with increased dexterity and acquire tool-use skills. From a neurologic point of view, discriminative touch includes the perception of touch, pressure, and vibration. **Haptic perception** is discriminative touch combined with the active memory of touch, texture, shape, temperature, volume/size, hardness, and weight that allows children to tell you that they have a penny in their hand even when they cannot see the penny. Haptic exploration begins as early as 2 months when a baby brings her hand to her mouth. The pairing of vision and touch sensations in the brain lays the foundations for the development of haptic perception. The emergence of haptic perception parallels the emergence of hand skills. Payne and Isaacs (2012) describe six hand movement patterns needed for haptic perception: (1) static contact, the ability to place an open hand on the object; (2) lateral motion, the ability to move extended fingers across the surface of the object; (3) unsupported holding, the ability to hold an object securely in the hand, without assistance; (4) enclosure, the ability to close the hand around the object, while the object is situated in the palm of the hand; (5) pressure, the bimanual task of holding an object with one hand while using a finger to exert downward pressure on the object; and (6) contour following, another bimanual task of holding an object with one hand while running fingers along the contours of the object.

When children have difficulty or inefficiency integrating touch information, they often have secondary difficulties in developing fine motor control and self-care skills. A common type of sensory processing disorder, *tactile defensiveness,* occurs when children react with protective or avoidance responses to what should be nonthreatening touch information. Children with tactile defensiveness may be very selective about the type of clothing they will wear and the type of foods they will eat, and may become very distressed in social situations around other children. Because it leads children to avoid touch and tactile exploration, tactile defensiveness can limit hand skill, self-care, and social skill development.

DEVELOPMENT OF POSTURAL CONTROL

Postural control is the ability to control the body's position in space and to remain erect in spite of changes in the surface being walked on (Payne & Isaacs, 2012). Postural reflexes and reactions developed in infancy support the development of postural control. The ability to walk upright indicates a mastery of the body's muscle system to overcome the influence of gravity. **Postural stability** is the ability to keep the body balanced and aligned. **Static postural stability** is the ability to maintain the preferred posture when the body is still. This is also called quiet stance postural control. This would include the ability to remain upright while sitting in a chair or to stand quietly when waiting in line without leaning against a support. In toddlers, static postural stability is brief, but dramatic improvements occur as children gain muscle bulk and behavioral control. By the age of 5, most children can stand quietly in line for 2 to 3 minutes and can sit quietly for 5 to 10 minutes.

In studies of postural stability, *stability* is defined as that point when the center of the body's mass is aligned over its base of support. **Stability limits** are the farthest that individuals can shift their mass off center without altering their base of support. Children with weak or immature nervous systems may be slow to develop static postural stability and have narrow stability limits. Children with Down syndrome provide an example of this, as they often are slow to sit independently, and when they do sit, they topple to the side easily if they attempt to reach for a toy. The difference in the resting tension in their muscles makes it harder for them to acquire motor skills, and an enriched play environment or preschool program like the one shown in **Figure 12-3** is recommended.

Although the balance and postural patterns of preschool children remain immature, children can engage in a wide variety of challenging motor tasks like ballet, swimming, and gymnastics. Throughout the preschool years, postural control becomes more adaptive as children develop the ability to integrate multiple perceptions and gain motor strength and flow.

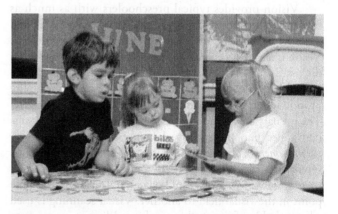

Figure 12-3   Early childhood education classrooms such as the one pictured can offer needed social and educational supports for children with Down syndrome to learn needed motor and social skills.

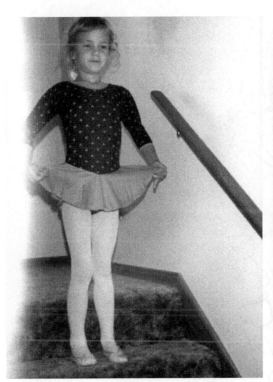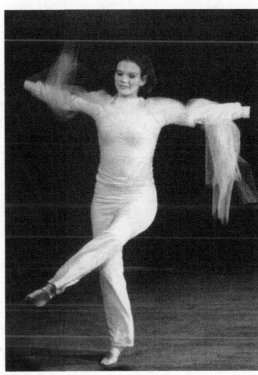

Figure 12-4   Movement flow improves in this dancer between the ages of 5 and 16.

Flow is the term used to describe smooth, fluid movements. Although toddlers may have static postural control in many positions, they are likely to also have limited ability to combine mobility and stability patterns functionally for a more active, dynamic form of postural stability. For example, when asked to kick a ball, a toddler will run up to the ball and stop. After stopping and establishing her balance, the toddler can then shift her weight to kick. Flow is likely to be the most noticeable difference between a preschool dancer and a dancer in adolescence. **Figure 12-4** shows a 5-year-old dancer next to a picture of the same dancer at age 16. The difference in quality of movement, even in these still photos, is evident.

By about age 5, many children can run fluidly and kick a ball without stopping or compromising their balance. This type of active, adaptive control is **dynamic postural stability**, and it is associated with the development of flow. **Dynamic Postural Stability** is the ability to maintain a stable base of support while performing an active, functional task that involves movement and postural shift. Dynamic postural control is a complex interaction of muscle strength, perception, and learning through practice. Children gain this skill earlier if it is practiced, as you see in the preschool hockey player or gymnast. **Figure 12-5** illustrates some of the improvements in running seen during the preschool years. The initial pattern shown is that of a new walker. The elementary stage shows an older preschooler, in whom flow is emerging and there is more economy of motor effort. Skills in the mature stage, characterized by flow and economy of movement, require practice and are refined into middle childhood.

Equilibrium reactions are complex patterns involving rotational movements along the body axis to maintain balance (Shumway-Cook & Woollacott, 2012). These reactions are considered neurologically mature because their presence indicates the integration of earlier primitive and transitional motor patterns. Equilibrium reactions in standing typically emerge between 12 and 21 months of age and are fully mature by age 4. The changes in equilibrium are reflected in the developmental progression of jumping skills. Early jumping mostly involves the legs, and no trunk rotation is observed. As **Figure 12-6** shows, in the elementary stage of development common to preschoolers, the upper body has become more active, and trunk rotation is emerging.

Rotational movement around the body axis characterizes equilibrium reactions. Such rotation requires active movement of multiple muscle groups acting together in a smooth, regulated fashion. This smooth rotation movement can occur only when the postural reflexes of infancy have been integrated and a more flexible means of control allows for simultaneous contraction of opposing muscle groups beyond preprogrammed reflex patterns.

Some children are slow to develop this smooth, coordinated control. Children with impairments in motor function, such as cerebral palsy or Down syndrome, will have difficulty developing these higher-level skills. Children without obvious motor impairments may still be "clumsy" and slow to refine their equilibrium reactions. In these cases, the limitation is not in developmental milestones but in flow and calibration of movement. **Calibration** of movement

Initial

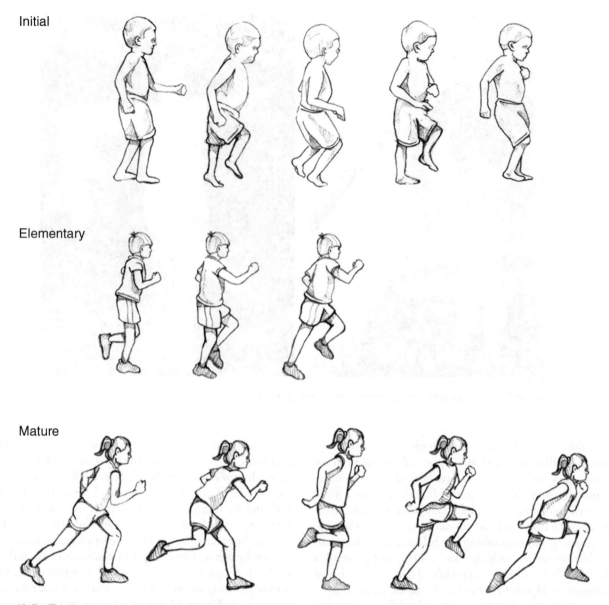

Elementary

Mature

Figure 12-5   This illustrates the developmental progression of running.

is the use of movements of appropriate force, speed, and directional control needed when attempting a task (American Occupational Therapy Association, 2014). Typically, at age 2 children have poor calibration and tend to use too much force with all tasks. By age 5 children have learned to adjust the force that they use in familiar tasks, although they still may use too much force in new and unfamiliar tasks.

Difficulties with calibration are evidenced by either too much or too little force being exerted or when the action is performed too quickly. Difficulties with calibration are common when *resting muscular tension* (muscle tone) is outside a typical range. When preschool children try to cuddle with pets, they often hold them either too lightly or too tightly, common errors in calibration (see **Figure 12-7**). Difficulties with calibration are easy to see in broken crayons, spraying juice boxes, and frequent tripping. Calibration

errors may also result in unintentionally hurting other children in play.

FINE MOTOR DEVELOPMENT

As mentioned in the discussion of infancy, fine motor development generally refers to those movements produced by the smaller muscles or muscle groups in the body. **Fine motor control**, in this text, includes the coordinated use of the eyes, hands, and muscles of the mouth. Although postural control is often nonvolitional, fine motor control is largely volitional (Bekkering & Pratt, 2004). Individuals must be conscious and self-directed to develop coordination and skill in the small muscle groups. Children with impairments in mental functions often have delayed fine motor skill development, even in the presence of an intact

Initial

Elementary

Mature

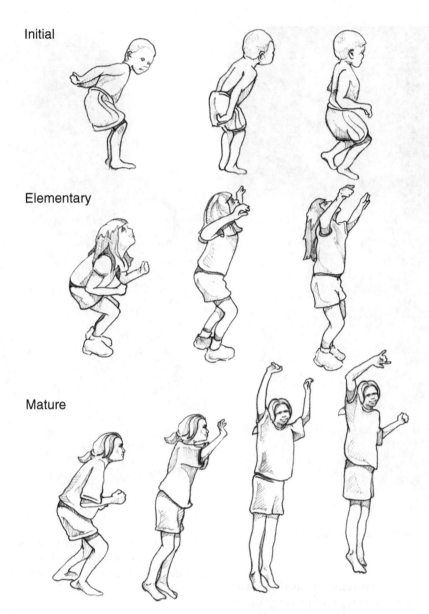

Figure 12-6   The developmental progression of jumping provides an example of the development of dynamic balance.

motor system (Dellatolas et al., 2003). It is not uncommon to see a child with profound cognitive impairments who does not develop the ability to hold a spoon or use a pencil even though there is no actual motor impairment limiting him. Additionally, children with vision impairments have difficulty developing refined hand skills due to the important role of vision in hand skill development (Brambring, 2007). These difficulties are greatest in the areas of tool use, which Brambring (2007) noted were acquired about 2.67 times later in blind children than in sighted children.

In Chapter 10, infant development of grasp and release was introduced. As infants move into the second year of development, they develop increasing proficiency in both grasp and release. Improving postural control allows the child to develop improved arm and hand control. With increasing control of finger extension, children begin to

demonstrate calibration in grading the degree of hand opening while releasing. This calibration allows for a more efficient object-release pattern. Henderson and Pehoski note that "efficient object release requires both the regulation of grip force with the timing of the placement of the object so the object is not 'dropped' but precisely placed" (2006, p. 152). The little girl in **Figure 12-8** is trying to add a block to a tower her older sister started. She does not yet have the graded calibration of force and timing for this task.

From the time that purposeful release is well established, children refine and specialize their grasp patterns based on the characteristics of the object they are grasping. As with other types of motor learning, it is normal to have a lot of variety and experimentation in emerging grasp patterns. There are two major types of grasp that are differentiated according to the position and mobility of the thumb joints (Henderson

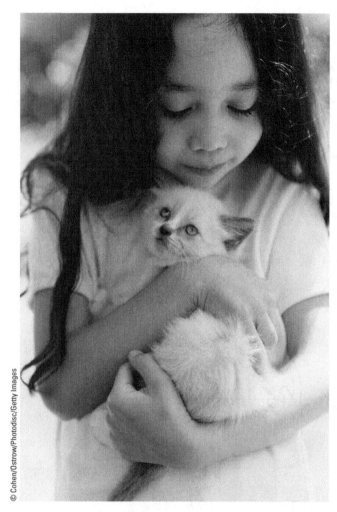

Figure 12-7   Calibration includes the ability to hold firmly without squeezing your pet.

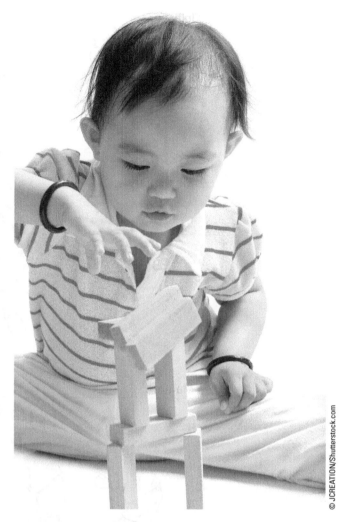

Figure 12-8   This baby is developing control over object release, but does not yet have adequate control to avoid "dropping" the block at this time. By the end of the preschool period, these skills will be mastered.

& Pehoski, 2006). **Power grasp** patterns are used for managing large or heavy objects. Some types of power grasp are *cylindrical grips, spherical grip, hook grip,* and *plate,* or *lateral, prehension* (see **Figure 12-9**). In the power grasp patterns, the full strength of the hand is used. These are the patterns used for holding and carrying, and in early toy play. Object size and shape play a major role in the selection of grip patterns.

Precision grasp patterns emerge only slightly later but continue to be refined through adolescence. In spite of their long period of refinement, most forms of precision grasp emerge in the preschool years. Distinctive features of the precision grasp patterns are the unsupported hand and active wrist extension (Shumway-Cook & Woollacott, 2012). Some examples of precision grasp are "chuck," or *tripod grips, pincer grasp* (the fingertips press against each other), and *lateral prehension* (pad-to-side; key grip) (see **Figure 12-10**). These forms of grasp are refined in the preschool years.

Together with the increase in hand activity and the expansion in types of play children engage in, there is a change in the physical structure of the hand from the soft, featureless infant hand to a hand with clearly defined arches and muscular areas. The development of this hand structure accommodates the development of precision grasp and manipulation. Three arches balance stability and mobility in the hand (see **Figure 12-11**). The proximal transverse palmar arch is rigid, but the other two arches, the distal transverse palmar arch and the longitudinal palmar arch, are flexible, and are maintained by activity in the hand's intrinsic muscles.

The muscles that make up the flexible arches shape the hand to grasp differently-shaped objects, direct the skilled movements of the fingers, and grade the power of grasps. All skilled movements begin with the shaping of the hand to accommodate the demands of the task. Concurrent with the development of palmar arches is the refinement of a calibrated release pattern and the development of voluntary isolated finger movements. The ability to move the fingers individually becomes important later in the preschool years as a support for the development of complex pre-academic fine motor tasks. Henderson and Pehoski (2006) report that finger isolation abilities are present in only 50 percent of children between the ages of 42 and 47 months of age, and continue to refine through 6 years of age.

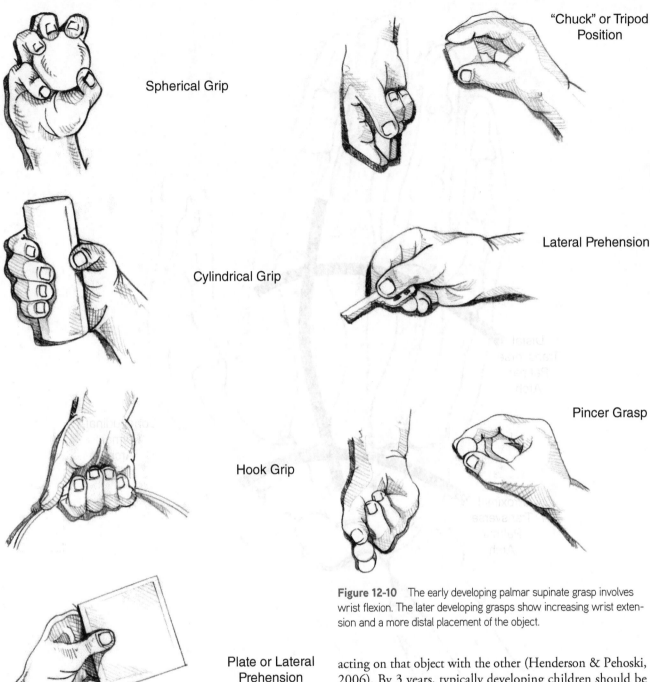

Spherical Grip

Cylindrical Grip

Hook Grip

Plate or Lateral Prehension

"Chuck" or Tripod Position

Lateral Prehension

Pincer Grasp

Figure 12-10   The early developing palmar supinate grasp involves wrist flexion. The later developing grasps show increasing wrist extension and a more distal placement of the object.

Figure 12-9   Various Types of Power Grasps

Complementary Two-Hand Use

At the same time that release-and-grasp patterns refine, children begin to use their hands in a complementary manner. By 1 year, infants can hold an object in each hand at the same time, and can move both hands in a "mirror" fashion. From 1 to 2 years, infants learn to hold an object in one hand while

acting on that object with the other (Henderson & Pehoski, 2006). By 3 years, typically developing children should be able to have both hands active at the same time, working in a complementary fashion. The process of using one hand as a lead hand and the other as an assist hand simultaneously to manipulate objects is called **bimanual coordination**.

This involves both the ability to motor plan a holding function with one hand and a doing function, and the ability to monitor the movements of both hands at the same time. This two-hand use pattern will open the door for the acquisition of many self-care skills including dressing, hair care, and self-feeding. Early in development, children frequently switch hands, with either hand taking the lead role in activity. Over the preschool years, most children come to consistently prefer one hand as the skilled hand. **Hand preference** is the consistent choice of the same hand for complex skilled tasks

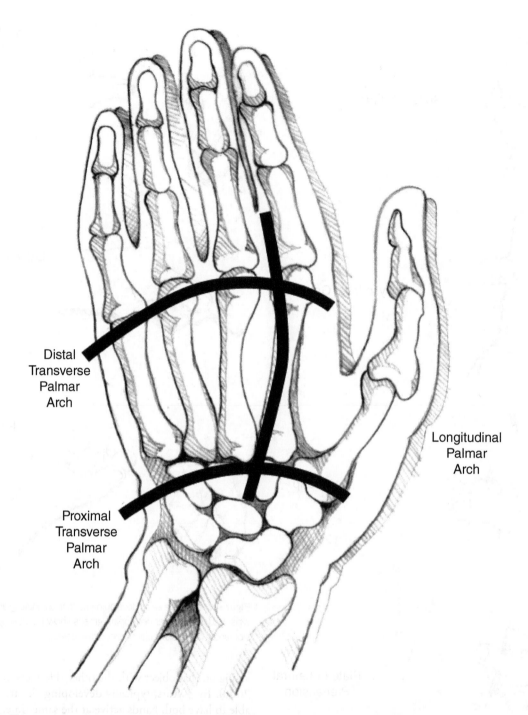

Figure 12-11   There are two transverse palmar arches, proximal and distal, and one longitudinal palmar arch.

and is believed to emerge as the cerebral hemispheres begin the process of lateralization. Hand preference is established in most children by the age of 4 (Henderson & Pehoski, 2006). True hand dominance (the exclusive use of one hand for a skilled task such as handwriting), however, may not develop until age 7. Failure to develop hand preference can also lead to delayed development of the skilled hand and specific tool grasps associated with writing and drawing.

Fine motor skill development has been studied by offering different blocks and other standard objects to children within specific age groups. Some researchers have argued against this approach to measurement of hand skills because of the relative proportions of the objects to the size of the child's hand. Hand skill development is complex and multifactorial, but the literature may have been underestimating the skills of the young children. They found that when the objects used in measuring hand function were scaled to the size of the subject's hand, there were very few differences in performance between child and adult subjects (Payne & Isaacs, 2012).

Failure to play with objects and engage in haptic exploration, whether due to a cognitive impairment or to environmental deprivation, can lead to inadequate development of the hand muscles and poorly defined palmar arches (Henderson & Pehoski, 2006). Children with limited variety of play are more likely to have difficulty adapting to the tool-use demands of school and to self-care. When there are no cognitive impairments, most preschool children catch up quickly when new tools are introduced. When fine motor hand tasks are presented in a developmentally appropriate, systematic format, preschool children can develop very fine hand control. An example of this would be the very young children who learn to play the violin using the Suzuki method.

DEVELOPMENT OF SELF-CARE SKILLS

Even in infancy, children are motivated to be active in their care. By 18 months, most children feed themselves part of each meal and will wash and dry their own hands, though they are not careful and do not check to see if dirt remains on the hands. Between 2 and 4 years of age, children develop many activities of daily living (ADLs). The main areas of self-care for a preschooler are sleeping, eating/drinking, toothbrushing, hand washing, nose-blowing, dressing, and bathing. This can be a frustrating time for parents, because the children want to do it themselves but are very inefficient and make many errors. Children need to have the quality of their performance in self-care checked throughout the preschool years. Activities of daily living are a focus of teaching and learning in the preschool years, but these activities often are also playful activities and serve as a rich source for sensory learning and exploration. **Figure 12-12** shows two young children engaging in bath time, while also interacting playfully and socially during the task.

The order in which children develop self-care skills varies with their culture and experience. Dressing skill often emerges early because it has meaning for the children and is part of the daily routine. Typically in complex skills like dressing, children learn part of a task before attempting the entire skill. **Table 12-3** presents a typical sequence of the acquisition of

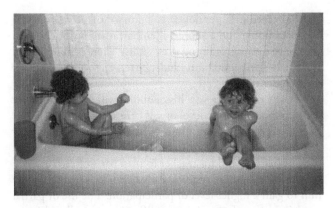

Figure 12-12 Self-care and sensory play skills often occur simultaneously in the preschool years.

dressing skills for children growing up in North America.

Children first learn skills that their parents highly value. For children in North America, the earliest self-care skills to develop in preschool years are oral hygiene, eating, dressing, and toilet hygiene. In addition to learning to take care of themselves, preschool children imitate and participate in instrumental activities of daily living (IADLs). Examples of emerging IADLs in the preschool years are setting the table, picking up toys, washing vegetables, and folding washcloths. In all these tasks, children can actively imitate and participate but will continue to need adult supervision. Preschool children often "practice" IADLs in their play activities, such as by playing house or pushing a toy lawn mower.

Although the sequence of skill acquisition may vary, by the end of the preschool years, children are independent in basic personal care, including toileting, and will be able to function with minimal supervision in the school setting. Some skills may be later to develop because of unusual demands. For example, children with very long or very curly hair may need assistance for several more years to wash, comb, and style their hair. A child's clothing in a cold northern climate may have more layers and more complex fasteners than the clothing typical of warmer climates. Chopsticks are also more complex to manage than Western utensils, and finger-feeding in this case may persist later into the preschool years.

Age	Typical Self-Dressing Sequence
TABLE 12-3	Typical Sequence of Acquisition of Dressing Skills for Children in North America

Age	Typical Self-Dressing Sequence
1 year	Holds out arms and legs, pulls off shoes and socks, and pushes arms through sleeves and legs through pants.
2 years	Removes unfastened coat, pulls down pants, finds armholes in T-shirt, and puts on front-buttoning coat/shirt.
3 years	Puts on T-shirt and shoes (may be on wrong foot), puts on socks, manages basic fasteners (zips and unzips, manages large buttons, snaps, buckles), unties and removes shoes, and removes pull-down garment.
4 years	Manages separating zipper, puts on shoes and socks correctly, dresses completely with few errors, and consistently finds front and back of garments.

Self-care independence is a source of pride for preschool children and a source of embarrassment for children who have delays in gaining these skills. There is much social pressure in preschool and kindergarten environments to be independent in self-care.

In the case of Trevor, his disability will make it difficult for him to achieve the level of self-care skills expected of his peer group. Rather than omitting these skills from his daily routine, the physical and occupational therapists can work with his parents and his teacher to plan parts of each activity that he can do, and to systematically build skills that will allow him to gain a higher level of participation. The use of partial participation and of activity modifications can allow him to be active and share in these developmentally valued tasks.

SCHOOL-READINESS SKILLS

One important outcome of successful preschool development is the acquisition of the specific skills needed to be successful in a school environment. Mastery of these skills is called **school readiness** (Daily, Burkhauser, & Halle, 2011). Children's academic and social competencies at age 5 have been recognized as important predictors of success within the educational system (Jeon et al., 2011).

There are no agreed-upon criteria for school readiness, but in general children must be healthy, both physically and

emotionally. Ideally, children should use language effectively, be largely independent in ADLs, and should be able to follow directions. Some skills that help children transition to the school setting are the ability to listen to stories without interrupting, to show understanding of general times of day, to recognize authority and to manage bathroom needs. A child's experiences during the preschool years can serve as a risk factor or a protective factor for school readiness. If a child has a significant disability, such as the one presented in the case of Trevor, the child may not be able to achieve the "ideal" of school readiness. The preschool focus on expressive communication, mobility, and self-care will help Trevor gain important skills and provide tools that educators can use when he is ready to begin traditional academic learning.

There has been a major focus in the United States on reducing risk through early childhood care programs and through therapies like occupational therapy, speech therapy, and physical therapy to help improve such children's potential for academic success. The skills that children must learn (such as matching shapes or colors, one-to-one correspondence, and other concepts) before learning more complex academic skills (such as reading, math, and spelling) are called **pre-academic skills**. Pre-academic skills are learned skills that help the child transition to the academic learning. Some pre-academic skills emerge as a part of typical early childhood development, others must be specifically taught. **Table 12-4** offers examples of the

TABLE 12-4	Pre-Academic Skill Development		
Age	**Visual Perception**	**Visual Motor**	**Cognitive**
2 to 2½ Years	Visual discrimination Sort by size or color Able to locate details and images in picture books Able to match circle, triangles, and squares	Use a paintbrush Imitate drawing a horizontal line Able to paste pieces of paper Able to fold a piece of paper with instruction	Able to attend to more than one thing at a time Memorize many favorite rhymes, songs, and stories Very interested in how things work Begins to incorporate others into his pretend play
2½ to 3 Years	Matches primary colors, such as blue, red, and yellow Can complete simple three-piece interlocking puzzles of familiar objects Able to point to at least six body parts in a picture Able to indicate pictures based on the descriptions "larger" or "smaller"	Begins snipping with scissors and progresses to making continuous snips Able to copy vertical and horizontal lines and circles with crayon or marker Able to pour from one container to another with little spilling Able to stack up to eight to nine small blocks	Can remember events that occurred up to 18 months earlier Knows where you are going in the car based on landmarks Begins to understand directional words, such as in, on, and under Uses self-talk to work through tasks and problems

Continues

TABLE 12-4 Pre-Academic Skill Development *(continued)*			
Age	**Visual Perception**	**Visual Motor**	**Cognitive**
3 to 3½ Years	Able to create a simple pattern when stringing beads Correctly names some colors Understands the concept of same/different Can match simple patterns	Can trace along a thick line Able to build a tower of more than nine blocks When writing is able to combine strokes to create a$^+$ Can use simple stencils and tracing tools given instruction	Able to learn to play games with simple rules Able to identify what items do not belong with the others Understands most of what is said, and 75 percent of speech is understandable Follows three-part commands
3½ to 4 Years	Matches 3-D objects to their outlines Correctly names five or more colors Able to complete a 10-piece form board puzzle Guesses a full picture by looking at half of it	Cuts a piece of paper in half Copies a few letters with horizontal and vertical lines Able to draw a person with three recognizable body parts Is able to color (mostly) within the lines	Can play simple card games with assistance Able to recall one to two aspects of a simple story Is able to categorize objects by size, color, shape, and type Understands "if, then" relationship
4 to 4½ Years	Able to match identical pictures Selects big, bigger, biggest; small, smaller, smallest Able to copy complex patterns with blocks Sorts objects by color, size, shape	Consistently able to follow moving objects with eyes Able to copy a square Able to place key in lock and open it Able to imitate finger-plays during songs, like the "Itsy Bitsy Spider"	Able to attend to more than one aspect of an object or picture at one time, such as shape and color Can recall three to four aspects of a story just heard Able to sing songs with 30 or more words Able to describe details of past events
4½ to 5 Years	Can arrange up to three pictures in sequential order Recognizes own name when written in uppercase letters Can find a hidden shape within a picture Can identify what is missing when something is removed from a four- to five-object array	Can cut out circles and squares Able to draw a face with eyes, nose, and mouth in correct place Draws simple objects that are recognizable Can draw between the lines in larger horizontal and vertical paths	Can attend for long period of time to difficult tasks Understands the basic concepts of time Can attend to the orientation and direction of objects, pictures, and letters Knows his or her address and phone number

sequence of sensorimotor-based pre-academic skill development through age 5. Pre-academic skills are taught as a of the early childhood school curriculum. Children who have not developed these skills should still enter school at the age of five, and should get the support there to reach their full potential.

Pre-academic skills include sensory, motor, cognitive, and language aspects. Note that in **Table 12-4**, knowing the name for colors may be listed as a visual perceptual skill, although this task requires both memory and language.

USING MATERIALS

Using materials requires the ability to use external things to complete a task. For the preschool child this can include using eating utensils, constructive toys, and personal hygiene tools like a toothbrush or hair comb. This also includes using writing utensils, an emerging skill for the preschooler. Typically developing children have the necessary mobility skills to move their bodies through space without difficulty. They walk, bend, and reach for objects; however, they may still need to stop other activities to perform the walking, bending, or reaching task well. By 5 years, the children's bilateral coordination skills are still maturing, and switching hands during a task or failing to use one hand as an assist to stabilize a task are common (Payne & Isaacs, 2012). In addition, by age 5, children typically know the use of everyday objects including household and self-care tools and are able to begin using these objects.

Some examples of materials used in elementary school are crayons, pencils, eating utensils, scissors, glue sticks, buttons, blocks, and coins. As noted earlier, children between the ages of 2 and 5 develop a hand preference and the ability to manipulate objects in one hand (the lead hand) while the other hand assists. Tool-use skills require this bimanual lead-assist pattern and are built on visual perception, somatosensory perception, and cognition. The play of typically developing preschool children includes many types of sensory experiences. These may be outdoor play activities like running and climbing or structured classroom activities. Because of the importance of vision during this stage in development, eye examinations and the use of prescription lenses to accommodate vision impairment is especially important.

Children must have developed complementary two-hand use, precision grasps, and the ability to shape the hand to the needs of the task to be effective with tool use. Associated with the development of tool use, in the development of in-hand manipulation. In-hand manipulation is "the process of using one hand to adjust an object for more effective object placement, or release; the object remains in that hand and usually does not come in contact with a surface during in-hand manipulation" (Exner, 1992, p. 35). It is this skill that allows you to dynamically adjust your grasp while using tools or performing a skilled task. Most children develop in-hand manipulation skills between the ages of 3 and 6 years, concurrently with the development of skill in force calibration and finger isolation.

There are three basic types of in-hand manipulation. The first of these, *translation,* "is a linear movement of the object in the hand from the finger surface to the palm or the palm to the fingers" (Exner, 1992, p. 39). *Shift movements* are the next type of in-hand manipulation. "Shift movements occur at the finger and thumb pads with the alternation of the thumb and finger movement" (Exner, 1992, p. 39–40). *Rotation* is the final type of in-hand manipulation. Rotation involves movements at or near the pads of the fingers that move an object around one or more of its axes. Children who have difficulty with hand shaping, isolating finger movements or difficulty with grip calibration are likely to have difficulty with tasks requiring in-hand manipulation. During the period where these skills are developing, variability in the methods or grasps used is common as children explore new motor control patterns (Henderson & Pehoski, 2006). With practice and experience, most children will settle on one preferred way of accomplishing a task. Children who lack variability in the learning stages may need careful assessment, because a lack of variation may reflect a muscle or motor control problem.

GRAPHOMOTOR SKILLS

Graphomotor skills are the collections of conceptual and perceptual motor skills involved in drawing and writing. Drawing, the art of producing a picture or plan with some implement (pen or pencil, for example), begins to develop first. Writing, the process of forming letters, numbers, and other significant figures, which incorporates language learning as well as sensory and motor skills, develops next. Early in the process of learning to write, children copy the letterforms as they would copy shapes. Prior to understanding the alphabet and its role in written language, this letter copying is more accurately described as drawing. When children with impairments in mental functions learn to write words by memorizing the shape of the word, the children are compensating for difficulty in processing written language by drawing on their graphic skills.

The prehension patterns required for graphomotor tasks are modifications of the tripod grasp, also called the three-jaw chuck, presented earlier in **Figure 12-10**. These *tripod grasps,* illustrated in **Figure 12-13**, emerge during the preschool years. Unlike the static grasp patterns described earlier, they become dynamic, utilizing in-hand manipulation skills to adjust the tool to meet the demands of the task. This skill will continue to be refined through middle childhood.

The sequence by which children learn graphomotor tasks usually begins with tracing (eyes direct hands to follow visual representation), then imitating (eyes watch and remember another's actions to repeat the action), followed by copying (eyes alternate glances between visual representation and own production) (Henderson & Pehoski, 2006). Although many technological tools allow children to compensate for poor graphomotor skill, the combination of visual and haptic perception, kinesthetic awareness, motor control, and memory needed for graphomotor tasks will be needed as well in many other realms of function, including the use of a computer keyboard or texting on a smartphone.

ATTENTION AND MEMORY

Many cognitive, reasoning, and memory skills develop in typically developing children by the age of 5. Competent global and specific mental functions are needed for children to perform well in a classroom setting. Devices and tools can help compensate for many motor and sensory deficits, but deficits in mental functioning are the most limiting in the home and school setting. In particular, selective attention is fundamental to all of the pre-academic skills listed in **Table 12-4**. Deficits in attention processes can lead to a negative trajectory in both academic and social skill learning (Hanania & Smith, 2010).

Attention functions develop throughout the preschool years, and involve increasingly finely tuned discriminations. For preschool children, attention is the foundation for all of the specific mental functions described in the ICF. In fact, some researchers argue that because the ICF

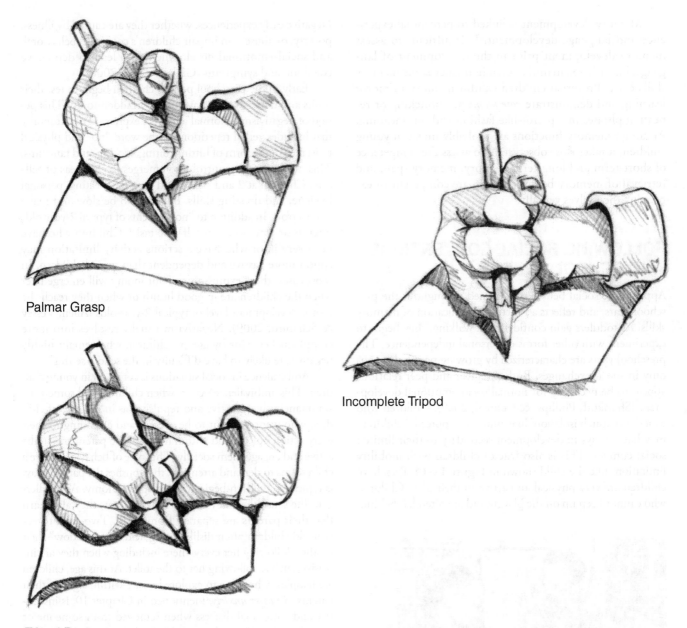

Palmar Grasp

Incomplete Tripod

Tripod Posture

Figure 12-13 The immature palmar grasp is widely seen in preschool. With practice in pencil use, children can develop the grasp that involves more pronation and wrist extension.

distinction between attention and executive functions is drawn from adult neuropsychological models, it is not useful in the consideration of cognition in young children (Visu-petra, Benga, & Miclea, 2007). In preschool children, positive cognitive functioning is based on the development of *executive attention* and *self-regulation*.

Executive attention refers to children's ability to regulate their responses, particularly in conflict situations where several responses are possible. Executive attention continues to develop through early adulthood, but undergoes a sensitive period of rapid development between 2 and 7 years of age (Holmboe & Johnson, 2005). Research in the area of executive attention in preschoolers looks at the pairing

of time between activation of attention and inhibition accuracy, and at the strategies children use to correct and self-regulate behaviors. Preschool children develop skills for self-regulation of attention and error detection. The control strategies that children use on tasks requiring touch responses were usually physical, like sitting on their hands or putting their hands in their pockets. Verbal self-regulation strategies do not seem to emerge until sometime after the fourth year of life (Backen Jones, Rothbart & Posner, 2003; Holmboe & Johnson, 2005). Attention, error detection, and self-regulation are necessary for learning, especially for academic learning. Failure to develop adequately in this area may lead to delays in other areas of independent function.

Memory development is linked to perceptual experience and language development. It is difficult to assess memory development prior to the development of language, but it is apparent that even in infancy some memory skills exist. Preverbal children exhibit memory in motor learning and demonstrate *rote memory,* mimicking or repeating phrases in a parrot-like fashion without meaning. Although memory functions are probably intact in young children, it takes close observation to assess the competence of short-term and long-term memory, memory span, and retrieval of memory before children are competent in expressing themselves verbally.

FOLLOWING SOCIAL CONVENTIONS AND SCHOOL RULES

Appropriate social behavior is learned throughout the preschool years, and reflects a functional application of memory skills. As toddlers gain confidence in walking, they begin to experiment with other forms of personal independence. The preschool years are characterized by growing personal autonomy in social exchanges. Both caregiver and peer relations appear to be necessary for normal socio-emotional development (Shonkoff, Phillips, & Council, 2000). Children who experience much isolation, like immune-suppressed children, may have delays in development secondary to their limited social contact. This is also true of children with mobility limitation, like the child shown in **Figure 12-14**. Preschool children are very physical and active in their play. Children who cannot keep up on the playground are often left behind.

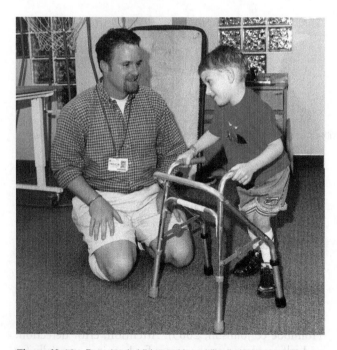

Figure 12-14 Preschool children with mobility limitations are likely to have proportionally more social interaction with adults and fewer with peers.

Negative early experiences, whether they are caused by illness, poverty, or abuse, can impair children's cognitive, behavioral, and social-emotional development and lead to depressive cognition and symptoms (Gibb & Abela, 2008).

Early in the preschool period, children begin to test their limits and do what they have been forbidden to do. This period of negativism is normal and is an expression of autonomy that includes verbal repetitions of the word "no" and physical resistance in the form of hitting, biting, kicking, and tantrums. This need to be in control also emerges in the areas of self-care. Children at 2 and 3 years old have basic eating, personal hygiene, and dressing skills, but tend to be slow and make many errors. In addition to "no," parents of typical 2-year-olds often hear "me do it" in self-care tasks. Children who have been very ill or who have a serious activity limitation may appear more passive and dependent than typical children. In most cases, these expressions of autonomy will emerge later when the children are in good health or when they reach the motor development level of typical 2-year-olds (Allen, Vessey & Schapiro, 2009). Negativism usually resolves into more compliant behavior by age 5. Children who remain highly negative are likely to have difficulty in the school setting.

Ambivalence in social situations is common in young children. This ambivalence occurs when children find something simultaneously attractive and repulsive, as in the case of children who want a parent to be present and attending to their every action but cry and withdraw when the parent tries to be active and engage them socially. This type of behavior, where a child seems to demand attention, then pushes the parent away, is typical as children begin to develop autonomy. As toddlers gain the sense that they can be independent, they also learn that their parents are separate from them. Two- and three-year-old children often dislike being held, but "shadow" their mother, following her everywhere including when they are intrusive, such as following her to the toilet. At this age, children are happiest when free to explore but are within sight of their parents. *Stranger anxiety,* mentioned in Chapter 10, is insecurity and emotional distress when removed from someone or something familiar and is an adaptive behavior in human infants who are dependent on others for all aspects of daily life. Related to this is separation anxiety. *Separation anxiety* refers to a young child's experience of anxiety due to separation from the primary care giver. For most children this anxious period resolves before the child turns 2. It is also normal for children who have conditions, such as blindness, whose early childhood period of dependency is extended and may manifest separation anxiety for a much more extended time than is typical sighted children. This type of separation anxiety is normative and not indicative of a persistent mental health problem. *Separation anxiety disorder* is a mental health condition in childhood that includes "a non-normative, pervasive anxiety state accentuated by separations from close attachment figures at developmental junctures where the need for proximity to attachment figures is no longer adaptive" (Milrod et al., 2014). This type of disorder has both genetic and social origins and is often a precursor to the manifestation of an anxiety disorder later in life.

PLAY

Play is intrinsically motivated, both culturally and personally meaningful, and bring and may manifest separation anxiety for a much more extended time than is typical sighted children. s pleasure. Play is a key support to learning and skill development in early childhood. The aspect of pleasure associated with play is important because pleasure is the basis of the innate drive to repeat the pleasurable activity. This inner drive toward mastery of skills through play is one of the basic premises of sensory integration theory, described earlier in this chapter (Lane & Bundy, 2012). Play evolves in tandem with the acquisition of developmental skills and becomes increasingly complex. Children learn through play and mastery of skills that they have some control over their world and can cause desired change. This belief in their personal power to change things is **self-efficacy**. Self-efficacy is an important school-readiness skill, as it enables children to be open to challenges and to believe that they can master new skills.

Play can be characterized in many ways, and different groups of scientists categorize play differently. This makes the scholarly literature on play a little challenging to navigate. First we will look at *forms of play*, specific types of activities that children engage in, and that become more complex as children develop. The National Institute for Play (2012) describes five forms of play that occur in the preschool years, and the Lego Foundation (2010) describes types of play. There is some overlap in their consideration so the two categorizations will be considered together here. The National Institute for Play categories are listed in parentheses where they overlap with the Lego Foundation categories. These are:

- **Attunement play** is a social exchange that establishes a connection, such as between newborn and mother. This is the one type of play that the Lego Foundation did not consider.
- **Physical (body) play** includes active rough-and-tumble activity and fine motor practice. Exercise activities related to children's developing whole-body and hand-eye-coordination also fall into this category.
- **Play with objects (object play)** includes those activities that incorporate objects. Object play occurs throughout the preschool period and can include tricycles, dress-up clothes, and building blocks. Play with objects begins when infants can grasp things and hold on to them intentionally. Early in the toddler years, children explore objects, and this object exploration gradually evolves to sorting and classifying objects, an essential pre-academic skill. Around the age of 4, children begin to recombine objects and develop an interest in building with objects. This interest in building has been described by some authors as *constructive play*, described later in this chapter, and is a specific form of play with objects. Play with objects is also particularly associated with "private speech," which reflects the integrated manner in which

cognitive, language, and play skills interrelate (The Lego Foundation, 2010). Play with objects or tools is called **constructive play** by some authors and includes any play activity that involves making or building things. Constructive play and imaginative play help develop imagination, problem-solving skills, fine motor skills, and self-efficacy, and prepare children with skills that they will need as they enter school.

- **Pretense/sociodramatic play (social play)** includes all forms of pretend play including dressing up and role-playing. Pretense play typically emerges during solitary play in the second year as children's language skills grow to support their imagination. Through the preschool years, children's pretense play expands and becomes more social, involving others into their pretend world.
- **Symbolic (imaginative) play** emerges late in the preschool period, as children gain language skills. Symbolic play is play with language. Symbolic play supports the development of children's abilities to express ideas, feelings, and experiences. This expression can be in any media including language, painting, drawing, music, and craft activities.
- **Games with rules**, the final form of play, emerge in a simple form in the preschool years and refine throughout life. Some of this type of play is in the form of play with electronic media devices aimed at young children. This form of play in the form of sports and organized group activity will be addressed in great detail in Chapter 13.

Each of the six types of play described supports the healthy development of young children. Although play has been neatly categorized, in reality, children's play nearly always includes more than one of these types of play at any given time. Play is also a central venue for the development of social competency and allows skill practice in social contexts. Within each form of play (except perhaps attunement play), children can choose to play alone, play with other children, or play with parents and other adults.

Mildred Parten (1932) developed a classification of children's participation in play based on the social features of the play activity. The earliest, least mature of Parten's classification of social play is **unoccupied play**. In this class of play, children are not actively playing; they may be observing, or even standing in one spot or performing random movements. Both attunement play and physical (body) play, described previously, could also be considered unoccupied play. **Solitary play** typically emerges around 2 years of age when children are focused on an activity that they enjoy without including others in the play activity. Solitary play can include any of the forms of play described earlier, except social play.

Onlooker play is the first truly social type of play in Parten's classification system. Onlooker play occurs when individuals engage in forms of social interaction, such as conversation about the play, without actually joining in the activity. An example of this would be a child talking to a group of children about their construction of a sand castle, without actually joining the activity. Children with autism spectrum disorders often have limited social play and may engage predominantly in unoccupied, solitary, and onlooker play.

Parallel play occurs when children play separately from others but close to them and mimicking their actions. For example, two children may be playing with sculpting clay. Although they are not working together, they may both build a similar animal with the clay because they copy each other. Parallel play can include any of the forms of play described earlier, except attunement play. Parallel play is seen in 2-year-olds, but continues to be seen throughout the preschool years as it serves as a transition to more mature forms of play. Children may simultaneously engage in parallel play and other forms of play as they experiment with social roles and learn prescribed social behaviors.

Associative play is a more mature form of play that reflects social connections. This type of play occurs when children enjoy the company of other children but have little organization to their activity. Following one another around in lines, borrowing, and demonstrating toys are examples of associative play—when the child is interested in the people playing but not in the activity they are doing.

The final form of social play Parten described is **cooperative play**. Cooperative play happens when children are interested both in the people they are playing with, and in the activity they are doing, and can include any of the forms of play listed earlier except attunement play. Typically, preschool play is organized and supervised by adults or older children. True cooperative play is most commonly equated with the category of games with rules and is most typically associated with middle childhood.

Much of preschool play is imitative and triggered by both toys and the manner in which the children see those toys used. Toys that mimic adult activities such as toy kitchens, telephones, and lawn mowers are very popular with this age group. **Figure 12-15** demonstrates typical imaginative preschool play.

The final form of play, games with rules, emerges in the late preschool years. From an early age, children are motivated to make sense of their world, and in exploring this, have an interest in rules. Preschool children's games with rules are usually structured by adults or older children, at least at first. Through these types of games, children learn many social skills including sharing, taking turns, and information sharing.

Preschool children do not distinguish easily between real and imagined events; for this reason they are especially vulnerable to the effects of television and movies because they cannot always understand when what they see is fiction (Paavonen, Roine, Pennonen, & Lahikainen, 2009). This is of concern because current statistics show that the average preschool-aged children in the United States spend more than four hours a day watching television at home and in day care settings (Christakis et al., 2013).

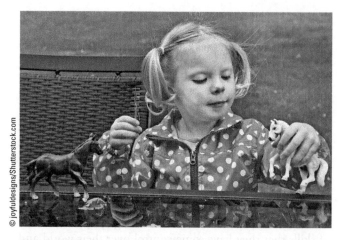

Figure 12-15 This little girl is combining both play with objects and pretense play. She is using her imagination and seems to have an internal dialog narrating a story for her horses. This shows the interrelationship between forms of play and the development of cognitive and language skills.

Preschool children learn best from active doing and active social interaction. The increased use of television and videogames to entertain young children has been identified as a concern because this type of entertainment is usually both passive and prescripted (thus not creative or interactive). The concern is that so much time is spent in passive entertainment, in which children do not develop needed skills, especially attention, task orientation, and personal autonomy skills that will be needed in the school setting. In addition to being passive entertainment, television can be a powerful influence in developing value systems and shaping behavior. The influence of advertising targeting children and the sedentary nature of television viewing have led to concerns about possible long-term lifestyle influences of young viewers (Hancox, Milne, & Poulton, 2004).

Unfortunately, much of today's television programming is violent. Social scientists have documented TV-induced fears in young children that have been caused by violent or explicit programming. These fears may even generalize and impact children's everyday life (Paavonen et al., 2009).

Many studies of television viewing among older children have shown television viewing to be associated with aggression, but there have been far less data on the association between television and aggression in the preschool years. Christakis and colleagues (2013) report that longitudinal studies of television viewing and violence in children before age 5 have revealed a potential risk factor for the subsequent development of bullying and aggressive behaviors in the early elementary school years. In general, before age 4, most children are unable to distinguish reality from fantasy and may view violence as ordinary. Also, violence as shown on television occurs with regularity but seems to have few consequences, which again supports that it is an ordinary occurrence. This results in both desensitization toward violence and an assumption that violence is useful in solving conflicts (Beresin, 2013).

In addition to television, electronic media, including touch screen technologies and computer games, are increasingly marketed to parents as learning tools and are widely used by preschool children. Although there have been many studies on the potential impact of television viewing on child development, the impact of touch screen technology use on the very young is largely unstudied, due in part to the newness of the technology. In a study by the Kaiser Family Foundation (2006), parents acknowledged that a primary reason that they chose electronic media as an activity for their children was to serve as an electronic babysitter, allowing the parents time to engage in other activities of their own. These parents said that they also used electronic media as a tool to help with discipline, both as a distraction when a child was in a negative mood and as a reward for good behavior.

Although the devices do often serve as babysitters, parents choose technologies, DVDs, and tablet-based "apps" based on their perceived educational benefits (Hutton, 2013). "[I]t appears that the primary reason many parents choose to bring media into their children's lives is not because of the educational benefits it offers kids, but because of the practical benefits it offers parents: uninterrupted time for chores, some peace and quiet, or even just an opportunity to watch their own favorite shows" (Kaiser Family Foundation, 2006, p. 5).

Although the reviews of the more passive media, television, and DVD viewing have been fairly negative for young children, there is some evidence that well-designed computer games can offer very engaging, creative, open-ended, or problem-solving challenges to children, and these interactive computer games seem to share some of the benefits of problem solving or constructional play with objects (The Lego Foundation, 2010).

SUMMARY

The preschool years are a time in which rapid social, emotional, and cognitive growth takes place. Children begin to develop unique personalities and can effectively express themselves to others. Play and social relationships play critical roles in preschool development, allowing for exploration, imitation, and practice of basic functional skills. There is more variability in the sequence of skill acquisition in this age group than in infancy, because the new skills acquired require practice and sometimes materials. By the end of the preschool period, children can independently manage basic self-care, follow social conventions, follow directions, and work in a group setting. Successful accomplishment of preschool tasks leaves children well prepared for the wider environment of school.

Play is a central occupation of preschool children and is integral to the development of all the other occupational behaviors expected of school-aged children. Rapid development of technologies and entertainment media aimed at very young children are mixed blessings. Newer interactive technologies appear to have some of the same positive learning opportunities that are associated with constructive play. However, many of these media-based tools offer story lines and scripts, and thus do not encourage free, creative exploration of ideas. Play of all types, including unstructured free play, is recognized as crucial for child development, and in particular for the nurturing of the imagination and creativity needed for today's preschoolers to meet the challenges of the twenty-first century.

Although it is easy to focus on objective skill performance in fine and gross motor skills as part of a therapeutic intervention program, it is essential that any professional working with preschool children interact playfully and support the development of all forms of play as part of the children's developmental needs.

CASE 1

Trevor ... Continued

Trevor, at age 3, was very dependent in all aspects of his life. Issues of decreased mobility, communication skills, and self-care skills have been discussed earlier in this chapter. In addition to these skills, Trevor will also need to develop play skills. With the broad availability of touch screen and joystick-operated gaming options, a child such as Trevor may be able to interact with his peer group through video and online games. One of the limitations of many AAC devices is that they do not interface with other

Continues

Case 1 *Continued*

electronic devices. This means that without special attention, Trevor may have to choose between talking with his friends and playing with his friends, because he needs a switch interface for both. It will be important for both occupational and physical therapists to support the development of play, including the use of adaptive tricycles, battery-powered ride-on cars, and expressive activities like art and music. As noted throughout this chapter, all areas of development interact with one another, and Trevor will need support in all areas to optimize his potential.

Guiding Questions

Some questions to consider:

1. There are many companies that make tricycles and other ride-on toys for children like Trevor. What other outdoor playground activities might we help adapt to let Trevor have a more typical childhood? Can you find an example on the Internet of an adaptation for another playground activity that might be appropriate for Trevor?

2. Think about the demands of caring for Trevor. How might that impact his parents and their lifestyle choices?

3. If Trevor had an older sibling, what do you think you might do to help make the relationship between the two siblings more positive? What do you think might be challenges in this situation?

CASE 2

Brandon

Brandon was born prematurely and was diagnosed with failure to thrive, gastroesophageal reflux, and retinopathy of prematurity resulting in extreme nearsightedness that cannot be fully corrected with glasses. Brandon is hypotonic and slow to gain developmental motor skills. He is now 38 months old. He does not move around much in play unless someone else is there, but will sit and play quietly by himself for long periods of time. Assessment results indicate that Brandon is (1) sitting well, (2) showing rotary transitions, (3) pulling-to-stand, and (4) cruising along furniture or holding onto people. He will stand independently, but becomes anxious and will not take steps when he is not holding on. He has adequate static postural control to maintain standing but has not yet developed dynamic postural control.

Brandon has good receptive and expressive language but has very immature social skills. He is very demanding and negative, and often difficult to control. Brandon is able to assist with many of his self-care activities, but does not do this consistently. His parents say they "pick their battles" and have had to focus on getting him to eat. For this reason, they have not insisted that he participate in dressing, toileting, or self-feeding.

Brandon has a wide variety of grasp patterns, including a pincer grasp, and he seems to enjoy touching and feeling things. His vision impairment has led to a lack of interest in many toys. He likes toys that light up and those that make sounds when touched. He has the basic hand skills needed to manage a spoon and begin self-feeding. He does not shape his hand in anticipation of the shape of the spoon and the muscular arches in his palms are poorly developed. Brandon has no established hand preference and is not effective in utensil use of eating or in taking off shoes, socks, or elastic waist shorts.

Continues

Case 2 *Continued*

Brandon receives special education preschool services and vision therapy, occupational therapy, and physical therapy in preschool. He seems to enjoy his preschool class, but prefers to interact with adults rather than with other children. Mobility and self-care are the major focuses of the intervention process so that Brandon can participate in home, preschool, and peer settings. Because of his nearsightedness, he has a lot of anxiety about moving away from others in his physical therapy sessions. It is the goal of the family that Brandon will be able to attend a regular kindergarten classroom with modifications for his visual impairment. To achieve this goal, Brandon's anxiety about movement and about interacting with his peers needs to be addressed. The team has decided to focus on the additional skills of self-feeding and toileting to help him move toward this goal. A physical therapist has been working on building his walking and transfer skills. Getting on and off of the toilet and using a rolling walker to get around school have been the first steps toward these goals. An occupational therapist has been working on his sensory processing skills, including his acceptance of new tastes and textures at mealtimes. By working on chewing and finger-feeding in playful context, the occupational therapist hopes to help Brandon gain confidence and motivation to do more for himself.

Guiding Questions

Some questions to consider:

1. Brandon has a serious vision impairment that has limited his social development. What types of social exchanges would you see between 3- and 4-year-olds in a preschool setting?
2. How might you modify Brandon's environment so that he has some positive experiences interacting with other children?
3. What classroom and technology adaptations can you think of that might help Brandon with the pre-academic tasks he will need in kindergarten?

Speaking of
Chronic Childhood Conditions

ANNE CRONIN, PhD, OTR/L, PEDIATRIC
OCCUPATIONAL THERAPIST

This is part of a transcript of an interview with a mother whose preschool child has cystic fibrosis and diabetes. Understanding typical development is important in understanding how to best support this family. Parents of preschool children with serious health problems are often very isolated from typical support systems:

Has your life changed to accommodate your special child?

[Laughs]. Do you even need to ask that one? Oh, totally. Completely. One hundred percent. My life isn't anything like it used to be. Well, I don't work. I have a degree in education, but I haven't worked since I had him. And we agreed I'd stay home with him for the first couple of years. But I see no forseeable way I can go back to work any time soon. Before, I was more active in outside activities. I have no outside activities now. I mean, he is exclusively what I do, and he has so many varied problems; he doesn't have just one. And they all kind of relate, and they all kind of don't . . .

Continues

Speaking of Continued

you know? He's got a lot of medical history. And he's all I do. I mean, literally. I keep the house clean, I get the meals on the table. But because of the asthma, particularly, I have to be real careful with the dust and things like that.

He was sick the minute he was born. I was in labor for three days, then ended up having a cesarean because he was starting to get into trouble. And he ingested meconium. So, from the minute he was born, he was sent to the NICU and I didn't hold him until he was a day old, two days old. I went home; he came home days later. At 3 weeks old, he had his first bowel obstruction. So, he was only home for about 10 days before he started getting into trouble. I think we were just numb. Because it was just from day one. We stayed that way. When the pediatrician said, "You know, I think he has cystic fibrosis . . . I want to test for that," I'd never heard of CF. My husband's a registered nurse. He had heard of it in his class. And we just went to the hospital. You're so bombarded with information and things. We really stayed numb until . . . even when he was diagnosed at 17 months with diabetes and he was so terribly sick, and then he developed other obstructions and then I think we got angry. We've had a lot of anger. We had a resident that wouldn't listen to us. And that almost resulted in my son's death. Because we kept telling her, there's something going on, and she kept saying no, it was a reaction elsewhere or something. She lied to us. She told us she had called the endocrinologist, and we talked to the endocrinologist and she didn't know there was a problem going on, which resulted in his second obstruction at that time being much more severe than the first one.

After you got used to the diagnoses, did your perspectives change?

It was something else, because you didn't hear anything good about CF. You heard all the bad stuff. And they told us life expectancy, and you know they told us all this stuff. So that was more stress. Not knowing.

Now, I don't think about it. It's just something else. It's just something I deal with. It's just a part of what I do. I'm the chairman, head, president, whatever of our support group here, and it's just something we do.

How was it for you when it was time to consider preschool?

We didn't do preschool because of the health threat of exposure to more children. When we did start school, I worried about the school schedule, the amount of stress that the teacher has on her, and the fact that he was a real special child and has a lot of special needs. I was concerned about his needs being met in a public school system. I was a public school teacher. I didn't want to put him in a public school. But I went in and talked to the principal, to the teacher, to the secretaries, about learning to do finger sticks, learning to do medicine.

If I were trying to describe what it feels like living with this disease/disability . . . is there something I haven't asked you that you think is important . . . that you would like the world to know . . . ?

I mean the whole picture, the whole overwhelming picture of his care is very different from day to day. Sometimes I feel so angry I can't think, but it's not at anything in particular. It's like there is a monster living inside this beautiful little boy, and we never know when it is going to all blow up.

REFERENCES

Allen, P., Vessey, J., & Schapiro, N. (2009). *Primary care of the child with a chronic condition* (5th ed.). St. Louis: Mosby.

American Occupational Therapy Association. (2014). *Occupational Therapy Practice Framework: Domain and process* (3rd ed.). Bethesda, MD: AOTA Press.

Backen Jones, L., Rothbart, M., & Posner, M. (2003). Development of executive attention in preschool children. *Developmental Science, 6,* 498–504.

Braddick, O., & Atkinson, J. (2013). Visual control of manual actions: Brain mechanisms in typical development and developmental disorders. *Developmental Medicine & Child Neurology, 55,* 13–18.

Brambring, M. (2007). Divergent development of manual skills in children who are blind or sighted. *Journal of Visual Impairment & Blindness, 101*(4), 212–225.

Bekkering, H., & Pratt, J. (2004). Object-based processes in the planning of goal-directed hand movements. *Quarterly Journal of Experimental Psychology: Section A, 57*(8), 1345–1368.

Belsky, J., & de Haan, M. (2011). Annual research review: Parenting and children's brain development: The end of the beginning. *Journal of Child Psychology & Psychiatry, 52*(4), 409–428.

Beresin, E. (2013). The impact of media violence on children and adolescents: Opportunities for clinical interventions. *DevelopMentor.* American Academy of Child and Adolescent Psychiatry. Retrieved from https://www.aacap.org/AACAP/Medical_Students_and_Residents/Mentorship_Matters/DevelopMentor/The_Impact_of_Media_Violence_on_Children_and_Adolescents_Opportunities_for_Clinical_Interventions.aspx

Burgess, J. N., & Broome, M. E. (2012). Perceptions of weight and body image among preschool children: A pilot study. *Pediatric Nursing, 38*(3), 147–176.

Christakis, D. A., Garrison, M. M., Herrenkohl, T., Haggerty, K., Rivara, F. P., Chuan, Z., & Liekweg, K. (2013). Modifying media content for preschool children: A randomized controlled trial. *Pediatrics, 131*(3), 431–438.

Daily, S., Burkhauser, M., & Halle, T. (2011). School readiness practices in the United States. *National Civic Review, 100*(4), 21–24.

Davis, E., Pitchford, N., Jaspan, T., McArthur, D., & Walker, D. (2010). Development of cognitive and motor function following cerebellar tumour injury sustained in early childhood. *Cortex: A Journal Devoted To The Study of the Nervous System & Behavior, 46*(7), 919–932.

Dellatolas, G., de Agostini, M., Curt, F., Kremin, H., Letierce, A., Maccario, J., & Lellouch, J. (2003). Manual skill, hand skill asymmetry, and cognitive performances in young children. *Laterality, 8*(4), 317.

Deoni, S., Dean, D., O'Muircheartaigh, J., Dirks, H., & Jerskey, B. (2012). Investigating white matter development in infancy and early childhood using myelin water faction and relaxation time mapping. *Neuroimage, 63*(3), 1038–1053.

Exner, C. (1992). In-hand manipulation skills. In J. Case-Smith & C. Pehoski (Eds.), *Development of hand skills in the child* (pp. 35–46). The American Occupational Therapy Association Press: Bethesda, MD.

Feldman, R. (2011) *Child development* (6th ed.). Upper Saddle River, NJ: Prentice Hall.

Ganz, J., Earles-Vollrath, T., Heath, A., Parker, R., Rispoli, M., & Duran, J. (2012). A meta-analysis of single case research studies on aided augmentative and alternative communication systems with individuals with autism spectrum disorders. *Journal of Autism & Developmental Disorders, 42*(1), 60–74.

Gibb, B. E., & Abela, J. Z. (2008). Emotional abuse, verbal victimization, and the development of children's negative inferential styles and depressive symptoms. *Cognitive Therapy & Research, 32*(2), 161–176.

Greenspan, S., Prizant, B. & Wetherby, A. (2004). *Hallmark developmental milestones.* Retrieved from http://www.firstsigns.org/healthydev/milestones.htm

Hanania, R., & Smith, L. B. (2010). Selective attention and attention switching: Towards a unified developmental approach. *Developmental Science, 1*(4), 622–635.

Hancox, R. J., Milne, B. J., & Poulton, R. (2004) Association between child and adolescent television viewing and adult health: A longitudinal birth cohort study. *Lancet, 364,* 257–262.

Henderson, A., & Pehoski, C. (Eds.). (2006). *Hand function in the child: Foundation for remediation* (2nd ed.). St. Louis: Mosby.

Holmboe, K., & Johnson, M. (2005). Educating executive attention. *Proceedings of the National Academy of Sciences of the United States of America, 102,* 14479–14480.

Hutton, J. S. (2013). Baby unplugged: A novel, market-based approach to reducing screen time and promoting healthy alternatives. *Clinical Pediatrics, 52*(1), 62–65.

James, K. (2010). Sensori-motor experience leads to changes in visual processing in the developing brain. *Developmental Science, 13*(2), 279–288.

Jeon, H., Peterson, C. A., Wall, S., Carta, J., Luze, G., Eshbaugh, E., & Swanson, M. (2011). Predicting school readiness for low-income children with disability risks identified early. *Exceptional Children, 77*(4), 435–452.

Kaiser Family Foundation. (2006). The media family: Electronic media in the lives of infants, toddlers, preschoolers, and their parents. Retrieved from http://www.kff.org/entmedia/7500.cfm

Kuhl, P., Conboy, B., Padden, D., Nelson, T., & Pruitt, J. (2005). Early speech perception and later language development: Implications for the "critical period." *Language Learning and Development, 1,* 237–264.

Lane, S., & Bundy, A. C. (2012). *Kids can be kids: A childhood occupations approach.* Philadelphia: F. A. Davis Co.

Lego Foundation. (2010). *The future of play: Defining the role and value of play in the 21st century.* Retrieved from http://www.legofoundation.com/en-us/research-and-learning/foundation-research/the-future-of-play/

Milrod, B., Markowitz, J., Gerber, A., Cyranowski, J., Altemus, M., Shapiro, T., & . . . Glatt, C. (2014). Childhood separation anxiety and the pathogenesis and treatment of adult anxiety. *The American Journal Of Psychiatry, 171*(1), 34–43. doi:10.1176/appi.ajp.2013.13060781

Monteiro Gaspar, M. J., Amaral, T. F., Oliveira, B. M., & Borges, N. (2011). Protective effect of physical activity on dissatisfaction with body image in children—A cross-sectional study. *Psychology of Sport & Exercise, 12*(5), 563–569.

Moon, W., Provenzale, J., Sarikaya, B., Ihn, Y., Morlese, J., Chen, S., & DeBellis, M. (2011). Diffusion-tensor imaging assessment of white matter maturation in childhood and adolescence. *AJR. American Journal of Roentgenology, 197*(3), 704–712.

National Institute for Play. (2012). *Play science—the patterns of play.* Retrieved from http://nifplay.org/states_play.html

Parten, M. (1932). Social play among preschool children. *Journal of Abnormal and Social Psychology, 27,* 243–269.

Payne, V. G., & Isaacs, L. D. (2012). *Human motor development: A lifespan approach.* New York: McGraw-Hill.

Paavonen, E. J., Roine, M. M., Pennonen, M. M., & Lahikainen, A. R. (2009). Do parental co-viewing and discussions mitigate TV-induced fears in young children? *Child: Care, Health & Development, 35*(6), 773–780.

Pizer, G., Walters, K., & Meier, R. P. (2007). Bringing up baby with baby signs: Language ideologies and socialization in hearing families. *Sign Language Studies, 7*(4), 387–430.

Shonkoff, J., Phillips, D. A., & Council, N. R. (Eds.) (2000). *From neurons to neighborhoods: The science of early childhood development*. Washington, DC: National Academy Press.

Shumway-Cook, A., & Woollacott, M. (2012). Motor control issues and theories. In *Motor control: Translating research into clinical practice* (4th ed., pp. 1–20). Baltimore: Lippincott, Williams and Wilkins.

Smith, L. (2006). Movement matters: The contributions of Esther Thelen. *Biological Theory, 1*(1), 87–89.

Strickling, C. (2010). Impact of visual impairment on development. *Texas School for the Blind and Visually Impaired*. Retrieved from http://www.tsbvi.edu/infants/3293-the-impact-of-visual-impairment-on-development

Vinter, A. A., Fernandes, V. V., Orlandi, O. O., & Morgan, P. P. (2013). Verbal definitions of familiar objects in blind children reflect their peculiar perceptual experience. *Child: Care, Health and Development, 39*(6), 856–863.

Visu-petra, L., Benga, O., & Miclea, M. (2007). Dimensions of attention and executive functioning in 5-TO 12-years-old children: Neuropsychological assessment with the NEPSY Battery. *Cognitie, Creier, Comportament/Cognition, Brain, Behavior, 11*(3), 585–608.

World Health Organization. (2001). ICF: International classification of functioning and disability. Geneva, Switzerland: World Health Organization.

CHAPTER 13

Childhood and School

Anne Cronin, PhD, OTR/L, FAOTA,
Associate Professor, Division of
Occupational Therapy,
West Virginia University,
Morgantown, West Virginia

Objectives

Upon completion of this chapter, readers should be able to:

- Describe the areas of greatest developmental growth in childhood, including the dimensions of school tasks and demands, cognitive/ behavioral self-regulation, self-care/self-management skills, and cooperative and competitive play;

- Discuss contemporary trends and problem areas in the health of children between the ages of 6 and 12 including issues of stress and mental health;

- Describe the impact of the family, the community, social media, and peers on the development of social behavior and identity formation in middle childhood;

- Identify common risk and protective factors in middle childhood;

- Explain the role of language and literacy skill development on the overall functional performance of children;

- Describe play and creativity in the context of middle childhood and skills acquisition; and

- Describe how children in middle childhood explore games with rules through structured activity, sport, and free play.

Key Terms

asynchronous development

body schema

bullying

cognitive map

cognitive monitoring

coincidence-anticipation
   (CA) timing

co-regulation

deafness

figure-ground perception

finger dexterity

hand dominance

hemispheric specialization

inclusion

kinesthetic perception

learned helplessness

leisure

low vision

metamemory

positive stress

psychomotor abilities

reaction time

self-concept

self-management skills

social capital

social competence

social knowledge

social referencing

spatial awareness

statutory blindness

temporal awareness

tolerable stress

toxic stress

virtual (digital) play

visual disorder

CASE 1

Elias

Elias was an active athletic 9-year-old. He had played team soccer every autumn, and softball spring since he was 6. Early last summer, Janet noticed her son Elias was limping. "The ache in his leg would come and go. We thought it was probably just growing pains." It turned out to be a tumor in his knee. Elias was diagnosed with Ewing's sarcoma, a rare and aggressive cancer. He started a 36-week regimen of chemotherapy right away. Janet says, "It was so overwhelming, but we felt confident in the care he was getting. Everyone was so positive. We never questioned it and never doubted the doctors."

Elias was in the hospital three weeks of each of the next nine months for chemo treatment, and sometimes with complications. His tumor responded well to the treatment, though, and he eventually had surgery to amputate his leg below the knee. Elias missed school and his friends. Because of the chemotherapy, his immune system was suppressed and he could have few outside visitors. He did have a teacher who came to visit him so that he could keep up with classes, but otherwise he felt left out and angry at the world.

Because of his chronic pain and difficulties with mobility and other daily tasks, Elias began to receive OT and PT in his home. The physical therapist was fun and made up games and silly obstacle courses that challenged Elias while making him laugh. His parents were ecstatic, because prior to these games, they insisted that it had been months since he had laughed.

The OT started working with Elias on dressing and self-care tasks, but found that he was poorly motivated and easily frustrated, lashing out at her in anger. He said that he did not see the point, that there was no reason to get dressed because there was nothing to do and nowhere to go. On impulse, the OT asked Elias where he would go if he could go anywhere he wanted. Elias chose Mars! On her next visit, Elias presented the OT of a drawing of himself on Mars, bald with one leg and a scowl on his face.

Continues

Case 1   *Continued*

Using Elias's interest in art, Elias and his OT began a long journey toward a healthier self-concept, improved motivation, and cooperation. His ADL and IADL skills improved, and his academic grades did too. Because the medical team had indicated that Elias would need bone-lengthening surgery every four to six months during his growth years, building resilience and coping strategies when he was in chronic pain were very important.

Through the use of humor and artistic expression, Elias was able to maintain and eventually improve his participation in everyday activities. He returned to school for fifth grade, at age 10, and was ready to go forward with his life.

Continues on page 299

INTRODUCTION

Before the relative wealth of the twentieth century, children began "working" in trades or in the family business in the age group of 6 to 12 years (Fass & Mason, 2000). The American acceptance of childhood as a distinct developmental period that was characterized by formal schooling emerged late in the nineteenth century (Fass, 2007). Access to public education and the financial (or governmental) resources to make education affordable transformed the "apprenticeships" of earlier generations into a description of this period as "school age." The world over, between the ages of 6 and 12, children gradually reduced the amount of time spent with their parents and spent more time outside of the home. This period, which we will call middle childhood, includes the seminal period of training and socialization that prepares children to become productive members of society. Although mandatory school enrollment is the norm in North America, in much of the world, education is still a luxury, and in middle childhood, children continue to play important economic roles for families (Leeder, 2003).

The main developmental thrust in skill growth common to middle childhood falls into the ICF models of "activities and participation" and "environmental factors" (World Health Organization, 2001), with the expansion of their independence in daily occupations and the development of formal occupational role behaviors. Children build real friendships in this age period, and their interactions with their peers become increasingly important to them.

Earlier in this text, you were presented with the historical debate concerning the varying roles of nature and nurture in human development. In infancy and early childhood, there is strong support for nature as the preeminent developmental force. In middle childhood, the evidence swings toward the nurture position, with children's performance contexts emerging as important influences on development.

Although the preschool years were characterized by incredible gains in communication and motor control, middle childhood, the time period from age 6 until the onset of puberty, is a time of gains in knowledge and participation in self-care, domestic life, interpersonal interactions, and civic life. Broad self-management skills emerge based on social demands and experiences in this life stage. **Self-management skills** refer to methods, skills, and strategies by which individuals can effectively direct their own activities toward the achievement of objectives, and includes goal setting, decision making, focusing, planning, scheduling, task tracking, self-evaluation, and self-intervention. In middle childhood, individuals gain the basic skills to care for themselves and function in society.

BODY FUNCTIONS AND STRUCTURES

The changes in the body that we will focus on the most in this chapter are in the increasing precision and refinement in motor control. This chapter considers the development of body structures and functions until the start of puberty. For most children, the growth rate slows and there are increases in both strength and physical endurance. This is the age group in which participation in organized sports becomes common.

BRAIN AND NERVOUS SYSTEM DEVELOPMENT

As the brain matures, its various parts develop more differentiation, and areas of the brain become specialized for certain kinds of information processing. As noted in Chapter 12, the left hemisphere of the cerebral cortex is very active in the preschool years, and from middle childhood on, is specialized in the management of language and movement.

From age 6, activity in the right hemisphere also increases as it becomes more specialized for the analysis of space and geometrical shapes and forms, elements that are all present at the same time. This specialization may occur differently in some people who are left-handed, but the pattern of specialization is less important, for this discussion, than the fact that hemispheric specialization occurs. **Hemispheric specialization** (also called brain lateralization) is the end result of the brain maturation that allows the hemispheres to work separately and more efficiently in school-age children (Groen, Whitehouse, Badcock, & Bishop, 2011). Many specialized functions, including the development of hand dominance are supported by hemispheric specialization.

In addition to the specialization of brain functions, the main structure connecting the two brain hemispheres, the corpus callosum, fully myelinates during middle childhood. This myelination allows for faster, more effective communication between the two hemispheres of the brain. The corpus callosum is the largest white matter structure in the brain and functions to coordinate information between the many areas of the brain, especially the cerebral hemispheres (Cantlon et al., 2011). The developing corpus callosum supports sensory and motor integration. Functional communication throughout the brain improves throughout this developmental period, and effective communication, especially linkages with the parietal and frontal lobes, are associated with measures of intelligence (Langeslag et al., 2013).

Much of the brain growth at this time is in the area of the brain called the frontal lobes. The frontal lobes are associated with specific mental functions including attention and higher-level cognitive functions such as abstraction, organization, planning, time management, cognitive flexibility, insight, and judgment. In preschool children, the frontal lobes are active and support the improvement of self-regulation and the ability to inhibit impulses. In the school-age years, the influence of the frontal lobes expands to allow improvements in cognitive flexibility (Hughes, 2011).

SENSORY CHARACTERISTICS

In middle childhood, the mechanisms for visual and auditory perception continue to refine. The typical classroom setting for children is very sensory-rich and assumes an ability to both perceive sensory input and to filter information so that they can attend to only that input that is important to the task at hand. **Figure 13-1** presents a typical elementary school classroom. Note that there are many types of visual stimuli. There will also be much auditory stimuli as children sit near one another at tables and the classroom fills with 20 or more students.

Senses such as touch that require close proximity between an individual and the object or event to be perceived are called *near senses.* The senses of touch, taste, and movement are considered near senses. The *far senses,* vision and hearing, enable individuals to perceive objects or events some distance away. In Chapter 12, we introduced some of the developmental differ-

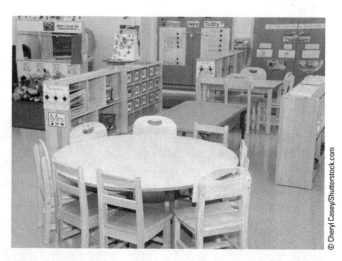

Figure 13-1   Classroom environments in the early grades are designed to attract attention and to help children learn to organize their behavior in the school setting. Although this works well for many children, children with difficulty processing sensory information may become overwhelmed in a sensory-rich classroom such as this one.

ences common to preschool children with vision impairments. The ability to see and understand the extended environment offers information that provides both security and affordances to support exploratory behavior. The far senses are vitally important to the ability to function in school and community settings. Children with visual and hearing impairments will need special accommodations to be able to learn and function well within the classroom environment.

Visual Development

One of the standard screening items for kindergarten children is a test of visual acuity. Vision is a predominant sensory input system used in the traditional school environment. For this reason, visual difficulties are important to identify early. *Static visual acuity,* as defined in Chapter 12, refers to the clarity with which people see stationary objects, when they are also stationary. Typically, visual acuity is tested by requiring a person to identify characters (such as letters and numbers) on a chart from a set distance. The visual system is fairly immature at birth. A newborn's visual acuity is approximately 20/400, developing to 20/20 in middle childhood (Pan et al., 2009). Similar to other neural systems, sensory systems mature in a use-dependent manner. Codina and colleagues (2011) described an example of this in reporting that by middle childhood, children who were born deaf had developed peripheral vision skills that were superior to those of their typically developing peers.

Visual disorders are abnormalities of the eye, the optic nerve, the optic tracts, or the brain that may cause a loss of visual acuity or visual fields. For most people, a loss of visual acuity can be corrected by special lenses or through surgery. Another type of visual disorder is a visual field disorder. A *visual field disorder* means that the ability to perceive visual stimuli in the periphery of what would be a typical visual field is limited. Because the peripheral visual field assists in adjusting reach and in responding to moving objects, a visual field loss can result in significant challenges to personal safety. In the United States, **statutory blindness** (also called legal blindness) requires that a person's best corrected visual acuity is 20/200 or less in the better eye, or a visual field limitation such that the widest diameter of the visual field, in the better eye, subtends an angle no greater than 20 degrees. The term *blindness* refers to a profound loss of vision. More common is a condition of *low vision*. **Low vision** denotes a level of vision that is 20/70 or worse and cannot be fully corrected with conventional glasses (U.S. National Library of Medicine, 2012a). Children with low vision have some useful sight, but will have difficulty with many academic tasks and with sports participation. These children face special challenges in school, where great emphasis is placed on learning through printed material. Children with severe visual impairment must rely on ear-hand coordination rather than eye-hand coordination. Ear-hand coordination develops one to two years later than eye-hand coordination in typically developing children, accounting for some of the motor delays seen in the school setting. In addition, people who are visually impaired develop compensations in a highly refined sense of touch.

Auditory Development

By middle childhood, the child is not only aware that an auditory stimulus is present, but has gained many skills in understanding and processing auditory information. The child is able to associate a variety of auditory stimuli with their sound source is able to search for and find the auditory stimulus. In addition the child can hear, remember, repeat, and recall words, phrase or sequences of numbers. Finally, the child utilizes auditory information to process language. Hearing loss exists when there is diminished sensitivity to the sounds normally heard in the speech frequencies. *Hearing impairment,* as defined in Chapter 5, is a broad term covering individuals with hearing loss ranging from mild to profound (deaf). Children with mild to moderate hearing losses can be easily accommodated in the regular classroom. Children with profound hearing loss often need both developmental and educational supports to fully participate with peers in middle childhood. **Deafness** is defined as a degree of poor hearing such that a person is unable to understand speech through hearing even in the presence of amplification (U.S. National Library of Medicine, 2012b). In recent years, many advances in the technology have become available to assist children with hearing impairments. One of these new technologies includes cochlear implants. A cochlear implant is a surgically implanted electronic device that serves as a processor that converts speech into electronic signals that the device transmits to the auditory nerve in the inner ear. This technology has been shown to support normal auditory cortical development in children with congenital deafness (Cardon, Campbell, & Sharma, 2012). Children with hearing impairments may be able to function in the regular classroom, with appropriate technology.

PHYSICAL DEVELOPMENT

Typical, well-nourished children grow 2 to 3 inches a year during the ages of 6 to about the age of 11 (American Academy of Pediatrics, 2012). During this time, body proportions gradually change as the relative size of the head decreases, and increases in skeletal and muscle mass replace "baby fat." During the preschool years, the greatest area of growth is the trunk, and the center of gravity is usually at about the mid-thoracic region (near the end of the ribs) when a child is standing. In the ages between 6 and 10, most of children's growth is in the limbs, and the center of gravity drops farther, to about the level of the umbilicus. This change in proportion is shown in **Figure 13-2**.

As the center of gravity drops, children's ability to balance and to maintain balance while running improves. As the center of gravity shifts, children are better able to balance during activities involving the manipulation of objects, as in sports (Payne & Isaacs, 2012). There has been much research on the refinement of postural control during childhood, demonstrating that postural responses grow faster and more reliable over time (Shumway-Cook & Woollacott, 2012). Many studies suggest a relationship between the development of cognitive and motor skills in childhood (Davis, Pitchford, & Limback, 2011). This relationship is strongest in young children and decreases with the age of the children. For example, Reilly, van Donkelaar, Saavedra, and Woollacott (2008) found that postural interference affected visual working memory in 4- to 6-year-olds, but not in 7- to 12-year-olds and adults. The motor skills of stability and alignment when standing or sitting and when moving and interacting with objects in their environment are essential skills for many of the activities that school-age children perform on a daily basis. The ability to adjust to postural challenges without interference with working memory is an essential support to classroom learning. **Figure 13-3** shows two 9-year-old boys playing in the sprinkler. The complexity and flexibility in their postural control is evident in this photo.

In addition to a lowering of their center of gravity, children during the middle childhood years make dramatic increases in muscular strength. With increasing strength, they will have gradual improvements in functional task performance. Several research studies indicate that grip strength increases by between 260 percent and 393 percent between the ages of 7 and 17 (Payne & Isaacs, 2012). In the preschool years, children can walk, bend, and reach for objects, but often have to stop other activity to manage this. Now children can walk, bend, and reach casually, grabbing an apple as they walk through the kitchen or high-fiving a friend as they pass in the hall. Motor skills continue to develop throughout childhood. In middle childhood, there is a dramatic increase in the ability to precisely calibrate movements to the demands of a task.

Although gender identity and gender roles are an important development focus during this age span, boys

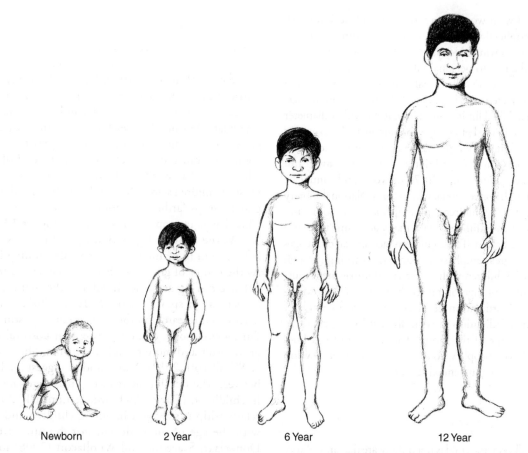

Newborn 2 Year 6 Year 12 Year

Figure 13-2 This drawing shows how body proportions change from birth through middle childhood.

and girls have few differences in motor performance in middle childhood (Feldman, 2011).

Children in this age range are often encouraged to gain a high level of mastery over physical skills, and often sample broadly among sports and other activities. Physical competence is one of the factors associated with popularity in both middle childhood and adolescence, so sports participation offers social benefits as well as health benefits. For children who become highly competitive and focused within a particular physical performance realm, whether it be dance or sports, there is a high risk for injury because the children's bones and joints are still growing and are more susceptible to injuries associated with excessive physical activity or training than they will be later in life (Hutchison, 2011).

Fine Motor Skills

As described in Chapter 12, the process of using each hand differently begins in the preschool years. Beginning with the haptic perception and in-hand manipulation that develops in the preschool years, the speed and dexterity of the movements increase throughout middle childhood. In familiar tasks, the variability of strategies used to perform the task decreases (Henderson & Pehoski, 2006). These refinements in movements are due to the continuing maturation of the CNS.

Similar changes are also seen in reaching and calibrating hand and arm movements resulting in improved accuracy. Visual processing skills are integral to the development of refined hand skills. Davis, Pitchford, and Limback (2011) consistently found that children's visual processing scores were highly correlated with their scores on tests of fine motor performance.

Finger dexterity is the ability to make precisely coordinated movements of the fingers of one or both hands to use or manipulate very small objects. Finger dexterity is required for handwriting, keyboarding, texting, and for using most game controllers. As children mature, the complexity of bimanual task demands increases. Increasingly, children in this age group are able to keep one hand stable while the other moves to complete a precise task. This increasing ability to do asymmetrical tasks is believed to reflect improved interhemispheric communication (Henderson & Pehoski, 2006).

The timing of motor actions refines as children develop temporal and spatial perception skills. This emergent skill is **coincidence-anticipation (CA) timing**, the ability to time a movement in response to another moving object. Experience with CA timing tasks is an important factor developing accuracy in this skill area. For children who engage in activities requiring this type of timing, the skill is well developed by the age of 12 (Kim, Nauhaus, Glazek, Young, & Lin, 2013). CA timing is necessary in many activities but is easily illustrated in

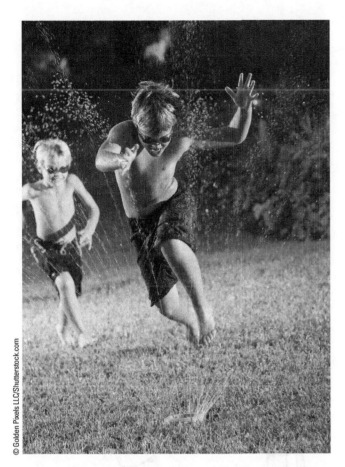

Figure 13-3   The confidence with which these boys move reflects the high degree of motor control they have developed as well as the ability to dynamically adjust their plan of action in response to visual information.

Figure 13-4, demonstrating normal developmental stages of catching. In the initial development of catching, the child is static, may turn away from the ball, and traps the ball in his arms rather than opening and positioning his hands for the catch. In the mature stage, which is typical of middle childhood, the eyes follow the ball into the hands, the arms adjust to the flight of the ball, and the hands grasp the ball in a well-timed motion. More complex CA timing is seen as children practice ball-related sports like softball, shown in **Figure 13-5**.

Hand Dominance

By the time children enter school, at the age of 5, a consistent hand preference is usually seen. **Hand dominance** is "the consistent and more proficient use of the preferred hand in functional and skilled tasks" (Henderson & Pehoski, 2006, p. 161). Hand dominance means that one hand has the most influence or control in the performance of skilled tasks. The establishment of hand dominance is considered an indicator of both hemispheric specialization and interhemispheric communication. Genetic factors play the most important part in determining hand dominance, but cultural and environmental

factors are also an influence (Hill & Khanem, 2009). In many societies, there is an effort to restrain left-handedness, sometimes altogether, and sometimes only in particular tasks. For example, in Kuwait, it is considered impolite to eat using your left hand. A left-handed person in Kuwait may end up having a pattern of mixed dominance, with the right hand dominant for eating and the left hand dominant for writing. This is a normal adaptation and has no negative developmental effects on individuals. Similarly, it is not unusual for a child to have one preferred hand for eating and writing and a different preferred hand for sports. There appear to be no overall differences in development of motor skills between children with right- and left-hand dominance (McManus, 2002).

Children who exhibit a consistent right- or left-hand preference are motorically superior to those who have a pattern of mixed-hand use (Mori, Iteya, & Gabbard, 2006). The literature suggests that hand dominance reflects hemispheric lateralization. Thus, those who are more strongly lateralized are likely to have a strong pattern of hand dominance. This reasoning proposes that inconsistent or mixed-handedness in children might be regarded as an indirect indicator of an immature central nervous system (Mori, Iteya, & Gabbard, 2006).

The development of a dominant "skilled" hand in bimanual patterns allows children to specialize and develop the refined dexterity needed for writing, keyboarding, and other school demands. When children have poorly established hand dominance, they may be seen to frequently switch hands and use either hand for similar tasks. For the skilled use of a dominant hand to develop, children must already have mastered postural control, eye-hand coordination, complementary bimanual function, and perceptual concepts (body image, laterality, and internal/external directionality).

MENTAL FUNCTIONS

Dramatic increases in both global and specific mental functions are seen in middle childhood. With their increased ability to inhibit behavior and the ability to internalize language, school-age children are able to engage in abstractions and mental calculations that were impossible earlier. This is also a period where the development of language and cognitive skills leads to the potential for creative and imaginative thought that is demonstrated in play and other daily occupations.

Attention Functions

The ability to attend and to self-correct and redirect when attention is diverted will be key skills as children progress through school. Although attention to novel and changing stimuli, like those common to video games, is easier to sustain, children in middle childhood learn to focus and concentrate their attention even in routine situations within a classroom. Typical 6-year-olds are easily distracted by sounds in the classroom. Children have to learn to selectively attend to relevant information and inhibit distracting irrelevant information

Initial

Elementary

Mature

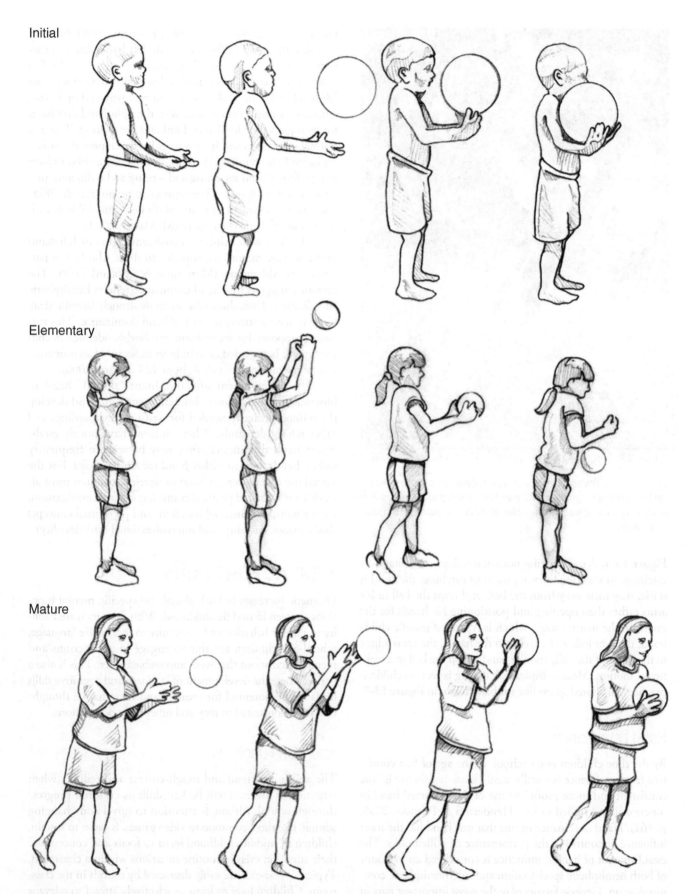

Figure 13-4 This drawing recreates the typical acquisition pattern for learning to catch a ball.

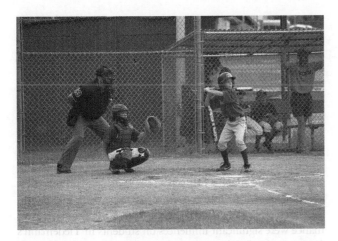

Figure 13-5 Softball requires highly developed coincidence-anticipation timing. Prior to achieving this skill level, children play "T-ball" and hit a stationary ball.

in situations, like classrooms, where multiple sensory inputs are competing. Children in the range of 5 to 12 years of age were found to be more susceptible to distractions from irrelevant information across a broad range of auditory and visual tasks than adolescents and young adults (Passow et al., 2013). Children with hearing impairments may have greater attentional challenges than typically developing children in this period because it is more difficult for them to find meaning in auditory information, making it more difficult to filter (Porter, Sladen, Ampah, Rothpletz, & Bess, 2013).

Attention deficit/hyperactivity disorder (ADHD) is a developmental disorder that manifests as behavioral difficulties, often first noticed in middle childhood, that are associated with inattention and impulsivity. ADHD is a disorder of behavioral inhibition and is often first noticeable when children start school. Many people hold misconceptions of ADHD, such as that it is not "real," it simply reflects poor parenting, or that it can be "fixed" by medications. Children with ADHD often have difficulty complying with classroom behavior expectations and have difficulty developing positive social relationships with peers. Executive attention, described in Chapter 12, is vital to learning in a classroom setting. Classroom attentional demands are increasing as children today are expected to sit indoors and at desks for long periods of time, with few breaks for physical activity. Children with ADHD who may have been successful in school a couple of decades ago might not be equally successful in today's school environment.

Memory Functions

Working memory, the ability to hold information in the mind to do verbal and nonverbal reasoning tasks plays a central role to learning in all of the environmental contexts of middle childhood as it supports attention, language comprehension, and language production (Whitely & Colozzo, 2013). Working memory involves the active, conscious processing and storage

of information. This is distinct from short term memory that is primarily associated with passive information storage along with automated subconscious processes. Working memory can be thought of as a sort of mental workspace that we can use to store important information while performing mental activities. Working memory in middle childhood is considered to have four primary aspects. The first of these is called the *phonological loop* and deals with sound or phonological information. The phonological loop supports speech perception and holds information as words for brief periods. It is also the mechanism that helps us rehearse and store verbal information. The second is the *visual spatial processor* that is used to store and process spatial and visual information. This aspect of working memory allows us to remember shapes, designs, and is involved in planning spatial movements, like planning one's way through a complex building. The *episodic buffer* has an important function as a 'backup' and storage area which communicates with both long term memory and the components of working memory. The final aspect is that of the central executive. The central executive drives the whole system and allocates data to the phonological loop and the visual spatial processor. The central executive is responsible for focusing attention (switching), coordinating the subsystems, controlling encoding and decoding strategies, and retrieving information from long-term memory (Michalczyk, Malstädt, Worgt, Könen, & Hasselhorn, 2013). The number of items that can be stored and manipulated at a time is the working memory "span." How much individuals can hold in their working memory span varies with age, innate ability, and the pace with which the information is presented. Barrouillet and colleagues (2009) found that children prior to age 7 were limited in their capacity to control their activity to switch their attention easily from memory processing to memory storage. After age 7, they showed dramatic improvements in working memory.

An important new cognitive development in this age group is metamemory. **Metamemory** is a type of metacognition that involves a conscious awareness of one's memory capabilities and the intentional strategies to aid memory (Karably & Zabrucky, 2009). As they progress through school, children must learn to store new information in their memories. Some common metamemory strategies used in this age group are:

- *Rehearsal:* repeating information to oneself over and over again.

- *Organization:* grouping together related items.

- *Mnemonics:* using a word, acronym, or other device to create a relationship between two or more items that are not members of the same category.

These metamemory strategies can be useful for occupational and physical therapists both in designing intervention programs that children can actively remember and learn to manage for themselves, and in supporting older clients who have memory challenges.

Psychomotor Functions

Psychomotor abilities (also called psychomotor functions) are specific mental functions of control over both motor and psychological events at the body level, including the capacity to manipulate and control objects (World Health Organization, 2001). Psychomotor abilities are demonstrated in skills such as hand-eye coordination and reaction time that involve an integration of cognitive and motor functions. It is our psychomotor abilities that allow us to use materials in daily occupations and to develop graphomotor skills. Occupational and physical therapists describe these types of psychomotor abilities as praxis. Praxis, also called *motor planning,* was defined in Chapter 6 as the mental ability to plan, organize, and sequence a new task. Skillful motor planning results in qualitative improvements in motor tasks, such as the ability to keep your hand and arm steady while moving your arm or while holding your arm and hand in one position, or the ability to move both arms smoothly at your sides while looking forward. Two of the developing skills in this age group that rely on psychomotor abilities were discussed earlier in this chapter are finger dexterity and coincidence-anticipation timing. Another example of a psychomotor ability is the ability to choose quickly between two or more movements in response to two or more different signals (lights, sounds, pictures). **Reaction time** is a psychomotor ability that allows the person to quickly move the arms and/or legs in response to a stimulus. The time delay between the presentation of a stimulus and the motor response to that stimulus is the reaction time. Reaction time and predictive response timing abilities increase from the ages of 5 to 12 years (Debrabant, Gheysen, Vingerhoets, & Van Waelvelde, 2012). There is much individual difference in reaction time, and it is a crucial feature that determines success in sports in this age group. In some cases, a slow reaction time may be related to poor temporal awareness. Throughout the primary school years, children experience a gradual improvement in reaction time. Improving reaction time supports the development of coincidence-anticipation timing, described earlier in this chapter.

Emotional Functions

During this developmental period, children gain the ability to recognize and discuss their feelings. They also begin to view themselves differently, less in terms of their physical attributes and more in terms of psychological traits. During middle childhood, children learn to hide or show emotions appropriately for their social context (Hutchison, 2011). School-age children have a strong desire to identify their place in the world as well, and as they mature, they develop a self-concept. A **self-concept** is the composite of ideas, feelings, and attitudes that the children have about their own identity, worth, capabilities, and limitations (Mosby, 2009). Children's self-concept develops as a result of personal and social evaluation of individuals. Self-concept grows in complexity throughout middle childhood, and by adolescence there may be several distinct spheres of self-concept. For example, in the academic sphere, children may

be aware that they excel in science but perform poorly in social studies. In the social sphere, children may be well accepted within their extended family but are on the social fringes at school. The values of important people in the child's life, cultural values, and for today's kids the values they see portrayed on television and the Internet, serve as standards that children measure themselves against as they develop their self-concept.

Teachers can have a significant impact on children's developing self-concept. Tiedemann (2000) found that parents' and teachers' gender stereotypes about children's mathematic abilities influenced children's self-concepts about their mathematic ability prior to having extensive math experiences in school. Teachers' gender expectations related to math performance were significant influences on students in Tiedemann's (2000) study. Gender expectations and beliefs are an important factor in the formation of self-concept (Hutchison, 2011).

As children start school, they begin to compare themselves with their peers, and they understand the expectations of teachers and parents. Children at this age often experience stress. Childhood stress can be caused by any situation that requires the child to adapt or change. Both day-to-day experiences and major life events can cause stress. When children grow up in chronic stressful conditions such as abuse or severe maternal depression there is evidence of changes within the developing brain and the probability of poor outcomes increases (National Scientific Council on the Developing Child, 2014). Three different types of stress are considered in the study of children; they are positive stress, tolerable stress, and toxic stress. **Positive stress** is the sense of pressure that results from challenging experiences that are short-lived. Positive stress is moderate and short-lived stress that results in learning and positive growth. **Tolerable stress** describes adverse life experiences that are more intense than those causing positive stress, but that are still relatively short-lived. Examples of tolerable stress would include death of a parent, a natural disaster, or a frightening accident. Tolerable stress is more difficult to assimilate and may require the support of a caring adult to overcome. Without support, tolerable stress can become toxic and lead to long-term negative health effects. **Toxic stress** is stress that results from intense adverse experiences that may be sustained over a long period of time. This is the type of stress associated with child abuse or chronic neglect. In these situations, children are unable to effectively manage the stress, and the stress response system gets activated for a prolonged amount of time. Toxic stress can lead to permanent changes in the development of the brain and can result in an exaggerated stress response later in life (National Scientific Council on the Developing Child, 2014).

Returning to the case that introduced this chapter, Elias is facing significant stress and significant challenges to his self-concept. At an age where many young boys are physically active and exploring sports participation, Elias is both ill and has lost a leg. Although he has good family support and good medical care, his self-image has been permanently altered. In addition to the loss of his leg and the social isolation caused by his condition, Elias must deal with both chronic pain and the side effects of his cancer treatment that make him feel tired and ill. This level of stress would be difficult to manage at any stage in life. Whether this becomes "tolerable" or "toxic" stress will depend on the support of the adults around him, both in his family and on his health care team. By engaging him with humor and building on his interests, both the PT and the OT are offering tangible support that should help Elias cope and respond to this difficult time as a period of "tolerable" stress.

For many children, school is the first time they experience achievement pressure and social stresses related to behavior regulation and peer aggression. In middle childhood, stress can come from outside sources (such as family, friends, or school), but it can also come from the child's own perceptions and expectations. In middle childhood, children begin to measure themselves against others and feel pressure because they perceive themselves to be less than they should be. This type of stress is typically positive stress because it results in children acting to become more secure in their place in the social world. Tolerable stresses in the preschool years are most likely to come from events, like injury or divorce. An episode of a serious or prolonged illness can also be the cause of a tolerable stress.

Toxic stress in young children can negatively impact brain growth and myelination. In addition, high levels of stress hormones can suppress the body's immune response and leave children vulnerable to a variety of health problems. Sustained high levels of stress hormones can result in lasting damage to areas of the brain responsible for learning and memory (National Scientific Council on the Developing Child, 2014).

Perceptual Functions

Perceptual functions were described earlier as specific mental functions of recognizing and interpreting sensory stimuli (World Health Organization, 2001). Perception is a mental function that draws from memory and language functions. As children gain cognitive skills and are exposed to new challenges, they also gain perceptual skills within all of the sensory systems. Some examples of perceptual functions follow.

Visual Perception

Visual perceptual skills develop extensively in middle childhood. Visual perception supports the development of reading and writing, as well as many instrumental activities of daily living (IADLs). **Table 13-1** presents some of the major aspects of visual perception that mature in middle childhood.

Figure-ground perception is a property of perception in which there is a tendency to identify a complex sensory field as an array of solid, well-defined objects standing out against a background. Figure-ground perception can occur in both of the far senses, allowing individuals to isolate important salient sensory cues while ignoring unimportant features of the array. This skill is refined between the ages of 4 and 13. Figure-ground perceptual abilities peak in adolescence and are important in many self-care and academic tasks. Visual figure-ground perception is necessary for completing school worksheets and determining front from back when dressing. Auditory figure-ground perception is the ability to single out the teacher's voice in a busy classroom, or to hear the ice cream truck coming down the street while you are watching TV. Because figure-ground perception requires attention, sensory input, and memory, it is poorly developed before middle childhood.

Kinesthetic Perception

Kinesthetic perception is the interpretation of information regarding the relative position of the body parts to each other, the position of the body in space, and an awareness of the

---

TABLE 13-1 The Maturation of Visual Perception

Skill	Definition	Approximate Time of Maturation
Perception of size constancy	The ability to recognize that objects maintain a constant size even if their distance from the observer varies. This allows children to accurately judge the size of objects.	This skill typically matures by age 11.
Perception of figure and ground	This allows children to locate and focus on an object embedded in a distracting background.	This skill typically matures at about age 8.
Perception of depth	This is the ability to judge distances and to recognize the three-dimensional nature of objects.	This skill typically matures at about age 12.
Perception of movement	This involves the ability to detect and track a moving object with the eye.	This skill typically matures at about age 10.

Adapted from Goggin, 2003. Reference Crediting: Goggin, N. (2003). KINE 3500 Lecture 4: Perceptual-Motor Development. Retrieved from http://www.coe.unt.edu/goggin/kine3500/350lec4.htm

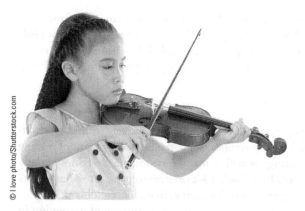

Figure 13-6   Playing the violin requires kinesthetic perception for both bowing and fingering the instrument. This skill needs to become unconscious for the young musician to play the notes correctly while attending to the musical score and the conductor.

body's movements (Goggin, 2003). Kinesthetic perception, like visual perception, includes many distinct perceptual skills. These include *stereognosis* (a form of haptic perception), the recognition of objects by manipulation, *proprioception*, the position of limb and body position in space, and *kinesthesis*, the perception of the extent of limb movements (Shumway-Cook & Woollacott, 2012). To develop proficiency in playing most musical instruments, a high degree of kinesthetic perception is needed. Elementary-school age is when most children are typically introduced to instruments, and many, like the 10-year-old shown in **Figure 13-6**, become proficient.

Kinesthetic awareness also allows for the large increase in skills seen in "ball" sports in this age group. The children can visually fixate on the ball, while being kinesthetically aware of their position and the movements needed.

HIGHER-LEVEL COGNITIVE FUNCTIONS

Higher-level cognitive functions are specific mental functions such as decision making, abstract thinking, planning and carrying out plans, mental flexibility, and deciding which behaviors are appropriate under what circumstances (World Health Organization, 2001). Anderson and Reidy (2012) established that executive function development begins in the preschool years and extends into middle childhood. Among the skills gained, there is a decline in time needed to process information and a corresponding increase in information processing capacity. In addition, children gain the ability to resist interference from irrelevant information and concentrate on information relevant to tasks at hand.

Cognitive monitoring is a higher-level cognitive function that involves self-examination of what you are currently doing, what you will do next, and how effectively the activity is serving to meet your intended purpose. Cognitive monitoring allows children to persist in school tasks like completing a book report or solving a math problem.

Participation in school environments requires a complex interaction of developmental skills. In some cases, adequate skill levels are present in isolation, but the combination of demands during the day leads to activity limitation. For occupational and physical therapists working in school environments, effective functional interventions will emphasize improving the children's participation in the school environment in all the areas that have been described.

Although it is not usually listed as part of the academic curriculum, a hierarchy of self-management skills is taught in most school settings that coincides with the metacognitive development of the children. Some of the most challenging aspects of school for young children are the self-regulation challenges, as they are asked to remain quiet in lines, to sit quietly with their peers, and to limit their use of classroom materials to specific assigned times. **Figure 13-7** shows children waiting in line as part of the school day.

Teachers use strategies to support this type of self-management skill development, such as posting a daily schedule of classroom activities, establishing classroom routines for common tasks such as collecting homework, and developing transition activities that prepare students for a change in classroom focus. As students gain skills, they are expected to be more independent on both individual and group tasks, including initiating and arranging time to complete the task, pacing task performance, and carrying out task steps in the correct sequence. Dramatic decreases are seen in impulsivity and increases in personal error detection during the ages from 6 to 10. The development of these self-management skills allows for the maturation of ADL skills described later in this chapter.

Cognitive maps are higher-level cognitive functions that we use to construct and accumulate spatial knowledge, allowing the "mind's eye" to visualize images and enhance recall and learning of information. Cognitive maps are mental representations of physical locations that help us find our way and remember important features of the environment. More simply, cognitive maps help you remember how to

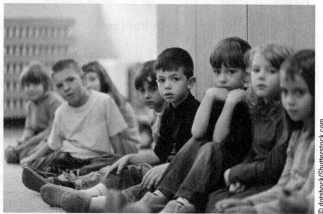

Figure 13-7   These 5-year-olds are learning to wait quietly as part of their introduction to school. This skill requires self-regulation and social awareness.

get around in your own house and, in a more complex situation, help you reason where the bathroom might be, based on past experience. Cognitive mapping emerges in middle childhood and continues to develop through adolescence. It is the conceptual tool that provides the foundation for geometry and the visual analysis of information in charts and graphs (Chown, Booker, & Kaplan, 2001). Cognitive maps are widely used in school and in IADL tasks to improve temporal organization, the orderly and logical sequencing of steps and sequences of a task from start to finish.

Experience of Time and Self Functions

Understanding basic time concepts is a component of most elementary curricula. **Temporal awareness** is a complex understanding of the passage of time. It is not about time in the academic sense but rather as it relates to the planning, sequencing, and altering of movements. Temporal awareness manifests in many ways, including the experience of the passage of time, in the experience of the movement of objects across space, and in the experience of timing in the sense of music and rhythms. As children encounter schedules and time sequences in their daily life, they become more aware of the temporal aspects of everyday life. Temporal awareness give the child a sort of "mental timer" that he or she can use to determine how fast to run to catch a ball or calculate whether you have enough time for a snack before catching the bus. Droit-Volet and Zélanti (2013) developed an experiment to test the time sensitivity of children as compared to adults. These scientists found that time sensitivity was present but fairly general in 5-year-olds, and that it developed based on age and experience throughout middle childhood. This study involved a complex time bisection task, but temporal awareness manifests functionally in repetitive motor activities, including skipping rope, playing the piano, and in the completion of ADLs and academic tasks within a specific time period. Practically, the ability to judge the relative time from a past event or until a future event in terms of the calendar year develops between 7 and 10 years of age (Feldman, 2011).

Spatial Awareness

Spatial awareness is the process through people become aware of the relative positions of their own bodies and objects around them. This awareness provides cues, such as depth and distance which are important for movement and orientation to the environment. By the age of 6, children have developed a **body schema,** a specialized form of spatial awareness that manifests as an internalized sense of the space that their body occupies and the space immediately surrounding our bodies (Holmes & Spence, 2004). The child's body schema combines somatic awareness with experiential memory of movement potential. In other words, the body schema is how children answer questions like, "Will I fit into that box?" or "Can I get to the door without brushing against that tree?" As children move and challenge their physical abilities, they gain cognitive information about the limits of their body, the body schema. Without the experience of self-controlled movement, this schema is probably slower to develop.

Body schema is the foundation for understanding spaces external to an individual. One of the primary strategies taught to parents of children with severe visual impairments is a variety of play activities to enhance the development of body schema. Typical children with poorly developed body schema often appear clumsy in middle childhood but are able to function in routine activities by compensating with their visual skills. Children with low vision do not have a backup system to use in compensation and can become quite fearful and resistive of both movement and large group activities without the support of a well-developed body schema.

Spatial awareness is also the understanding of both near and far space around an individual and is assessed by the accuracy in locating items within that space. Spatial awareness in a 6-year-old may be limited to planning how to toss a paper into a wastebasket. By the age of 10, children are not only aware of space in a dynamic manner but are beginning to plan using cognitive maps of the space.

Children organize their actions into a logical series of steps, and this is a *cognitive map* that leads them from task initiation, continuing each step of the activity in a logical and effective way until they complete the task. When they initiate an activity (for example, setting the table), school-age children mix logical order with impulse, perhaps putting out the plates before the placemats, observing, and then moving the plates to place the mats under them. With practice, the sequence improves, and the order of task completion increasingly makes sense.

ASYNCHRONOUS DEVELOPMENT

The term **asynchronous development** describes a situation in which the normal developmental progression is highly uneven. In intellectually gifted children, the gap between the children's intellectual capability and their age-appropriate social and physical skills can lead to frustration and emotional distress. This problem is especially apparent in the preschool years as young children become frustrated when their limited physical capabilities prevent them from acting on their ideas, or from producing the physical products that they imagine.

Asynchronous development occurs whenever the physical and cognitive developments are markedly uneven. An example pediatric therapists often see is a child with severe motor impairments, like cerebral palsy, and intact abilities to reason. When these children see and understand what goes on around them but lack the ability to communicate with others, to explore and experiment, and to act on their ideas, they become withdrawn and often angry. In both highly gifted children and children with good cognitive skills and severe motor impairment, the children are at greater risk for developing social and emotional problems.

Typically developing children learn self-efficacy through play, as they explore and experiment with the world around them. Children with an asynchronous pattern of development are more likely to feel helpless, and to experience distress and anxiety in response to everyday experiences. Without the motor skills to communicate, these children do not learn routine social exchanges and may be limited to squeals or grunts to get attention. They know that this is not normal but know no options to gain skill in communicating. Megan, a nonverbal 8-year-old with severe athetoid cerebral palsy, has a wide array of eye gestures that her family has learned to read to communicate with her. She does not have any verbal language, and her eye communication system does not work well with outsiders. After her initial attempts at communication with peers failed in the preschool setting, Megan did not try to initiate interaction and was very passive in all the daily classroom activities. Megan learned that she was not effective and could not actively engage others. Megan had learned that she was helpless.

Learned helplessness is a pattern of behavior that occurs when a person is faced with unsolvable problems. When children feel they have little or no ability to improve upon their situation, they may give up as Megan did. Learned helplessness perpetuates itself: As children try less, they have less opportunity for success. So, returning to the example of Megan, if she refuses to try to interact with her age peers, over time her isolation will increase and she will not gain the developmental skills she will need to succeed in school and in social interactions (Feldman, 2011). Dependency, whether caused by physical impairments, by medical treatment regimes, or by overprotective parents, creates social and emotional barriers for children (Allen, Vessey, & Shapiro, 2009). Learned helplessness can occur in any individual, but children with asynchronous patterns of development are at far greater risk of developing this debilitating behavior. Much of what teachers and therapists of children with asynchronous development do is focus on ways that children can perform and participate at levels acceptable to them.

ACTIVITIES AND PARTICIPATION

In the ICF, the category of "activities and participation" includes learning, communication, mobility, self-care, interpersonal relationships, and community life (World Health Organization, 2001). Although children engage in a great variety of complex daily occupations and have many skills and interests, children have relatively little control about how their time is structured (Rodger & Ziviani, 2006). Hofferth and Sandberg (2001) reported that children spend an average of 55 percent of their time performing ADL activities (this includes sleeping, eating, and self-care), 15 percent in school or day

care, and the remaining 30 percent in discretionary activities. In a follow-up study, Hofferth (2009) reported that since the 2001 report, video game play and television viewing increased, and other play, sleep, sports, and outdoor activities declined. She summarized this finding in the statement "every additional hour per week spent playing video games or watching television resulted in 7 to 10 fewer minutes playing, sleeping, reading, and studying" (p. 127). In this chapter, we will focus on those specific aspects of activities and participation that are a focus of developing children. These important developmental challenges are in the areas of communication, interpersonal interactions, and the major life area of education and the area of community, social, and civic life.

ACTIVITIES OF DAILY LIVING

Independence in basic self-care activities is usually achieved in middle childhood. Typically developing children entering school at age 5 will be toilet trained and self-sufficient in eating and simple hygiene. These children will be able to manage their clothes generally, but may frequently need help with fasteners or some other aspect of the dressing task. In this chapter, we will address the mastery of activities of daily living (ADLs), the emergence of skills in instrumental activities of daily living (IADLs), and the development of play and social interaction skills to allow participation in a wide range of social activities outside of the home.

Rodger and Ziviani (2006) note that the amount of time that is allocated to ADLs varies greatly across age and cultural groups. In general, as children mature, they spend less time in basic ADL activities. Although children develop few new ADL skills, their performance of these skills gains sophistication as they mature. **Table 13-2** shows a progression of ADL skill performance from early school age to preadolescence common in Western cultures.

Elias, who is being treated for cancer will have extended periods of illness and immobilization. This will not only interfere with his ability to explore new roles and new ADL skills, it may lead to some regression. In response to his pain and fatigue, adult caregivers are likely to do things for Elias that he had been doing on his own. This is a natural way of nurturing and supporting him. Even though it is a form of nurturing, it will be important to include Elias in decisions about what he will and won't do for himself. If having an adult helper causes him discomfort, either because of his loss of privacy or his loss of independence, it would be best to explore modifications to those tasks that allow him to do them partially. Although this may not be physically necessary, it may provide him with important emotional support.

COMMUNICATION FUNCTIONS

In typically developing children, communicative language development includes expressive and receptive language skills that parallel the children's developing cognitive skills. In

TABLE 13-2 Self-Care Skill Progression

ADL Tasks	Middle Childhood	Preadolescence
Bathing/Showering	Takes bath or shower with parental reminder, may require supervision in early years.	Independent in initiating and performing bathing or showering.
Eating	Able to eat all types and textures of food using familiar utensils.	No change.
Hair Care	Able to effectively brush hair.	Able to effectively wash, brush, and style hair.
Meal Preparation	Can fix a simple cold meal, such as a bowl of cereal or a sandwich.	Varies with practice, but potentially able to prepare complete meal.
Dressing	Able to dress and undress independently; may require assistance with fasteners and in putting shoes on the right feet in the early years; needs parental guidance choosing correct clothing for environmental context.	Dresses independently; is able to dress appropriately for the weather and other environmental contexts; has developed a sense of clothing preferences that are expressed in clothing choice.
Personal Hygiene	Able to manage basic personal hygiene and toileting tasks independently.	Gains new skills based on culture and gender; may apply deodorant, floss teeth, apply makeup.
Communication/Safety	Can convey important information and seek help from appropriate adults; remembers to keep in touch via cell phone when this is expected by parents. Can dial and initiate a telephone call (without using speed dial).	May choose to communicate with peers rather than parent. Increased skill in using text messages and computers as reading level increases.
Personal Device Care	Will require supervision with managing assistive devices such as glasses, contact lenses, hearing aids, and orthoses.	With instruction and practice, will be able to manage assistive devices such as glasses, contact lenses, hearing aids, and orthoses.
Sleep/Rest	Needs parental supervision and prompting to manage bed times and wake-up times.	Is able to take responsibility for waking self up in the morning for school; may continue to need bedtime prompts.

middle childhood, children can engage in constructive conversation with a variety of relevant questions. Their conversations are designed to reflect culturally prescribed rules, including manners and traditions for interacting with elders and members of the opposite sex. Children are gaining experience and understanding of social contexts, and in the later part of middle childhood, they begin to grasp the double meanings of words, which enables them to understand metaphors, riddles, and puns (American Speech and Hearing Association, 2012).

In middle childhood, children also become skilled at initiating and maintaining conversations. One of the skills children learn in this period is how to introduce and respond to conversational "icebreakers." An icebreaker is something attractive or fun, that attracts people and leads them into conversation. An icebreaker can be as simple as wearing a team jersey for a sports team that you follow, so that other fans feel free to talk and share their feelings about your team. An icebreaker can be more deliberate, such as telling a joke or asking a leading question. Children model the strategies of the adults around them in introducing and maintaining conversations, and gain skill not only in "icebreaking" but also in taking turns and controlling impulses to interrupt ongoing conversations.

In studies of adult men and women, men tend to be direct and forceful in their speech and to interrupt others. Women are more likely to express support for others' ideas and to be collaborative in their speech (Shinn & O'Brien, 2008). Although these gender differences are apparent in parents' communication with other adults and with their children, recent studies show no consistent gender differences in communication patterns among school-age children. Shinn and O'Brien (2008) comment that "the lack of gender differences found in the present study may be due to the fact that children in middle childhood have moved away from early stereotypes of gender roles but have not yet experienced gender intensification" (p. 66).

As the social experience of children expands through exposure to the school environment, children learn to tailor their communications to their audience. They learn to speak appropriately to teachers, classmates, and other adults. Although difference in communication across genders may not be evident, there are communication differences within peer groups. Murphy and Faulkner (2006) found that popular girls were most likely to use directives, elaborated disagreements and descriptors, rule reminders, and specific clarification requests. Unpopular girls were the least likely to use these strategies. Popular and unpopular boys showed levels intermediate to those of the girls. Murphy and Faulkner (2006) also reported a higher frequency of domineering communication acts for both popular girls and popular boys than for their unpopular partners. This study suggests that in middle childhood, popularity rather than gender was a stronger influence on communication patterns.

In the school setting, children are increasingly exposed to the written word, and they gain both increased spoken vocabulary and written communication skills over time. Because difficulties with written communication are a common reason for children to be referred to occupational therapy, it is important to remember that written communication is fundamentally a language-based skill. Improving the hand skills in children with a language delay may improve fine motor control but will not necessarily have any impact on their written communication.

SCHOOL FUNCTION

In middle childhood, one of the most influential social institutions is the children's school environment. For most children, the middle childhood years include extended periods of time away from home in a school setting. In the school setting, children gain experience with adults who are not part of their family and with people from differing backgrounds. Through their experiences in school and among others in their community, children gain a sense of personal identity and self-concept. As participants in school, children learn to engage in all school-related responsibilities and privileges, and in learning the course material. They must also learn to work cooperatively with other students, taking direction from teachers.

INTERPERSONAL RELATIONSHIPS

In middle childhood, children begin to build a sense of identity that extends beyond their external physical traits. In their interactions with age peers, children begin to evaluate their own abilities and behaviors by comparing them to others. From this comparison, called social referencing, children develop a coping tool for dealing with ambiguous situations. Social referencing is first noted in infancy babies look at the facial expressions of others to help themselves decide what to do. By the time they are in school, children learn to imitate the behaviors of others in new and novel situations. This allows them to have tools to ease into interpersonal relationships and social exchanges across contexts and situations. Children

who are developmentally different may use social referencing to speculate on their own strengths and weakness and the long-term impact of their impairment or developmental difference. Elias will be observant of his classmates' responses to him, and these responses will fuel his own changing self-concept. Similarly, when Elias returns to school with a prosthetic leg, his classmates will look to each other and to the adults in the school to gauge their reaction to Elias. Social referencing is a significant influence on the development of a context-appropriate self-concept and on determining socially acceptable behavior.

Related to social referencing is social knowledge. Social knowledge is learned through interpersonal relationships and experience in social contexts. Children's ability to understand and interpret peer relationships becomes increasingly important to this age group. Dodge, Murphy, and Buchsbaum (1984) were pioneers in this area of research, describing five steps in acquiring social knowledge:

1. Decoding social cues

2. Interpreting social cues

3. Searching for a response

4. Selecting an optimal response

5. Taking action

Social knowledge is involved in all aspects of peer relations, classroom cooperation, friendships, and aggression. By middle childhood, children have learned to be cautious in their responses to physical disability. Although preschool children might easily walk up to a person with a leg amputation and ask "where did you put your leg?," by middle childhood children are more likely to remain quiet and only look at the person when they feel unobserved. The social knowledge that an amputation is unfortunate and undesirable will make Elias's transition back to school and to peer group participation more challenging. Dodge and colleagues (2003) have performed 20 years of research on social-knowledge skill as an influence on aggression and friendship behaviors. They found that early peer rejection predicts growth in aggression, especially in boys. The children in **Figure 13-8** have compensated for their varying ages to successfully negotiate social referencing and friendship formation.

Friends and other peers are important influences in middle childhood. Friends offer emotional support, social knowledge, and improved communication skills (Yu, Ostrosky, & Fowler, 2011). In their early friendships, children learn emotional self-regulations, communication skills, and gain social knowledge (Guralnick, Neville, Hammond, & Connor, 2007). Friendships provide a sense of belonging and security and lessen the stress of navigating school and growing social expectations (Rubin, Bukowski, & Parker, 2006). Additionally, cooperation with peers and close friendships in middle childhood are related to enduring happiness and well-being (Berndt, 2004; Holder & Coleman, 2009).

Friendships in the preschool years are changeable and largely determined by the access children have to one

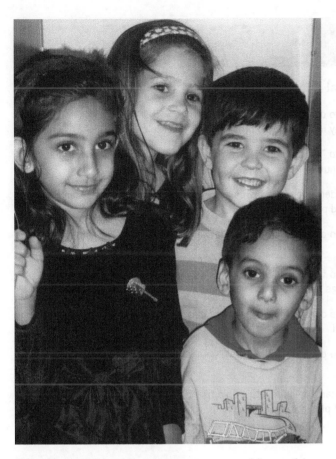

Figure 13-8   Children of varying ages can successfully negotiate social referencing and friendship information.

another. In middle childhood, friendships become more adultlike, based on mutual affection in a relationship that is voluntary, not based on "playdates" arranged by parents or a role assigned by a teacher (Bowker, Rubin, Burgess, Booth-LaForce, & Rose-Krasnor, 2006).

This is the time of intense peer contexts, including play in "forts," secret hideouts, summer camps, and clubs. During middle childhood, children develop a distinct peer culture in which the rules differ from those common in their interactions with adults. In the earlier discussion of communication, the distinctive peer-specific patterns of communication based on popularity reflect this peer culture. Social competence emerges as the smooth, sequential, appropriate use of social skills like humor, reading nonverbal behavior, and understanding social conventions in a dynamic way across contexts (Feldman, 2011). Social competence is associated with popularity.

A final construct relevant to children's growing social network is *social capital*. Social capital is the presence (or absence) of some tangible resource that is valued within a social network, something that will afford the owner of the resource preferential treatment. For example, a young girl whose family owns a business that offers horseback riding lessons may be sought after as a friend among her classmates who love horses. Being pretty, athletic, extroverted, or any other naturally occurring

attribute valued by the culture can be social capital. Social capital is a sort of currency, a social value that makes others want to be part of your social circle, to be a friend. Social capital, then, can increase friendship opportunities.

In Chapter 15, issues associated with having a disability during childhood will be discussed. One common experience of many children with disabilities is that they lack access to many common types of social capital. This means that they will have to work harder to be noticed and to be accepted into a social group. Sometimes an important consideration for therapists working with children who are developing differently is to help those children develop some type of social capital. The social capital might be a tablet computer that assists with communication in a school classroom when most students do not have their own computer. Social capital could be fluency with a local interest, such as a sports team or recreational activity. Building therapy activities in a manner that builds or develops social capital can help extend the positive impact of the therapeutic intervention into the school and community setting.

MAJOR LIFE AREAS

The ICF category of "activities and participation" includes a subcategory focused on the activities of carrying out the tasks and actions required to engage in education, work, and employment, and to conduct economic transactions. This category, called "major life areas," becomes of interest as children move from the home environment into school and the community (WHO, 2001).

School Tasks and Demands

Although the focus of public education is to acquire academic skills, children develop many other crucial functional skills in the school environment. As children progress through school, they have less teacher direction and a greater demand for independence in their assignments and in managing their time. Although much attention is focused on the academic portion of school, the school curricula are often very specific on subject areas like mathematics, reading, and science while offering no official curricula goals in school participation. School participation includes interactions in instructional settings, effective organizational strategies, involvement in testing activities, and peer interactions. Although individuals vary greatly in the sequence and timing of self-management skill acquisition, by the age of 11, most children are in self-care, mobility, and social function as illustrated in **Table 13-3**.

School Activity Performance

In middle childhood, postural control should include the necessary trunk control and balance needed to perform expected occupations. The balance skills expand as sports and other athletic pursuits become more common. This is a time when children may develop specialized skills in dance, gymnastics,

TABLE 13-3   Development of Mobility and Social Function in Middle Childhood

Mobility	Social Function
Able to move effectively between standing and sitting in a variety of situations and on rough and uneven surfaces.	Able to demonstrate comprehension of verbal instructions and to convey information to others that is clear in meaning.
Able to get in and out of vehicles, including cars and buses.	Able to "keep working" with an age peer on a single task for at least 30 minutes.
Able to move at the same speed and distance as the crowd in corridors and out of doors.	Considers the preferences and interests of friends when planning shared play activities.
Able to pick up and carry large objects (such as a chair) from one room to another.	Able to demonstrate good safety awareness in familiar situations.
Able to manage stairs and ladders within routine environments.	Able to function independently in a variety of familiar community settings without assistance.
Can use a house key to unlock and open a typical door to a house or apartment.	Able to control their behavior and avoid problem behaviors during school.
Child can play hopscotch or jump rope, or other games that involve hopping.	Able to play competitive table games, and follow the rules.
Is able to engage in intense physical activity for extended periods, as in sports participation.	Child can communicate with a friend using the telephone, computer, or cell phone without adult help.

martial arts, and team sports. School aged children are expected to reach to grasp objects that they need when they are on the floor, in a desk, or across a counter in the school cafeteria. In middle childhood, bilateral-coordination skills mature, and increased dexterity and improved in-hand manipulation are seen as students shift and adjust their pencils, open condiment packets, and develop skill with musical instruments. These new skills may continue to be conscious but become habits with practice and no longer need cognitive direction.

Many complex bimanual skills are needed in the school setting. These include carrying both single objects and trays full of objects, opening and closing all types of doors, moving through a line (such as a cafeteria serving line), gathering needed objects in a reasonable time, managing a backpack or book bag full of books, and safely carrying fragile objects.

Children in school settings are expected to have a well-developed hand dominance and good finger dexterity. Handwriting is a part of most academic programs, and the expectation that children have both the motor skills and the strength to write long paragraphs and essays is common in classrooms of 10- and 11-year-old children. Many children now begin to use the computer at the same age that they learn to write, with text messaging possible at the same time, as shown in **Figure 13-9**. Children can manage the computer mouse and game controllers long before they can type effectively. Children in this age are often very fast and accurate with text messaging and other forms of fine motor skills associated with the use of electronic communication devices. Although touch-

typing is not taught in most primary curricula, the tactile kinesthetic awareness needed for effective typing is becoming increasingly important in the school setting.

CARRYING OUT DAILY ROUTINE

By the age of 8, children's school participation includes carrying out daily routines. Children begin to learn simple routines in early childhood and become increasingly able to organize their time and materials to initiate and complete tasks independently. To gain these skills in a functional manner that generalizes between situations, children must begin to abstract and generalize ideas and consider new features of the environment and how they might affect performance of a desired task. Although many routines can be taught in a rote fashion, they will remain isolated to the conditions under which they were taught if the children are not able to manipulate information, integrate new features, and solve problems as they present themselves. These are higher-level mental manipulations that emerge in middle childhood and continue to develop into adulthood.

Many instrumental activities of daily living (IADLs) emerge in middle childhood. Most children of this age help with household and classroom chores. At first they serve as assistants, like the young girl helping her father with the laundry in **Figure 13-10**, and by preadolescence have several independent IADL skills. Children begin to do chores, and many also begin to earn their own money. In middle childhood, children begin to learn to manage money, plan, and shop.

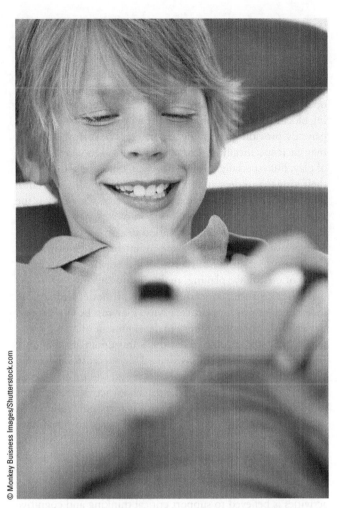

Figure 13-9   Both text messaging and many gaming systems require excellent dexterity skills. The use of texting and social media with parental support has been found to strengthen children's literacy skills.

Young people today consider mobile phone/Internet literacy an essential skill for everyday life. Mobile phones are now seen as an essential part of social communication, and they are seen in tools in developing and maintaining friendships. This requires not only fine finger dexterity, but planning and memory for tasks like keeping the phone charged, bringing the phone with you, sending text messages, checking messages, and other telephone maintenance tasks. This new IADL should be considered when planning strategies to help school-age children function effectively with their peers.

Between the ages of 9 and 12, most children develop the initiative and sense of personal responsibility to assume full care of pets and to be held responsible for chores at home and in the community. By the end of middle childhood, typically developing children can manage money and social interactions to make a purchase and collect the correct change. Another IADL that may develop is the ability to be responsible for the care of pets. In **Figure 13-11**, a young girl poses with her horse. She has not only learned to ride, but she also has learned to care for her horse.

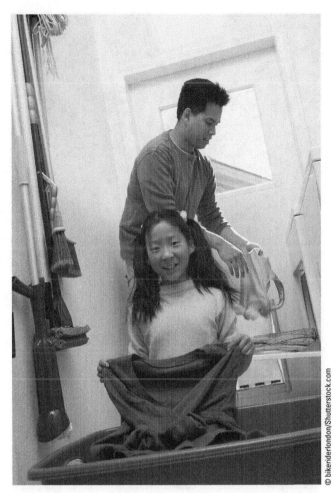

Figure 13-10   IADL skills emerge with practice and supervision, beginning in middle childhood. With practice and supervision, children can become very skilled in these tasks.

Chapter 7 includes a description of service animals as supports for people with disabilities. Most organizations will not consider providing a service animal for children less than 12 years of age, because they may not yet have developed the maturity to care for the animal and to maintain its training.

PLAY AND LEISURE

Leisure is free time spent away from school, work, and domestic chores that involves self-direction and self-discovery. With their growing ability to engage in occupations, children in middle childhood are first able to appreciate leisure time. Many of the typically developing children's leisure pursuits will involve some form of play. As we described in Chapter 12, play is a self-directed, enjoyable, and intrinsically motivated activity in which individuals engage. It is often said that play is the work of children. What is meant by this is that when making things during play, whether scripts for action figures or cardboard castles, children are also building "the cognitive platform for their future skills" (Gauntlett & Thomsen, 2013). Playfulness is

be parallel and less rule-driven, with conflicts solved by compromise rather than competition (Feldman, 2011).

Play with objects continues to be effective as a skill development tool in middle childhood, but the objects or the use of the objects become more sophisticated, often utilizing open-ended constructional tools like art materials and building blocks. Play with objects may or may not be adult-directed play. By providing appealing art materials or costumes, adults may elicit specifically desired play activities. Through all forms of play, but especially through play with objects, children show their growing understanding of the world and culture around them, and are able to demonstrate creativity. Creativity is the ability to make or otherwise bring into existence something new, whether a new game, a solution to a problem, or an artistic expression. Creativity, like play, is intrinsically motivated.

Gauntlett and Thomsen (2013) describe three components of creativity: playing, making, and sharing.

There is some concern that play in modern urbanized societies does not support creativity. Play can be constrained by several factors, including the development of a risk-averse society, the separation of individuals from the natural world, and the focus on early educational achievement. In some cases, children have highly structured days that include a school day and then a series of structured after-school activities chosen to build skills in sports or other pursuits. Although children in middle childhood have the ability and interest in scheduling their own time and their own activities, many parents continue to organize their activities in an attempt to give them "the best," or more pragmatically, to assure that they are supervised while the parents are at work. Engagement in creative play activities is believed to support critical thinking and cognitive flexibility later in life (LaMore et al., 2013).

VIRTUAL PLAY

Virtual (digital) play is play involving digital technologies activity that is chosen as a form of leisure (rather than as a school or learning activity).

Increasingly, children are utilizing digital technologies in their play. These technologies not only are interactive, but they also allow types of play that were not previously possible, such as online gaming, in which a group of friends can interact from their own homes through a massive multiplayer online game (also called MMO). An MMO is a multiplayer game format that is capable of supporting large numbers of players simultaneously. These games can be found for most network-capable platforms, including the personal computer, video game console, or smartphones. Unlike the passive experience of watching television, these MMOs allow players to cooperate and compete with one another, practicing the same social behavior skills in which they might engage in face-to-face games. These MMOs can be engaged in individually but are often social and communal and nearly always involve competition and intellectual challenge.

Game devices and smartphones are very common play and social platforms in this age group. Children carry them

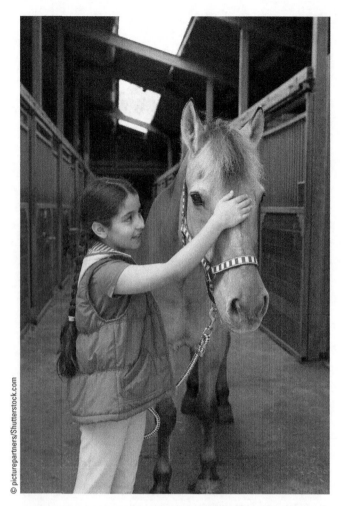

Figure 13-11   Children learn from the opportunities in their daily life. This girl has learned to responsibly care for an animal while gaining social and physical skills as she explores equestrian sports.

strongly related to cognitive development and emotional well-being. Play has a central role in the development of linguistic and other representational abilities as introduced in Chapter 12. In addition, playful interactions support the development of metacognitive and self-regulatory abilities (Whitebread, 2010). Play in middle childhood includes all of the forms of play described in Chapter 12, but it also includes the expanded arenas of sports, nature exploration, and unstructured leisure time. In middle childhood, children's play activities become very gender segregated. In play environments, boys and girls may actively avoid one another. This gender segregation occurs in most human societies at this age (Feldman, 2011). This segregation means that friendship patterns tend to be same-sex friendships, and gender differences in play become evident (Berndt, 2004). It has been consistently observed that boys tend to have larger networks of friends, tend to play in groups, and engage more in aggressive rough-and-tumble play. Boys' games often have winners and losers, and there is a striving for hierarchy and dominance within the group; arguments are often a part of these games. Girls tend to focus on one or two "best friends" who are of relatively equal status. Girls' play was more likely to

with them to most of their activity environments, including in the car, on public transportation, and on playgrounds. Television and DVD viewing are types of virtual leisure that have become primary preferred activities of many school-age children (McHale, Couter, & Tucker, 2001; Wright et al., 2001). These are passive forms of entertainment and should not be considered play unless they include some interactive or creative element.

GAMES WITH RULES

The form of play described as "games with rules" is broad and includes solitary as well as social activities. A game is structured activity that may be playful, or may be part of an athletic or educational competition. Games, even solitary games, involve rules that involve two or more sides, competition, and agreed-upon criteria for determining a winner. Rules are subject to variations and changes, and children often negotiate rules in order to create the game they wish to play. Games with rules can be virtual or face-to-face. A category of games with rules in which there is extensive participation in this age group is in the category of sports. Children between the ages of 6 and 17 have the highest degree of sports participation of any age group in the United States (Sporting Goods Manufacturers Association, 2013). Participation in sports is highly valued in Western cultures, not only in supporting healthy lifestyles, but also in teaching sportsmanship and goal-focused behaviors. Sports teach useful lessons, such as the value of practice and the value of persisting in the face of failures.

As noted earlier in this chapter, children in this age group are very physically able, but have immature skeletal systems. This means that serious sports injuries may have more lasting effects than they would have later in life.

FREE PLAY

There is extensive evidence that time dedicated to free unstructured, child-directed play stimulates learning and creativity (The Lego Foundation, 2010). For many children, middle childhood is a period for passionate and obsessive interests that they can pursue given periods of unstructured time. Fascinations with animals or sports are commonly described in this age group. Although there are lists of favored hobbies and free-time activities, these tend to be very regional and culturally influenced. In her study of activity preferences in children, Griffiths (2011) noted that "some of the children in the sample felt under pressure to demonstrate that they 'did something' during their free time, possibly to please me (in my role as researcher/adult), others apologetically confessed that they 'did nothing.'" Further elaborating on this, the author reported that the children "revealed some intriguing and quirky interests which they did not consider to be 'proper' ways to spend time" (p. 197). An example of these potentially "improper" activity choices is "hanging out with my cousin." When Griffiths asked what they did together, "the initial

response of 'not anything really'" transformed into rich discussion of how they "tell each other stories about scary things and stuff" (p. 197). The picture of activities that emerged from Griffith's study included interacting in important relationships with others (this could be parents, friends, and so on), interaction and exploration in their immediate physical environment, indoor activities (such as computer gaming), and outdoor activities (social games involving group play, and camping, walking, and hiking). Free play, whether solitary or social, is associated with the development of creativity and enhanced learning (The Lego Foundation, 2010).

ENVIRONMENTAL CONTEXTS AND CULTURE

The social skills needed in peer play contexts will be different from those needed among peers at school and in peer interactions involving teachers, coaches, and counselors who structure activities. The expanding performance arenas of middle childhood offers exposure to new environmental and cultural contexts. Through social referencing, children use their peer group and friendships to model their social and interpersonal behavior as they explore new performance contexts. This tendency to model peers in middle childhood has lent the greatest support for *inclusion* in the school setting. **Inclusion** in education means that all students in a school, regardless of their strengths or weaknesses in any area, are part of the regular school community. There is evidence to support the theory that children with cognitive impairments and other developmental differences develop more appropriate and positive social interaction when placed with typically developing peers. There has been some evidence that inclusive education practices do result in improved social behavior for many children (Vogler, Koranda, & Romance, 2000), but the bulk of the evidence is quite mixed or openly negative (Graham & Slee, 2008). Although inclusive education was originally promoted as optimal for all children, there is evidence that children with impairments placed in the regular classroom often have fewer social interactions and a low friendship status in peer groups (Cheney, Osher, & Caesar, 2002; Ridsdale & Thompson, 2002). This is especially true with children who have compromised ability to perceive nonverbal communication in others, particularly children with hearing impairments, autism, and some types of learning disabilities (Stoutjesdijk, Scholte, & Swaab, 2012). Bullying and victimization are common in middle childhood, with almost 85 percent of girls and 80 percent of boys experiencing some form of harassment in school at least once (Feldman, 2011). *Bullying* can include many things, and can occur at any time in the life span, but most bullying in middle childhood occurs in school. **Bullying** is a form of aggressive behavior perpetuated by either an individual or a group that involves the use of force or coercion directed repeatedly toward particular victims. Peer reports agree that bullying includes hitting and pushing, threatening people, and forcing people to do things they don't want to do (Boulton, Trueman, & Flemington, 2002). In this research, "fewer pupils, but still more than half, agreed that 'name calling,' 'telling nasty stories about other people,' and 'taking people's belongings' were types of bullying" (Boulton, Trueman, & Flemington, 2002, p. 353). During middle childhood, bullying and victimization are often directed at children who are loners and those who are fairly passive (Feldman, 2011)

Both friendship and bullying patterns have changed recently with the wide availability of cell phones and the Internet for children of all ages. *Cyberbullying* is deliberately using digital media to communicate false, embarrassing, or hostile information about another person. Cyberbullying can include abuse using email, text messaging, "tweeting," blogging, video messages, and posting to social networking sites. Cyberbullying has gotten public attention because it has led to suicides and other tragedies in both adolescents and young adults. Although more prevalent in older individuals, cyberbullying is a growing concern for people caring for school-age children. Hannah (2010) estimated that 25 to 30 percent of children and adolescents have experienced cyberbullying. Because cyberbullies can pose as someone else, this is the most anonymous form of bullying (Bolton & Graeve, 2005).

Poverty

There is a significant correlation between child poverty and higher risk for physical, cognitive, social, emotional, and behavioral problems, and higher rates of poverty, crime, and poor health in adulthood (West Virginia Center for Budget and Policy, 2013). Poverty places children at greater risk for many difficulties, and in some cases, decreased opportunities for play. In middle childhood, poverty can lead to poor motor skills, and more accidents and injuries. It can also lead to substandard nutrition that is another health risk factor. Children living in poverty are more likely to have cognitive difficulties, such as poor academic performance, especially in the early grades. Poverty also is associated with high levels of personal stress and puts children at risk for mental health problems. All of the patterns become more significant as the degree of poverty becomes greater (West Virginia Center for Budget and Policy, 2013).

Adult Social Contexts

Although growth in peer relationships and friendships is one of the central developmental tasks of middle childhood, the family remains a central and vital source of support and influence on children. As noted earlier in this chapter, children have increasing interest in and opportunities for being alone. The children are growing in independence and are not as closely supervised as they were in the preschool years. As children move through the years of middle childhood, they transition from having their time and activities almost completely controlled by their parents to having increasing control of their daily occupations.

This period, during which both the parents and the children share control of everyday behaviors, is called co-regulation. **Co-regulation** is when one person (for example the child) takes an action (buying a nutritious lunch) in response to another person's action (a parent's request). In this example, the child responds to the parent's guidance, but at school what she chooses for lunch is really her choice, not her parent's choice.

As they participate more in school, sports, and community activities, school-age children meet and may be influenced by adults other than their parents. Many of these interactions will be positive, but children in this period are highly impressionable, and may become victims for sexual predators. Although caution is urged in both the content and time spent engaged in electronic play, the medium of the Internet in particular has afforded some new and positive opportunities for children's social development. The parameters of Internet play (anonymity, interactivity, and connectivity) provide a nonthreatening format in which to explore roles and personal identity (Maczewski, 2002; Subrahmanyam, Greenfield, Kraut, & Gross, 2001). Many organizations associated with specific conditions or special interests have Internet sites and web-based forums. Although research has not caught up with the explosive development in this area, it appears that the Internet may provide an audience of peers with similar experiences and a forum for self-expression and peer support (Jones, Zahl, & Huws, 2001).

SUMMARY

The period of middle childhood is characterized by the understanding of one's self and one's culture beyond the home. The greatest developmental demands of this period are associated with active participation in school and community environments. Children gain in independence and competence in IADLs and begin to develop unique interests and express themselves creatively through play and hobbies. This is a time when children explore their social world, and they increasingly explore the virtual communities available to them through cell phone use and social networking. As they branch out into the world beyond the family,

they may encounter new risks, including bullying, stress-related problems, and potentially, sports injuries.

Children with developmental differences or impairments are at a particular disadvantage because they now learn to measure themselves against their peers rather than by the more lenient adult measure of how far they have come. As children enter puberty, they have formed ideas about themselves and what their own strengths and weaknesses are that they will carry into adolescence. Through play and school friendships that endure, children learn to negotiate the complex interpersonal world of their community.

CASE 1

Elias . . . Continued

Elias will return to school after a year of surgeries and cancer treatments. With the prosthetic limb, Elias will have some difficulty participating in sports at school. In addition, he is likely to be self-conscious because of the appearance of the prosthesis, and being able to blend in with his peer groups rather than engage in activities that make it more apparent.

Guiding Questions

Some questions to consider:

1. In the long run, Elias should be able to return to playing many sports. Do you think this is something that should be addressed now, or do you think he should be discouraged from exploring sports until he has adjusted to the return to school? Why?
2. If you do an image search for "pediatric prostheses," you will see many types of artificial limbs. Some cosmetically look like the limb they are replacing, and some look like high-tech hardware. Which is better? Why do you think this?

Children's Cancer Research Fund (2012). Andrew's Story: Surviving Ewings Sarcoma. Retrieved from http://www.childrenscancer.org/main/andrews_story_surviving_ewings_sarcoma/

CASE 2

Chloe

Chloe, 6½ years old, had been diagnosed at birth with a lumbar (L1/L2) myeloeningocele and received a shunt for hydrocephalus. Chloe is in a regular first-grade class of 20 students. She gets assistance in school with toileting and with managing her lunch tray. The classroom assistant sits with Chloe while the other children participate in gym and play on the playground.

Chloe has a hip-knee-ankle gait orthosis that only occasionally comes with her to school. She does have a standing frame at school and is transported to and from school in a wheelchair with a pressure-relief cushion. She needs moderate assistance at school for transfers, and maximum assistance for tub transfers at home. Chloe is able to transfer from the chair to the floor, but only does this with much prompting because she is afraid of falling.

Chloe assists with dressing, but continues to have difficulty with zippers, small buttons, and shoelaces. She uses a knife, fork, and spoon during meals, with some spillage. She is unable to peel an orange or banana, and has difficulty opening Tupperware containers and the school milk boxes. Chloe is catheterized and is dependent in bowel and bladder care.

Chloe enjoys school and seems to make friends easily. She has been slow to develop writing skills, and writes with an immature static tripod grasp. At this time she can print her name and only a few additional letters

Continues

Case 2   *Continued*

of the alphabet. On standardized testing, Chloe had difficulty with the visual-perceptual skills of visual-spatial relations and visual-sequential memory. Although assured by the first-grade teacher that they would promote Chloe with her class, Chloe's parents are concerned by her poor writing, reading, and math skills.

Chloe says that she likes school, and wants to read better so she can stay in the reading group with her friend Julie. Chloe and her parents want her to be able to stay in the regular classroom (rather than special education). She has been referred for both OT and PT through the school system.

Guiding Questions

Some questions to consider:

1. The teacher would like ideas and support from the OT and PT in adapting classroom activities to integrate and include Chloe more. What ideas do you have to help Chloe?
2. Considering her limitations, which of these would be the top priority in helping Chloe do the schoolwork in the regular classroom? Why?

Speaking of
School Challenges

HANNAH McMONAGLE,
PARENT OF A YOUNG MAN WITH ASPERGER'S SYNDROME

The focus in schools today is that of academics, good grades, and sports. These are the things that my son Gregory does well. Gregory does well in academics, but he has difficulty making friends. When things happen that are out of order or unplanned, or he is losing a game, he will fly into a tantrum and wave his arms and cry very loudly. He will confront any teacher or group of teachers without a qualm. Teachers report that he is uncooperative and confrontational, and often will refuse to participate.

Last year Gregory was tested by many specialists and was diagnosed with Asperger's syndrome. The occupational therapy report showed that he had difficulty with certain tasks in school. His writing is often illegible, and his organization is poor in terms of how the work is set out. He often misses part of the written instructions. My own impression is that he has some form of learning disability and is often unable to get his thoughts on paper in any kind of coordinated fashion.

At his school I requested an IEP (special education support), and the school principal asked why I wanted it, as Gregory had very high standardized test scores. I was very annoyed by this comment and pointed out to her that my concern was that academics was only one part of the education. My concern was the education of the whole child; the schools seem to forget that social skills are a very important part of education.

Gregory sees everything in terms of black and white. Many of the social expressions that we take for granted, Gregory is unable to read. For example, if you tell him to sink or swim, he would interpret this literally. One day I was talking to Gregory and said, "I could have died," and his mouth fell wide open.

He is unable to look people in the eye and will look down and away when he is introduced to someone. In church he is unable to hold hands with anyone other than his brother or myself. If he is upset about something, he will shout loudly no matter where he is. He will not initiate conversation with other kids, but will stay on the fringe and might be drawn in after several sessions.

Gregory's grades are good, but will he be able to ever leave home and take care of himself? Will he be able to shop, ask for help, and manage the social expectations of college or a job? What is an education worth if it does not lead him toward a productive adult life? Why should the kids with obvious physical impairments but no difficulty with the social environment at school qualify for special help more easily than Gregory, whose limitations are invisible?

REFERENCES

Allen, P., Vessey, J., & Schapiro, N. (2009). *Primary care of the child with a chronic condition* (5th ed.). St. Louis: Mosby.

American Academy of Pediatrics. (2012). *Physical development of school age children.* Retrieved from http://www.healthychildren.org/English/ages-stages/gradeschool/puberty/pages/Physical-Development-of-School-Age-Children.aspx

American Speech and Hearing Association. (2012). *Typical speech and language development.* Retrieved from http://www.asha.org/public/speech/development/

Anderson, P., & Reidy, N. (2012). Assessing executive function in preschoolers. *Neuropsychology Review, 22*(4), 345–360.

Barrouillet, P., Gavens, N., Vergauwe, E., Gaillard, V., & Camos, V. (2009). Working memory span development: A time-based resource-sharing model account. *Developmental Psychology, 45*(2), 477–490.

Berndt, T. J. (2004). Children's friendships: Shifts over a half century in perspectives on their development and effects. *Merrill Palmer Quarterly, 50*(3), 206–223.

Bolton, J., & Graeve, S. (2005). No room for bullies: From the classroom to cyberspace teaching respect, stopping abuse, and rewarding kindness. Lincoln, NE: Boys Town Press.

Boulton, M. J., Trueman, M., & Flemington, I. (2002). Associations between secondary school pupils' definitions of bullying, attitudes toward bullying, and tendencies to engage in bullying: Age and sex differences. *Educational Studies 23*(4), 353–370.

Bowker, J., Rubin, K. H., Burgess, K. B., Booth-LaForce, C., & Rose-Krasnor, L. (2006). Behavioral characteristics associated with stable and fluid best friendship patterns in middle childhood. *Merrill-Palmer Quarterly, 52*(4), 671–693.

Cantlon, J. F., Davis, S. W., Libertus, M. E., Kahane, J., Brannon, E. M., & Pelphrey, K. A. (2011). Inter-parietal white matter development predicts numerical performance in young children. *Learning & Individual Differences, 21*(6), 672–680.

Cheney, D., Osher, T., & Caesar, M. (2002). Providing ongoing skill development and support for educators and parents of students with emotional and behavioral disabilities. *Journal of Child and Family Studies, 11,* 79–89.

Children's Cancer Research Fund. (2012). *Andrew's story: Surviving Ewing's sarcoma.* Retrieved from http://www.partnersinhope.org/andrew-january2014.html

Chown, E., Booker, L., & Kaplan, S. (2001). Perception, action planning, and cognitive maps. *Behavioral and Brain Sciences, 24,* 882–884.

Codina, C., Buckley, D., Port, M., & Pascalis, O. (2011). Deaf and hearing children: A comparison of peripheral vision development. *Developmental Science, 14*(4), 725–737.

Cardon, G., Campbell, J., & Sharma, A. (2012). Plasticity in the developing auditory cortex: Evidence from children with sensorineural hearing loss and auditory neuropathy spectrum disorder. *Journal of the American Academy of Audiology, 23*(6), 396–411.

Davis, E. E., Pitchford, N. J., & Limback, E. (2011). The interrelation between cognitive and motor development in typically developing children aged 4–11 years is underpinned by visual processing and fine manual control. *British Journal of Psychology, 102*(3), 569–584.

Debrabant, J., Gheysen, F., Vingerhoets, G., & Van Waelvelde, H. (2012). Age-related differences in predictive response timing in children: Evidence from regularly relative to irregularly paced reaction time performance. *Human Movement Science, 31*(4), 801–810.

Dodge, K., Lansford, J., Burks, V., Bates, J., Pettit, G., Fontaine, R., & Price, J. (2003). Peer rejection and social information-processing factors in the development of aggressive behavior problems in children. *Child Development, 74,* 374–394.

Dodge, K. A., Murphy, R. M., & Buchsbaum, K. (1984). The assessment of intention-cue detection skills in children: Implications for developmental psychopathology. *Child Development, 55,* 163–173.

Droit-Volet, S., & Zélanti, P. (2013). Development of time sensitivity: Duration ratios in time bisection. *Quarterly Journal of Experimental Psychology, 66*(4), 671–686.

Fass, P., and Mason, M. (2000). *Childhood in America.* New York: NYU Press.

Fass, P. (2007). Children of a new world: Society, culture and globalization. New York: New York University Press.

Feldman, R. (2011) *Child development* (6th ed.). Upper Saddle River, NJ: Prentice Hall.

Gauntlett , D., and Thomsen, B. (2013). *Cultures of creativity: Nurturing creative mindsets across cultures.* The Lego Foundation. Retrieved from http://www.legofoundation.com/en-us/research-and-learning/foundation-research/cultures-of-creativity/

Goggin, N. (2003). *KINE 3500 Lecture 4: Perceptual-motor development.* Accessed 4/23/2012 from http://www.coe.unt.edu/goggin/kine3500/350lec4.htm

Graham, L. J., & Slee, R. (2008). An illusory interiority: Interrogating the discourse/s of inclusion. *Educational Philosophy & Theory, 40*(2), 277–293.

Griffiths, M. (2011). Favoured free-time: Comparing children's activity preferences in the UK and the USA. *Children & Society, 25*(3), 190–201.

Groen, M. A., Whitehouse, A. O., Badcock, N. A., & Bishop, D. M. (2011). Where were those rabbits? A new paradigm to determine cerebral lateralisation of visuospatial memory function in children. *Neuropsychologia, 49*(12), 3265–3271.

Guralnick, M., Neville, B., Hammond, M., & Connor, R. (2007). The friendships of young children with developmental delays: A longitudinal analysis. *Journal of Applied Developmental Psychology, 28,* 64–79.

Hannah, M. (2010). Cyberbullying education for parents: A guide for clinicians. *Journal of Social Sciences, 6,* 530–534.

Henderson, A., & Pehoski, C. (Eds.). (2006). *Hand function in the child* (2nd ed.). St. Louis: Mosby.

Hill, E., & Khanem, F. (2009). The development of hand preference in children: The effect of task demands and links with manual dexterity. *Brain & Cognition, 71*(2), 99–107.

Hofferth, S. L., & Sandberg, J. E. (2001). How American children spend their time. *Journal of Marriage & Family, 63*(2), 295.

Hofferth, S. (2009). Media use vs. work and play in middle childhood. *Social Indicators Research, 93*(1), 127–129.

Holder, M. D., & Coleman, B. (2009). The contribution of social relationships to children's happiness. *Journal of Happiness Studies, 10,* 329–349.

Holmes, N., & Spence, C. (2004). The body schema and the multisensory representation(s) of peripersonal space. *Cognitive Processing, 5*(2), 94–105.

Hughes, C. (2011). Changes and challenges in 20 years of research into the development of executive functions. *Infant & Child Development, 20*(3), 251–271.

Hutchison, E. (2011) *Dimensions of human behavior: The changing life course* (4th ed.). Thousand Oaks, CA: Sage Publications.

Jones, R., Zahl, A., & Huws, J. (2001). First-hand accounts of emotional experiences in autism: A qualitative analysis. *Disability and Society, 16,* 393–401.

Karably, K. & Zabrucky, K. (2009). Children's metamemory: A review of the literature and implications for the classroom. *International Electronic Journal of Elementary Education, 2,* 32–52.

Kim, R., Nauhaus, G., Glazek, K., Young, D., & Lin, S. (2013). Development of coincidence-anticipation timing in a catching task. *Perceptual and Motor Skills, 117*(1), 1361–1380.

LaMore, R., Root-Bernstein, R., Root-Bernstein, M., Schweitzer, J., Lawton, J., Roraback, E., Peruski, A., VanDyke, M. and Fernandez, L. (2013). Arts and Crafts: Critical to Economic Innovation. *Economic Development Quarterly, 27*(3), 221–229. Langeslag, S. E., Schmidt, M., Ghassabian, A., Jaddoe, V. W., Hofman, A., van der Lugt, A., & . . . White, T. H. (2013). Functional connectivity between parietal and frontal brain regions and intelligence in young children: The Generation R study. *Human Brain Mapping, 34*(12), 3299–3307.

Leeder, E. (2003). The family in global perspective: A gendered journey. Thousand Oaks, CA: Sage Publications.

Lego Foundation. (2010). *The future of play: Defining the role and value of play in the 21st century.* Retrieved from http://www .legofoundation.com/en-us/research-and-learning/foundation -research/the-future-of-play/

Maczewski, M. (2002). Exploring identities through the Internet: Youth experiences online. *Child and Youth Care Forum, 31,* 111–129.

McHale, S., Crouter, A., & Tucker, C. (2001). Free-time activities in middle childhood: Links with adjustment in early adolescence. *Child Development, 72,* 1764–1778.

McManus, C. (2002). Right hand, left hand: The origins of asymmetry in brains, bodies, atoms and cultures. Boston, MA: Harvard University Press.

Mori, S., Iteya, M., & Gabbard, C. (2006). Hand preference consistency and eye-hand coordination in young children during a motor task. *Perceptual & Motor Skills, 102*(1), 29–34.

Mosby. (2009). *Mosby's Medical Dictionary* (8th ed.). Oxford, UK: Elsevier Inc.

Murphy, S. M., & Faulkner, D. (2006). Gender differences in verbal communication between popular and unpopular children during an interactive task. *Social Development, 15*(1), 82–108.

Michalczyk, K., Malstädt, N., Worgt, M., Könen, T., & Hasselhorn, M. (2013). Age differences and measurement invariance of working memory in 5- to 12-year-old children. *European Journal of Psychological Assessment, 29*(3), 220–229.

National Scientific Council on the Developing Child. (2014). *Excessive stress disrupts the architecture of the developing brain: Working Paper 3.* Updated Edition. Retrieved from www .developingchild.harvard.edu

Pan, Y., Tarczy-Hornoch, K., Cotter, S., Wen, G., Borchert, M., Azen, S., & Varma, R. (2009). Visual acuity norms in preschool children: The Multi-Ethnic Pediatric Eye Disease Study. *Optometry and Vision Science, 86,* 607–612.

Passow, S., Müller, M., Westerhausen, R., Hugdahl, K., Wartenburger, I., Heekeren, H. R., & . . . Li, S. (2013). Development of attentional control of verbal auditory perception from middle to late childhood: Comparisons to healthy aging. *Developmental Psychology, 49*(10), 1982–1993.

Payne, V. G., & Isaacs, L. D. (2012). *Human motor development: A lifespan approach.* New York: McGraw-Hill.

Porter, H., Sladen, D. P., Ampah, S. B., Rothpletz, A., & Bess, F. H. (2013). Developmental outcomes in early school-age children with minimal hearing loss. *American Journal of Audiology, 22*(2), 263–270.

Reilly, D. S., van Donkelaar, P., Saavedra, S., & Woollacott, M. H. (2008). Interaction between the development of postural control and the executive function of attention. *Journal of Motor Behaviour, 40,* 90–102.

Ridsdale, J., & Thompson, D. (2002). Perceptions of social adjustment of hearing-impaired pupils in an integrated secondary school unit. *Educational Psychology in Practice, 18,* 21–34.

Rodger, S., & Ziviani, J. (2006). Occupational therapy with children: Understanding children's occupations and enabling participation. Carlton, VIC: Blackwell Publishing.

Rubin, K., Bukowski, W., & Parker, J. (2006). Peer interactions, relationships, and groups. In W. Damon, R. M. Lerner, & N. Eisenberg (Eds.), *Handbook of child psychology: Vol. 3. Social, emotional, and personality development* (6th ed., pp. 571–645). New York: Wiley.

Rubin, K., Wojslawowicz, J., Rose-Krasnor, L., Booth-LaForce, C., & Burgess, K. (2006). The best friendships of shy/withdrawn children: Prevalence, stability, and relationship quality. *Journal of Abnormal Child Psychology, 34,* 143–157.

Shinn, L., & O'Brien, M. (2008). Parent–child conversational styles in middle childhood: Gender and social class differences. *Sex Roles, 59*(1/2), 61–67.

Shumway-Cook, A., & Woollacott, M. (2012). *Motor control: Translating research into clinical practice* (4th ed.). Baltimore: Lippincott, Williams and Wilkins.

Sporting Goods Manufacturers Association. (2013). *2013 sports, fitness, and leisure activities topline participation report.* Retrieved from http://www.sfia.org/reports/301_2013-Sports,-Fitness ,-and-Leisure-Activities-Topline-Participation-Report

Stoutjesdijk, R., Scholte, E. M., & Swaab, H. (2012). Special needs characteristics of children with emotional and behavioral disorders that affect inclusion in regular education. *Journal of Emotional & Behavioral Disorders, 20*(2), 92–104.

Subrahmanyam, K., Greenfield, P., Kraut, R., & Gross, E. (2001). The impact of computer use on children's and adolescents' development. *Journal of Applied Developmental Psychology, 22,* 7–30.

Tiedemann, J. (2000). Parents' gender stereotypes and teachers' beliefs as predictors of children's concept of their mathematical ability in elementary school. *Journal of Educational Psychology, 92*(1), 144.

U.S. National Library of Medicine & U.S. Department of Health and Human Services National Institutes of Health. (2012a). Vision impairment and blindness. Retrieved from http://www.nlm.nih.gov/medlineplus/visionimpairmentandblindness.html

U.S. National Library of Medicine & U.S. Department of Health and Human Services National Institutes of Health. (2012b). Hearing disorders and deafness. Retrieved from http://www.nlm.nih.gov/medlineplus/hearingdisordersanddeafness.html

Vogler, E., Koranda, P., & Romance, T. (2000). Including a child with severe cerebral palsy in physical education: A case study. *Adapted Physical Activity Quarterly, 17*(2), 161–175.

West Virginia Center for Budget and Policy. (2013). *Child poverty in West Virginia: A growing and persistent problem.* Retrieved from http://www.wvpolicy.org/child-poverty-in-west-virginia-a-growing-and-persistent-problem

Whitebread, D. (2012). *The importance of play.* The Lego Foundation. Retrieved from http://www.theideaconference.com/#/knowledge-hub

Whitely, C., & Colozzo, P. (2013). Who's who? Memory updating and character reference in children's narratives. *Journal of Speech, Language & Hearing Research, 56*(5), 1625–1636.

World Health Organization (WHO). (2001). *ICF: International classification of functioning and disability.* Geneva, Switzerland: World Health Organization.

Wright, J. C., Huston, A. C., Vandewater, E. A., Backhands, D., Scantlin, R. M., Kotler, J. A., Caplovitz, A., Lee, J., Hofferth, S., & Finkelstein, J. (2001). American children's use of electronic media in 1997: A national survey. *Journal of Applied Developmental Psychology, 22,* 31–47.

Yu, S., Ostrsosky, M., & Fowler, S. (2011). Children's friendship development: A comparative study. *Early Childhood Research and Practice, 13.* Retrieved from http://ecrp.uiuc.edu/v13n1/yu.html

CHAPTER 14

Adolescent Development

Anne Cronin, PhD, OTR/L, FAOTA,
Associate Professor, Division of
Occupational Therapy,
West Virginia University,
Morgantown, West Virginia

Objectives

Upon completion of this chapter, readers should be able to:

- Identify the nervous system's developmental trends in adolescence, and relate this to health and social behavior decision making;

- Identify typical adolescent performance in areas described in the ICF as activities and participation including the concept of occupational roles;

- Differentiate between performance skills and performance patterns of typically developing adolescents;

- Identify the variety and scope of communication strategies used to support adolescent activities and participation;

- Describe patterns of adolescent engagement in the major life areas of education and work;

- Discuss the impact of social media and other digital technologies on the social and emotional well-being of adolescents;

- Describe the roles of the differing types of interpersonal interactions common in adolescents, and the roles of these relationships in the individuals' development; and

- Define resiliency and its importance in adolescent development.

Key Terms

anorexia nervosa

bulimia

career

depression

eating disorder

epiphysis

gender identity

identity formation

limbic system

neural connectivity

obesity

occupational roles

performance skill

prefrontal cortex

reference group

resilience

romantic relationship

semantic memory

sexual orientation

sexuality

sleep hygiene

striatal system

substance abuse

temporal discounting

vocation

work

CASE 1

Vincent

Vincent is 16 years old and sustained multitrauma secondary to a head-on motor vehicle accident (MVA). His right leg was seriously injured and he is now non–weight bearing with a right femur nailing. He has ongoing abdominal pain and joint pain secondary to the accident. Vincent lives with his parents and a younger sister (13) in a trailer with three steps to enter. He attends high school, played varsity basketball, and is in the drama club. Vincent was a passenger in the car when the accident happened; the driver was his girlfriend. At the accident scene, both he and she were tested and had a high blood alcohol level. Vincent's girlfriend was shaken up, but not hurt. Vincent spent four days in the acute care hospital, and has just been transferred from acute care to the rehabilitation unit.

At this time, he needs moderate assistance (setup and standby support) in upper-body dressing, eating, and grooming. He needs total assistance in lower-body dressing and toileting. He is not sleeping well due to pain and nightmares. He has some mild confusion, is oriented to name and place only and requires occasional verbal prompts in problem-solving and memory tasks. Prior to the accident, he was independent in all ADL and IADL tasks. He does not initiate conversation and lacks initiative to participate in rehab.

Vincent is upset that he will not be able to finish out the basketball season with his friends; he has been an average student, and is worried that he will never catch up and will not get the grades to be allowed to continue to participate in sports. His girlfriend has visited him in the hospital, but she is so distressed by his condition that the visits have not been positive for him. Vincent has been told that his full recovery will take at least six months. His parents and sister have been supportive, but the family emphasizes that Vincent needs to be able to do more for himself, because even if he stays home from school, there will be no one at home to care for him.

Continues on page 324

INTRODUCTION

Adolescence is the developmental stage that bridges child-hood and adulthood. Typically adolescence is considered the teenage years, but it is more complex than that. Technically, adolescence begins at puberty, which can be as early as 10 years old for some girls. Puberty is the process of physical changes by which a child's body matures into an adult body capable of sexual reproduction to enable fertilization. Although the physical and physiological changes associated with puberty are recognized as the "official" markers of the beginning of adolescence, the psychological and social changes that take place in young people are often the most evident signs of adolescence onset. For some young people, long-standing cultural traditions serve as formal markers of the beginning of the adolescent period. Some religious faiths recognize entry into adolescence with a formal rite of passage. In the eyes of the faith, these rites are more accurately viewed as an official acknowledgment of the transition from childhood to the status of being considered a man or a woman. This passage gives young people rights to attend prayer services that are restricted to adult members of the faith.

For example, young boys of the Jewish faith have their *bar mitzvahs* (see **Figure 14-1**) and young girls their *bat mitzvahs* when they turn 13. Lengthy study precedes this formal religious ceremony. These young people often wear symbolic, ceremonial dress to mark the occasion. Festivities and celebration, frequently quite elaborate, resembling a wedding reception, follow the formal religious service.

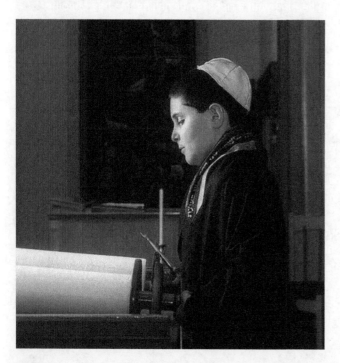

Figure 14-1 The Jewish bar mitzvah and bat mitzah are rites of passage that acknowledge 13-year-olds as adults in the eyes of the synagogue and the Jewish community.

Some Christian denominations have periods of study and religious ceremonies that also typically occur at this age. *Confirmation* recognizes that adolescents have matured to the point of being able to make independent, informed, personal decisions about their faith. This ceremony is an acknowledgment by the church that the adolescents are no longer dependent upon parents to make important decisions for them. They are old enough to make decisions of faith for themselves. These religious rituals are some of the few remaining rites of passage in contemporary society that acknowledge how young teens are regarded differently by society or at least by the members of their faith community.

Specifying the end of adolescence is more problematic due to the lack of a clear marker or indicator of the achievement of adulthood. There is no physical or physiologic change to mark the conclusion of adolescence. Adolescence is important psychologically as a key period in identity development. Historically, markers of adulthood in the United States included living independently from parents or other adult caregivers, marriage and starting a family, or full acceptance into a profession or vocation. One of the proposed indicators of attainment of adulthood is economic independence from parents or other adults. This rite of passage could take place when young people assume responsibility for their own financial support by entering the workforce, or by making the necessary arrangements to support themselves financially on educational loans or through a combination of employment and educational loans.

In this period, individuals first intentionally build and reflect on occupational roles. **Occupational roles** are patterns of behavior that individuals actively identify with and that offer guidance about expected behaviors and responsibilities in specific defined situations. Occupational roles are often culturally defined. Some roles are necessary and inherent, such as the role of son or sibling. Other roles are actively chosen by individuals, such as musician or athlete. Roles may overlap, as in the case of a sibling that is also a caregiver, and roles may conflict, as in the case of an employee who must cut back her work hours so that she has more time to complete needed school work and master her student role. Occupational roles are separate from, but often related to, career aspirations in this age group. For example, excelling in the student role may assure that individuals will be able to attend college and begin training for their desired career.

In adolescence, young people begin to seriously plan for their transition into adult life and into the workforce. As societies become increasingly complex and technologically developed, the requirement for advanced education and training extends the period of time that is necessary to sufficiently prepare to enter the workforce. As requirements for higher education and training continue to expand, economic independence occurs later in young people's lives. As we will discuss later in this text, the point of transition between adolescence and adulthood has grown less clear in recent years, and some psychologists have proposed an additional developmental stage of early (or emerging) adulthood.

BODY FUNCTIONS AND STRUCTURES

Most of adolescent physical growth occurs during the first two thirds of the adolescent period. During and following puberty, gender differences in strength and body composition develop. The maturation of sexual functions occurring during this time period will not receive specific attention in this text. Our emphasis is on motor control and functional performance in daily life occupations.

BRAIN AND NERVOUS SYSTEM DEVELOPMENT

The process of brain growth and myelination continues into adolescence resulting in increased neural connectivity (Carlisi, Pavletic, & Ernst, 2013). The combination of myelination and neural pruning that began earlier in life continues through adolescence, with the result that by the end of adolescence, the proportion of gray matter in the brain (unmyelinated brain tissue) to white matter (myelinated brain tissue) decreases. **Neural connectivity** refers to physical links between areas of the brain that share common developmental trajectories. Brain studies show that areas with high neural connectivity activate together during a task. In addition, the *prefrontal cortex* of the brain matures during adolescence.

The **prefrontal cortex** is the anterior part of the frontal lobes of the brain. The prefrontal area of the brain is an area of high neural connectivity, including strong connections with the *limbic system* and the *striatal system*. The **limbic system** is a complex set of structures in the midbrain area that lies just under the cerebral cortex. The limbic system is primarily responsible for the brain activities that underlie our emotional life, and with the formation of memories. The prefrontal cortex, with its high neural connectivity and links to the limbic system, is a central brain area associated with metacognition and executive functions (Carlisi, Pavletic, & Ernst, 2013).

The **striatal system**, also known as the neostriatum or striate nucleus, is located in the cerebral cortex and is heavily interconnected with subcortical areas in the midbrain. The striatal system influences the planning and modulation of movement pathways, supports the executive function processes, and is activated by stimuli associated with reward and novel or intense stimuli. The increased risk-taking behavior seen in many adolescents is believed to be contributed to by an increased receptivity of the striatal system (Galván & McGlennen, 2013). One of the reasons neuroscientists have focused so much research on the adolescent brain is that this is a sensitive period of development characterized by increased risk taking and sensation seeking at the same time that many human physical capabilities are at their peak (Carlisi, Pavletic, & Ernst, 2013). Many of the health and social problems adolescents experience are results of their own good (or bad) decision making and a

propensity for risk taking. This is a paradoxical issue: At the healthiest and most physically adept period in the life span, young people make deliberate choices that damage their health. "Unintentional injury was the leading cause of death (in U.S. adolescents), followed by homicide, suicide, cancer, and heart disease. Together, these causes account for 84.3 percent of deaths in this age group, although nearly half of all adolescent deaths are attributable to unintentional injury" (USHHS, 2011). Of deaths within the category of unintentional injury, 44.1 percent can be attributed to motor vehicle accidents. Other sources of unintentional injury common to adolescents are substance abuse and engaging in high-risk physical activities.

The most common adolescent behaviors that cause poor health and disability, rather than death, are not wearing a helmet when riding a bicycle, riding with a driver who has been drinking alcohol, failure to wear a seat belt, driving after consuming alcohol, and texting or emailing while driving (USHHS CDC, 2012). As can be deduced from this list, faulty decision making is at the heart of many adolescent health problems. A common decision-making pattern seen in adolescence, reflecting immature executive functions, is temporal discounting. **Temporal discounting** (also called the invincibility fallacy) occurs when young people discount the potential long-range impacts of decisions, focusing instead on immediate rewards. Temporal discounting underlies social problems such as unwanted pregnancy, low educational achievement, and criminal actions, which also reflect poor impulse control and poor executive reasoning. In the case of Vincent and his girlfriend, temporal discounting is evident. Drinking alcoholic beverages is illegal at their age. In itself, this decision reflects rebellion and risky behavior. The consequences of drinking and driving are far more severe. Even though they both survived the collision, Vincent has lost his valued place on the team and must undergo an extensive and painful rehabilitation process. His girlfriend has lost her driver's license, and will not be allowed to get a new one until she is 18 years old. In addition, she faces steep fines and a court appearance for her actions and must repay her parents for the cost of repairing the car. Because both young people could have died or caused the death of others, their consequences seem moderate. Although Vincent may have learned a lesson, drinking and driving remains one of the major causes of death for American adolescents.

PHYSICAL DEVELOPMENT

Puberty, driven by changes in the endocrine system, is a period in which changes in secondary sex characteristics appear and the reproductive system reaches maturity. In girls, secondary sex characteristics include the budding of nipples and breasts, followed by growth of pubic hair and growth of genitalia. In males, secondary sex characteristics include the physical growth of the testicles, followed by growth of pubic hair. Later, axillary hair and facial and body hair appear. The onset of menses is the definitively identified event signifying puberty in females, typically occurring in American females at around 12 years. For males, the highlight of puberty is less obvious but may be considered the first ejaculation of mature sperm, sometime during middle adolescence (Feldman, 2011).

The most common method of assessing physical maturity in adolescents is known as the *sex maturity rating scale (SMR)*, developed by Tanner (1962), and otherwise referred to as *Tanner stages.* The SMR is a method of using visual inspection of genitalia or breasts and pubic hair to evaluate stages of pubertal development. Tanner Stage I is considered *pre-adolescence,* evidenced by absence of pubic hair, flat breasts in females, and absence of pubic hair in males. Tanner Stage II is considered *early adolescence,* and is characterized by sparse pubic hair, small, raised breasts in females, and enlargement of testes with darkening of pubic hair in males. Stages III and IV are considered *middle adolescence.* Coarsening and curling of pubic hair characterize Stage III. Tanner Stage III in girls is characterized by enlargement and raising of the breasts, whereas in males there is an increase in penis size. Stage IV in girls is characterized by the areola and nipple forming a separate contour from the breast and in males by continued growth of the penis. Stage V for both sexes is characterized by adult genitalia (Tanner, 1962). Puberty-related changes in the body occur based on genetics and are very individual. Young people who begin to puberty at earlier (or later) ages than their peers are considered "off-time". Adolescents who are "off time in their pubertal development experience more stress than do on-time adolescents" (Susman & Rogol, 2004, p. 30). This stress seems to be greatest for girls who develop early. Developing off time is associated emotional distress, poor body image, higher levels of depression, and substance abuse. With the maturation of sexual function, there is also the emergence of sexuality. **Sexuality** is the state of being sexual, including not only sexual physical acts but also the more complicated elements of emotion, physiologic drive, pregnancy, birth control, and sexually transmitted disease.

Skeletal growth in this period is often asynchronous. It is common that hands and feet mature before arms and legs and that the legs reach peak growth before shoulders and chest. This is contrary to the general developmental trends of cephalocaudal and proximodistal growth described earlier in the text. Adolescence also involves a period of rapid bone growth. An **epiphysis** is the end portion of a long bone, initially separated from the shaft (diaphysis) by a section of cartilage. From infancy, the cartilage in the epiphysis gradually ossifies so that the end of the bone and the shaft of the bone fuse together. Growth occurs in the epiphyseal region. The peak velocity for growth in height occurs at a mean of 13.5 years in boys and 11.5 years in girls. Pubertal growth accounts for about 20 percent of final adult height, a total averaging 9 to 11 inches in females and 6 to 11 inches in males. An average adolescent growth spurt lasts 24 to 36 months, and during this time the epiphyseal portion of the bone is especially vulnerable. As the growth spurt ends, the

epiphyseal junction ossifies and individuals attain their adult height. In males, the epiphyseal junction remains open for about two years longer than it does in females. This is reason that males, on average, are 4 to 5 inches taller than females.

A major reason for concerns about competitive athletic training in children and teens is that the cartilage of the epiphysis is flexible and susceptible to damage (Malina, 2011). The rapid skeletal growth in adolescence may result in certain variations becoming increasingly evident or even pathologic, such as the case of idiopathic scoliosis. *Idiopathic scoliosis* is a curvature of the spine that manifests itself in the prepubertal years and requires aggressive management during the adolescent period of rapid skeletal growth (Horne, Flannery, & Usman, 2014). DiFiori et al. (2014) published a position statement on behalf of the American Medical Society for Sports Medicine on youth sports participation and overuse injuries. A comprehensive literature review led to several conclusions. First, history of prior injury is heavily correlated with subsequent injury; therefore, screening exams may be helpful in determining risk. Second, sport readiness is a key factor in determination of risk, including both cognitive and psychomotor elements. Third, menstrual dysfunction is a risk factor for female athletes. Finally, early sport specialization and associated specialized intensive training should be avoided in children and young adolescents, except for some specific sports such as gymnastics.

Weight gains during adolescence follow patterns similar to those for height but are also greatly affected by environmental factors. Typically, males develop broader shoulders, straighter hips, and longer limbs during adolescence. Females tend to develop narrower shoulders and broader hips and lean body masses decrease from about 80 to 74 percent while average body fat levels increase from 16 to 27 percent by the end of adolescence. Conversely, in males, body fat levels decrease among males during adolescence, dropping to an average of 12 percent body fat by the end of puberty (Stang & Story, 2005).

Obesity is the term used for ranges of weight that are greater than what is generally considered healthy for a given height. Body mass index (BMI) is the standard used to judge weight. An adult who has a BMI between 25 and 29.9 is considered overweight. An adult who has a BMI of 30 or higher is considered obese. In the United States, 1 in 5 adolescents is overweight, and 1 in 20 is classified as obese. Lack of exercise, the easy availability of fast foods, and the increased use of electronic devices and the Internet for both leisure and social activities are cited as reasons for obesity in both middle childhood and adolescence. Obesity greatly increases the impact of many health conditions and may limit participation in some valued occupations. The support of healthy lifestyle decisions can be integrated into interventions for young people to help address this insidious problem.

SLEEP

Research data suggest adolescents actually need more sleep than younger students, and daytime sleepiness is pronounced throughout the day even after sufficient sleep (Loessl et al., 2008). Through most of the life span, humans have a built-in day, which averages about 24 hours, that predicts typical sleep/wake cycles. This internalized process is called a *circadian rhythm*. Before adolescence, these circadian rhythms direct most children to naturally fall asleep around 9 p.m. Puberty changes teens' circadian rhythm, delaying the time they start feeling sleepy—often until 12 p.m. or later. In addition to changes in the circadian rhythm, there are also substantial changes in structure and patterns of sleep across adolescence (Colrain & Baker, 2011). These changes in sleep patterns are caused by many factors, including increasing school demands, extracurricular activities and are associated with the changes in brain structure and organization described earlier in this chapter. This behavior change is driven by changes in sleep wave forms in response to changes in brain structure and organization.

Sleep problems often worsen as individuals progress from early to late adolescence (Loessl et al., 2008). Unfortunately, many schools have an early morning starting time. As a result, the trend is that adolescent students are often sleepy or sleep-deprived in classes. The increased need for sleep, together with the difficulty falling to sleep, leads many young people to stay up late at night. Changes in sleep patterns during adolescence are a normal part of development, but, because of the societal expectation of early morning school participation many adolescents get insufficient sleep. Sleep deprivation is associated with the development of mood disorders, obesity, impaired higher cognitive functions, increased risk for traffic accidents, and substance abuse (Colrain & Baker, 2011).

There is evidence that using good *sleep hygiene* skills can manage the problem of sleep deprivation. **Sleep hygiene** includes the habits, environmental factors, and practices that

may influence the length and quality of sleep. Strategies to encourage sleep and reinforce the maintenance of a circadian pattern that is consistent with the daily demands of adolescents are described in **Table 14-1**. In addition to these approaches, a healthy lifestyle with a nutritious diet and regular exercise will reinforce the sleep hygiene strategies described.

MOTOR PERFORMANCE SKILLS

As adolescents continue to mature, they become better able to move their bodies with greater precision, demonstrating coordinated flow and calibration of movements. Adolescent females typically make modest developmental gains in their gross and fine motor skills until approximately 15 years of age. After this point, they generally do not experience any additional improvement in their motor skills unless they are specifically training for a sport or hobby that requires these skills. Adolescent males, on the other hand, continue to improve, particularly in the areas of strength and endurance throughout the entire period of adolescence, even into their early 20s (Feldman, 2011).

Typically developing adolescents are expected to have the ability to bend, to flex, and to rotate their trunks without any restrictions or stiffness. By adolescence, young people's bilateral coordination skills have fully matured. They routinely use two hands or one hand and another body part to accomplish any desired task that requires stabilizing and manipulating objects. They open small makeup containers and the rings of a three-ring binder without problems. Adolescents have the grasp-and-release patterns, the isolated finger movements, and the in-hand manipulation skills to pick up, shift, and adjust their pens or pencils in their hand

TABLE 14-1 Sleep Hygiene Strategies
Go to bed at the same time each night and rise at the same time each morning.
Remove all TVs, computers, and other "gadgets," including computers and smartphones, from the bedroom.
Avoid large meals before bedtime.
Make sure the bedroom is a quiet, dark, and relaxing environment.
Avoid chocolates, candies, and caffeinated drinks for at least a few hours prior to bedtime.
Physical activity, such as walking, exercise, and strength training may help promote sleep, but not within a few hours of bedtime.
Avoid pulling an "all-nighter" to study.
Do not sleep more than two to three hours past a usual wake time on weekends.
Expose yourself to bright light upon awakening in the morning.
Limit napping. A short nap is okay, but limit it to 30 or 45 minutes.
Adapted from Prohealthcare-http://www.prohealthcare.org/services/SleepCenter/good-sleep-habits-for-teens/

to take notes in class, to rotate their pencils in their hand to use the eraser end of the pencil, to pull a key out of a pocket or purse and insert it in the ignition, and to put coins into soda machines without difficulty.

By adolescence there is a clearly quantitative aspect to motor skill performance, manifested by a complex interaction of such parameters as strength, speed, power, reaction time, and endurance. The name performance skill is often applied to these refined motor patterns. There are differences among individuals in these parameters based on environmental factors, such as training and practice, as well as innate factors, such as gender and body type. **Figure 14-2** illustrates a spontaneous game of football. This sport involves complex motor coordination skills as well as, perceptual awareness, and the ability to alter motor plans dynamically to follow the game's action.

Changes in motor performance skills correlate with physical growth. For example, it is suggested that changes in balance ability occur as the high center of gravity in children is displaced progressively lower through adolescence. Overall, this tends to coincide with steadily improving static and dynamic balance throughout the adolescent period. The phenomenon of "adolescent awkwardness" has been difficult to document through quantitative study. The current conclusion is that this phenomenon exists in some individuals, mostly males, at the time of peak height velocity. Adolescent physical changes may not occur in a smooth, regular schedule; adolescents may go through awkward stages, both about their appearance and physical coordination (Medline Plus, 2014). Changes in strength during adolescence have been documented, with the greatest gains in abdominal and grip strength. For males upper trunk strength increases throughout adolescence. Grip strength

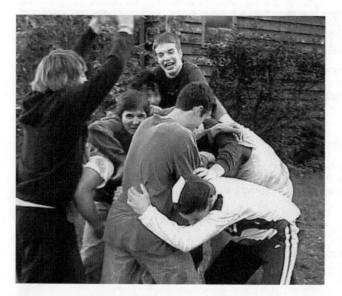

Figure 14-2 Contact sports, such as football, reflect both cultural and developmental trends. These young men are demonstrating highly refined movement skills in the rowdy form of social interaction.

in both males and females increase tremendously during adolescence, but the increase for males in much higher.

SPECIFIC MENTAL FUNCTIONS

Reyna and colleagues (2012) describe three major patterns in the development of mental functions in adolescence that will be presented in this chapter: (1) memory, (2) reasoning, and (3) judgment.

Memory becomes more complex with the expansion of specialized types of memory. **Semantic memory** is the memory of concept and word meanings. It involves the recollection of facts and general knowledge about the world. Semantic memory expands throughout adolescent development. As teens gain experience of the world, they increasingly are able to give meaning to otherwise meaningless words and sentences. Through this process of semantic memory, adolescents are increasingly able to learn about new concepts by applying their knowledge learned from things in the past (Reyna et al., 2012).

Metacognition and higher-order reasoning undergoes rapid expansion during adolescence. This area of development has received a lot of attention because "a large number of adolescents stagnate cognitively and fail to thrive academically" (Reyna et al., 2012, p. 124). Recent studies suggest that higher-order cognitive skills, including working memory and inhibition of impulses, develop throughout adolescence and into early adulthood. With this development of higher order skills there is also an increased complexity to reasoning. Reyna and colleagues (2012) noted that adults and adolescents tend to have two, sometimes conflicting, versions of reality in their minds. There is the quick take of what is essential about something the individual has experienced or observed, and the less nuanced, more literal, representation of reality. The quick take, called the "gist representation" by Reyna and associates reflects the subjective meaning of the event to the individual. The literal, or "verbatim thinking" is more specific about considering facts or situations in detail. Unlike reasoning later into adulthood, adolescents lack experience and are prone to base risky decisions on verbatim details rather than on the gist of the situation. Adolescents' perceptions of the relative risks and benefits of any decision tend to vary with their psychosocial context, as reflected in effects of gender, age, and cultural background and more than adults, their decisions are vulnerable to the contextual cues they receive when faced with a risky choice.

Judgment is the ability to make considered decisions or come to sensible conclusions. There is also evidence these skills can be trained and accelerated. In this way, teens' educational environment plays a role in organizing the brain through what students are taught and how they are encouraged to think. Cognitive training interventions can be effective in assisting individuals with problems in these areas, and are widely recommended for people with attention deficit/hyperactivity disorder and other conditions associated with impaired working memory and impulse control (Reyna et al., 2012).

Adolescence and early adulthood are characterized by increased risk-taking behaviors (Galván & McGlennen, 2013). Earlier, the developmental changes in the prefrontal cortex, limbic, and striatal systems were discussed. Recent research indicates that the striatal system becomes more sensitive, and thus more reward seeking, before the prefrontal cortex is fully ready to regulate risk and reward-driven behavior negatively impacting judgment. This results in the cognitive dichotomy that is seen in adolescence. A teen is "capable of controlled, analytical, rational processes but often relies on more automatic, intuitive, heuristic processes" (Galván, 2012, p. 268). This means that adolescents are vulnerable to the emotional and environmental temptations around them. Although they have the ability to demonstrate high-level problem solving in an emotion-neutral situation, when a situation is emotionally charged, adolescents are more likely to be swayed by their emotions. Emotion-driven reward seeking is at its highest in the adolescent period, resulting in poor judgment in emotion-laden situations. Adolescence and early adulthood are characterized by errors in judgment and increased risk-taking behaviors (Galván & McGlennen, 2013). Judgment and emotional processing will improve as the prefrontal cortex fully matures.

ACTIVITIES AND PARTICIPATION

This period in the life span is really the first in which individuals have the foundational skills to participate in all of the areas described in the ICF as "activities and participation" (World Health Organization, 2001). These areas are presented in **Table 14-2**. By adolescence, most individuals have gained a high level of skill in the activity of learning and applying knowledge. As ordinary ADL and IADL skills become routine, adolescents develop elaborate process skills to allow the transfer and adaptation of previously learned tasks to new environments.

In many of the areas of activities and participation described in the ICF, adolescents are highly skilled and independent. These areas include learning and applying knowledge, general tasks and demands, communication, and mobility. Continued development occurs in the areas of self-care, domestic life, interpersonal interactions and relationships, and community, social, and civic life.

The adolescent expansion into new areas of activities and participation are supported by advances in process skills. Process skills were introduced in Chapter 6 and are problem-solving and decision-making strategies that are

---

TABLE 14-2   ICF Descriptions of Areas of Activities and Participation

- LEARNING AND APPLYING KNOWLEDGE (basic learning and applying knowledge)

- GENERAL TASKS AND DEMANDS (general aspects of carrying out single or multiple tasks, organizing routines, and handling stress)

- COMMUNICATION (communicating by language, signs and symbols, including receiving and producing messages, carrying on conversations, and using communication devices and techniques)

- MOBILITY (moving by changing body position or location or by transferring from one place to another; by carrying, moving, or manipulating objects; by walking, running, or climbing; and by using various forms of transportation)

- SELF-CARE (caring for oneself, washing and drying oneself, caring for one's body and body parts, dressing, eating, and drinking, and looking after one's health)

- DOMESTIC LIFE (carrying out domestic and everyday actions and tasks. Areas of domestic life include acquiring a place to live, food, clothing, and other necessities, household cleaning and repairing, caring for personal and other household objects, and assisting others.)

- INTERPERSONAL INTERACTIONS AND RELATIONSHIPS (carrying out the actions and tasks required for basic and complex interactions with people—strangers, friends, relatives, family members, and lovers—in a contextually and socially appropriate manner)

- MAJOR LIFE AREAS (carrying out the tasks and actions required to engage in education, work, and employment and to conduct economic transactions)

- COMMUNITY, SOCIAL, AND CIVIC LIFE (actions and tasks required to engage in organized social life outside the family, in community, and in social and civic areas of life)

Adapted from World Health Organization, 2001. Reference Crediting: World Health Organization (WHO), (2001). ICF: International classification of functioning and disability. Geneva, Switzerland: World Health Organization.

selected based on prior knowledge and experience. Process skills include finding solutions to situations by identifying issues, developing options and solutions, evaluating potential effects of solutions, and executing a chosen solution. Adolescents use the process skill of knowledge throughout the day as they choose the right tools before initiating a task, and they know what task objects are needed for different activities that compose a part of their day. They also have the knowledge to use the tools and materials that they have chosen for different tasks according to their intended

purpose. Although they may occasionally substitute objects, like a washcloth for a toothbrush, or a knife for a fork, they know the purpose of the task objects that they use for various tasks and in most cases use them appropriately and safely. Examples of process skills in school, home, and community settings are listed in **Table 14-3**.

In this section, we will present some of the significant achievements in the ICF category of "activities and participation" as listed in **Table 14-2**. These skills will offer examples of common achievements, but readers will need

---

TABLE 14-3 Adolescent Process Skills

Examples of Activities Engaged in by Typically Developing Adolescents

Process Skills	School	Home	Work in Community	Play/Leisure and Social Settings in the Community
Energy—Refers to sustained effort over the course of task performance				
Paces	Working on in-class assignments with a consistent, steady rhythm.	Not rushing through or "taking forever" to complete a task like homework or chores.	Taking the required time to fill orders and check on customers who need refills in a coffee shop.	Pacing one's running speed to compete in a cross-country track event.
Attends	Taking notes on key points during a class lecture.	Responding to family conversations with incorporation of information presented by others.	Attending to the safety of people in the pool rather than to non-job-related activity.	Paying attention to the football play rather than being distracted by the talk from the opposing team.
Knowledge—Refers to the ability to seek and use task-related knowledge				
Chooses	Selecting the correct notebooks and textbooks from a locker prior to the next class.	Choosing the lawn-mower and edger to mow and trim the lawn.	Choosing four plates, napkins, and four sets of utensils to set the table for four people.	Choosing a Frisbee from a closet full of games and sporting goods equipment.
Uses	Using pens, rulers, compasses, and paper for their intended purposes.	Using a toothbrush and dental floss for their intended purposes.	Using the designated dish sponge to clean the dishes but not using it to clean the floor.	Using a basketball and net to shoot hoops with friends.
Handles	Supporting a full beaker of solution with two hands to prevent it from spilling or being dropped.	Carrying a dinner plate from the table to the kitchen sink with two hands.	Supporting a pitcher of water with two hands when refilling customers' drinking glasses.	Using two hands and lifting from under the piece when transporting unfired green-ware to the kiln to be fired.
Heeds	Completing an in-class assignment without missing any part of it.	Loading all of the dinner dishes into the dish-washer, filling the soap dispenser, and starting the dishwasher.	Upon seeing a customer leave, going to the table, clearing it, wiping it clean, and resetting it with napkins and silverware.	Continuing to play tennis, alternating between forehand and backhand sides of the court until the conclusion of the game.

Continues

TABLE 14-3   Adolescent Process Skills   *(continued)*

Process Skills	School	Home	Work in Community	Play/Leisure and Social Settings in the Community
Inquires	Asking questions of a teacher only when the information has not been given previously.	Not needing to ask about the washer settings once they have been fully explained.	Asking the supervisor for clarification when a customer asks a question about something that has not been previously explained.	Asking the coach questions only about plays or techniques that have not previously been explained.
Temporal organization—Refers to beginning, logical ordering, continuation, and completion of the steps and action sequences of a task				
Initiates.	Starting to work on a test, following directions from the teacher.	Beginning homework without a reminder.	Seeing a customer enter the shop and proceeding to ask if he needs help locating something.	Beginning routine stretches at the beginning of practice without being told.
Continues.	Continuing to complete each step in a biology or chemistry lab without stopping to do something else.	Continuing to vacuum a room completely without being distracted by the surroundings.	Continuing to make and bake pizzas without losing concentration on the task.	Continuing to play basketball despite heckling from spectators.
Sequences.	On a block schedule, attending classes in the correct order for the given day.	Following the steps of a recipe in the order specified by the instructions.	Collecting payment and giving change before filling food order so food does not get cold.	Following Robert's Rules of Order to run a club meeting.
Terminates.	Stopping work when the assignment has been completed rather than stopping prematurely or persisting unnecessarily.	Signing off Internet messaging on the computer after spending a reasonable amount of time online.	Stopping work on cleaning the tiles around the pool once the full perimeter has been covered.	Leaving a party in progress with sufficient time to return home by the set curfew time.
Searches/locates.	Locating pen and paper in a full backpack.	Looking for a knife and cutting board in the kitchen drawers, and for peanut butter in the cabinet.	Searching for clothing items or shoes in the stockroom to find the size needed by a customer.	Searching the school directory to locate club members' telephone numbers and email addresses.
Gathers.	Collecting pencil, notebook, textbook, and calculator for geometry class.	Collecting shirt, pants, underwear, socks, and shoes from closet and drawers.	Picking up items at the end of the register and placing them in grocery bags.	Putting bat, glove, batting gloves, sweatbands, cleats, towel, and uniform in bat bag to take to a softball game.
Organizes.	Setting up supplies and space in art class so water and paint will not be knocked over inadvertently.	Arranging notebooks and snacks on desk in a way that minimizes the likelihood of a spill.	Arranging beverage cups in a portable rack to carry into the stadium to sell.	Setting up easel, canvas, paints, palette, brushes, and stool to prepare to paint a landscape.
Restores.	Shutting down the Internet on the library computer after doing a search in the library.	Putting folded, clean clothes away in closet and drawers.	Returning salt, pepper, and sugar containers to the table after refilling.	Returning helmets, shoulder pads, balls, and protective equipment to the locker room.

Continues

TABLE 14-3 Adolescent Process Skills *(continued)*

Adaptation—Relates to the ability to anticipate, correct for, and benefit by learning from the consequences of errors that arise in the course of task performance

Process Skills	School	Home	Work in Community	Play/Leisure and Social Settings in the Community
Navigates.	Moving around the cafeteria without bumping into tables and chairs or people.	Moving around the kitchen without bumping into counters or cabinets.	Walking around the store without bumping into clothing displays or clothing racks.	Avoiding getting too close to players from the opposing team when playing soccer.
Notices/ responds.	Noticing that an error was not fully erased and finishing the correction process completely.	Noticing that the laundry hamper is full and starting the washing machine.	Blowing the lifeguard whistle upon noticing a young child running around the pool.	Noticing that the pitcher is throwing outside pitches and moving closer to the plate to hit the ball.
Accommodates.	Noticing that the teacher follows the textbook and moving the textbook into closer view.	Realizing that buttoning was off by one hole and unbuttoning and rebuttoning shirt.	Adjusting the umbrella to maintain shade on the lifeguard stand.	Turning down the volume on the car radio upon noticing a detour and slowed traffic.
Adjusts	Realizing that there is no chalk in the tray and going to a neighboring classroom to get a piece of chalk for the club meeting.	Noticing that the vacuum is not picking up dirt and lint as it should and stopping to change the filter bag.	Upon seeing an empty water glass, fetching the pitcher to refill the glass.	When a trash bag becomes full, going to get a new bag during a community cleanup effort.
Benefits.	Discovering that the teacher's study guide covered most of the test questions and using the next test guide to improve performance.	Separating saturated colors from whites after turning the laundry pink as a result of mixing them.	After leaving a pizza in the oven for too long, setting the timer as an auditory reminder to remove the pizza after 20 minutes.	Sending out meeting reminders before the next meeting after realizing that attendance was low due to a lack of publicity about the meeting time.

to understand that the skills young people in adolescence develop are tailored to their life experience, culture, occupational roles, and resources. For example, in the United States, it is common for adolescents to learn to drive a car. For many American teens, this is a major life step toward adulthood. In many other parts of the world, driving a car is not a significant part of the adolescent experience.

COMMUNICATION FUNCTIONS

Adolescents who are developing typically engage in social interaction experiences throughout their days at school, at home, and in the community. Interactions with peers in the hallways of school, on the sidelines of a practice field, or at a party require appropriate physicality. Communication is both verbal and non-verbal. Teens communicate when they make physical contact when shaking hands or hugging each other

upon seeing each other after a time apart. Communication pragmatics were described in Chapter 5 as the rules and conventions for talking. Pragmatics in non-verbal communication includes the social rules for interacting physically. Most adolescents respond to social context and apply this context to their communication strategies. For example, they know when touching is appropriate and when it is not. They use eye gazes to communicate and interact with others. Eye contact communicates interest in a person and the discussion, and contributes to sustaining an interaction.

They also demonstrate communication pragmatics as they learn to use effective gestures to indicate, demonstrate, or add emphasis to their discussion and to coordinate the movement of their body in relation to others. These coordinated physical maneuvers include adjusting the space between themselves and others to demonstrate respect for other people's comfort zones. Adolescents communicate a great deal through body language postures. Leaning forward and sitting back with crossed arms and legs convey messages of acceptance and interest in the first case and rejection and disinterest in the second. Adolescents generally practice appropriate physicality first with peers of the same sex and adults like their parents, teachers, and their friends' parents.

Gradually, they gain confidence in the physical aspects of their communication and interaction and develop a level of comfort interacting with peers of the opposite sex. Pinning a boutonniere on a lapel or a corsage on a date's dress for the first time, as in **Figure 14-3**, illustrates the challenge of becoming comfortable with the physicality aspects of touch and proximity that occur on a first date.

Healthy communication in relationships require adolescents to focus their speech and behavior on the ongoing social action and contribute to the social process. They have the ability to change focus to the ongoing social action multiple times as they pass or pause to speak briefly with different friends or groups. Adolescents relate by acknowledging receipt of social messages; giving indications of interest; offering assistance, encouragement, and compliments; displaying concern about other people's feelings; using appropriate humor; and offering ideas, opinions, and suggestions. These actions result in the establishment and maintenance of rapport. The close friendships and dating relationships associated with adolescence provide the perfect opportunity for young people to build and practice these relationship-building and relationship-maintaining skills. Friends help their peers through successes and disappointments, celebrations, and heartbreaks.

In addition to face-to-face communication, teens today routinely engage in various forms of social media. Research has shown that participating in social media benefits adolescents

by enhancing communications and social connections (Ito et al., 2008). According to a recent poll, 22 percent of teenagers log on to their favorite social media site more than 10 times a day, and more than half of adolescents log on to a social media site more than once a day (Common Sense Media, 2012). Romer, Bagdasarov, and More (2013) found that heavy TV use in adolescents is associated with poorer school performance, but moderate use of the Internet (one to four hours per day) does not interfere with school and is positively associated with participation in clubs and sports. Increasingly, adolescents are using digital and social media to reinforce existing relationships, both with friends and romantic partners. This social media use can either support or be a source of distress to young people. Boyd and Hargittai (2013) comment that "since the rise of the Internet, we have seen a wide variety of concerns regarding young people's technological engagement, including privacy, pornography, hacking, cyberbullying, sexting, addiction, sexual victimization, identity theft, self-harm content, file sharing, and violent content" (p. 248).

These serious concerns have been explored extensively (Boyd & Hargittai, 2013; Ito et al., 2009), and the risks to youth have not been found to be substantiated. Although there are risks, they are no greater than the risks of encountering fraud or a sexual predator in traditional social exchanges. Boyd and Hargittai (2013) argue that parental fears associated with social media can contribute to a "culture of fear" that may prompt young people to be more isolated and less engaged with public life.

MOBILITY

By the later part of the teen years, young people are able and expected to function independently in the community. With this expectation, there is also an expectation that they master community mobility. Community mobility includes the effective use of any form of mobility commonly used in the area. This includes independent use of busses, taxis, and trains. The ability to legally drive a car and have access to an automobile, whether that occurs in the form of a shared family vehicle or one that is provided to the adolescent primarily for his or her use, is a significant milestone for adolescents in the United States. Driving allows adolescents to become part of the daily family transportation circuit, taking siblings to appointments and making trips to the grocery store when needed. The young man in **Figure 14-4** proudly displays his newly earned driver's license.

Returning to the case of Vincent, he is in a wheelchair most of the day now. When in the chair, he is able to propel himself slowly but is unable to lift or bend forward to pick up an object from the floor due to pain. Vincent will be going back home and to school after rehab. Mobility is a particular concern because of the stairs going into the home and limited space in the home for a wheelchair. He does not want to have to go back to school in the wheelchair and

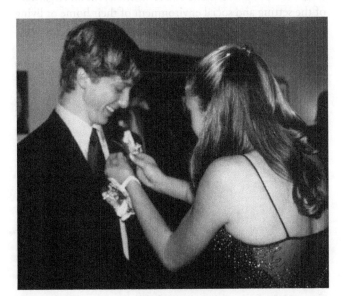

Figure 14-3 Experiencing the social conventions of dating for the first time can be awkward initially, until physical contact with the opposite sex becomes more familiar and comfortable.

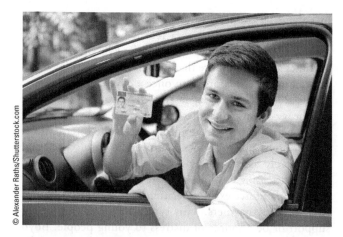

Figure 14-4 For many adolescents, getting a driver's license is the first step toward independence.

is worried about how he will get to school. He cannot drive and cannot get on or off the regular school bus by himself. Because he had only had his driver's license a few months before the accident, he feels the loss of his independence very keenly.

As with this loss of mobility, the loss of independence in dressing and bathing is very distressing for him. He feels that he has regressed back to the level of dependency of a preschool child. He resents his dependency, and this emotional challenge will make it harder for the occupational and physical therapists to help him recover.

SELF-CARE

By the age of 12, children have acquired most of the ADL skills that they need to become autonomous. They are responsible for feeding, bathing, grooming, toileting, and dressing themselves. If parents or caregivers have purchased most of their clothes for them up until this time, there may be a noticeable change in motivation to make their own selections and choices of clothes. With the recent trend of adolescent and adult clothing styles influencing the design of children's clothes, parents may have exercised limits on the styles of clothing that they bought for their children. During adolescence, the choice of dress is often one of the first ways that young people express their autonomy from parental control.

Good hygiene skills, such as routine tooth brushing, hair care, daily bathing, and hand washing before meals are generally acquired earlier in childhood. By the time that individuals become adolescents, verbal reminders are not routinely needed unless these habits were not sufficiently established previously. As boys and girls begin to physically mature and body odor becomes an issue, proper hygiene may need reinforcement in the form of verbal reminders until the use of deodorant becomes a habit. As girls experience the first few months of their menstrual periods, instruction in feminine

hygiene and the proper disposal of used feminine hygiene products is needed. Once these new hygiene skills have been established, young adolescents are expected to continue them independently without adult supervision.

Preoccupation with these areas of occupational performance is related to self-esteem. Satisfaction with one's physical appearance and body image is consistently the variable most related to self-esteem (Clay, Vignoles, & Dittmar, 2005). Social acceptance by peers, academic achievement, and athletic success also correlate with self-esteem, but appearance has the greatest influence. Adolescents care about how they look. Although girls as a rule tend to develop interests in fashion, hairstyles, and fragrances a little earlier than most boys, but both boys and girls become interested in their appearance and their physical attractiveness during adolescence.

Choosing the way one looks from an appearance standpoint is an early expression of experimentation with self-definition. Some adolescents move through a series of group identities, trying different ones on for size to determine if a group is a good match for them personally. It is not uncommon for adolescents to use the style of their hair and their choice of dress to communicate their identification with a particular group, the members of which tend to look and dress in a particular distinctive style. Appearance also contributes to the development of their social identity. Many girls learn to wear makeup as adolescents, as illustrated in **Figure 14-5**.

DOMESTIC LIFE

Most adolescent Americans live in homes with one or both parents and other members of their family. However, some may live in other social arrangements, such as with grandparents, in foster care, or in an institutional setting, such as a group home or a residential school. Regardless of the setting and social environment of their home or living arrangement, most adolescents have multiple occupational

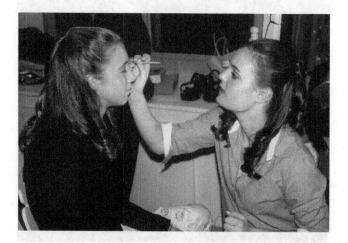

Figure 14-5 Some adolescent girls find the grooming task of applying makeup to be important every day, and even more so on special occasions like school dances.

roles and have responsibility for some instrumental activities of daily living (IADL). Young adolescents may be responsible for keeping their room neat, making their bed, taking out the trash, cutting the grass, setting the table, washing dishes, doing their own laundry, and helping with the housecleaning. Many adolescents learn to prepare simple cold and hot meals using the microwave, stove, and oven. Adolescents whose parents both work and those who have younger siblings may be responsible for preparing simple dishes, such as hot dogs, pizza, and macaroni and cheese for their siblings.

If adolescents take medicine routinely, they are increasingly expected to assume greater responsibility for their own medication management. There is a general relinquishing of responsibility on the part of parents, and assumption of responsibility on the part of the adolescent that takes place over time. Shopping is considered an IADL, but for the most part, the type of shopping that is done by adolescents is more correctly categorized as a leisure activity. Adolescent shopping is often nonobligatory and engaged in during discretionary time. Some adolescents may have the responsibility of doing the grocery or drugstore shopping for their families, but it is not typically the responsibility of adolescents to perform those tasks unless they have assumed more adultlike roles within the family. As adolescents age, they typically become more involved in IADLs.

In some parts of the world, adolescents are recognized in society as adults and are expected to assume adult roles. The typical older adolescent has the skills to do this adequately. In industrial societies where adolescence is an extended period of preparation for the assumption of adult role, adolescents contemplating moving out of the family home and at the same time they develop a greater interest in performing tasks that they see as necessary for living independently. Even if they have not performed clothing care and meal preparation tasks earlier in their lives, they may seek out adult assistance for acquiring these skills in the months or year prior to an anticipated move from the family home.

INTERPERSONAL INTERACTIONS

Underlying the growing number and type of interpersonal interactions of average teens is **identity formation**, the establishment of a distinct personality of individuals that helps them identify their newly forming place in society and life (Feldman, 2011). This process of identity formation defines individuals to others as well as to themselves. In adolescence, identity formation centers around questions like "Who am I?," "Where do I belong?," and "What do I want to be?" Reflected in identity formation is the individuals' self-concept (What am I like?) and their self-esteem (How well do I like myself?). Identity formation is an individual process, but the process is structured by the sociocultural context within which the teens live and interact. Identity formation can be especially challenging for teens who feel different from others because of their cultural, ethnic, gender, or sexual identity.

Resilience is a term used to describe a person's ability to cope with stress and adversity. Resilient coping may result in individuals "bouncing back" to a previous state of normal functioning, or simply not showing negative effects (Masten, 2009). Research on resiliency has shown that the presence of a caring adult is an extremely important asset in the life of young people. Resiliency becomes an increasingly important trait as adolescents move into adulthood. For individuals on a traditional development path, early adulthood followed by middle adulthood are the two life periods that are associated with the highest stress.

Resilience may be an obvious "bouncing back" from a negative or stressful experience, such as an illness or death in the family. Resilience may also be a more subtle response. Teens who quietly but steadfastly choose not to conform to society's expectations, whether it is an extreme lack of interest in fashion or a difference in gender orientation, show resilience (Ungar, 2010). Resilience in both children and youth is dependent upon those who are marginalized being able to communicate and "talk back" to those who would tell them that their capacity to cope is an individual problem (Bottrell, 2009). Resilience can be supported through training in individual coping strategies, may be built through support from the family and the community, and it may be supported by policies like "antibullying" initiatives in schools.

A component of identity formation is the establishment of **gender identity**, the understanding of oneself as a man or a woman. Hutchison (2011) notes that "all cultures have norms about gender roles, and social institutions incorporate expectations about how females and males are to behave" (p. 237). Although the United States may have some flexibility in gender standards, with similar expectations for members of both genders, very distinctive gender roles are prescribed in much of the world. Clashes between flexible gender expectations of the mainstream United States and the more fixed standards of many immigrant groups can be a source of conflict in families with strong ethnic ties to another culture.

As part of the identity formation that occurs during adolescence, teens begin to find out what types of people they are sexually attracted to. **Sexual orientation** describes an enduring pattern of attraction that may be emotional, romantic, sexual, or some combination of these to other people. Those people may be of the opposite sex, the same sex, or both sexes. Exploration of personal, gender and sexual identity is widespread in adolescence. In spite of this exploration, this is still a time of high peer pressure and expectations of social conformity. It is perhaps because of this that relatively few adolescents "come out" and identify themselves as gay, lesbian, bisexual, or transgendered (GLBT) in adolescence. Although historically most of the information on the experience of GLBT teens has been anecdotal, recent studies have shown that these young people who are in the sexual minority face more fighting in early adolescence (Russell, Everett, Rosario, & Birkett, 2014). GLBT teens experienced more nonphysical victimization, including having personal property stolen, and nonphysical bullying, although this trend is not as strong as the trend toward increased fighting. Russell and colleagues (2014) found the fighting declined with age overall, but the nonphysical forms of school victimization persisted throughout the high school years. GLBT teens can become socially isolated and develop depression. Russell and Toomey (2012) noted more suicide ideation and a greater suicide risk among adolescent men with a same-sex sexual orientation than there was among their peers. These authors reported that this trend reflected the developmental trends of adolescence, including identity development and a personal sense of failure.

In addition to developing a sexual identity, adolescence is a time when young people evaluate their ethnic background and explore ethnic identity. This might be expressed as an interest in family heritage, such as seen in the fifth-generation American who develops a passion for all things Irish, or it might be the self-identification with a particular minority or ethnic group. This could mean that young people whose families emigrated from Mexico would form an exclusive social group, or it could be that high school students from town do not interact much with students from rural communities. Hutchinson (2011) notes that by late adolescence, individuals may have been exposed to ethnic discrimination, and this exposure will influence identity formation. In general, young people from ethnic minority groups tend to develop a strong ethnic identity.

RELATIONSHIPS

In the adolescent period, there is a great expansion both in the type and numbers of relationships that young people maintain. They are exploring new relationship types, as they grow to understand their sexuality. At the same time, they have broad school and community connections with both adults and peers. During this developmental period the adolescent's relationship with his or her parents are often re-negotiated to reflect changing abilities and needs, but the family remains an important source of affirmation and support for most teens. Friends and other peers have an important influence in this period, but parents continue to be a significant influence. The parent/child relationship is very important throughout the teen years, and teens who have positive relationships with parents tend to also have positive relationships with peers.

Informal Social Relationships

Friends offer maturing individuals with the opportunity to compare and evaluate their growing abilities in a meaningful way. This is a time when young people start to look

beyond the family and question the authority and the relevance of information adults provide. As a **reference group**, friends serve as sources of information, role models, and audiences for new behaviors. Reference groups present a set of social standards against which teens can judge themselves (Feldman, 2011). Younger adolescents tend to select reference groups that are similar to themselves in gender and interests. Building on opportunities for social participation through involvement in activities in the community, adolescents may form friendships that broaden and may include members of the opposite sex by the middle part of adolescence (Hutchison, 2011). As the adolescents mature, their reference groups become more varied in the gender, age, and interests of the members.

Throughout adolescence, teens spend increasingly more time with their peers and without parental supervision. Peer pressure is the influence of a social group that is valued by the individual. Peer conformity, the behavioral response to peer pressure, is at its height in early adolescence. Although peer pressure is often presented as a negative influence, it can be both positive and negative. On the positive side, peer pressure can motivate prosocial behaviors such as academic success and healthy lifestyles. Peers often listen to, accept, and understand the frustrations, challenges, and concerns associated with being a teenager. Some of the negative influence of peers can be associated with risky or reckless behavior and feelings of rejection. Teens who feel isolated or rejected are more likely to engage in risky behaviors to try and impress others or to "prove themselves" to their peers. Adolescents with disabilities may choose to blend in with peers rather than take recommended actions to manage their health. Young people with serious conditions like diabetes may fail to maintain the medical regime needed for the management of the condition. Similarly, adolescents with orthopedic conditions, such as cerebral palsy may resist the use of splints or braces, because they are not part of the group standard. This desire to conform with peers and the desire to fit in can be a significant impediment in providing health care support for adolescents because of their desire to blend in.

In recent years, teens have increasingly begun to use technology as a tool in social networking. With instant messaging, text messages, and personal news streams like Twitter that allow peers to "follow" their friends, adolescents without access to technology may be excluded from many peer communications. Common Sense Media (2012) reports that "Nine out of 10 (90%) 13- to 17-year-olds have used some form of social media. Three out of four (75%) teenagers currently have a profile on a social networking site, and one in five (22%) has a current Twitter account (27% have ever used Twitter)" (p. 9). Accessing the Internet via webcam and "video chatting" with online friends while texting or instant messaging, as the young women in **Figure 14-6**, are not uncommon.

Although adults have expressed many concerns about the growth of social media, adolescents overwhelmingly report that social and digital media have improved their

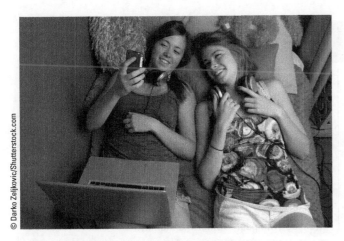

Figure 14-6 Electronic technologies have changed the way teens interact socially. These young women are video chatting while also reading texts from friends.

relationships. "More than one in four teens say that using their social networking site makes them feel less shy (29%) and more outgoing (28%); one in five says it makes them feel more confident (20%), more popular (19%), and more sympathetic to others (19%); and 15% say it makes them feel better about themselves. By comparison, only 5% say social networking makes them feel less outgoing; 4% feel worse about themselves, less confident, and less popular after using their social networking site; and 3% feel shyer" (Common Sense Media, 2012, p. 10).

Although there are many benefits associated with social media use, there are also risks. O'Keeffe and Clarke-Pearson (2011) identified the following categories of risk associated with social media use: peer-to-peer; inappropriate content; lack of understanding of online privacy issues; and outside influences of third-party advertising groups. Peer-to-peer risks such as cyberbullying were introduced in Chapter 13. Cyberbullying often grows more potentially damaging in adolescence and can cause profound psychosocial outcomes including depression, anxiety, severe isolation, and in extreme cases, suicide (Hinduja & Patchin, 2010).

Sexting can be defined as "sending, receiving, or forwarding sexually explicit messages, photographs, or images via cell phone, computer, or other digital devices" (Berkshire District Attorney, 2010). These sexually explicit images become distributed rapidly via cell phones or the Internet. One survey revealed that 20 percent of teens have sent or posted nude or seminude photographs or videos of themselves (National Campaign to Prevent Teen and Unplanned Pregnancy, 2008). Sexting is a social activity that is often not shared beyond a small peer group and is not found to be distressing to the parties involved. When sexting is unwelcome, it may be viewed as child pornography and result in felony charges, school suspension for perpetrators, and emotional distress with accompanying mental health conditions for victims (O'Keefe & Clarke-Pearson, 2011).

The main risk to adolescents online today are unintentional effects caused by improper use of technology, sharing too much information, or posting false information about themselves or others (Barnes, 2006). Although distinct from sexting, similar issues and concerns occur with posting sexually explicit images. Many sites allow users to block images that are tagged as "not safe for work" or "explicit," and individuals can set their browsers to block these images, but it is possible to be faced with an unwanted image if the person who posted it did not tag it for explicit content. More distressing are Internet shock sites, websites that are intended to be offensive or disturbing to its viewers (Herrmann, 2007). Most shock sites may be thought of as "Internet traps," or sites that you are linked to unexpectedly or unintentionally. These sites prey on unskilled, unsophisticated Internet users such as some young teens.

Family Relationships

Caring, supportive family relationships have been shown to be a source of resiliency and to serve as protective factors for positive youth development (Hutchison, 2011). As younger adolescents begin to push for greater independence, parents have the challenge of allowing them to experience greater autonomy, but within limits. These boundaries are frequently the source of friction between parents and their adolescent children as the determination of what is considered reasonable and safe is often quite different when viewed from the perspective of adults than from the perspective of 12- to 15-year-old adolescents.

Relationships with the family during this period support and reflect teens' internal process of identity formation. For many individuals, this process begins with the recognition of how they want to be like (or unlike) a parent, and how they feel about what the family expectations are about their future. This begins a process of separation from parents that may become complete in adolescence or may extend well into the adult years. This process of individuation is described by Hutchison (2011) as having four components. Complete individuation requires achieving all of the components presented in **Table 14-4**.

Mealtimes, transportation and travel times, visits, vacations, and weekends or weekday evenings at home are typical times for social participation within the family. Many adolescents continue to enjoy going out to eat, going to the movies, or watching television together with their families.

Intimate Relationships

Intimacy is the ability to trust, and the ability to share private thoughts and feelings with selected others. Associated with intimacy are romantic relationships and sexual activity. Hutchison (2011) describes a **romantic relationship** as a relationship between partners that is both emotionally and sexually oriented. Many of the romantic relationships that develop in adolescence last for only a few weeks or months, and though they may seem unimportant to adults, these early relationships are important to developing the capacity for long-term, committed relationships in adulthood (Sorenson, 2007). In early

TABLE 14-4 Individuation from Family of Origin

Functional Independence	This is when the person can function in the everyday performance of tasks without parental assistance.	Functional independence in ADLs typically develops in middle childhood. Independence in IADLs typically develops in adolescence.
Attitudinal Independence	This is developing one's own set of values and beliefs, which may mirror those of their parents or be unique.	In adolescence, the differentiation will have a broader focus like political or religious beliefs. Attitudinal independence may fully develop in adolescence or may continue to evolve into adulthood.
Emotional Independence	This occurs when individuals are not dependent on their parents for approval or emotional support.	In adolescence, individuals may share personal trials or stresses with peers rather than family. Emotional independence may fully develop in adolescence, but it typically continues to evolve into adulthood.
Conflictual Independence	This stage occurs when individuals recognize their separateness from parents without negative emotions like guilt or resentment.	Early in adolescence, it is common that parents are ridiculed for the ways their children perceive them as "embarrassing" or "out of touch." An example of conflictual independence occurs when young people "agree to disagree" with a style or fashion rather than ridiculing it.

adolescence, most youth are very preoccupied with romantic issues and the idea of having a romantic partner. Although some younger adolescents "go out," this usually does not involve dating in the traditional sense. Groups of younger adolescents may arrange to meet at the movies, or a boy and girl may talk on the telephone or hang around together at school.

Relationships become a focus of social life during middle to late adolescence when three-fourths of teens report having had a relationship, dated, or "hooked up" with someone. In fact, many youth in middle to late adolescence report spending more time with their romantic partner than with friends and family (Sorenson, 2007). The socially prescribed timing and expectations for forming romantic relationships vary from culture to culture. As dating becomes more common and more frequent, identification with the role of someone's boyfriend or girlfriend often contributes to a teenager's identity. True intimacy becomes more common in a relationship in later adolescence. These more serious dating relationships may mature into committed adult relationships, or the individuals may move on to other relationships. Although many teens do not become sexually active, they are probably thinking about sex as they seek to establish their own identity. Sexual experiences including masturbation and intercourse are significant life experiences and valued activities for many adolescents.

Adolescents who are attracted to other members of the same sex may need more time to develop their identity and gain greater acceptance of their sexual orientation outside of the intense peer scrutiny of adolescence. As noted earlier, early in the adolescent period, young people who express LGBT tendencies are more like to be exposed to physical violence, verbal abuse and bullying. It can be argued that LGBT adolescents live in a culture that is less judgmental than previous eras,

but acceptance of gender orientations other than heterosexuality varies greatly in different areas of the country and the world.

Teens in rehabilitation settings, dealing with illness or disability may be hesitant to talk about their concerns related to sexuality and sexual activity. Although many occupational and physical therapists are uncomfortable addressing the sexuality of adolescents, it is important to recognize that sexual activity is a routine part of life.

MAJOR LIFE AREAS

In the adolescent years, individuals first engage in the full spectrum of major life activities, engaging in education, work, and employment. Although many adolescents will have had money and done some shopping, in adolescence, youths begin to manage their own money, use banking services, and learn to conduct economic transactions without the oversight of their parents. Many of the occupational roles of adolescents are associated by their participation in major life areas.

Education

In the United States and many other parts of the world, young people are required to participate in formal education. The occupational role of student varies not only by nationality, but also by other less concrete factors such as peer influences and socioeconomic status. At ages 11 through 14, students are expected to be attending middle school (also called junior high school). During these years, students transition from being in a single classroom with one generalist teacher to having multiple teachers who teach courses in specific subject areas. In the role of middle school student, individuals are expected to conform to a code of behavior and a code of dress. The student occupational role at all grade levels includes the expression of respect for teachers and a commitment to pursue assigned tasks at the top of their ability. Middle school students are expected to change rooms and teachers to benefit from teachers who have advanced training and specialized knowledge. The high school years, ages 15 to 18, are less structured, and students are encouraged to pursue interests and to prepare themselves for adult life. With each subsequent year of schooling, the expectations of student occupational role become greater. They are expected to pay attention in class, to take appropriate notes to help them learn the content, to complete all assigned classwork and homework, to study for tests, and to learn the information identified as essential content of the curriculum.

Formal educational participation includes engagement in academics, nonacademics—such as interactions in the lunchroom and school hallways—and extracurricular activities. Participation in education at the middle and high school level is arguably the most influential performance pattern in the life of most adolescents. During the 9 to 10 months when school is in session, adolescents' time is organized around school, transportation, extracurricular activities, and homework schedules. Teens' perception of their success or failure in their occupational role as students will impact their decision making about their future life paths.

As they progress through school, adolescents learn the consequences of studying and preparing for class and tests and those of insufficient preparation. Study habits are generally well established by this time, but these habits may be challenged or proven ineffective, as courses become more challenging and more demanding. High school students may be able to continue independently in their preparation for tests, but they may discover that for some courses there are distinct advantages to forming alliances with classmates, such as study buddies or study groups. As students grow older, they begin making the connection between their coursework and their future as college students or workers.

High schools are generally larger schools and draw from larger geographic areas than the schools the teens attended earlier. For this reason, there is more likely to be cultural diversity and cultural tensions in the high school setting. The sense of feeling outside of the mainstream culture is believed to be a contributing factor in the low high school graduation rates of members of social minorities (Hutchison, 2011). Some alternatives to traditional high schools provide less critical and more supportive environments for learners with special challenges. Homeschooling is a viable option for motivated students and for students who learn differently. Alternative schools are available for high school students who are parents and need child care, and for students who have had difficulty conforming to the behavior standards of a traditional high school.

Family social background is associated with academic attainment and career aspirations (Schoon & Polek, 2011).

A **career** is an organized path pursued by individuals for an extended period leading to a profession or means of livelihood. Adolescents become career-literate through observation of significant others, media portrayal of careers, and part-time employment or volunteer experience in the community. They may aspire to a career, and begin both exploration of and preparation for this career in high school. However, in most industrialized countries true career development occurs after the completion of high school in the early adulthood stage of life. Research has shown that young people from disadvantaged backgrounds often do less well in school, leave school earlier, and have lower goals for future work or career pursuits.

WORK AND EMPLOYMENT

Work, in our context, refers to a trade or other means of livelihood. Work may be a job to earn money while in school that has no long-term bearing on vocational or career goals. The term **vocation** refers to the affective aspect, or "calling," associated with finding one's life's work. In the adolescent years, individuals consider their possible futures, seeking a path toward adult life involving both work and vocational interests. Schools offer *vocational guidance,* a service based on the use of tests, academic aptitudes, and interests to find out what career or occupation may best suit a person. In much of the world, adolescents' first responsibility is work, and participation in education is a luxury that is encouraged when possible. Although this is not typical in the United States, some families in the United States need their teens to work to contribute to the family. For other adolescents, such as the young man in **Figure 14-7**, work is voluntary, but offers a path to increased skill development, personal responsibility, and increased independence.

The young person's first experience in the role of employee often happens in adolescence. Many teens get part-time jobs while they are in school. Even without a formal "job," most adolescents take on responsibilities for which

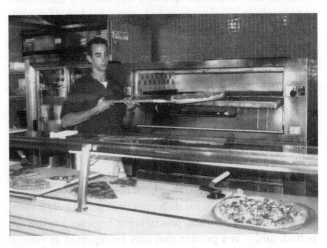

Figure 14-7 Many adolescents over 16 work part-time in service-related jobs.

they are paid, but that do not put them in the mainstream workforce. Jobs such as babysitting for young children, doing yard work for neighbors, pet-sitting, delivering newsletters, being paid by community organizations for refereeing athletic activities, or staffing a concession stand are common occasional jobs for adolescents. These short-term work opportunities allow young people to make some of their own spending money and exposes them to the social and cultural expectations of their work place. This reflects an expansion of their social contexts and a step toward adult work roles.

In the United States, the Fair Labor Standards Act (FLSA) sets 14 years of age as the minimum age for employment and limits the number of hours worked by minors under the age of 16 in regular employment settings. These laws are very specific—people who are 14 and 15 years old cannot work more than 3 hours on a school day or 18 hours in a school week. They can, however, work up to 8 hours on a non-school day or 40 hours in a non-school week, which permits them to hold jobs during school vacations and breaks. They are also limited in regard to the times when they are allowed to work (7 a.m. to 7 p.m.), except during the summer months from June 1 through Labor Day, when evening hours are extended to 9 p.m. (U.S. Department of Labor, n.d.).

For people aged 16 years and above, the maximum work hours are generally the same as for adults. There is still a requirement that students cannot work more than 4 hours on a school day unless they are enrolled in the work experience education program at their high school. Students who are involved in work experience education are allowed to work up to 23 hours per week, any portion of which may be during school hours (U.S. Department of Labor, n.d.). Nearly 70 percent of teens in this age category report working in a job outside the home (Braveman & Page, 2012).

Vocational choice in adolescence is influenced by (1) the reality factor, the constraints in the actual work world like the amount of required travel or the expectation of shift work; (2) the individual's aptitudes and access to educational opportunities; (3) the emotional appeal (or lack of appeal) that the individual has for a work environment, such as a desire to work with animals or a desire to build machines; and (4) the individual's values, learned from family and society about the importance of work and the acceptability of certain types of work (Braveman & Page, 2012). identify a vocation or. Not all individuals choose a career, or they may choose a career that is not financially supportive. As an example, some young people today are very involved in online role-playing games, and spend more than 20 hours a week engaged in progression within their gaming community. They may choose employment that supports their basic needs, but focus their interests and enthusiasm for their pursuit of gaming. The vocational and career-planning process is just beginning in this age period, and it is a process that may be repeated at various times throughout adulthood as interests, skills, and life demands change.

COMMUNITY, SOCIAL, AND CIVIC LIFE

The ICF category of "activities and participation" includes a subcategory focused on the actions and tasks required to engage in organized social life outside the family, in community, social, and civic areas of life (WHO, 2001). This category, called "community, social, and civic life" becomes of interest as youths take on independent roles in society through venues such as sports, leisure activities, and social activism. Adolescents grow increasingly engaged in organized social life outside the family, in community, social, and civic areas of life. For most teens, these community, social, and civic roles are voluntary and reflect individual passions or interests. As adolescents grow more independent and are less involved in supervised extracurricular activities, they often have unsupervised "free time." Caldwell and Witt (2011) estimate that "free time" makes up about 40 percent of the nonworking day. How they spend this time has implications for development and for their health. Participation in social groups that are a part of their lives contributes extensively to their self-definition and the development of an occupational identity. In addition to group participation, adolescents can fill their free time in unhealthy or negative ways, such as being involved in vandalism or using illegal drugs. In this section, we will give special consideration to sports participation. This activity is highly valued and is also a significant reason that adolescents are seen in health care and rehabilitation settings.

Sports Participation

Athletic achievement is one of the most publicly recognized and heralded in popular culture. Information about athletic accomplishments is spread throughout the school and community. Athletes, especially those who excel, become a focus of attention due to their special sport team jackets or dress on game days, having attention focused upon them at pep rallies, on the public address system, and in school and community newspapers. Eime and colleagues (2013) offer substantive evidence of both psychological and social health benefits of participation in sport, especially team sport, by adolescents. Moreau et al. (2014) reported results of a qualitative study of nine adolescents undergoing a sports challenge. The authors found six driving factors underlying sports as a tool to promote psychosocial development in adolescents. The six factors named are (1) encouragement of cooperation among peers, (2) the presence of a facilitator with a positive attitude, (3) challenges to the adolescents' comfort zone, (4) the relationship between enjoyment and effort, (5) the importance of training innovation, and, finally, (6) the shared risk as a cohesive bond. Sports participation can be a formal competitive pursuit, but it also can be an informal leisure activity. Community-based sports teams such as the one pictured in **Figure 14-8** are common recreational activities for teens. Interest in sports as spectators is also a common reason for social gatherings.

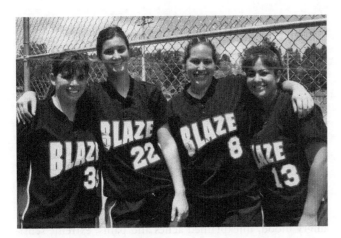

Figure 14-8 Team sports allow many adolescents to develop physical abilities and to make close friends.

Although youth sports participation has many positive aspects, health care professionals should be knowledgeable about risk factors and characteristics of common injuries to provide appropriate guidance to athletes, parents, and coaches. Many physical therapists participate in community-based sports screening programs that serve the purpose of providing anticipatory guidance for injury risk and prevention.

In addition to participating as athletes, adolescents are also often involved in sports as spectators or fans. Individuals who are not athletes may be actively involved in sports through volunteer work at games, through participation in the school band, or through organized social events involving group viewing of either televised or live games. School and community sports events help the young person make social connections and feel a part of the larger community.

Expanded Contexts for Leisure

Leisure time in adolescence is influenced by context and access to the necessary space and equipment. For example, access to a golf course and a set of clubs permits adolescents to develop an interest in playing golf. Adolescents who have access to oceans, bays, rivers, lakes, and other bodies of water have another group of leisure activities made available to them. They enjoy boating, canoeing, fishing, and a variety of water sports like waterskiing, jet skiing, and duck hunting. Likewise, if they have access to countryside and forests, they often grow up enjoying hunting for birds, deer, and other game. Leisure activities are also influenced to a great extent by social context.

Often young people's leisure time is not planned in advance. This use of time usually involves informal play activities that are engaged in spontaneously for the experience of the moment. These include activities like listening to music, hanging out with friends, picking up a book or magazine to read for pleasure or a musical instrument for the sheer enjoyment of playing, watching television, shopping, dining out with friends, going to movies, watching movies, playing video games or computer games, or communicating

with friends via digital media. Most of these activities involve little or no advanced planning and just happen in the moment. Because adolescents do not need adult supervision for their leisure, their involvement in structured extracurricular activities may be less than it was in childhood.

Some leisure pursuits are structured and are actively chosen by the teen. Special interests such as music and drama can be pursued both through school and community venues.

Some leisure pursuits are more structured. The availability of leisure activities guided by caring adults can provide a supportive push for young people to learn skills and competencies that will help them grow and attain future goals. Eime and colleagues (2013) provide examples of programs that emphasize how adult-provided structure, organization, and leadership contribute to adolescent development. These authors found that adolescents who "participate in structured extracurricular activities are less likely to engage in antisocial behavior, more likely to have a higher level of academic achievement, and more likely to have positive psychosocial functioning" (p. 17).

HEALTH AND IMPAIRMENT

For most people, adolescence is a healthy period in the life span. From the life course development model, adolescence is a crucial period in which many influences shape health and patterns of behavior and make lifestyle choices that affect both their current and future health. Adolescents are increasingly independent, and are expected to take greater responsibility for habits and lifestyle choices. Experimentation with adult behavior reflects normative adolescent development; however, early initiation of normative adult behavior such as drinking and sexual activity can be health damaging. Environmental factors such as family, peer group, school, and community characteristics also contribute to adolescents' health and risk behaviors.

Child Health USA (2011) reported that, in 2007, accidents involving motor vehicles were the leading cause of death (44.1 percent), and homicide by firearm was the second leading cause of injury death (18.2 percent). It is likely that a significant proportion of the motor vehicle accidents were alcohol related. Alcohol and other forms of substance abuse are a significant health concern for professionals working with adolescents. One-fifth of deaths among adolescent males were homicides, compared to 7.8 percent of deaths among females (Child Health USA, 2011).

Eating disorders, such as **anorexia nervosa** and **bulimia,** also tend to manifest themselves in the adolescent period of physiologic and psychologic change. Currently, eating disorders are understood in the context of a life course developmental model, which must take into account genetic risk factors, other biologic risks, and environmental factors (Gicquel, 2013). Anorexia nervosa is defined in the *Diagnostic and Statistical Manual* 5 (DSM-5) as a disorder primarily affecting adolescent girls and young woman characterized by a pathologic fear of becoming fat and manifesting as excessive restriction of food intake. Bulimia is defined in DSM-5 as abnormal binge eating followed by induced vomiting or purging, occurring at least on a weekly basis (American Psychiatric Association, 2013). Eating disorders have high mortality and morbidity and require intensive intervention for successful treatment. Early identification and treatment improve outcomes (DeSocio, 2013). Management of eating disorders involves multiple dimensions, which includes physiologic monitoring of health status, psychotherapy, and occasionally prescription drugs in the case of bulimia. Family-based treatment for anorexia and cognitive behavior therapy for bulimia and binge eating have shown success (Hay, 2013).

Substance abuse, also known as drug abuse, is a pattern of substance (drug) use in which individuals consume a substance in amounts or with methods neither approved nor supervised by medical professionals. Adolescents experiment with and overuse common substances such as alcohol and tobacco. They also experiment with illicit substances such as synthetic and the non-medical use of medications. Substance abuse in adolescence is a significant public health challenge. Not only are there the health risks associated with substance abuse, suicide is also very common in adolescent alcohol abusers. One in four suicides in adolescents is related to alcohol abuse (O'Connor & Sheehy, 2000). Similarly, 12.8 percent of adolescent male deaths were attributed to suicide, compared to 7.4 percent of adolescent female deaths (Child Health USA, 2011).

Depression is a condition of mental disturbance, typically with lack of energy and difficulty in maintaining concentration or interest in life, also called a *mood disorder*. Depression in teens can look very different from depression in adults, and is more likely to include irritable or angry mood, unexplained aches and pains, extreme sensitivity to criticism, and withdrawal from some, but not all, people. As many as 28 percent of adolescents experience symptoms that meet the mental health criteria for major depression over the course of adolescence, making it a significant health problem (National Institutes of Mental Health, 2012). Other health issues common to adolescents include sexually transmitted diseases, unplanned pregnancy, and obesity.

SUMMARY

With childhood behind them and adulthood in front of them, the developmental challenges of adolescence are to discover oneself and one's abilities; to arrive at a self-definition, or identity, that incorporates these assets; and to determine the societal roles that are suitable physically and psychologically. The means for accomplishing these developmental challenges is engagement in occupation in context. Adolescents who are developing typically use this period of their lives to participate in a variety of self-defining activities on a daily or routine basis. The composite result of these many and varied occupational experiences are personal development. These activities develop adolescents' mental, sensory, and neuromusculoskeletal functions and other underlying physiologic functions. Adolescents who are provided with the opportunities to choose and experience a wide array of occupations set in a wide range of naturally occurring contexts will be provided with the conditions to promote optimal development.

CASE 1
Vincent... Continued

Vincent is likely to receive both physical and occupational therapy as part of his recovery. The therapists will have to listen to him and respect his feelings to help him move forward. In this case, both occupational and physical therapy will contribute to Vincent's return to his daily occupations.

Facing the disruption of his life plans and his emerging self-identity, Vincent will need ongoing emotional as well as physical support to recover and to successfully transition to adult life roles.

CASE 2

Mark

Mark was 15 years and 8 months and in the first semester of his sophomore year in high school when his parents brought him to the outpatient adolescent substance-abuse treatment program. Mark was suspended from school for having marijuana on school grounds. During his initial interview with the occupational therapist, Mark shared that his parents were both professional people with very busy work schedules. He also said that he had a sister who was away at an elite state university, majoring in premed. Unlike his "perfect" sister, he had struggled with school for as long as he could remember. He confirmed the report in his chart that he had started drinking beer during the end of seventh grade, had been using Vicodin when he could get it, and he had been using marijuana on a daily basis for about a year.

Mark said that he had been shy in elementary and middle school, and he had trouble fitting in when he started high school last year. He "wasn't one of the smart kids, or preppie kids, or jocks." He had been asked by some "skaters" to join them after school. He tried to get the hang of skateboarding but "was terrible at it." He said that he had never been very coordinated. His dad tried to get him interested in playing football and baseball when he was younger, but even though he played several years of Little League ball, he was "always the worst player on the team" and finally had chosen to quit.

When things didn't work out for him with the skater crowd, Mark started hanging out with two students who were the ones who introduced him to "smoking weed." Getting high relaxed him and made him feel better about life. He admitted that his schoolwork wasn't good, because in his opinion "it was completely boring." He hated school because every subject that he took required reading. His parents had come to expect poor report cards from him, and their comment was always the same, that they "didn't expect As and Bs. They just didn't want to see Ds and Fs."

He told me that when he was younger, he used to enjoy collecting and organizing baseball cards and playing video games, but now he spent most of his free time hanging out with his friends or in his room listening to music and watching television. His parents gave him an allowance of $25 a week, but his allowance was not tied to any responsibilities around the house. They had never forced him to do chores because they had a cleaning service that came in weekly, and his mom had always done the family's laundry. He had no goals except to get his driver's license in seven months. He had no idea of what kind of work he might want to do someday, and he had never tried to get involved in any extracurricular activities at the school.

Mark was living every day in the present and had no vision of his future. Although he was from a quite affluent family, he tended to see his family as more of a stressor than a resource. He had not had many opportunities to experience success academically, athletically, or socially. His self-definition was very limited and negative. He had no defined leisure interests that contributed to his feeling productive or accomplished, or about which he expressed feelings of pleasure or enjoyment.

Treatment at the outpatient program included individual and group therapy with the substance-abuse counselors and weekly individual and multifamily group counseling with the family therapist. The OT on the program team helped him explore new interests and restore prior interests, develop the self-confidence to cope with challenges in his life, and experience success in occupational challenges like preparing a meal. The occupational therapist helped Mark look at the way that he had been spending his time, to consider whether the activities that he had done regularly contributed to feelings of productivity, pleasure, and restoration, and if not, what replacement activities appealed to him. Organizing a weekly schedule helped him consider how to develop healthy habits that would sustain a life in recovery.

Continues

Case 2 *Continued*

Through the process of OT and family therapy, and despite Mark's initial resistance, he and his parents were helped to recognize the benefit of being given reasonable responsibilities at home, like doing his own laundry, taking out the trash, and keeping his room and bathroom clean. Mark successfully completed the program and was able to level with his parents about his feelings of inadequacy growing up in a home where the expectations were so high for academic and athletic success. When Mark left the program, he stated emphatically that he wanted to stay away from drugs. After attempting to make it on his own without attending aftercare and relapsing on two occasions, Mark admitted that support was essential to his recovery.

The occupational therapist who had worked with Mark happened to run into Mark at the mall food park about a year after he left the program. The general rule in therapy, to avoid risking a breach of confidentiality, is not to speak to former clients when you happen to cross paths in the community, but in this case Mark approached me. Although still a little shy, he told me that he still had problems with school, but that he was getting help from a tutor and that his grades were getting better. He had gotten his driver's license during the summer, taken a part-time job at a store that sold backpacking and hiking gear to help pay for the cost of his insurance, and had taken several good hiking trips. He smiled sheepishly as he bragged that he had also "gotten pretty good at ironing" his own shirts and pants. Before we said good-bye, he said, "When I was in treatment you made me start thinking about my life. I wasn't really ready to hear everything that you had to say at the time, but now a lot of the things that you talked about keep coming back to me! Thanks!"

Guiding Questions

Some questions to consider:

1. Occupational therapists work with people who have difficulty functioning due to mental health problems. Mark's very limited participation in the ICF activities of "domestic life" was unusual for someone his age. In addition to helping with meals and laundry, what other domestic skills should Mark master before he moves out on his own?
2. Sibling relationships are often supportive, but Mark's comments suggested that he views his own abilities negatively because of his sister's successes. What strategies can you think of that could help Mark build a more positive self-identity?

CASE 3

Jeremy

Jeremy was a 13-year-old eighth-grader who was very active in school and community sports. He began playing organized sports at the age of 5 in a community T-ball league and has played baseball ever since. When Jeremy got to middle school, he started playing football. The coaches quickly identified him as being a talented athlete. In the fall of his eighth-grade year, the basketball coach asked Jeremy if he was interested in trying out for the basketball team. Despite never having played organized basketball, Jeremy earned

Continues

Case 3 *Continued*

a spot on the team and excelled due to his athleticism and quickness. During the last two weeks of the basketball season, Jeremy began complaining of bilateral knee pain. Jeremy was a very competitive athlete and did not want to lose playing time, and he certainly did not want the other boys to think that he could not handle the rigors of basketball practice, so he did not initially tell his coach or his parents about the pain. When the pain became persistent and hurting even when he was at rest, he decided to tell his parents.

When Jeremy's mother found out about the pain, she immediately took him to their family doctor, who diagnosed him with "growing pains." With his parent's fear alleviated by the diagnosis, Jeremy continued to play despite the pain. Then, in late winter, after the basketball session was over, his pain began to subside. Despite playing baseball in the spring and summer, he had no further complaint of knee pain. In mid-August, during the second week of football practice, Jeremy's pain began to gradually return. By the time the season started in early September, he could hardly run. He complained to his parents that he had pain when he walked down hills and down steps. He also had pain when he tried to sprint or jump. His parents decided that it was time to take him to see a local orthopedic surgeon whom they knew from church.

Jeremy played baseball from April to July, football from August to November, and basketball from November to February. Jeremy was having pain not only during activity but also after exercise, suggesting a more chronic condition. Jeremy's doctor ordered plain radiographs, because Jeremy was still growing and had open epiphyseal plates. The radiographs revealed a slight separation of the epiphysis at both tibial tuberosities, which was a sure sign of Osgood-Schlatter disease.

Jeremy and his mother were confused about why he had no pain over the summer. His doctor explained that this condition was exacerbated primarily by the jumping and eccentric loading that was common in both basketball and football wide receivers. He also explained that Osgood-Schlatter disease was very sensitive to the volume of exercise performed, and that Jeremy may have been well within his exercise envelope while playing baseball but exceeded his limits with basketball and football. Following this diagnosis, Jeremy was referred to physical therapy.

The physical therapist instructed him in proper quadriceps stretching and closed kinetic chain eccentric strengthening exercises. The physical therapist also emphasized the importance of being honest with his parents about when and how much pain he was having. In physical therapy, Jeremy learned the importance of recognizing the early signs and symptoms of overuse and how to manage his acute pain by relative rest and ice. Jeremy was seen a second time two weeks later to evaluate his progress and make sure that he was doing his exercises correctly. At the time of the second visit, he was not having any pain and was back to playing football. Jeremy decided that he would stick to baseball and football, which were his two favorite sports, and give up basketball. Following this intervention, Jeremy was able to play baseball and football without further problems. He excelled in baseball, and in his senior year of high school, he was offered a chance to play college baseball at a local Division III college.

Guiding Questions

Some questions to consider:

1. Jeremy did not tell anyone about his pain because he did not want to appear weak to his friends and teammates. Do you think that this is reflective of American culture and its expectations of toughness in young men? Or is it something that any serious athlete might do? Explain your answer.
2. The physical therapist put a lot of effort into helping Jeremy understand the condition. Because Jeremy was only 13, the therapist could have focused only on educating Jeremy's parents. What do you think were the benefits of directing this education toward Jeremy?

Speaking of
Those Teen Years

ANDREA EARLE MULLINS, MS, OTR/L,
OCCUPATIONAL THERAPIST, GRAFTON SCHOOL

Working with adolescents is something I enjoy immensely. I work with people in all stages of adolescence, from 12- and 13-year-old young adolescents to young adults of 19 and 20. I am an occupational therapist at a private, not-for-profit school and residential treatment program for children and adolescents who have experienced sufficient difficulties functioning in their home or public school environment to justify their placement at our facility.

My experience growing up with a family friend who has a *pervasive developmental disorder* was the driving force behind my interest in this area of practice. I especially remember the challenges he faced during adolescence in developing friendships and participating in social activities. I so wanted to work with young people with these types of challenges that I was willing four years ago to accept a job in this setting in a nontraditional occupational therapy role, as a behavior specialist. My focus in that role was on designing individualized *positive behavior support* programs to help students and staff people learn techniques that promote adaptive behaviors and improve overall quality of life. A little over a year ago, I transitioned into the "traditional" occupational therapy role in this program. I found that my experience as a behavior specialist was completely compatible and highly complementary to my training as an occupational therapist.

The students I work with are diagnosed with a variety of disabilities, including autism, Asperger's disorder, mental retardation, and various psychiatric disorders like bipolar disorder, attention deficit disorder, and major depressive disorder. One of my main roles as an occupational therapist is to help these students engage in the process of forming their own unique identity. I have worked with many teenagers who have missed out on so many important stages of social and self-growth. Many of the students with whom I work do not have active family involvement. Many are under custody of the state department of social services. Most of them are extremely limited in their social engagement with "typically developing" peers. Although they have disabilities, these adolescents, like all young people, need satisfying social roles for the future.

I engage students in activities that provide them with the opportunities to discover their interests and preferences, and they begin to define their own unique identities. As we do this, an amazing process often unfolds. For example, I worked for over a year with a young woman in her late adolescence. When I first began working with "Sue," she was not able to identify any personal interests other than watching TV. She had lived in foster care and group homes for most of her life and had not been exposed to many basic activities that life has to offer. She had never actively explored her values, interests, and beliefs. People who worked with Sue told me that she was "lazy," "bossy," and "unmotivated." We started to explore her interests and values in a very nonthreatening way. We completed interest checklists and gradually began to explore various choices. When Sue expressed an interest in animals, we began to work with our therapy dog at the end of each session, performing grooming tasks and taking the dog for walks. I always tried to make sessions fun and enjoyable. We discovered that Sue had many interests that she had never previously had the chance to experience or explore. Over the course of the next several months, she began volunteering at a local animal shelter. Since then she has progressed to a level of independence that is allowing her to work toward a career in dog grooming. As she discovered her unique talents and gifts, she began to open up in many ways, expressing an enthusiasm for life that she had never shown before. Her progress has unfolded into all areas of her life. Today she is working on becoming a leader and advocate for other people with disabilities.

REFERENCES

American Psychiatric Association. (2013) *Diagnostic and statistical manual of mental disorders* (5th ed.). Arlington, Virginia: American Psychiatric Publishing.

Barnes, S. (2006). A privacy paradox: Social networking in the United States. *First Monday, 11,* 9.

Berkshire District Attorney. (2010). *Sexting.* Pittsfield, MA: Commonwealth of Massachusetts. Retrieved from http://www.mass.gov/berkshireda/crime-awareness-and-prevention/sexting/sexting.htm

Bottrell, D. (2009). Understanding "marginal" perspectives: Towards a social theory of resilience. *Qualitative Social Work, 8*(3), 321–339.

Boyd, D., & Hargittai. E. (2013). Connected and concerned: Variation in parents' online safety concerns. *Policy & Internet, 5*(3), 245–269.

Braveman, B., & Page, J. (2012). *Work: Promoting participation and productivity through occupational therapy.* Philadelphia. PA: F.A. Davis.

Caldwell, L., & Witt, P. (2011). Leisure, recreation, and play from a developmental context. *New Directions For Youth Development, 2011, 130,* 13–27.

Carlisi, C. O., Pavletic, N. N., & Ernst, M. M. (2013). New perspectives on neural systems models of adolescent behavior: Functional brain connectivity. *Neuropsychiatrie De L'enfance Et De L'adolescence, 61*(4), 209–218.

Child Health USA. (2011). *Adolescent mortality.* Retrieved from http://mchb.hrsa.gov/chusa11/hstat/hsa/pages/229am.html

Clay, D.,Vignoles, V., & Dittmar, H. (2005). Body image and self-esteem among adolescent girls: Testing the influence of sociocultural factors. *Journal of Research on Adolescence, 15,* 451–477.

Colrain, I., & Baker, F. (2011). Changes in sleep as a function of adolescent development. *Neuropsychology Review, 21,* 5–21.

Common Sense Media. (2012). *Social media, social life: How teens view their digital lives.* San Francisco, CA: Common Sense Media.

DeSocio, J. (2013). The neurobiology of risk and pre-emptive interventions for anorexia nervosa. *Journal of Child and Adolescent Psychiatric Nursing, 26*(1), 16–22.

DiFiori, J. P., Benjamin, J., Brenner, J., Gregory, A., Hayanthi, N., Landry, G., & Luke, A. (2014). Overuse injuries and burnout in youth sports: A position statement from the American Medical Society for Sports Medicine. *Clinical Journal of Sport Medicine, 24*(1), 3–20.

Eime, R. M., Young, J. A., Harvey, J. T., Charity, M. J., & Payne, W. R. (2013). A systematic review of the psychological and social benefits of participation in sport for children and adolescents: informing development of a conceptual model of health through sport. *International Journal of Behavioral Nutrition & Physical Activity, 10*(1), 98–118.

Feldman, R. (2011) *Child development* (6th ed.). Upper Saddle River, NJ: Prentice Hall.

Galván, A., & McGlennen, K. M. (2013). Enhanced striatal sensitivity to aversive reinforcement in adolescents versus adults. *Journal of Cognitive Neuroscience, 25*(2), 284–296.

Galván, A. (2012). Risky behavior in adolescents: The role of the developing brain. In V. F. Reyna, S. B. Chapman, M. R. Dougherty, J. Confrey (Eds.), *The adolescent brain: Learning, reasoning, and decision making* (pp. 267–289). Washington, DC US: American Psychological Association.

Gicquel, L. (2013) Anorexia nervosa during adolescence and young adulthood: Towards a developmental and integrative approach sensitive to time course. *Journal of Physiology-Paris, 107*(4), 268–277.

Hay, P. (2013). Assessment and management of eating disorders: An update. *Australian Prescriber, 36*(5), 154–157.

Herrmann, S. (2007). *BBC News: Shock tactics.* Retrieved from http://www.bbc.co.uk/blogs/theeditors/2007/06/shock_tactics.html

Hinduja, S., & Patchin, J. (2010). Bullying, cyberbullying, and suicide. *Archives of Suicide Research, 14,* 206–221.

Horne, J., Flannery, R., & Usman, S. (2014). Adolescent idiopathic scoliosis: Diagnosis and management. *American Family Physician, 89*(3), 193–198.

Hutchison, E. (2011) *Dimensions of human behavior: The changing life course* (4th ed.). Thousand Oaks, CA: Sage Publications.

Ito, M., Horst, H., Bittani, M., Boyd, D., Herr-Stephenson, B., Lange, P., Pascoe, C., and Robinson, L. (2008). *Living and learning with new media: Summary of findings from the Digital Youth Project.* Chicago, IL: John D. and Catherine T. MacArthur Foundation Reports on Digital Media and Learning.

Ito, M., Baumer, S., Bittanti, M., Boyd, D., Cody, R., Herr, B., Horst, H., Lange, P., Mahendran, D., Martinez, K., Pascoe, C., Perkel, D., Robinson, L., Sims, C., & Tripp, L. (2009). *Hanging out, messing around, geeking out: Living and learning with new media.* Cambridge: MIT Press.

Loessl, B. B., Valerius, G. G., Kopasz, M. M., Hornyak, M. M., Riemann, D. D., & Voderholzer, U. U. (2008). Are adolescents chronically sleep-deprived? An investigation of sleep habits of adolescents in the Southwest of Germany. *Child: Care, Health & Development, 34*(5), 549–556.

Malina, R. M. (2011). Skeletal age and age verification in youth sport. *Sports Medicine, 41*(11), 925–947.

Masten, A. S. (2009). Ordinary magic: Lessons from research on resilience in human development. *Education Canada, 49,* 28–32.

Medline Plus. (2014). *Adolescent development.* Retrieved from http://www.nlm.nih.gov/medlineplus/ency/article/002003.htm

Moreau, N., Chanteau, O., Benoit, M., Dumas, M.-P., Laurin-lamother, A., Parlavecchio, L., & Lester, C. (2014) Sports activities in a psychosocial perspective: Preliminary analysis of adolescent participation in sports challenges. *International Review for the Sociology of Sport, 49*(1), 85–101.

National Campaign to Prevent Teen and Unplanned Pregnancy. (2008). *Sex and tech: Results of a survey of teens and young adults.* Washington, DC: National Campaign to Prevent Teen and Unplanned Pregnancy. Retrieved from http://thenationalcampaign.org/resource/sex-and-tech

National Institutes of Mental Health. (2012). *Depression in children and adolescents*. Retrieved from http://www.nimh.nih.gov/health/topics/depression/depression-in-children-and-adolescents.shtml

O'Connor, R., & Sheehy, N. (2000). *Understanding suicidal behaviour*. Leicester: BPS Books (pp. 33–36).

O'Keeffe, G., & Clarke-Pearson, K. (2011). The impact of social media on children, adolescents, and families. *Pediatrics, 127,* 800–804.

Payne, V. G., & Isaacs, L. D. (2012). *Human motor development: A lifespan approach* (8th ed.). New York, NY: McGraw Hill.

ProHealth Care. (2012). *Good sleep habits for teenagers*. Retrieved from http://www.prohealthcare.org/services-sleep-center-good-sleep-habits-for-teens.aspx

Reyna, V. F., Estrada, S., DeMarinis, J., Myers, R., Stanisz, J., & Mills, B., (2011). Neurobiological and memory models of risky decision making in adolescents versus young adults. *Journal of Experimental Psychology: Learning, Memory, and Cognition, 37*(5), 1125–1142.

Romer, D., Bagdasarov, Z., & More, E. (2013). Older versus newer media and the well-being of United States youth: Results from a national longitudinal panel. *Journal of Adolescent Health, 52*(5), 613–619.

Russell, S. T., Everett, B. G., Rosario, M., & Birkett, M. (2014). Indicators of victimization and sexual orientation among adolescents: Analyses from youth risk behavior surveys. *American Journal of Public Health, 104*(2), 255–261.

Russell, S. T., & Toomey, R. B. (2012). Men's sexual orientation and suicide: Evidence for U. S. adolescent-specific risk. *Social Science & Medicine, 74*(4), 523–529.

Schoon, I., & Polek, E. (2011). Teenage career aspirations and adult career attainment: The role of gender, social background and general cognitive ability. *International Journal of Behavioral Development, 35*(3), 210–217.

Sorenson, S. (2007). Adolescent romantic relationships. *Facts and Findings*. Retrieved from http://www.actforyouth.net/resources/rf/rf_romantic_0707.pdf

Stang, J., & Story, M. (Eds.) (2005). *Guidelines for adolescent nutrition services*. Retrieved from http://www.epi.umn.edu/let/pubs/adol_book.shtm

Susman, E. J., & Rogol, A. (2004). Puberty and psychological development. In R. M. Lerner & L. Steinberg (Eds.). (2004), Handbook of adolescent psychology (2nd ed., pp. 15–44). Hoboken, NJ: Wiley.

Tanner, J. M. (1962). *Growth at adolescence*. Oxford: Blackwell.

Ungar, M. (2010). Families as navigators and negotiators: Facilitating culturally and contextually specific expressions of resilience. *Family Process, 49*(3), 421–435.

U.S. Department of Health and Human Services, Health Resources and Services Administration, Maternal and Child Health Bureau (USHHS). (2011). Adolescent mortality. *Child Health USA 2011*. Rockville, Maryland: U.S. Department of Health and Human Services.

U.S. Department of Health and Human Services, Health Resources and Services Administration, Center for Disease Control (USHHS CDC). (2012). Youth Risk Behavior Surveillance—United States 2011. *Morbidity and Mortality Weekly Report, 61*(4), 1–162.

U.S. Department of Labor (n.d.). *Youth and labor*. Retrieved from http://www.dol.gov/dol/topic/youthlabor/workhours.htm

World Health Organization (WHO), (2001). *ICF: International classification of functioning and disability*. Geneva, Switzerland: World Health Organization.

CHAPTER 15

Family and Disablement Issues throughout Childhood

Anne Cronin, PhD, OTR/L, FAOTA,
Associate Professor, Division of
Occupational Therapy,
West Virginia University,
Morgantown, West Virginia
and

Susannah Grimm Poe, Ed.D.,
Associate Professor, Department of
Pediatrics, WVU School of Medicine,
WG Klingberg Center for Child
Development, Morgantown,
West Virginia

Objectives

Upon completion of this chapter, readers should be able to:

- Differentiate developmental disorder from developmental delay;

- Identify and describe key health and disability conditions that emerge in childhood;

- Define normalization as both a parenting strategy and as an outcome in family functioning when dealing with children and youth with chronic health conditions;

- Explain how the health traditions model and the uncertainty in illness theory can be used to better meet the needs of children and families living with a disability;

- Offer strategies to address and support culturally effective health care in providing intervention services to children and youth;

- Explain how characteristics of children impact the nature of both parent and sibling relationships; and

- Explain strategies to support the participation of children and youth with disabilities in community and leisure activities.

Key Terms

anxiety disorders

attention deficit/hyperactivity disorder (ADHD)

autism spectrum disorder (ASD)

developmental delay

developmental disability

Health Traditions Model

hippotherapy

intellectual disability (ID)

learning disability (LD)

mental health disorder

multitrauma

normalization

parenting stress

Part B of the Individuals with Disabilities Education Act

post-traumatic stress disorder (PTSD)

Special Olympics

white coat syndrome

CASE 1

Logan

When he was 6 and ready to transition into first grade, Logan was referred for an occupational therapy evaluation of sensory processing and classroom participation skills. He had a history of prematurity, language delay, and generalized delays in development. Logan had received behavioral support, occupational therapy services, and speech therapy through community and school settings since the age of 2. During the assessment, it was noted that Logan had typical range of motion and muscle tone. His sitting posture was functional, and he had effective, age-appropriate grasp-and-release patterns. In spite of this, Logan had difficulty with school-related fine motor tasks and persisted at these activities for only very short periods of time. During clinical observation, Logan was noted to use both hands together in a lead assist pattern only inconsistently and needed cues to look at tasks. He had specific preferences in play that were repetitive and did not challenge him to develop new skills. Logan did demonstrate some repetitive self-stimulatory behaviors, such as staring at the lights and rocking his body, especially when he felt stressed. He had difficulty with tasks requiring joint attention (that is, attention to the same item or topic as another person), and in task performance had difficulty orienting and understanding the specific elements of tasks. For example, he did not persist at a drawing task because the task itself did not make sense to him. Logan had significant language delays, and during this observation it appeared that he had difficulty understanding, retaining, and retrieving spoken instruction or directions.

Logan has had differences in development since his birth, but with a supportive family and preschool setting, he had gained many needed skills. The demands of the school setting that he will face in the upcoming year are of concern because the performance skills needed to be successful in first grade are exactly those skills he is weakest in: expressive communication, attention, working memory, sensory processing, and problem solving during task performance. Often in points of transition, such as the one Logan faces, both the child and the family are confronted with difficult challenges in both understanding and supporting the needs of each individual child with a disability.

Continues on page 349

INTRODUCTION

Some people are born with a disability. Birth defects and prematurity, introduced in Chapter 11, are major causes of both physical and mental congenital disability. In this chapter, we will consider some additional types of impairments that result in disability other than those present at birth. For example, some children become injured or ill and are left with a disability as a result. Other children develop the signs of a disability gradually as they mature. In the U.S. Census of 2010, about 5.2 million (8.4 percent) children had some kind of disability. About 3.6 percent of children under the age of 6 had a disability, and most of these disabilities were caused by congenital or developmental problems (Brault, 2012).

About 4.5 million children (12.2 percent) between the ages of 6 and 14 have a disability. Of these, about 2.3 million children had difficulty doing regular schoolwork (6.2 percent), including 1.6 million who reported receiving special education services (Brault, 2012). In this chapter, the emphasis will be on those conditions that are not usually diagnosed in infancy, even though children who were diagnosed with chronic problems in infancy often continue to have performance limitations through childhood and form a significant part of any pediatric physical or occupational therapists caseload.

In general, throughout the life span, the proportion of the population that has a disability increases. This increase is illustrated in **Figure 15-1**. If you separate out the childhood years, the pattern is similar. The big increase in disability occurs in the age group of 6 to 14 years because statistics now include cognitive, learning, and mental health problems that were not captured in the earlier data. **Table 15-1** shows the 2010 U.S. Census data that are specific to children.

One objective of this chapter is to introduce professionals in occupational and physical therapy to developmental disabilities that are first diagnosed in childhood. Another objective is to show how that diagnosis can affect a child's family. Because therapists have such a critical role in the rehabilitation of children with developmental disorders, it is necessary that they understand not only their part in helping the child but also the role of the family and the support systems within the community.

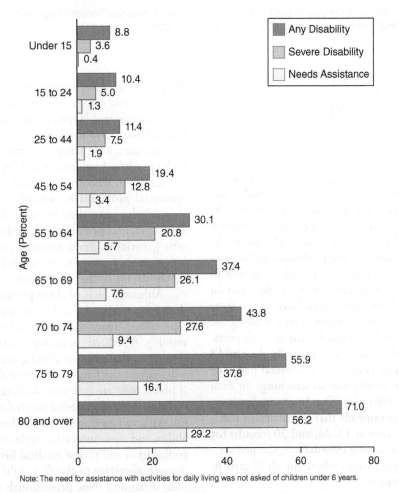

Note: The need for assistance with activities for daily living was not asked of children under 6 years.

Figure 15-1   The incidence of disability in the population increases with age.

Source: U.S. Census Bureau. Survey of Income and Program Participation, June–September 2005.

TABLE 15-1   Census Data Showing Disability in Children

Category	Number Estimate	Percentage Estimate
Under 15 years	62,176	100
With a disability	5,218	8.4
Under 3 years	12,676	100
With a disability	289	2.3
3 to 5 years	12,961	100
With a disability	465	3.6
6 to 14 years	36,540	100
With a disability	4,464	12.2
Learning disability	692	1.9
Attention deficit/hyperactivity disorder	1,867	5.1
Intellectual disability	154	0.4
Other developmental disability	540	1.5
Other developmental condition	1,654	4.5
ADL limitation	370	1.0

Adapted from Brault, 2012. Reference Creditng: Brault, M. (2012). Americans with Disabilities: Household economic studies. U.S. Census Bureau. Retrieved from http://www.census.gov/people/disability/publications/sipp2010.html

DEVELOPMENTAL DIFFERENCES AND THE FAMILY

The first indicator that a child may have a developmental problem may occur when milestones are not reached at the expected times. Some children may have additional indicators that cause concern, such as the presence of atypical body structure or facial features, escalating behavior problems, coordination or muscle tone problems, difficulties with vision or hearing, repetitive play, or lack of interest in socializing with peers. When parents realize a child is not on the same developmental path as other children of the same age, they understandably want to know what is causing the delay and what to do to help the child catch up with peers. The first professional they talk with is usually the child's primary care physician or pediatrician. General pediatricians routinely perform developmental screenings on each child during every well-child visit. The American Academy of Pediatrics (2014) recommends that pediatricians complete a developmental screen at 13, 24, and 36 months for all children. With this screening information, the pediatrician can discuss with the parents where the child tests in each domain of development.

Developmental screenings are designed to compare the performance of children to their same-aged peers. Because learning experiences vary across cultures and across socioeconomic status, there is a wide range of performance that is considered "typical" even among typically developing children. Screening tests are designed to be conservative and include a wide range of normal, and so may not always pick up subtle developmental delays in the preschool years.

Children who are identified as having possible developmental problems are usually referred to those professionals who specialize in early development, including developmental pediatricians, pediatric neurologists, pediatric geneticists, developmental psychologists, speech and language therapists, occupational therapists, or physical therapists, for further evaluation.

Although each of these professionals may assess children for a diagnosis, each may approach the children in a "specialized" manner, one that relies on their special area of training. A pediatric neurologist is concerned with the functioning of the brain on development, whereas a geneticist will explore the family history of disorders and determine if blood tests are necessary to detect chromosome abnormalities. A developmental psychologist looks at the level of life skills and awareness the children have, including social ability and communication style, whereas a developmental pediatrician will review medical history and order any tests deemed necessary to clarify a child's medical condition. In ideal situations, these professionals work together as a team to provide all the information necessary to establish a clear and accurate diagnosis.

Although many parents and professionals are reluctant to label a child with a diagnosis early in life, there is benefit in an early diagnosis for all developmental disabilities. A diagnosis is a professional decision, or label, reflecting the supposed nature and cause of developmental differences presented by a child. The diagnosis may provide an answer for a parent who has been concerned that something is wrong with a child's development.

As noted in Chapter 11, the period of uncertainty, when a parent suspects a problem but no explanation or diagnosis has been offered, is very stressful for parents. Having a diagnosis can provide parents with the road map they need to begin treatment. The earlier specific interventions are started, the better the outcome. Greater changes in neurodevelopmental function can occur in younger children. Due to the inherent neuroplasticity of the brain of young children, early intensive intervention has been shown to help reduce impairments. For example, powered mobility devices can give young children with cerebral palsy the independent mobility to keep up with peers, or a cochlear implant can give children with deafness the chance to communicate typically.

Unfortunately, not all conditions are easy to identify in early childhood. In the case of a child such as Logan, whose story introduces this chapter, there is a long history of developing differently but he also functions well in many areas. His delays have qualified him for special services including speech therapy, physical therapy, and occupational therapy, but his diagnostic label has remained vague, "developmental delay."

Developmental delay and developmental disability are separate but often related labels given to children who fail to reach developmental milestones at the expected times. Developmental professionals use the term **developmental delay** to describe children who are slow in development but who have the potential to catch up. For example, a child born prematurely, without complications, may not initially meet all milestones at the expected time but usually catches up around the age of 2 years. **Developmental disability**, however, implies a more pervasive and chronic delay and is used as an umbrella term for a variety of diagnoses, including intellectual disability, cerebral palsy, and autism. Developmental disabilities are lifelong physical and associated mental/intellectual disorders of the developing nervous system that manifest prior to age 22. They may include delay or limitations of function in one or multiple domains, including motor performance, cognition, hearing and speech, vision, and behavior.

For Logan's family, the distinction between developmental delay and developmental disability is important. As he faces school, it has become clear that although he continues to gain skills, he is gaining them at a slower rate than his age peers. Logan's pediatrician suggested to the family that he has autism, a chronic, lifelong disability. Logan's family is distraught and seeking alternative explanations and second opinions because they say that they "won't give up on him." For this family, the change of words from delay to disability signifies a lack of hope for the future. Not every family will respond as Logan's has, but it is important to understand how big of an impact that words we may use casually may have on families.

IMPACT OF DEVELOPMENTAL CONDITIONS ON FAMILY FUNCTION

Positive developmental outcomes are built on repeated interactions between growing children and their environmental contexts. A child's family is an important influence on the child's development and a strong predictor of emotional well-being (Allen, Vessey, & Shapiro, 2009). Having a child with any type of chronic health or developmental condition places additional demands on families. Some of these demands can negatively impact family quality of life (Hsieh et al., 2013). The greatest challenges are reported by parents of children with severe disabilities who indicate that they do not always receive all the specialized services and help that they require, have help from family and friends, have access to services and specialized programs, or know where to look for help (Browne et al., 2013).

Although the early adjustment may be challenging, most families who have children with serious illnesses or disabilities eventually view their children and their lives as normal and manage the related demands successfully (Deatrick et al., 2006). Some families describe this as finding a "new normal." Many studies of families with children who have a variety of conditions have described a parenting style that focused on the routine rather than one centered on child vulnerability, caregiving, and caregiver burden. This parenting style of **normalization** includes proceeding with an expectation of normalcy, and is a positive style of family response to childhood chronic illness.

Parents consistently identify normalization as a valued goal and develop strategies to create and sustain a family life they experience as normal and satisfying. In this way, normalization is both a process and an outcome, and these two aspects of the concept may overlap and often are not differentiated precisely in the literature (Gjengedal, Rustoen, Wahl, & Hanesta, 2003; McDougal, 2002; Rehm & Bradley, 2005). Parenting for normalization combines the efforts family members make to create a normal family life (process), their perceptions of the consequences of these efforts (outcome), and the meanings they attribute to their management efforts (Knafl, Darney, Gallo, & Angst, 2010).

Families who normalize childhood chronic illness recognize the seriousness of the illness while continuing to view their child and family as unchanged in important ways—using a "normalcy lens." Accepting a viewpoint that sees a child and family as normal helps the family learn to manage illness or disorder-related demands in a way that sustains usual patterns of family and child functioning. The basic attribute of normalization as a parenting style are presented in **Table 15-2**.

TABLE 15-2 Defining Attributes of Normalization as a Parenting Style

1. Acknowledging the condition and its potential to threaten family function and family lifestyle.

2. Interacting with others based on a view of the child and family as normal.

3. Adopting a "normalcy lens" for defining the child and family.

4. Engaging in parenting behaviors and family routines that are consistent with the "normalcy lens".

5. Developing a treatment regimen that is consistent with the "normalcy lens".

Adapted from Deatrick et al., 1999.

A positive outcome of a family focus on normalization is family participation. Family participation in the care of a child enhances development, especially in the areas of social participation and emotional well-being (Axelsson, Granlund, & Wilder, 2013). Participation is sometimes difficult to measure, because simply being present during an activity does not qualify you as a participant. Maxwell and Granlund (2011) suggested that the conception of participation in the ICF includes a psychological perspective that emphasizes the subjective experience of engagement. Children learn to be active participants through interaction in both environmental and social contexts. The more severe a child's impairment, the more adaptation the family will need to make to enhance participation. Axelsson, Granlund, and Wilder (2013) remark, "the child's closest network, the family, has the task to construct routines that uphold consistent and satisfying daily activities for the child to participate and engage in" (p. 523). This may include the development of specific routines around daily activity, such as pairing exercise routines with bathing and evening ADLs, or it may influence the family's choice of leisure and recreation activities.

The specific types of activities that children prefer are impacted by family and social factors (Axelsson, Granlund, & Wilder, 2013). The single biggest child characteristic that was associated with levels of family participation was cognition. Cognition affects participation broadly. Children with lower levels of cognitive function participated in family functions less and engaged in fewer unstructured "child-driven" activities. For example, Logan was able to participate effectively in community play activities when he was younger, but now that his age peers are participating in organized sports, his difficulties understanding rules and following the sequence of play have become more apparent. Although his motor skills are not impaired, his delays in cognition impede his ability to participate successfully in team sports.

Though normalization is a positive adaptive strategy that puts the developmental challenges into the background of consciousness some of the time, most chronic conditions involve periods of stability and periods of exacerbated problems. Families may seek normalization, but at times the overwhelming pressures of the medical or behavioral condition dominate family functioning. Understanding the multiple stressors families face is central to being effective in supporting both a child and the family.

The *uncertainty in illness theory (UIT)* (Mishel, 2006) was introduced in Chapter 11. This theory posits that uncertainty results when an individual (or individuals) cannot conceive of a way to accept the impact of an illness or disorder. In Mishel's term, this means that the individual cannot form an adequate cognitive schema to interpret the meaning of illness-related events. This leads to distress because the family members have no control over the challenges that come up. Mishel proposes that uncertainty leads to psychological distress if coping responses are insufficient to resolve uncertainty or to manage any negative emotional arousal when uncertainty cannot be resolved (Stewart, Mishel, Lynn, & Terhorst, 2010). Parents can appraise uncertainty as either dangerous or beneficial. Many things can trigger uncertainty. **Table 15-3** includes examples of things that might trigger uncertainty. It is important to note that many of the things on this list are not illness or disorder related. For example, if a family has been told that the window for learning to talk ends at age 6, they may become increasingly distressed as their nonverbal child approaches her 6th birthday.

Mishel (2006) reports that most adults initially appraise uncertainty as dangerous, and then they begin to consider whether or not they have the skills and resources to reduce the uncertainty. Most parents want some degree of control, but may find their child's care needs too medically complex or overwhelming for them to manage on their own. Parents commonly respond to uncertainty through two forms of information management. The first is the aggressive pursuit of information about the child's condition. The second approach is avoidance of social situations where the child's condition stands out or is likely to be remarked upon (Santacroce, Deatrick, & Ledlie, 2002). Uncertainty can also manifest in aspects of the child's condition. Garner and colleagues (2013) found that parents

TABLE 15-3 Potential Triggers of Uncertainty

Normative Triggers	Disease-Related Triggers
Anniversaries and birthdays	Changes in the treatment regimen
Interactions with extended families	Communications with health care providers
Stories in the media	Onset of illness
Illness of a caregiver	Waiting on test results
Loss of a support service (such as a night nurse)	Increased child dependence on technology

Adapted from Allen, Vessey, & Shapiro, 2009. Reference Creditng: Allen, P.J., Vessey, J.A., & Shapiro (2009). Primary Care of the Child with a Chronic Condition, 5th edition. St. Louis, MO: C.V. Mosby.

of children with externalizing behavioral conditions (such as attention deficit/hyperactivity disorder or autism spectrum disorders) reported fewer positive interactions with their children and had the highest "ineffective parenting scores" in their research. These authors did not explore possible explanations for this finding, but it is possible that the uncertainty inherent in parenting a child with atypical and unpredictable behavior may lead to psychological and emotional distress in the parent.

Parents who are unable to, or are uncomfortable with, managing their children in social situations such as medical or therapy appointments may avoid these challenging encounters. Frequent cancellations of appointments or lack of participation in parent-centered school activities may be an avoidance strategy as described in UIT. A parent's overuse of the avoidance strategy can lead to a lack of adherence to the medical treatment regimen or home therapy programs. It can also lead to social isolation and decreased support from the community.

COMMON DEVELOPMENTAL DISABILITIES

The most common developmental disabilities, excluding those introduced in Chapter 11, are autism spectrum disorders, learning and intellectual disabilities, and attention deficit/hyperactivity disorder. Each of these disabilities can vary from mild to severe, and children can have more than a single diagnosis. In most cases, these conditions are diagnosed in early childhood.

AUTISM SPECTRUM DISORDER

Autism spectrum disorder (ASD) is a complex developmental disorder that is marked by challenges in two main areas: social communication and repetitive and unusual routines or behaviors (American Psychological Association, 2013).

These difficulties can result in functional limitations in effective communication, social participation, social relationships, academic achievement, or occupational performance. The onset of the symptoms of ASD manifest in the early developmental period, but deficits may not become fully manifest until social communication demands exceed the child's limited capacities (APA, 2013). For example, a young child who is cared for at home may just seem shy or quiet among peers as a toddler, but when he reaches school-age, his lack of interest in socialization will become more obvious. The American Psychological Association describes autism as "the most severe developmental disability" (2014). Phrases such as this, although well founded, may exaggerate the reactions of some families toward accepting this diagnostic label. This is especially true because people with ASD are quite varied, and the "spectrum" includes people who range in severity from high to low functioning. The determination of the severity is based on the degree of social communication impairments and restricted repetitive patterns of behavior, and severity is given a "level of functioning " score at diagnosis, with Level One requiring the least intervention and Level Three requiring the most. The diagnosis can also be further explained by the addition of a qualifier, when applicable, that indicates the presence of any known genetic cause, for example, the level of language and intellectual disability and the presence of medical conditions, such as seizures, anxiety, depression, and/or gastrointestinal (GI) problems. Within the diagnosis of autism come varying levels of disability—for example, one child with autism may have interest in other children and will play near others, whereas another child may prefer to be alone and will withdraw from peers. One child may have enough functional words to ask for what he wants, whereas another may be completely nonverbal and wait to have her needs met. Some children with autism will be affectionate with familiar people whereas others pull away from any touch. It is difficult to measure functional intelligence in people with ASD, and recent studies have explored a variety of measures in addition to standard intelligence tests. In a study of 75 children, Charman and colleagues (2011) found that

55 percent of the children tested had an intellectual disability. This finding suggests that ASD is less strongly associated with intellectual disability than earlier studies would indicate. In people with milder symptom severity and higher intelligence, limited quality of social relations are common and associated with high anxiety levels (Eussen et al., 2013).

LEARNING DISABILITIES AND INTELLECTUAL DISABILITIES

A **learning disability (LD)** is a neurologically based impairment that affects the brain's ability to process and respond to information. Although used more broadly in some parts of the world, in the United States, this label is used when children's level of achievement is substantially below what is expected by their intelligence level (Child Trends Databank, 2014). This is a lifelong condition that has a great impact on the individuals' ability to learn in a traditional academic setting. In addition to academic learning problems, this condition may also result in specific difficulties with written and spoken language, coordination, self-regulation, and social interaction (Lane & Bundy, 2012).

The label of *learning disability* refers to the symptoms (educational difficulties) rather than the cause of condition. In this way, the term is an umbrella term, which may include many specific causal factors. LD occurs in about 7 percent of U.S. school-age children living at or above the poverty line, and in 10 percent of the children living below it, with boys being more likely to be identified with this condition (Child Trends Databank, 2014). LD affects many aspects of life, including education and employment, family life, and daily routines. Children with LD are far more likely than other children to be enrolled in special education and to use health care services (Child Trends Databank, 2014). **Figure 15-2** shows a young boy struggling with his schoolwork. Children like him may need extra support both at home and at school to succeed in academic learning.

INTELLECTUAL DISABILITY

Intellectual disability (ID) is the current terminology suggested to replace the term *mental retardation* in the United States. ID is a more serious impairment than LD, and involves a below-average cognitive ability with three characteristics: intelligent quotient (IQ) of 70 or below; significant limitations in the ability to adapt and carry on everyday life activities such as self-care, communication, and participating in academic and social environments; and the onset of the disability occurs before age 18 (The ARC, n.d.).

Like LD, *ID* is an umbrella term describing the presentation of the condition, but which may include many specific causal factors. ID can be caused by both environmental and/or biological factors. When it occurs as part of

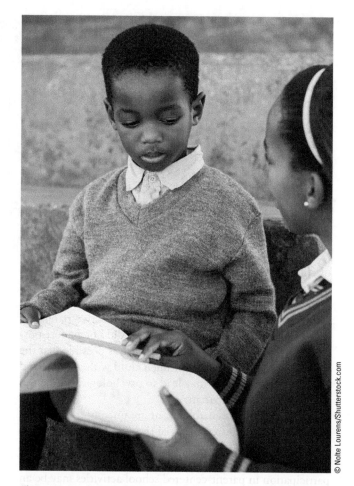

Figure 15-2   Children with dyslexia may not be able to learn in school without special educational support.

a genetic syndrome, such as Down syndrome, children may be diagnosed in infancy. When there is not a clear genetic syndrome or the impairment is less severe, the identification of ID occurs as a child experiences delayed developmental milestones in multiple domains.

ID is most often classified in terms of performance on IQ tests. The classifications and IQ score ranges are presented in **Table 15-4**. Table 15-4 also includes the four official levels of ID and the category of *borderline intellectual functioning*. Borderline intellectual functioning (also called below-average IQ) is a categorization of cognitive impairment. It is not uncommon that children in the preschool years are given this label, and is recategorized as mild ID later as more academic problems emerge.

Lane and Bundy (2012) caution against overreliance on IQ in labeling levels of ID. IQ scores do not always take into account the individual's strengths and weaknesses across multiple domains, or for cultural bias in the tests. **Table 15-4** also includes a general statement about expectations for independent functions. Most individuals with ID are able to live independently with some support and accommodation. The individuals in the severe and profound range often have concomitant diagnoses such

TABLE 15-4   Classification of ID by Level

Classification	Incidence	IQ Score	Functional Performance
Borderline Intellectual Functioning	Not a category of ID	70–85	Full independence in all domains.
Mild ID	85% of all people with ID	50–70	Full independence in most domains; may need assistance or accommodation for some adult expectations (such as employment, money management, and child rearing).
Moderate ID	10% of all people with ID	35–55	Partial dependence; most independent in ADL but needs support with IADL; greatest dependence is seen in those with more limited language; will need ongoing assistance to function in the community.
Severe ID	4% of all people with ID	20–40	Limitations in basic ADLs; requiring direct caregiving support in all daily tasks.
Profound ID	1% of all people with ID	<20	

as microcephaly or cerebral palsy that further restrict their ability to function without support.

ATTENTION DEFICIT/ HYPERACTIVITY DISORDER

Attention deficit/hyperactivity disorder (ADHD) is one of the most common neurobehavioral disorders with about 11 percent of 4- to 17-year-old children diagnosed in the United States (CDC, 2013a). Like LD, this disorder is typically diagnosed in childhood, but can be a lifelong condition. Symptoms include difficulty orienting to and persisting at tasks, difficulty controlling behavior, and hyperactivity (overactivity). People with ADHD often have difficulty conforming in traditional academic settings, have difficulty with their peers, and have difficulties that interfere with friendships (CDC, 2013a).

There is no one definitive test that can diagnose children as having ADHD. Standard protocols can be used in diagnosis, but many other conditions result in behaviors similar to those typical to children with ADHD. For example, ADHD can be confused with hyperkineses of developmental delay, a condition that occurs when a child is acting at his or her developmental age rather than chronological age. For example, if a child who just celebrated his 5th birthday has the adaptive behavior skills, language, and cognition of a 2-year-old, his behavior is going to be more like a 2-year-old. He can look impulsive or inattentive, but that is because he has not yet developed the performance patterns typical of most 5-year-olds. Also, inattention and restlessness can be caused by medical problems such as allergies, thyroid disorders, and high blood lead levels. Problems in routines and ADL patterns resulting in sleep shortages or hypoglycemia can also cause ADHD-like symptoms. It is especially important for

rehabilitation professionals to recognize that other serious conditions such as autism spectrum disorder, fetal alcohol syndrome, and depression can all include symptoms of inattention and impulsiveness. If a child has indications that a more serious condition might be present, the therapist should confer with the child's primary care physician to see if additional testing is warranted. Because early diagnosis and early treatment are so important, arriving at an accurate diagnosis is important for both the child and the family.

It is perhaps related to difficulties with behavioral inhibition, but "children with ADHD, compared to children without ADHD, were more likely to have major injuries (59% vs. 49%), hospital inpatient (26% vs. 18%), hospital outpatient (41% vs. 33%), or emergency department admission (81% vs. 74%)" (CDC, 2013a). This means that physical and occupational therapists are likely to have clients with ADHD in traditional hospital and rehabilitation settings.

COMMON ACQUIRED OR EMERGENT CONDITIONS IN CHILDREN AND ADOLESCENTS

If a young person acquires a disabling condition during this period, it is most commonly either a condition with a genetic component, mental illness, or the effect of an accident or other trauma. Two broad categories of conditions, emotional/behavioral disorders and multitraumatic injuries, will be presented here. Any condition that keeps children from experiencing the challenges and social exchanges that characterize childhood can have a lasting impact on self-image and educational success.

EMOTIONAL AND BEHAVIORAL DISORDERS

Mental health disorders (also called mental illnesses) are any conditions characterized by impairment of an individual's normal cognitive, emotional, or behavioral functioning, and caused by social, psychological, biochemical, genetic, or other factors, such as infection or head trauma. The term *mental illness* applies to children; however, this diagnostic label is seldom used with young people. More commonly, you will see labels such as *emotional disturbance* and *behavioral disorder* to describe atypical psychosocial development. One of the reasons for these alternative terms is to reduce stigma, but another compelling reason is that many otherwise typically developing young people act, at times, in a manner that would be considered deviant in adults.

For children to be identified as having a mental health disorder, it must be determined that the problem significantly impacts daily function and that it is not a transient reaction to a life event. Although it is not talked about much, mental illness is one of the most common chronic problems seen in young people today. The CDC estimates that 13 to 20 percent of children living in the United States (up to 1 out of 5 children) experience a mental disorder in a given year (CDC, 2013b). In fact, nearly half of all lifetime cases of mental disorders begin by age 14 (National Institute of Mental Health, 2014). The CDC statistics include a wide variety of mental health disorders. These data include all children diagnosed with conditions listed in the American Psychiatric Association's *Diagnostic and Statistical Manual of Mental Disorders* (5th ed.; 2013). The statistics included in this section on mental health disorders includes children with ASD and ADHD described earlier as neurodevelopmental conditions. Because many children with ASD and ADHD also have anxiety and mood disorders, the statistics on the disorders are difficult to separate. The most prevalent mental health disorder in children and adolescents is anxiety disorder.

Anxiety Disorders

Great advances have been made in understanding anxiety in recent years, and this understanding has made it possible to identify and treat problems earlier. Anxiety is a normal reaction to stress. Everyone experiences anxiety. But when anxiety impairs everyday life in ways that limit social involvement, routine activities, or functioning, it is considered an anxiety disorder. Anxiety disorders include unusual fears or phobias, obsessive-compulsive thoughts and behaviors, panic attacks, and an irrational dread of everyday situations. If one or all of these occurs over a period of more than six months, it has become a mental health disorder. There are a wide variety of **anxiety disorders**, including separation anxiety disorder, generalized anxiety disorder, post-traumatic stress disorder, and specific phobias, to name a few.

Childhood and adolescent anxiety disorders are best viewed from a developmental perspective that assumes that normal and abnormal manifestations of fear and anxiety are part of one and the same continuum (Beesdo et al., 2009). The developmental nature of anxiety is evident in that only two types of anxiety disorders are usually seen in the preschool years, selective mutism and generalized anxiety disorder. From about age 6 on, the range of anxiety disorders diagnosed expands to that similar to the range found in adults. It has been suggested that anxiety disorders are not really separate disorders, but rather more of a spectrum of disorders. What is seen in child development is that often children will have one disorder for a while, then switch to another, or just add another on (Muris & Broeren, 2009). About 8 percent of teens have an anxiety disorder, with symptoms commonly emerging around age 6 (National Institute of Mental Health, n.d.). In the same study, it was noted that only 18 percent of teens with anxiety disorders received mental health care. This is important to consider because addressing mental health issues as well as any other issues that bring children to therapy will greatly improve the success of your intervention and children's quality of life.

Children with many of the types of developmental conditions described earlier—autism, learning disability, and ADHD—commonly also have difficulties with anxiety. Children with chronic illness who have experienced trauma and or pain, including pain following orthopedic surgeries, often develop strong fears when in health care settings. Although the fears may not reach the level of a full-blown phobia, **white coat syndrome** is a fear of doctors and others (wearing white coats) in health care settings is a manifestation of anxious behaviors based on prior negative experiences. For these young people, fear and anxiety prevent them from accepting vital care. Although occupational therapists are more likely to see children and adolescents clinically for anxiety-related problems, both occupational and physical therapists must understand and recognize the negative impact anxiety can have on therapy interventions.

MULTITRAUMATIC INJURIES

Multitrauma (also called *polytrauma*) is a medical term describing the condition of people who have been subjected to multiple traumatic injuries, such as a serious head injury in addition to a serious burn. In children and adolescents, multitraumas are often associated with motor vehicle accidents or natural disasters. The most common types of trauma seen in children are burns, traumatic brain injuries, and limb amputations. These conditions are unexpected and result in an extended period of care that extends from onset and acute care to community reentry. The injuries received may heal, but often leave individuals with a lifelong disability (Lane & Bundy, 2012).

Initially, the focus of the medical team in cases of multitrauma is on survival. Once survival has been assured, the focus then shifts to supporting functional outcome, emotional well-being, and the long-term quality of life for pediatric traumatic injury survivors and their families. Although there is some variation in recovery patterns based on types of trauma, Martin-Herz, Zatzick, and McMahon (2012) report that it may take two or more years following return to home from trauma rehabilitation before a family feels it has regained the quality of life it enjoyed prior to the injury. In addition to the initial trauma, there is an overall post-injury acute stress disorder rate of 40 percent (Holbrook et al., 2005a). This is a form of **Post-traumatic stress disorder (PTSD)**, a severe anxiety disorder that can develop after exposure to any event that results in psychological trauma. For some families, the acute stress from the trauma persists into a long-term pattern of PTSD. Both acute stress and PTSD have a negative impact on quality of life and may restrict participation in academic and other daily life activities (Holbrook et al., 2005b)

FAMILY CULTURE AND CULTURALLY RESPONSIVE HEALTH CARE

Browne and colleagues (2013) demonstrate that when children have delayed developmental milestones or diminished behavioral and emotional strengths, parents reported higher levels of family stress. This stress is greater in children with conditions that result in dysregulated or unpredictable behaviors, such as are seen in conditions like ASD, ADHD, and anxiety disorders. These families often report internal conflict, discord, and interpersonal hostility (Browne et al., 2013). It was also noted that the most stressed parents "were not accessing any additional proactive or preventative services, but had increased utilization expenditures for 911 emergency and ambulance calls" (Browne et al., 2013, p. 181). This is consistent with the avoidance patterns of coping described earlier in the uncertainty in illness theory (UIT) (Mishel, 2006). Parents who are excessively stressed in their role as parents may withdraw rather than seek help. This has a negative outcome for both the children and the family. In comparison, families that make persistent and early accommodations in the social and occupational areas differ very little from families with typically developing children in their physical and mental health. This continues to be true particularly when their children reach school age and older, even when the disability remains. Occupational and physical therapists often have long-term relationships with families of children with special needs. Because of this, therapists are in a good position to offer parenting support and to assist a family in making accommodation for their child that will not restrict family function or the willingness to seek appropriate medical care.

Culture influences many health beliefs and care giving practices. Some common areas in which health beliefs would be especially important to explore with families are alternative medicine and non-physician healers, and gender specific roles in caregiving relationships.

Alternative approaches to medical care are widely used both as independent treatment strategies and as supports in combination with more traditional medical approaches. Health care providers should respect the health beliefs of parents even when these beliefs are not consistent with the beliefs the clinician holds. Many traditional practices and alternative medicine approaches are entirely benign, and may offer comfort and emotional support to the family. Helping families understand the medical aspects of their child's care, and how benign alternative strategies might be introduced can be important. If an alternative or traditional intervention approach chosen by the family is not benign, or has the potential to interfere with recommended interventions, the clinician can help the discussion and serve as an advocate for the family as they plan their child's care.

In some cultural contexts women are expected to defer important decisions to and, in some instances, to communicate through the male figure. This pattern is especially challenging in that it is primarily mothers, rather than fathers, who attend during clinic visits and therapy sessions. There is much potential for miscommunication and misunderstanding when the information between clinician and father is conducted through a deferential third party. Additionally, in some cultures, the family is the main social unit and family members are actively engaged in all aspects of child care. Similarly,

Similarly, cultural beliefs will impact the parents' interpretation of the disability, their response to both the disability and the health care providers, and the amount and type of family support that is offered. For example, physical disfigurement may be culturally viewed as more devastating in a girl than in a boy. The girl may be segregated socially to hide her disfigurement whereas a boy's disfigurement may not be as isolating. Conversely, a significant mobility limitation, such as spina bifida, may be easier for parents to accept in a girl than in a boy. A common issue therapists face is a parental trend toward lowering expectations for a child with special needs. Although the child may have the ability to participate in tasks, the family may overcompensate and excuse the child from ADL and IADL tasks that would be expected of other children at their developmental level.

An approach to understanding the diverse health beliefs and social expectations of families is the **health traditions model**. As illustrated in **Figure 15-3**, the health traditions model incorporates physical, mental, and spiritual values to consider health holistically and to explore what people do from a traditional perspective to maintain, protect, and restore health (Spector, 2004).

The ethnic, religious, and cultural heritage of each family's health-related beliefs must be respected and melded with modern methods of health care for the best outcome. Some family beliefs are easy to accommodate. For example, in central Europe, special care is often taken to keep the necks and throats of young children warm, to ward off respiratory diseases. In **Table 15-5**, this would reflect the use of proper clothing to maintain physical health. Wearing neck scarves, although not a widespread pattern of clothing children wear

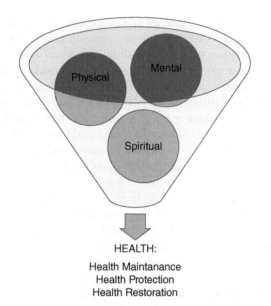

HEALTH:

Health Maintanance
Health Protection
Health Restoration

Figure 15-3   Contributors to Health within the Health Traditions Model

in the United States, is easy to accept and incorporate into an ADL plan. Similarly, people from a Chinese heritage will avoid giving their child cold drinks to protect their health, because of a belief that the cold liquid may predispose them to colds or flu. The cold liquids that are favorites of Americans, and are prevalent in hospital as well as school settings, may be very upsetting for Chinese parents.

It is also important to consider that health management in many cultures centers on community-based resources and the cultural lifestyle. Families with traditional belief systems may try to treat health and disability conditions on their own or through peers, rather than seek medical

advice. This is especially true if the condition is common or is experienced by other family members. In the poverty culture associated with Appalachia in the United States, there is a deep distrust of outsiders and people in authority. Families may hide children with disabilities from health care providers, rejecting the free early intervention services they are entitled to, in order to keep strangers away from their homes and families.

In most cases, culturally sensitive clinicians can understand and work within the families' belief systems. Although there are medical and educational supports for families dealing with many of the conditions listed in this chapter, some parents will not engage with these services. Nonadherence to medical treatment has been recognized as a prevalent problem that can negatively affect children's outcome (Rapoff, 2010). In many cases, family members are interested in supporting their children, but need additional support or accommodations from the health care team. Peplow and Carpenter (2013) studied the adherence to a physical therapy program in parents of children with cerebral palsy. These authors found that there were large differences in the parents' preferred learning styles. They also found that parents in the study identified the need to adapt the exercises in response to differing situations and different parenting styles. Families in the study noted that ensuring the child did the prescribed exercises required a considerable commitment of time and effort, and had a significant negative impact on family relationships. This study illustrates the conflict between occupational and physical therapy service delivery within the medical model (in which the professional is viewed as the expert and decision maker) and the needs of families. Families may defer to or fail to question home therapy programs, even when they

TABLE 15-5	Examples of the Interrelated Facets of the Health Traditions Model		
	Physical	**Mental**	**Spiritual**
Maintain Health	Proper clothing Proper diet Proper exercise Proper rest	Meditation/relaxation Community participation in rituals/recreation	Following lifestyle practices guided by spiritual beliefs Meditation/contemplation
Protect Health	Special food/herbs taken in combination or special food/herbs avoided in combination	Avoid people/foods/activities believed to cause illness Homeopathic/Ayurvedic supplements	Religious worship Prayer Meditation/contemplation Wearing amulets or other symbolic objects
Restore Health	Homeopathic/Ayurvedic remedies Special foods	Rest Traditional (alternative) healers Homeopathic/Ayurvedic remedies	Spiritual rituals/special prayers Exorcism Traditional (alternative) healers

Adapted from Spector, 2004, p. 76. Reference Creditng: Spector, R. (2004). Cultural Diversity in Health and Illness, 6th edition. Upper Saddle River, NJ: Pearson-Prentice Hall.

are aware that they may not be able to adhere to the program. Occupational and physical therapists need to develop intervention programs that are meaningful and relevant to all individuals involved.

PARENTAL STRESS AND COPING

Many contextual factors influence how the family copes with the care of a disabled child. In this case, the ICF classification model can be applied to a family in reflecting the interrelatedness of context and function (World Health Organization, 2002). The gender of a parent influences interaction patterns even in typically developing children (Zaman & Fivush, 2013). Similarly, studies have consistently reported that children from single-parent households often fare worse behaviorally than those from two-parent households. Mokrue, Chen, and Elias (2012) studied ethnic minority children and found that girls in single-mother households demonstrated more negative behavior than those in two-parent households. Behavior problems for boys in single-mother households did not differ from those in two-parent households. So in this study, both the gender of the parent and of the child was important.

Parenting stress is a well-established construct defined as the perceived discrepancy between the demands of parenting and the resources available to meet those demands (Spinelli, Poehlmann, & Bolt, 2013). The birth of a medically fragile infant or an infant with a developmental difference will increase parental stress. Parental stress comes not only from the needs of caring for a disabled child or lack of partner support. Kao and colleagues (2012) report that parents express concern that they do not have enough time to attend to typically developing siblings because of one child's disability. Economic pressures are another source of stress. Many parents feel that they must remain at home to care for a child and are unable to earn money to support the family.

Parent functioning and resiliency to stress has been consistently shown to be a major determinant of child adjustment in all child populations (Giallo & Gavidia-Payne, 2006). High levels of parenting stress have been linked to lower child competence, more early childhood anxiety symptoms, and behavioral problems (Spinelli, Poehlmann, & Bolt, 2013). A pattern of increased maternal stress has been documented for the first 3 years of an infant's life when an infant has medical complication or when an infant is one in a multiple birth.

Although there have been many social and economic changes that have altered patterns of parental caregiving, the bulk of child care responsibilities in the care of a child with disabilities continues to fall upon the mother in most cases (Mitchell, 2007). Mothers with a disabled child have much lower rates of paid employment than mothers of nondisabled children. PTSD symptoms also are noted in parents who are dealing with life-threatening childhood conditions such as cancer. Allen, Vessey, and Shapiro (2009) note that when there is an acute threat to a child's life, "PTSD-associated symptoms are normative and protective in that they restrict parental awareness of upsetting events, dampen potentially overwhelming distressing emotions, and allow parents to make treatment decisions and take other steps to preserve child and family life" (p. 77). Mothers are most likely to be in the home, and they are most likely to attend clinic visits with their child. For this reason, the bulk of the studies of parents of children with special needs have focused on mothers.

Although many studies have been done on mothers, there is no reason to believe that mothers and fathers experience different levels of parenting-related stress simply because of gender. Those parents who are temperamentally more vulnerable to stress are likely to have more stress, and more persistent stress in caring for special needs (Mezulis, Hyde, & Abramson, 2006).

CHARACTERISTICS OF CHILD

As children acquire new developmental skills, the child and parent interactions develop over time as a result of mutual influences (Sameroff, 2009). When a child's development is atypical, parent-child interaction patterns will be impacted. Adamson and colleagues (2012) looked at these changing interactions through the development of joint attention skills. Typically, joint attention emerges in the first year of life, but its emergence may be delayed by developmental disorders. Following joint engagement, early language acquisition transforms interaction patterns, including communication dynamics and the establishment of shared topics as a point of reference. For example, if a mother and child are walking down the sidewalk and each spot a dog ahead on the sidewalk, they will engage in joint attention by looking at each other to make sure the other sees it, followed by conversation about the dog, moving from joint attention to dynamic communication. Children who don't look to another for confirmation lack joint attention, and so social communication is restricted. Adamson and colleagues (2012) compared joint attention and early communication skills in parent-child interactions in three groups. They looked at the interaction patterns in families with typically developing children, with children with Down syndrome, and with children with ASD. They found that, in general, parent-child interactions became richer and more complex as the children gained skills. The children with Down syndrome gained skills more slowly, so the rate of change in the interactions was also slowed. For children with ASD, the initial patterns did not become more complex and the enrichment of parent-child social exchanges was disrupted by the child's failure to acquire joint attention skills. In this example, parents of children with ASD are at greater risk for social detachment from their child. When a child does not initiate interaction or does not reliably respond to the parents' efforts at interaction, as often seen in children with ASD, parents may become frustrated with lack of engagement and may stop trying.

Cultural values play into the impact of child characteristics on the parent-child relationship. Wang, Michaels, and Day (2011) report that attitudes toward people with severe intellectual disabilities are more negative in the People's Republic of China than in many other areas in the world. These authors suggest that the negative attitudes of neighbors and extended family may contribute to increased levels of maternal stress. They note that in Chinese society, parents attach high value to the academic achievement of their children, and as a result, the stress level of mothers of children with severe intellectual disabilities was generally higher than the stress level reported in studies of parents of children with autism in the United States. A common parental coping style is avoidance, and this negative style can lead to further isolation of a child from developmental opportunities and therapeutic support. As the global community becomes more diverse, cultural sensitivity and responsiveness to parents' perceptions of distress will become an increasingly important part of health care practice.

Child characteristics can impact parent-child relationships in other ways. Wilton (2011) found that the parent-child interaction through language was an essential aspect of supporting optimal development in children with visual impairments. When parents offer rich, detailed descriptions as they label objects in play, they aid children in forming mental images. This allows children to better compensate for their lack of visual information.

Another way that a child's disability may limit typical forms of interaction, whether they be motor, sensory, or cognitive, is the parent's failure to recognize a child's developmental gains. For example, parents of nonambulatory children with little means of getting needs met besides reliance on their parents may have difficulty in viewing their child as a separate person. Co-regulation was described in Chapter 13 as the performance of tasks in which both the parents and the children share control. It is through co-regulation that most children learn to do chores, organize their time, and regulate their behavior. It is through co-regulation with parents that children gain the skills that they will need to function effectively in social contexts. Some parents become overprotective of children with a disability and do not allow them the independence necessary for normal separation, even when the children are ready, or they transmit their fear to the children, making them afraid of separation. Parents may become too overwhelmed with daily care to set consistent behavioral limits for children and, as a result, the children develop behaviors so demanding that they soon are controlling the home. In both cases the developmental process of co-regulation does not occur optimally.

Child factors are also an influence on both child and family responses to disability when the condition is acquired rather than developmental. Childhood injuries not only result in physical impairments, but they also put children at risk for emotional distress and post-traumatic stress disorder symptoms (PTSD) (Morris, Lee, & Delahanty, 2013) as discussed earlier in the discussion of multitrauma.

Childhood PTSD can result in social impairments and difficulties in the parent-child relationship. Morris, Lee, and Delahanty (2013) stressed the importance of considering the parent-child dyad when dealing with children who have experienced trauma. These researchers found that the way parents appraised an event had a direct impact on children's responses to the traumatic event.

Although much of the focus of this section has focused on problems, it should be emphasized that studies report that many families experience positive outcomes associated with parenting children with disabilities. Some of these commonly noted positive outcomes are increased tolerance, patience, compassion, and altruism; strengthening of family relationships and cohesion; and positive relationships with school and community members (Lee & Gardner, 2010).

SIBLINGS

Siblings are fellow travelers through the life span. They share experiences and have a store of private knowledge about family and lifestyle. In childhood, siblings can be captive audiences, available companions, and rivals. They are the measuring sticks by which all achievements are judged. Through sibling relationships, the social, emotional, and psychological development of each child is honed. Well-meaning parents sometimes try to protect siblings by not talking to them about another sibling's disorder (Kao, Romero-Bosch, Plante, & Lobato, 2012). They may play down the impact of the impairment and try to minimize interruptions to the siblings' routine. At any age, nondisabled children need to understand what their sibling's disability is and what to expect in the future. They need to be shown the strengths and weaknesses of their sibling, and realize that the sibling is not completely defined by the disability. They may need help in learning ways to interact with the sibling, not just as a caretaker but also through typical peer relations. Providing supportive education for siblings and incorporating the feelings and needs of siblings into the process of planning interventions can support a child who is a therapy client by providing a more positive and supportive developmental context.

The family environment plays an important role in how siblings adjust to a diagnosis of a developmentally delayed brother or sister. For example, siblings from families reporting consistent and regular family routines had fewer adjustment difficulties than siblings from families reporting fewer routines (Giallo & Gavidia-Payne, 2006). These authors suggest that shared family activities may serve as a resilience factor for siblings, allowing them to regularly share positive experiences, receive social support, and deal with problems. Another protective factor for siblings is the use of effective communication and problem-solving strategies within the family. Giallo and Gavidia-Payne (2006) suggest that because there is evidence that some siblings may be highly sensitive to stress and conflict in the family, poor family communication and problem solving may exacerbate or contribute to any adjustment difficulties siblings experience.

Research indicates that the majority of siblings are well adjusted, especially when considered longitudinally, yet a small number of siblings are at risk of developing significant adjustment difficulties (Giallo & Gavidia-Payne, 2006). One of the strongest predictors of negative sibling adjustment difficulties is parent distress. Studies have shown that siblings of children with disabilities are particularly sensitive to family conflict and parent mood (Giallo & Gavidia-Payne, 2006). This finding further supports the need for clinicians to attend to the feelings and concerns of parents of children with special needs.

Birth order and the nature of a disability can also have some impact on the relationship between siblings, especially in the realm of caretaking. In families of typically developing children, older siblings often assume some of the care for younger siblings. This role is also evident in families of younger children with disabilities, but the normative caretaking role of an older sibling is magnified. In particular, older sisters of a sibling with an intellectual disability are expected to provide more care to a younger brother or sister with an intellectual disability (Lobato, 1990). However, in families where the older child is intellectually disabled, for example, the younger children often assume the child care role for the older disabled sibling; thus the role relationship is transposed. This is particularly true if the sibling with a disability has fewer functional competencies (Stoneman, Brody, Davis, Crapps, & Malone, 2003).

How siblings respond to these increased caregiving expectations vary. Many studies suggest that this is a source of resentment and discontent in the sibling relationship. The reaction of typically developing siblings will be influenced by broad factors, such as cultural expectations, and by more intimate factors such as family routines and resources. Kao and colleagues (2012) interviewed Latino siblings of children with disabilities. In this study, the siblings described restricted opportunities to participate in social activities because of their brother or sister. Although this experience may be common to many siblings, it may be more salient for Latino siblings growing up in the United States, because here children spend much more time in extracurricular and peer group activities than with their families.

Cultural values and expectations play a role in the sibling experience. In comparing the responses of Caucasian and Latino siblings, Kao and colleagues remarked that "in contrast to previous sibling interview studies, the child's need for caregiving was a prominent topic in the Latino sibling and parent narratives. Siblings were actively involved in helping and supervising the child and they appeared to be integral parts of each other's lives, consistent with Latino cultures, where sibling relationships are given more importance and sibling caregiving is routine" (2012, p. 550).

To this point in the discussion, we have considered children with a disability generically. There is clear support that siblings have more conflicting and distressing thoughts about a brother or sister who has cognitive, behavioral, or mental health problems. Tsao, Davenport, and Schmiege (2012)

studied both siblings of children with autism and siblings of children with cognitive disabilities. In both sibling groups, negative sibling relationships were associated with worries about the future of the child with a disability, perceptions of parental favoritism toward the child with a disability, and feelings of rejection toward the child with a disability. In contrast to Kao's study, where caregiving and family-centered chores were highly emphasized, it was noted that, perhaps because of parental guilt over the time spent with the sibling with special needs, siblings of children with autism report doing less domestic work than siblings of typically developing children (Tsao, Davenport, & Schmiege, 2012).

Mazaheri and colleagues (2013) focused their study on siblings of individuals with a specific type of cognitive impairment, Prader-Willi syndrome. They reported that 92 percent of siblings reported moderate to severe symptoms of post-traumatic stress reactions. This was a higher incidence of post-traumatic stress symptoms than normative data (healthy siblings), or siblings of children/young adults with cancer. Siblings in the Prader-Willi study reported "increased arousal, avoidance, hypervigilance, feelings of anger, sadness when reminded of their sibling's illness, startle responses, sleep problems, and pessimism about the future" (Mazaheri et al., 2013, p. 870). These findings about siblings with ASD and cognitive impairments were included to make it clear that there is a complex interplay between all family members, each individual's resources in terms of temperament and support, and the functional impact of the child's disability. The experience of living with a sibling with a disability is highly unique, and physical and occupational therapists should try to support positive sibling interactions, but to do so they must take the time to understand the individual needs of each party.

Siblings with a positive attitude can offer a "child's view" of their world to their brother or sister with special needs. Because children with special needs often spend far more of their time with adults than do typically developing peers, this child's view can be crucial in supporting the development of the child. Many childhood experiences, such as the one pictured in **Figure 15-4**, can be best offered through the sibling relationship.

EXTENDED FAMILY MEMBERS

By extended family members, we include any close relation who is actively involved with the care of children in the family. Members of the extended family that are most likely to be involved with children having disabilities are grandparents. Grandparents can be important providers of routine child care to children with disabilities and as such can greatly impact both parental and child well-being. Like parents, grandparents must adjust to a child's disability, and if their adaptation is not positive, grandparents can add stress or emotional burden to the family (Lee & Gardner, 2010; Mitchell, 2007). If grandparents adjust positively and accept a grandchild with a disability, they can become an essential resource and support for the family.

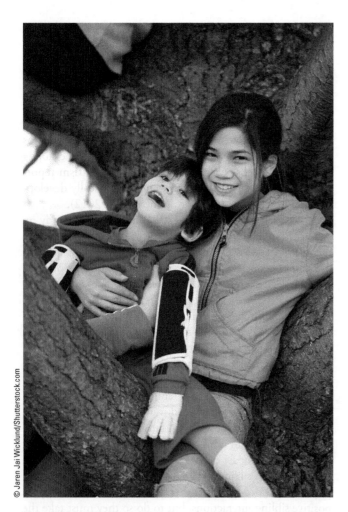

© Jaren Jai Wicklund/Shutterstock.com

Figure 15-4 Siblings provide unique supports and opportunities, like climbing trees, for brothers and sisters with special needs.

When a grandparent participates in the day-to-day care of a child, that participation can help parents maintain a positive attitude and reduces the physical exhaustion inherent in caring for a child with special needs. Grandparents who are involved with the care of a child and who strive to understand the demands of the diagnosis develop a comfort with the child that normalizes the intergenerational relationship. In addition, when grandparents are involved, it is more likely that other family members will join in the care of the child (Green, 2001).

It was noted earlier that mothers of children with a disability have low rates of paid employment. Russell (2003) noted that many mothers wanted to work but were prevented by a lack of available and appropriate child care. A major source of grandparent support is in the provision of informal child care that allows parents respite from their ongoing vigilance, and can also be an important source of support that enables parents, especially mothers, to undertake paid employment (Mitchell, 2007).

When grandparents cannot be involved due to age or disability, parents often feel caught in the middle of the need to care for both their child and their parents. Parents in Green's study (2001) often expressed the need to balance the needs

of the two generations and assure family members that they could manage both. Although grandparenting help had a positive effect on family well-being, sources of support outside the family were not found to have as positive an impact on parental adjustment and were often associated with lower levels of well-being than that obtained with grandparenting support (Green, 2001).

PARENT-TO-PARENT SUPPORT

When a child is diagnosed with a disability, friends and family members who once provided companionship and support to the parents may no longer be able or willing to act in that capacity, either because they are uncomfortable around the child or because they are grieving for the child and family (Hartman, Radin, & McConnell, 1992). As a result, parents of newly diagnosed children may lose important support just when they are trying to come to terms with their own grief. In some cases, parents feel they must reverse roles and respond to the sadness of those friends and family members in an attempt to console and comfort them.

Very often the most valued source of new support becomes the parents of other children with disabilities. This informal support fosters the parents' acceptance and understanding of the needs of the children and their siblings. Parent to Parent USA (P2PUSA) is a national nonprofit organization committed to promoting access, quality, and leadership in parent-to-parent support across the country. This organization utilizes the Internet to offer parent-to-parent support as a core resource for families with children who have a special health care need, disability, or mental health issue. Through this or similar programs, veteran parents can also guide a parent to the most helpful programs and services available and share the skills they have learned in accessing those systems. The connection that such relationships offer helps parents of newly diagnosed children regain a sense of community.

Many states provide a more formal source of assistance through Family Support Networks (FSN). A coordinated system run by parents of children with special needs, FSNs provide psychosocial support, peer training, and in some instances financial assistance to other families of children with special needs. Network staff can also help parents of newly diagnosed children identify and collaborate with treatment professionals who could benefit the children.

Members of these support networks can serve as positive role models by sharing their own parenting experiences. According to Hartman et al. (1992), the most significant role modeling provided by parents of children with disabilities occurs when more veteran parents demonstrate enjoyment of their children and pride in their accomplishments. They show, by example, that it is possible for families to survive their grief and live relatively happy and productive lives. With support, most parents of newly diagnosed children begin to see themselves as more capable and feel less dependent on others for answers. They begin to identify their own needs and use newly acquired skills to solve problems (Hartman et al., 1992). Eventually these parents will be the veterans and, as they grow in confidence and abilities, this system of support can provide an opportunity for them to reciprocate by helping other parents. Internet support groups can also provide a sense of community and can be especially important for parents of children with rare disorders who live in rural or isolated areas or who are reluctant to meet others face-to-face.

MAJOR LIFE AREAS

Although the impact on the major life areas of parents that was described in Chapter 11 persists, as the child matures into a young adult there are steadily increasing disability-related impacts on education, work and employment, and economic life. Their opportunities are influenced by others in their communities including teachers, lawmakers, and members of community organizations that the parent and child interact with.

In childhood, participation in major life areas is usually directed by adults, reflecting the process of co-regulation described earlier. In addition to the supervision and direction of parents, an increasing number of other adults interact with the older child. By adolescence the typical youth functions both at home and in the community in a variety of social roles. Legislation and social policy may influence how children participate in these extended social roles, as was noted in the discussion of employment legislation in Chapter 14. Although we usually think of children in the context of their families, they are influenced indirectly through government, social, educational and economic policies that extend far beyond the boundaries of the family. This influence can be reflected through specific legislation, such as the *Individuals with Disabilities Education Act*, or more indirectly through the availability of public transportation and after-school programming in the community.

EDUCATION

In 1975, the U.S. Congress passed the Education for All Handicapped Children Act of 1975 *now updated and renamed the Individuals with Disabilities Education Act (IDEA)*. The intent of this act was to provide adequate education for "handicapped children," assist states in providing these services, and evaluate the effectiveness of implemented programs in the United States (Mills, 1996). It was created to address the problem of 8 million disabled children with unmet educational needs in the public school system, and another 1 million children with special needs who did not even attend school due to their disabilities (Mills, 1996). The act requires that public schools create an *Individualized Education Program* (IEP) for each student who is found to be eligible under both the federal and state eligibility/disability

standards. Under IDEA, special education and related services (including occupational, physical, and speech therapy) should be provided as needed to meet the unique learning needs of eligible children with disabilities, preschool through age 21.

The current legislation ensures special education and support services to children with disabilities throughout the nation. IDEA governs how states and public agencies provide early intervention, special education and related services to eligible infants, toddlers, children and youth with disabilities. Infants and toddlers with disabilities (birth-2) and their families receive early intervention services under IDEA Part C. Children and youth (ages 3–21) receive special education and related services under IDEA Part B. IDEA provides resources for parents of young children with developmental delays and other disabilities in early intervention, as it was described in Chapter 11. Designed to be both preventative and ameliorative for children with developmental delay, early intervention programs are mandated by federal legislation and are available in all states. Sometimes these early interventions successfully help children meet milestones appropriately, and services are discontinued. But when children require continued intervention, the staff will work with the family to transition the children into the next level of educational support, usually a preschool special needs program.

Special Education

At age 3, children with special needs transition out of the early intervention (Part C) services provided through IDEA. *Special education* is instruction designed to support the learning needs of students who are not able to benefit from educational services in the regular classroom or who need special supports in order to learn. Children with persistent problems who are expected to need additional support to succeed in the educational environment will be enrolled into Part B services. **Part B of the Individuals with Disabilities Education Act** provides assistance for education of all children with disabilities in their educational pursuits through special education services. *Special education* may be classroom based or individualized to addresses the students' individual differences and needs. IDEA mandates that special education plans be designed to meet individual learning needs. Unless the children's IEP requires another location, the children must be educated in the school they would attend if they did not have a disability. Furthermore, the children must receive the special education instruction in the *least restrictive environment (LRE)*, and the state must ensure that children with disabilities are educated with unimpaired children to the maximum extent possible. Special classes, separate schooling, or other removal of children from a regular educational environment can occur only if the nature or severity of the disorder is such that the child cannot be educated in regular classes with the help of supplementary aids and services, in which case the setting for special education services may include instruction in a classroom, in the children's home, in a hospital or other institution, or in another setting.

WORK AND EMPLOYMENT

Beginning in middle childhood and increasing throughout adolescence, young people are increasingly involved in work both in the home and in the community, as was described in Chapter 14. Individuals with intellectual disabilities will be slower to develop work skills and may need more support to be productive in a work environment. Vocational exploration, vocational counseling, and vocational training are part of the educational experience for all students, and IDEA mandates an attention to developing skills to support a student's transition from school to the community.

COMMUNITY, SOCIAL, AND CIVIC LIFE

As discussed in Chapter 14, leisure and play activities are of central importance for building children's competence, self-determination, and personal identity. Children's participation in meaningful leisure activities correlates with their well-being (Adolfsson, 2011) and quality of life, especially if they live with disability (Shikako-Thomas et al., 2012). Not surprisingly, children and youths with disabilities express a desire to participate actively in the same types of activities as their counterparts without disabilities (Shimoni, Engel-Yeger, & Tirosh, 2010). Which activities individual children prefer is influenced by their age, gender, parental education, and place of residence (urban versus rural) (Schreuer, Sachs, & Rosenblum, 2014). In general, the activities girls prefer are less physically challenging than those boys prefer.

Physical activity can make a contribution to the development of children's coordination, understanding of rules, and cooperation with others. Many children with special needs will require adaptation to be successful. Coaches and other leaders must be trained to understand the physical and attentional limits of children with special needs as well as how they communicate, and consider ways to give all children a specific role in the game that will emphasize their abilities. It is important to give all children a chance to lead others, if possible. When children are unable to compete physically in sports or other recreational events, they may find meaningful occupation in supporting a favorite team as "water boy" (or girl) or as manager. Scouting programs, such as the Girl Scouts of America, encourage fitness and social participation through a variety of merit badges. The criteria for earning badges can be individualized to meet the abilities of interested girls with physical limitations or other special needs. Opportunities for community involvement and recreational opportunities are growing in most areas for children with disabilities. Almost every community has Special Olympics programs, and traditional organizations like church groups and 4-H groups encourage the participation of children with disabilities. **Special Olympics** is an international organization dedicated to empowering children (and adults) with developmental and intellectual disabilities to become more physically fit,

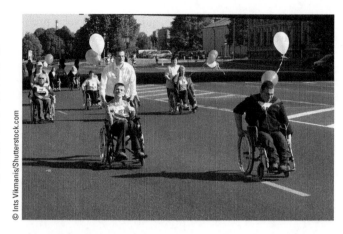

Figure 15-5 Some community sports activities, such as this race, allow people with physical impairments to team up with an able-bodied partner for the event.

respected, and productive through sports training and competition (Mooar, 2002). **Figure 15-5** shows a special race event where competitors in wheelchairs are paired with able-bodied partners and the two individuals compete as a team.

For highly motivated wheelchair athletes, programs are available in larger communities. There are many adaptations of popular games including indoor games such as table tennis and volleyball and outdoor sports such as skiing and boating that make these activities possible for young people with disabilities. These programs offer the opportunity for people with physical disabilities to participate competitively in team sports. Occupational and physical therapists often serve as advocates and help develop programs of these sorts within a community. **Figure 15-6** shows a team of wheelchair athletes competing in the popular European sport, handball.

There are some specialized recreational and educational programs for people with disabilities. **Hippotherapy** is one of these special programs. In hippotherapy, the movement of the horse is used as a tool in treatment by physical therapists and occupational therapists. In hippotherapy, individuals engage in activities that are both fun and challenging as a therapist modifies the horse's movement and evaluates sensory input. The horse's walk provides vestibular input through movement,

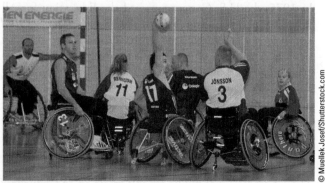

Figure 15-6 Teams of wheelchair athletes can play competitively in many sports with minor adaptations to the equipment and the rules.

which is variable, rhythmic, and repetitive, and the resulting movements of the rider are similar to the movements of the pelvis while walking (McGibbon, Andrade, Widener, & Cintas, 1998). Specific riding skills are not taught in hippotherapy, but the foundation is laid to improve neurologic function and sensory processing.

Other widely available programs for people with special needs are aquatic therapy programs (Hutzler, Chacham, Bergman, & Szeinberg, 1998) and yoga therapy programs (De Leon, 2009). Advanced certification is available for health professionals interested in aquatic therapy, hippotherapy, and yoga therapy.

SUMMARY

The achievements of children with developmental difficulties, chronic illness, or physical disability are most often different from those expected for more typically developing children. Just as there is wide variation in what typically developing children can achieve in adulthood, there is also wide variation in what children with a developmental disability can attain. In many cases, the children's diagnosis and accompanying deficits can help predict the outcome.

For example, children with autism who don't gain useful speech before age 6 may never have communicative language. In addition to a person's individual strengths and weaknesses, the support the family plays is the most important role in a child's outcome. Family characteristics and patterns of interactions can influence not only children's or adolescents' development of cognitive abilities but also their social competency and the development of functional skills.

CASE 1

Logan...Continued

Although Logan's family did not accept the use of the label *autism* related to their son, they found that he continued to need much support to develop skills for the school environment. Although the family did not seek services specifically for autism, they did pursue occupational therapy, speech therapy, auditory "listening" therapy, and an intervention that used periods of time spent in a hyperbaric chamber. Authors Bowker, D'Angelo, Hicks, and Wells (2011) found that most families of children with ASD used several strategies to address the condition. These authors also found that factors other than scientific evidence influenced the family's choice of treatments for their child. These factors include parenting style, family lifestyle choices, access to specific services and treatments, the impact of media, and testimonials from other families.

If the diagnosis of ASD had been presented to Logan's family earlier, they may have been better able to accept it. When Logan was age 6, the family ended up in conflict with the school because the school felt the most appropriate educational placement for him was with an autism specialist teacher, and the family was unhappy with this placement. Physical and occupational therapists working in a school setting may be involved in negotiating this type of placement decision and helping build communication linkages between families and school personnel.

Guiding Questions

Some questions to consider:

1. Logan's parents accepted that Logan was "different" and needed special education. They had come to accept the diagnostic label of developmental delay. Why do you think that they then reacted so negatively to the diagnosis of autism?
2. Logan's family needed continued support and trusted you in your role with Logan. How could you support the family, while guiding them toward evidence-based strategies to help Logan become more successful in his daily occupations?

CASE 2

Curtis

Curtis is 9 years old, and his parents have been told that he has attention deficit/hyperactivity disorder and developmental coordination disorder. Curtis is the third of five children and lives with his mother. Curtis's mother has her own business cleaning offices and small businesses, and the kids (twin boys aged 7, a 12 year old and a 14-year-old older sister) are cared for by the older sister (with emergency support from the next-door neighbor, when the kids are not in school and their mother works). Curtis's father is not in touch and does not help with the bills.

Curtis is in the third grade where he has difficulty sitting still and difficulty organizing his schoolwork. He is a "C" student although he has an above-average IQ. The teacher comments, "This child is very sweet and means well but has no self-control. His legs and feet move like a jackhammer all day. He is always out of the seat talking to others and so distracted from everything."

Curtis has many unusual behaviors in addition to his distractibility. He becomes fearful and sometimes aggressive with unexpected touch, especially in group situations like recess and gym. He dislikes getting his hands messy in any activity. School lunch, art, and science labs have been difficult this year. He is a messy dresser, looks disheveled, does not notice when his pants are twisted, or if his shirt is half untucked. On the playground, Curtis craves fast, spinning, or intense movement experiences. He loves to swing as high as possible and for long periods of time and is always running, jumping, hopping, and so on, instead of walking.

Although very active physically, Curtis frequently slumps, lies down, or leans his head on his hand or arm while working at his desk. He falls a lot and seems to have more difficulty catching himself from falling than his classmates. He has poor gross motor skills. Problem areas include jumping, catching a ball, jumping jacks, climbing a ladder, and poor endurance. In gym class, Curtis has difficulty learning sports skills and performs far below his age peers. This is an area of concern for his mother because so many of his friends have joined sports teams. Curtis's sports ability seems very low, and he is losing opportunities to socialize with his friends by not participating.

Curtis is fully independent in personal hygiene and dressing, but often needs prompting to initiate these tasks. He has difficulty managing his time both in the classroom and at home. He does not have any regular household chores and increasingly challenges his older sister when she tries to enforce rules at home. Curtis's mother has started him in outpatient PT and OT to supplement the support he gets at school.

Guiding Questions

Some questions to consider:

1. Curtis is having difficulty at home, at school and in the community. School-based therapists must focus on school related function in their goals. Outpatient PT and OT will be working from a medical model, looking at functional deficits across settings. What type of things do you think that the outpatient therapists may treat, that cannot be addressed by the school therapists?
2. Curtis dislikes school and has started describing himself as "stupid." What might you, as a therapist working with Curtis do to help him build a more positive view of himself?

Speaking of
My Special Gift

CARRIE COBUN, PARENT OF A YOUNG
LADY WITH SPECIAL NEEDS

Becoming a mother was a dream I've had since I was a little girl. I couldn't wait to become an adult, get married, and have children. My dreams of the perfect "Gerber" baby were no different from any other mother's. My dreams were abruptly shattered when my one and only daughter, Amanda Beth, was born 17 years ago . . .

Mandy was different from the very beginning, but like most new mothers, I loved her for just the way she was and refused to believe, initially, that anything could possibly be wrong with her. I had taken excellent care of myself during the pregnancy and had no reason to believe she would not be perfect. I will skip the painful details of being told the news of "brain damage that was severe in nature" and "you know she'll never be anything but a baby," and just say that the past 17 years have been a mix of joy, intense grief and sadness, celebrations, and hope.

Mandy was diagnosed as having spastic quadriplegic cerebral palsy when she was approximately 2 years of age. Her type of cerebral palsy involves spastic muscles, involuntary movements, a seizure disorder, intellectual disability, visual impairments, and the inability to communicate using verbal language. Mandy is unable to walk and uses a wheelchair. In addition to all of that, she has had numerous gastrointestinal problems, which many children do who are unable to walk and move independently.

She has had numerous surgeries on her bowels as well as a spinal fusion due to a 65 percent curvature of her spine. She always amazes me when she is hospitalized because she endures so much pain and complains much less than adults do!

What have I learned from Mandy? She has never spoken a single word but has taught me more than anyone I know. She has taught me the true meaning of unconditional love. She touches everyone whom she meets and never fails to make those around her smile. When I take her out in the community, whether it's to the mall or Wal-Mart, rarely do we walk by someone who doesn't look upon her with a smile. This is a picture of Mandy and me together (see **Figure 15-7**). She is truly an angel.

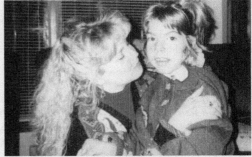

Do I have immense challenges that I face each and every day in raising a daughter with special needs? You bet I do! My chal-

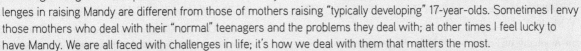

lenges in raising Mandy are different from those of mothers raising "typically developing" 17-year-olds. Sometimes I envy those mothers who deal with their "normal" teenagers and the problems they deal with; at other times I feel lucky to have Mandy. We are all faced with challenges in life; it's how we deal with them that matters the most.

As Mandy continues to grow into a young adult, the challenges seem to grow with each passing day. I have days where I feel I just can't do it anymore. I feel guilty when I have those feelings, but I realize I am only human. Mandy continues to get heavier, and lifting her is becoming a problem. But the heavier toll is the emotional one that parenting a child with special needs often brings to the primary caregiver. There are days where I feel I am being pulled in a million different directions. *Everyone* seems to want me for something related to Mandy, and Mandy needs 24-hour total care. I do my best to allow her as much independence as possible, but I also understand what she can and cannot do.

I have learned many things over the course of the past 17 years from Mandy and those who have cared for her. I have met some of the most wonderful professionals practicing in West Virginia. I have also met some professionals who are in need of intense training in learning how to communicate with parents and their children. I have learned the most from other parents who have children similar to my own. They live the same life as I, and they have been my real teachers.

Continues

Speaking of   *Continued*

If I were to offer advice to other parents or professionals caring for children with special needs, I would say this to them: Take care of yourself! It took me many years to "let go" of believing that only I could care for Mandy. Over the past several years I have become much better in letting others care for her. In this crazy world in which we live, anything could happen to me. I have to be sure there are others who can care for her as well as I can. With this realization comes another problem: How do parents access quality, affordable care for their children and young adults? This is becoming a major issue for parents across the country. The same problem exists within our elderly population. We expect our children and elderly to receive quality care but pay their caregivers very minimally. Until our state and federal governments make quality respite care a priority on their agendas, it will continue to be difficult to find caregivers for our children.

In summary, my life with Mandy has been filled with joys and challenges. I wouldn't trade Mandy for the world, but I do wish that there were more opportunities for her and for our family to live a more "normalized" life with the supports we need. I still believe that Mandy is a gift to me from God, and I will strive to do my best for her as long as I am able.

REFERENCES

Adamson, L., Bakeman, R., Deckner, D., & Nelson, P. P. (2012). Rating parent-child interactions: Joint engagement, communication dynamics, and shared topics in autism, Down syndrome, and typical development. *Journal of Autism & Developmental Disorders, 42*(12), 2622–2635.

Adolfsson, M. (2011). *Applying the ICF-CY to identify everyday life situations of children and youth with disabilities. Dissertation in Disability Research, Series No. 14; Studies from Swedish Institute for Disability Research, No. 39.* Retrieved from http://www.diva-portal.org/smash/get/diva2:443678/FULLTEXT01.pdf

Allen, P. J., Vessey, J. A., & Shapiro, N. (2009). *Primary care of the child with a chronic condition* (5th ed.). St. Louis, MO: C.V. Mosby.

American Academy of Pediatrics. (2014). Recommendations for pediatric preventive health care. *Pediatrics, 133*(3), 568–570.

American Psychological Association (APA). (2014). *Psychology topics: Autism.* Retrieved from http://www.apa.org/topics/autism/

American Psychiatric Association (APA). (2013). *Diagnostic and statistical manual of mental disorders* (5th ed.). Arlington, VA: American Psychiatric Publishing.

Axelsson, A. K., Granlund, M. M., & Wilder, J. J. (2013). Engagement in family activities: A quantitative, comparative study of children with profound intellectual and multiple disabilities and children with typical development. *Child: Care, Health & Development, 39*(4), 523–534.

Beesdo, K., Knappe, S., & Pine, D. (2009). Anxiety and anxiety disorders in children and adolescents: Developmental issues and implications for DSM-V. *Psychiatric Clinics of North America, 32*(3), 483–524.

Bowker, A., D'Angelo, N., Hicks, R., & Wells, K. (2011). Treatments for autism: Parental choices and perceptions of change. *Journal of Autism & Developmental Disorders, 41*(10), 1373–1382. doi:10.1007/s10803-010-1164-y

Brault, M. (2012). *Americans with disabilities: Household economic studies.* U.S. Census Bureau. Retrieved from http://www.census.gov/people/disability/publications/sipp2010.html

Browne, D., Rokeach, A., Wiener, J., Hoch, J., Meunier, J., & Thurston, S. (2013). Examining the family-level and economic impact of complex child disabilities as a function of child hyperactivity and service integration. *Journal of Developmental and Physical Disabilities, 25*(2), 181–201.

Centers for Disease Control and Prevention (CDC). (2013a). *Attention deficit/hyperactivity disorder: Data and statistics.* Retrieved from http://www.cdc.gov/ncbddd/adhd/data.html

Centers for Disease Control and Prevention (CDC). (2013b). *Morbidity and mortality weekly report: Mental health surveillance among children United States 2005–2011.* Retrieved from http://www.cdc.gov/mmwr/preview/mmwrhtml/su6202a1.htm?s_cid=su6202a1_w

Charman, T. T., Pickles, A. A., Simonoff, E. E., Chandler, S. S., Loucas, T. T., & Baird, G. G. (2011). IQ in children with autism spectrum disorders: Data from the Special Needs and Autism Project (SNAP). *Psychological Medicine, 41*(3), 619–627.

Child Trends Databank. (2014). *Learning disabilities.* Retrieved from http://www.childtrends.org/?indicators=learning-disabilities

Deatrick, J. A., Thibodeaux, A. G., Mooney, K., Schmus, C., Pollack, R., & Davey, B. H. (2006). Family management style framework: A new tool with potential to assess families who have children with brain tumors. *Journal of Pediatric Oncology Nursing, 23,* 19–27.

De Leon, V. (2009). Yoga can be an effective therapy for children with special needs. *The Spokesman-Review,* October 26, 2009. Retrieved from http://www.spokesman.com/stories/2009/oct/26/stretching-mind-and-body/

Eussen, M., Van Gool, A., Verheij, F., De Nijs, P., Verhulst, F., & Greaves-Lord, K. (2013). The association of quality of social relations, symptom severity and intelligence with anxiety in children with autism spectrum disorders. *Autism: The International Journal of Research & Practice, 17*(6), 723–735.

Garner, R. E., Arim, R. G., Kohen, D. E., Lach, L. M., MacKenzie, M. J., Brehaut, J. C., & Rosenbaum, P. L. (2013). Parenting children with neurodevelopmental disorders and/or behaviour problems. *Child: Care, Health & Development, 39*(3), 412–421.

Giallo, R., & Gavidia-Payne, S. (2006). Child, parent and family factors as predictors of adjustment for siblings of children with a disability. *Journal of Intellectual Disability Research, 50*(Part 12), 937–948.

Gjengedal, E., Rustoen, T., Wahl, A., & Hanesta, B. (2003). Growing up and living with cystic fibrosis: Everyday life and encounters with the health care and social services—A qualitative study. *ANS: Advances in Nursing Science, 26*(2), 149–159.

Green, A. (2001). Grandma's hands: Parental perception of the importance of grandparents as secondary caregivers in families of children with disabilities. *International Journal of Aging and Human Development, 53,* 11–33.

Hartman, A., Radin, M., & McConnell, B. (1992). Parent-to-parent support: A critical component of health care services for families. *Issues in Comprehensive Pediatric Nursing, 15,* 55–67.

Holbrook, T. L., Hoyt, D. B., Coimbra, R., Potenza, B., Sise, M., & Anderson, J. P. (2005a). High rates of acute stress disorder impact quality-of-life outcomes in injured adolescents: Mechanism and gender predict acute stress disorder risk. *Journal of Trauma: Injury, Infection, and Critical Care, 59*(5), 1126–1130.

Holbrook, T. L., Hoyt, D. B., Coimbra, R., Potenza, B., Sise, M., & Anderson, J. P. (2005b). Long-term posttraumatic stress disorder persists after major trauma in adolescents: New data on risk factors and functional outcome. *Journal of Trauma: Injury, Infection, and Critical Care, 58*(4), 764–769 and discussion 769–771.

Hsieh, R., Hsueh, Y., Huang, H., Lin, M., Tseng, W., & Lee, W. (2013). Quality of life and impact of children with unclassified developmental delays. *Journal of Paediatrics & Child Health, 49*(2), E116–E121.

Hutzler, Y., Chacham, A., Bergman, U., & Szeinberg, A. (1998). Effects of a movement and swimming program on vital capacity and water orientation skills of children with cerebral palsy, *Developmental Medicine and Child Neurology, 40,* 176–181.

Kao, B. B., Romero-Bosch, L. L., Plante, W. W., & Lobato, D. D. (2012). The experiences of Latino siblings of children with developmental disabilities. *Child: Care, Health & Development, 38*(4), 545–552.

Knafl, K., Darney, B., Gallo, A., & Angst, D. (2010). Parental perceptions of the outcome and meaning of normalization. *Research in Nursing and Health, 33*(2), 87–98.

Lane, S., & Bundy, A. C. (2012). *Kids can be kids: A childhood occupations approach.* Philadelphia: F.A. Davis Co.

Lee, M., & Gardner, J. (2010). Grandparents' involvement and support in families with children with disabilities. *Educational Gerontology, 36*(6), 467–499.

Lobato, D. J. (1990). *Brothers, sisters, and special needs: Information and activities for helping young siblings of children with chronic illness and developmental disabilities.* Baltimore: Brookes.

Martin-Herz, S., Zatzick, D., & McMahon, R. (2012). Health-related quality of life in children and adolescents following traumatic injury: A review. *Clinical Child & Family Psychology Review, 15*(3), 192–214.

Maxwell, G. & Granlund, M. (2011). How are conditions for participation expressed in education policy documents? A review of documents in Scotland and Sweden. *European Journal of Special Needs Education, 26,* 251–272.

Mazaheri, M. M., Rae-Seebach, R. D., Preston, H. E., Schmidt, M. M., Kountz-Edwards, S. S., Field, N. N., & ... Packman, W. W. (2013). The impact of Prader-Willi syndrome on the family's quality of life and caregiving, and the unaffected siblings' psychosocial adjustment. *Journal of Intellectual Disability Research, 57*(9), 861–873.

McDougal, J. (2002). Promoting normalization in families with preschool children with type 1 diabetes. *Journal for Specialists in Pediatric Nursing, 7*(3), 113–120.

McGibbon, N., Andrade, C., Widener, G., & Cintas, H. (1998). Effect of an equine-movement therapy program on gait, energy expenditure, and motor function in children with spastic cerebral palsy: A pilot study. *Developmental Medicine and Child Neurology, 40,* 754–762.

Mezulis, A. H., Hyde, J., & Abramson, L. Y. (2006). The developmental origins of cognitive vulnerability to depression: Temperament, parenting, and negative life events in childhood as contributors to negative cognitive style. *Developmental Psychology, 42*(6), 1012–1025.

Mills, D. (1996). Beyond weapons: The case for including a dangerousness exception to the "stay put" provision of the Individuals with Disabilities Education Act (IDEA). *Journal of Juvenile Law, 17,* 94–106.

Mishel, M. (2006). *What do we know about uncertainty in illness?* Japanese Society for Nursing Research. Retrieved from http://www.jsnr.jp/meeting/docs/31_02.pdf

Mitchell, W. (2007). Research review: The role of grandparents in intergenerational support for families with disabled children: a review of the literature. *Child & Family Social Work, 12*(1), 94–101.

Mokrue, K., Chen, Y. Y., & Elias, M. (2012). The interaction between family structure and child gender on behavior problems in urban ethnic minority children. *International Journal of Behavioral Development, 36*(2), 130–136.

Mooar, P. (2002). Experiences as sports coordinator for the Philadelphia County Special Olympics. *Clinical Orthopedics, 396,* 50–55.

Morris, A., Lee, T., & Delahanty, D. (2013). Interactive relationship between parent and child event appraisals and child PTSD symptoms after an injury. *Psychological Trauma: Theory, Research, Practice, and Policy, 5*(6), 554–561.

Muris, P., & Broeren, S. (2009). Twenty-five years of research on childhood anxiety disorders: Publication trends between 1982 and 2006 and a selective review of the literature. *Journal of Child & Family Studies, 18*(4), 388–395.

National Institute of Mental Health (NIMH) (2014). Any disorder among children. Retrieved from http://www.nimh.nih.gov/statistics/1ANYDIS_CHILD.shtml

National Institute of Mental Health (NIMH). (n.d.). Anxiety disorders in children and adolescents—Fact sheet. Retrieved from http://www.nimh.nih.gov/health/publications/anxiety-disorders-in-children-and-adolescents/index.shtml

Peplow, U. C., & Carpenter, C. (2013). Perceptions of parents of children with cerebral palsy about the relevance of, and adherence to, exercise programs: A qualitative study. *Physical & Occupational Therapy in Pediatrics, 33*(3), 285–299.

Rapoff, M. A. (2010). *Adherence to pediatric medical regimens* (2nd ed.). New York, NY: Springer.

Rehm, R., & Bradley, J. (2005). Normalization in families raising a child who is medically fragile/technology dependent and developmentally delayed. *Qualitative Health Research, 15*(6), 807–820.

Russell, P. (2003) *"Bridging the gap" developing policy and practice and childcare options for disabled children and their families.* Council for Disabled Children, London.

Sameroff, A. (Ed.). (2009). *The transactional model of development: How children and contexts shape each other.* Washington, DC: American Psychological Association.

Santacroce, S., Deatrick, J., & Ledlie, S. (2002). Redefining treatment: How biological mothers manage their children's treatment for perinatally acquired HIV. *AIDS Care: Psychological and Socio-Medical Aspects of AIDS/HIV, 14,* 247–260.

Schreuer, N. N., Sachs, D. D., & Rosenblum, S. S. (2014). Participation in leisure activities: Differences between children with and without physical disabilities. *Research in Developmental Disabilities, 35*(1), 223–233.

Shikako-Thomas, K. K., Dahan-Oliel, N. N., Shevell, M., Law, M., Birenbaum, R., Poulin, C., et al. (2012). Play and be happy? Leisure participation and quality of life in school-aged children with cerebral palsy. *International Journal of Pediatrics*, doi:10.1155/2012/387280

Shimoni, M., Engel-Yeger, B., & Tirosh, E. (2010). Participation in leisure activities among boys with attention deficit hyperactivity disorder. *Research in Developmental Disabilities, 31*(6), 1234–1239.

Spector, R. (2004). *Cultural diversity in health and illness* (6th ed.). Upper Saddle River, NJ: Pearson-Prentice Hall.

Spinelli, M., Poehlmann, J., & Bolt, D. (2013). Predictors of parenting stress trajectories in premature infant–mother dyads. *Journal of Family Psychology, 27*(6), 873–883.

Stewart, J., Mishel, M., Lynn, M., & Terhorst, L. (2010). Test of a conceptual model of uncertainty in children and adolescents with cancer. *Research in Nursing & Health, 33*(3), 179–191.

Stoneman, Z., Brody, G. H., Davis, K., Crapps, J. M., & Malone, D. M. (2003). Ascribed role relations between children with mental retardation and their younger siblings. *American Journal on Mental Retardation, 95,* 537–550.

The ARC. (n.d.). *What I want to learn about . . . Intellectual disability.* Retrieved from http://www.thearc.org/page.aspx?pid=2543

Tsao, L., Davenport, R., & Schmiege, C. (2012). Supporting siblings of children with autism spectrum disorders. *Early Childhood Education Journal, 40*(1), 47–54.

Wang, P., Michaels, C. A., & Day, M. S. (2011). Stresses and coping strategies of Chinese families with children with autism and other developmental disabilities. *Journal of Autism & Developmental Disorders, 41*(6), 783–795.

Wilton, A. P. (2011). Implications of parent-child interaction for early language development of young children with visual impairments. *Insight: Research & Practice in Visual Impairment & Blindness, 4*(3), 139–147.

World Health Organization. (2002). *ICF: International classification of functioning and disability.* Geneva, Switzerland: World Health Organization.

Zaman, W., & Fivush, R. (2013). Gender differences in elaborative parent-child emotion and play narratives. *Sex Roles, 68*(9/10), 591–604.

CHAPTER 16

Early Adulthood

Anne Cronin, PhD, OTR/L,
Associate Professor, Division of
Occupational Therapy,
West Virginia University,
Morgantown, West Virginia

Objectives

Upon completion of this chapter, readers should be able to:

- Understand factors contributing to the attainment of adult status in contemporary society;

- Characterize the functional impact of neural and cognitive maturation in early adulthood;

- Identify cultural and socioeconomic variations in expectations for occupation and co-occupation in young adults;

- Relate the issues surrounding Arnett's argument that the developmental stage of "emerging adulthood" should be introduced between adolescence and early adulthood;

- Understand the complexities of achieving vocational education, job flexibility, and economic constraints as they impact entering the workforce;

- Appraise past and current relationship patterns between young adults and their families of origin;

- Discuss the issues and challenges associated with becoming a parent in early adulthood; and

- Describe how adult occupations create meaning in lifestyle and performance patterns.

Key Terms

achieving stage

boomerang generation

cardiovascular fitness

cohabitation

continuous career path model

co-occupation

coping

crystallized intelligence

developmental theory of
   vocational choice

discontinuous career paths

emerging adulthood period

executive stage

formal relationships

generation Y

health equity

marriage

occupational identity

parenting

religiosity

responsible stage

self-disclosure

self-regulation

sensory modulation disorder (SMD)

spirituality

stress

supported employment

work-life balance

CASE 1

DeAndre

DeAndre, 24, served in the army in Afghanistan. While deployed, DeAndre sustained a traumatic brain injury (TBI) and an incomplete spinal cord injury at the L4 to L6 regions. After three weeks in the Veterans Affairs Polytrauma Network Site, DeAndre was discharged to home and to the care of the Department of Veterans Affairs outreach "vet centers." DeAndre wants to pick up his life again, but he continues to struggle with chronic pain, deconditioning, and post-traumatic stress disorder related to the spinal injury. At this time, DeAndre is living with his parents near a small rural town. He left for the army when he was 18, and on coming home found that his old friends had moved on or had changed. After six years of close companionship in the military, he feels isolated and abandoned.

DeAndre sometimes has difficulty with attention, problem solving, memory, and perception. He finds it difficult to concentrate, and sometimes gets sidetracked and forgets to finish what he started. As a result of the TBI, DeAndre has moderate limitations in his right visual field and has some neglect of the right side of his body. He also has had difficulty walking, but is improving. He now uses a walker and is able to physically complete all ADLs. He still needs help organizing tasks and needs prompting to check his right side to compensate for his visual problems.

DeAndre has moved back in with his parents. He gets home health therapy because he is unable to drive a car due to physical and visual perceptual limits. He is able to physically manage his medications and his home exercise program, but often needs prompting to remember these tasks. DeAndre's parents currently do all of the home management and financial management tasks for DeAndre.

Although he feels positive about the potential for walking again, DeAndre continues to have significant mood swings and is often angry and irritable in his therapy sessions. He hates that he needs his parents' help, and that at 24 he needs to be "taken care of like a baby."

Continues on page 374

INTRODUCTION

For many adolescents struggling to move beyond the years of turbulence, the idea of adulthood is an exciting one. Adulthood normally represents a time of increased independence, the opportunity to pursue personal goals without the intensity of supervision and structure of previous years. For young people today, the transition to adulthood is more complex than it was for earlier generations. In the 1960s, it was common for people to finish their basic schooling, get a job, marry, and have children. Then when sociologists and psychologists posed the question, "When is someone an adult?," the answer was clear.

Now, the definition of what makes one an adult is much looser. The end of adolescence and the beginning of adulthood are socially defined and influenced by context and social expectations. For example, a 15-year-old mother will be expected to take on adult roles and responsibilities for the care of her child, even though she has not finished school and may not be able to support herself financially. Although technically an adolescent, a young mother may be functioning as an adult. At the opposite end of the spectrum, a 30-year-old graduate student who has not married, does not have a full-time job, lives at a subsistence income level, and spends much of her time in role-playing games on the Internet is technically an adult, but may be functioning more like an adolescent.

In the past, a discussion of early adulthood has focused on establishing a family and a career. This characterization no longer reflects the developmental experience of today's young adults, what the social press calls generation Y and the net generation. **Generation Y** is the generation born in the 1980s and 1990s, a generation that grew up with the expectation that women would enter the workforce and with digital and electronic technology. While this generation continues to value the establishment of a family and a career, the path to these goals is less clear and the timing of events, such as marriage before having a child, are more fluid. This developmental period is difficult to characterize because social change has left so little as normative or socially expected. The paths individuals take toward adult responsibilities are diverse in timing and content across individuals (Berk, 2010).

In response to the changes in the life experience of modern young adults, Arnett (2000) suggested the literature include a new life stage, the stage of emerging adulthood. The **emerging adulthood period**, in Arnett's description, is a phase of the life span between adolescence and full-fledged adulthood that primarily applies to individuals who do not have children and who do not have sufficient income to become fully financially independent (Arnett, 2000). Young adults who have the economic resources to do so will usually explore alternatives in education, work, personal beliefs and values, and love more intensively than they did as teenagers (Arnett, 2007). The emerging adulthood stage allows for a prolonged period of identity and occupational development. Because of the many transitions and increased autonomy

associated with adulthood, this is an age group where occupation takes on new meaning. Occupations, such as the expectation of raising children, have diverse social and cultural meanings. These meanings influence individuals' views of the occupation within the context of their own life. Occupations such as parenting, marriage, and employment shape the context for interpersonal relationships throughout adulthood. For this reason, decisions made in early adulthood may have a long-lasting impact on individuals.

Personal experiences, both private and interpersonal, make some seemingly routine or mundane activities stand out as meaningful and may lend depth to the meanings individuals attach to shared cultural patterns of responding to life, such as ceremonies and celebrations. Christiansen and Townsend (2010) note that "people understand the meaning of their lives by considering their occupations as part of their life story. It seems that occupations gain meaning over time by becoming part of an individual's unfolding autobiography…" (p. 13).

The years characterizing the transition to adulthood are characterized by dramatic life changes. Individuals often begin to think of themselves in this age span as shaping a "life story," and they make decisions that reflect both their backgrounds and their aspirations. At this age span particularly, we begin to think in terms of historical cohorts, and *history normative* aspects of development. Although little changes in the biological and physical aspects of the early adulthood experience, the older literature describing early adulthood is no longer completely relevant to gaining an understanding of today's early adulthood experience. The events, both historical and personal, that impact young people during early adulthood are of critical importance given the personal, financial, and social costs associated with unsatisfying careers, unsuccessful marriages, and parenting problems. If problem-solving skills and decision-making ability are influenced by life experience, then the transitioning to adulthood can be conceptualized as a period when major life decisions are made without much life experience upon which to base them.

The lack of life experience is both an advantage and a disadvantage for this age group. Today's young adults are seen as creative innovators who are facing societal challenges with energy and enthusiasm. Philip Lauri, the creative director of Detroit Lives!, is quoted by Shore (2012) as commenting: "We are reinventing the American Dream. We haven't had that opportunity in 100 years." Today's young adults view themselves as creative innovators with determination and commitment to positively change the social system. Related to this, young adult occupations, roles, and the meanings they assign to all aspects of participation in adult life are likely to change and refine over time as they gain experience and skill. Early adulthood is a period where many people gain multiple occupations and roles. Throughout adulthood, occupations and roles change to reflect the beliefs of individuals about what they can and cannot perform, about the choices that they make, and about their own evaluation of their performance in the many occupations that make up their lifestyle.

This chapter will provide an overview of the various issues commonly associated with the period of emerging adulthood and the more traditional life tasks associated with early adulthood. Theoretical ideas on career selection, marriage, and parenting will be discussed with an emphasis on highlighting factors that contribute to both success and adjustment problems. As in other periods in the life cycle, societal participation as a young person is highly influenced by the manner in which one has negotiated developmental challenges faced at earlier periods. The coming together of numerous challenges during early adulthood establishes the foundation for the assumption of adult responsibilities.

WHAT IS EARLY ADULTHOOD?

The typical age span associated with early adulthood is 21 to 34 years of age. The traditional milestones used to define "adult" (completing formal schooling, leaving home, getting married, having a child, and establishing financial independence) no longer capture the average experience of today's young people (Settersten & Ray, 2010). The popular media has many descriptive labels for people in this age span, including "the net generation," "generation Y," "the boomerang generation," "kidults," and "twixters."

In this chapter, we will broadly consider the age of transition to adulthood as encompassing ages 18 through 40. At age 18, young people face the transition away from state-mandated schooling, and may choose to pursue additional schooling, vocational training, take an entry-level job, or continue to live with their parents. This is the first big transition in the path toward adulthood. The stage of emerging adulthood, introduced in this chapter, begins at the point in adolescence that these lasting life decisions are made. This period is distinct demographically because it is a period characterized by an exceptionally high level of demographic change and diversity. The mid-20s are years of frequent change and transition in occupation, educational status, and personal relationships. Because many decisions, including marriage, children, and career, are postponed in the current social and economic environment, becoming established into adult roles may extend as late as 40 years of age.

BODY FUNCTIONS AND STRUCTURES

Early adulthood is for most people a period of peak physical and mental performance. There does continue to be brain maturation in this period, but most other body structures are fully mature.

BRAIN AND NERVOUS SYSTEM DEVELOPMENT

Overall, nervous system function is at its peak performance level in early adulthood. During this period, the prefrontal cortex fully matures, bringing well-developed executive function skills into everyday life. Most scientists now indicate that the brain is "adult" around age 25. An adult brain has less plasticity than the developing brain. *Neurogenesis,* the process by which new nerve cells are generated, was described earlier in Chapter 9. There is growing evidence that there continues to be neurogenesis, the generation of new neurons, in adult brains. Specifically, in early and middle adulthood, new neurons continue to be formed in the lateral ventricles and the hippocampus, although the rate of neurogenesis and the associated neuroplasticity is far less than that of younger people (Steinberg, 2012). The continued possibility of neurogenesis gives hope that even damaged brain regions can be functionally repaired.

The research on adult neurogenesis has been done with animal models, and for this reason, it is unclear what the functional impact of this finding is in humans (Kempermann, Wiskott, & Gage, 2004). Based on computer modeling, researchers have suggested that new neurons increase memory capacity (Becker, 2005), reduce interference between memories (Wiskott, Rasch, & Kempermann, 2006), or add information about time to memories (Aimone, Wiles, & Gage, 2006). These findings offer promise for the support of new learning and functional recovery for adults in occupational and physical therapy interventions. Another neurobiological advance that occurs in early adulthood, with the maturation of the prefrontal cortex, is a greater capacity for refined behavioral self-regulation. Self-regulation refers to individuals' capacity to alter their behaviors in accordance to some standards, ideals, or goals either stemming from internal or societal expectations (Baumeister & Vohs, 2007). Through the process of self-regulation, young adults are able to inhibit spontaneous responses in favor of less immediate ones from which they will benefit more. The ability to self-regulate behavior and suppress impulses supports achievement in the tasks of young adulthood. Specifically, self-regulation places one's "social conscience" over selfish impulses, allowing people to do what is right and not what they want to do (Baumeister & Bushman, 2011). In addition, the self-regulatory process prevents impulses that could be costly to individuals in the long run, even when they experience short-term benefits (Baumeister & Vohs, 2007).

SENSORY FUNCTIONS

Sensory acuity is at a peak level in early adulthood. Baldwin and Ash (2011) report high levels of sensory acuity in young adults, and propose that this high level of sensory function provides a significant support to working memory functions. Adults who had deficits in sensory acuity or sensory processing in childhood will continue to have these differences as they enter adulthood. Sensory processing was introduced in Chapter 12 as a complex set of neurobiologic functions that enable the brain to understand what is going on both inside the body and in all of the environmental contexts in which individuals engage. Individuals whose nervous system is unable to organize sensory signals into appropriate responses may have a condition called *sensory processing disorder* (SPD). This condition emerges in early childhood and may persist throughout the life span. **Sensory modulation disorder (SMD)**, is a subtype of SPD in which individuals react in atypical ways to sensory input, often resulting in the perception of typically innocuous sensations as irritating, unpleasant, or painful. This condition is associated with functional limitations, including a difficulty in both children and adults to maintain an appropriate level of arousal or alertness. SMD in adults is often accompanied by anxiety, depression, and maladaptation (Bar-Shalita, Vatine, Parush, Deutsch, & Seltzer, 2012). During this period of transitions and life changes, young adults with SMD may be especially vulnerable.

COGNITIVE FUNCTIONS

Beginning around age 18, people's thinking becomes more personal, integrative, and practical in response to real-life experiences and commitments. Young adults are better able than ever before to consider different points of view at the same time. With this new ability, they are able to form relationships with peers based on observing that they care about the same things and that they share the same values. They can also understand constructive criticism, appreciating that other people are intending to be helpful, even if the effect is painful at the moment. Adult thinking is embedded in individuals' personal social, employment, family, and environmental contexts. Schaie and Willis (2000) proposed seven stages of age-related cognitive development: acquisitive, achieving, responsible, executive, reorganizational, reintegrative, and legacy creating. These stages are illustrated in **Figure 16-1**, showing their corresponding span of prevalence in the life span. The focus in this chapter will be on Schaie and Willis's "achieving stage."

The **achieving stage** is Schaie and Willis's stage of early adult thought where previously acquired knowledge is used to establish oneself in the world. During this stage, young adults must apply their intelligence to attaining long-term goals regarding their careers, family, and contributions to society. In addition, they must confront and resolve several major issues,

and the decisions they make—such as whether to go to college, what job to take, and when to marry—have implications for the rest of their lives (Feldman, 2010). As young people master the social and cognitive skills needed for independent adult function, they move into situations where they need to apply these skills in situations that require social responsibility, thus moving into Schaie and Willis's responsible stage.

Typically, the **responsible stage** occurs when a family is established and an adult is responsible for a spouse and children. Schaie and Willis emphasized that the transition between stages was not dependent upon the age of individuals; rather it was based in the opportunities that people had to develop and practice relevant skills. Although the achieving and responsible stages are most associated with early adulthood, it is possible that in some contexts, young adults may also move into the executive stage.

In the **executive stage**, individuals broaden their focus from the personal domain to the community or societal level (Feldman, 2010). Notice that the executive stage is out of line with the achieving and responsible stages in **Figure 16-1**. This is intentional to reflect that not all people function at the executive level. Function at this level requires both opportunity and intrinsic ability.

In the case that opened this chapter, DeAndre had chosen an adult path and was clearly in the achieving stage. He had always dreamed of a military career. Now, still early in young adulthood, his injuries have ended his military career and he no longer has a clear path. In addition, he is dealing with pain and a loss of functional skills. Although he will be able to function independently again, he is dependent on his parents at this time. When young adults face a trauma or life experience that derails them, which takes them off the expected path, it is especially emotionally challenging. DeAndre is having to relive the dependency of childhood and the identity exploration of adolescence. To move forward, he will need both emotional and physical support.

Stress and Coping

With the increased flexibility of thought and the expansion into so many new environments and occupations, for many people early adulthood holds many significant stressors. **Stress** is the body's response to anything that disrupts daily routines and occupations. Signs of stress can be emotional,

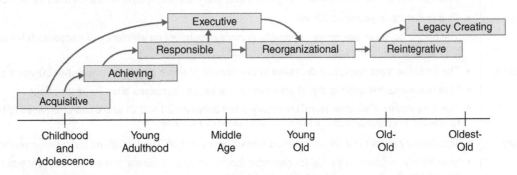

Figure 16-1 Schaie and Willis's (2000) Seven Stages of Age-Related Cognitive Development.

psychological, and physical. The individuals' resilience to stress has been developing through childhood and adolescence. By the time stressors of early adulthood emerge, most people have the resources to respond to both positive and tolerable stresses as described in Chapter 13.

Coping is a positive stress response that involves expending conscious effort to solve personal and interpersonal problems in a manner that overcomes or minimizes stress or conflict. With the maturing of executive functions and higher-level reasoning, young adults gain skills in coping that will help them move through adulthood. As they mature and think more about future consequences, young adults have an easier time modulating risk taking and making informed decisions about the future. As early adults are faced with, and address the stressors of adult life they develop more extensive coping patterns.

Fluid and Crystallized Intelligence

Fluid intelligence was introduced in Chapter 6 to define one aspect of intelligence. Fluid intelligence is the ability to process novel information and to think logically and solve problems in novel situations, independent of acquired knowledge. This form of intelligence is closely associated with working memory and is negatively impacted when tasks are time-pressured (when the person is forced to work quickly). Fluid intelligence peaks in early adulthood, and by the age of 30, begins a slow decline (Li, Baldassi, Johnson, & Weber, 2013).

Crystallized intelligence, an aspect of intelligence, is of growing importance in adulthood. It is the ability to apply knowledge gained through practice of skills, educational learning, and experience. It is not actually memory or knowledge, but it does rely on accessing information from long-term memory and using stored memories to aid in deciding how to respond to given situations. Crystallized intelligence improves throughout early and middle adulthood. In the study of early adulthood, we will consider both fluid and crystallized intelligence, but in this chapter our focus will be on fluid intelligence and the use of intellect to influence everyday performance and functional abilities.

PHYSICAL FUNCTIONS

For most people, early adulthood is a period of peak physical status and optimal health. Between the ages of 19 and 26, individuals typically reach the optimal speed of reaction time and attain adult growth of the skeletal, respiratory, and cardiovascular systems. This is a time of cardiovascular fitness for many individuals. **Cardiovascular fitness** refers to the combined efficiency of the heart, lungs, and vascular system in delivering oxygen to the working muscle tissue so that prolonged physical work can be maintained (Payne & Isaacs, 2012). **Table 16-1** provides an overview of biophysical changes during the transitional years.

TABLE 16-1 Physical Changes in Early Adulthood	
System	**Changes**
Skeletal system	• Skeletal bone growth is complete around 25 years of age. • Bone continues to be deposited faster than it is broken down up until about 35 years of age.
Neuromuscular system	• Muscular performance is at peak performance between 20 and 30 years of age. • Reaction times generally peak just before onset of young adulthood and remain constant until the late 20s.
Integumentary system	• After adolescence, skin begins to lose moisture, gradually becoming drier with age. • First signs of gray hair and baldness may appear in young adulthood.
Cardiovascular system	• Adult size and rhythm are established by 16 years of age. • Total blood volume of young adult is 70 to 85 ml per kilogram of body weight. • Blood pressure rises slowly from early childhood, and cholesterol levels increase from the age of 21 years.
Respiratory system	• This is mature in young adulthood. • The body's ability to use oxygen optimally is more dependent on efficiency of cardiovascular system and the needs of skeletal muscle than on maturity of lungs.
Gastrointestinal system	• The digestive tract displays a decrease in the amount of some digestive juices after 30 years of age. • Ptyalin (an enzyme used to digest starches) in the saliva decreases after 20 years of age. • The third molars ("wisdom teeth") normally erupt between 20 and 21 years and often need to be removed to prevent irreparable damage to proper occlusion of the jaws.
Genitourinary system	• Total urinary output in a 24-hour period ranges between 1,000 and 2,000 ml for average young adults. • Statistically, the optimal period for reproduction in females (in terms of greatest frequency of successful pregnancies) is between 20 and 30 years of age.

Social and affective pressures that characterize adolescence and early adulthood tempt individuals to abuse their newly acquired physical and cognitive skills. This paradoxical issue, where healthy and physically adept young people make deliberate choices that damage their health, begins in adolescence and continues into young adulthood. Draut (2005) notes that many young adults spend less time in exercise or sports activities and pay less attention to their health than they did during adolescence. The fact that they can bounce back from considerable stress and exertion may lead many young adults to push their bodies too far.

HEALTH CHALLENGES

Motor vehicle accidents and suicides are the leading causes of death in this age group, as they were in adolescence. As with adolescents, obesity is an important emerging health problem in this life stage. According to Ogden and colleagues (2012), almost 41 million women and more than 37 million men aged 20 and over were obese in 2009–2010. Obesity is greater among some sectors of the population than others; for example, non-Hispanic blacks have the highest age-adjusted rates of obesity (49.5 percent) compared with Mexican Americans (40.4 percent), all Hispanics (39.1 percent), and non-Hispanic whites (34.3 percent) (Flegal, Carroll, Kit, & Ogden, 2012). People living in rural communities and people with developmental disabilities also have higher rates of obesity than those seen in the general population.

Obesity is a complex chronic condition caused by multiple genetic, biological, psychological, social, lifestyle, and dietary factors. Being overweight or obese is associated with a poor body image and a lower perceived quality of life in young women. The body image problem is largely a problem of women, as women tend to be more concerned about their weight than men, and men tend to be more satisfied with how they look even if they are overweight or obese (Saloumi & Plourde, 2010).

HEALTH RISKS

Poor personal lifestyle choices seem common during late adolescence and early adulthood and can have adverse long-term consequences when they impact one's health status. Among the most dangerous and problematic of health-compromising behaviors is unprotected sex. Hutchison (2011) states that "the potential for sexually transmitted infections, including HIV, is related to frequent sexual experimentation, substance abuse (particularly binge drinking), and smoking or use of other tobacco products" (p. 281).

In 2010, the National Survey on Drug Use and Health reported that, in 2010, the rate of illicit drug use among young adults aged 18 to 25 was higher than any other age group at 21.5 percent. Among young adults, the rates were 18.5 percent for marijuana, 5.9 percent for nonmedical use of psychotherapeutic drugs, 2.0 percent for hallucinogens, and 1.5 percent for cocaine (Substance Abuse and Mental Health Services Administration [SAMSHA], 2011).

What factors influence substance abuse in early adulthood? The National Institute on Drug Abuse (2010) reports that peers have a large influence on an individual's behavior in choosing to use or abuse drugs recreationally. Risk factors for developing an addiction include family history of addiction, being male, peer pressure, lack of family involvement, anxiety, depression, and loneliness, and taking a highly addictive drug (Mayo Foundation for Medical Education and Research, 2014). Peer pressure in early adulthood is tied to social and leisure activities. As illustrated in **Figure 16-2**, meeting friends for "happy hour" is sociable for many young people and allows people to build networks of acquaintances that may help them make valued career and romantic connections. This also may encourage individuals to drink to excess or to use illicit drugs to be accepted into the group.

Access to health care is another problem for many young adults. Although they are typically similar in health status and injuries to adolescents, young adults are far less likely to receive regular medical care. **Health equity** refers to the study of differences in the quality of health and health care across different populations. In the United States, people in early adulthood have been the group most likely to lack employer-supported health insurance and include the greatest proportion of uninsured people (Goldberg, Hayes, & Huntley, 2004). In 2012, the largest American subgroup to have no health insurance consisted of those transitioning to adulthood. Since that time changes in health care legislation in the United States has made health insurance more accessible through healthcare exchanges. Millman (2014) reported that by March of 2014 as many as 45 percent of those enrolling in new health plans were between 18 and 34 years old. Studies conducted since the implementation of the Affordable Care Act in the United States has reported improved health and quality of life for young adults. Interestingly, the biggest advantage for young adults seems to

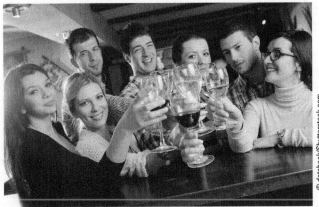

Figure 16-2 Friends are an important influence in early adulthood. This influence can be positive, but also may include peer pressure to drink alcohol or imbibe in illicit drugs.

be increased access to dependent health insurance coverage. Carlson, Lennox Kail, Lynch, and Dreher (2014) report that more than half of the difference in health improvement can be attributed to changes in dependent coverage.

ACTIVITIES AND PARTICIPATION

In young adulthood, people move into new settings and have a greater degree of freedom to choose the areas in which they will participate than ever before. To assume adult roles in society, mastery of some occupations is necessary. For example, to achieve adult status, individuals must have effective strategies for managing ADL and IADL tasks. These tasks may be performed using adaptations and compensations, but adults are expected to manage the process themselves. The *Occupational Therapy Practice Framework* (AOTA, 2014) includes the following self-care activities as integral to independent function: bathing and showering, grooming, bowel and bladder management, dressing, eating and feeding, functional mobility, personal device care, personal hygiene and grooming, sexual activity, and toilet hygiene. By this time, most people have mastered both ADLs and IADLs, and the largest areas of growth are in the areas of domestic life and the acquisition of materials and services needed to support their lifestyle.

DOMESTIC LIFE

Categories of domestic life activities described in the ICF (World Health Organization, 2001) are acquisition of necessities, acquisition of goods and services, household tasks, caring for household objects, and assisting others. Although participation in domestic life activities started early in childhood, the mastery of domestic life occupations is a central focus of early adult social expectations.

Acquisition of necessities

"Acquisition of necessities" as described in the ICF includes several aspects. The first of these, acquiring a place to live, is a central issue in early adulthood. Many young people move away from their home of origin after completing high school. Some move to college and university dormitories, some to apartments, and some to housing provided by their employer. It is not uncommon for individuals to move four or more times yearly during the first part of early adulthood. Early adulthood is the most highly mobile period in contemporary life, and each decision to move is a potentially stressful one.

The pattern of leaving home for college and then returning to live with parents after college is a growing trend because of the economic challenges of paying for an education, starting a family, and gaining meaningful employment. Although DeAndre, whose case was presented earlier, returned to his parents' home because of impairments acquired through his military services, he is likely to see this move as negative unless he can find a way to contribute to the family as an adult. As was noted in Chapter 4, the fastest-growing sector of the homeless population in the United States, are young adults. This includes young people without good social support systems, including those who have been in the military, in foster care, and in the criminal justice system. It also includes young mothers who had children before gaining the needed educational credentials to be competitive in the workplace. These young women have particular difficulty because they are qualified for only menial service industry positions, positions that do not offer health insurance or child care. Veterans like DeAndre who have experienced TBI and PTSD often have persistent difficulties conforming to the behavioral expectations in the workplace, and many such veterans also become homeless.

Acquisition of Goods and Services

"Acquisition of goods and services" involves shopping for, purchasing, and transporting material things needed to support domestic life. In adolescence, most people begin shopping for themselves, but only for incidental things such as clothing or snacks. Young adults need to make major purchases that require careful thought and comparison shopping. Some examples of these larger, more involved purchases might be the purchase of a computer, furniture, or a motor vehicle.

Automobiles can play a major role in the acquisition of goods and services, both as an expensive commodity that the young adult may need to acquire and as a transportation support for the acquisition of other goods and services. Most young people are able to drive a car by late adolescence, but the cost of purchasing, insuring, and maintaining a vehicle is often prohibitive. Davis, Dutzik, and Baxandall (2012) report that, "From 2001 and 2009, the average annual number of vehicle-miles traveled by young people (16- to 34-year-olds) decreased from 10,300 miles to 7,900 miles per capita—a drop of 23 percent. The trend away from steady growth in driving is likely to be long-lasting—even once the economy recovers. Young people are driving less for a host of reasons—higher gas prices, new licensing laws, improvements in technology that support alternative transportation, and changes in generation Y's values and preferences—all factors that are likely to have an impact for years to come" (p. 1). The trend away from driving is paired with an increase in the use of public transportation. **Figure 16-3** shows a busy train station full of commuters and students that reflects this trend.

Household Tasks

Young adults who continue to live in their parents' home or live in a college dormitory may be able to postpone the

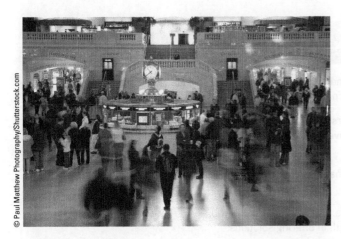

Figure 16-3 Increasingly, young adults are relying on all forms of public transportation rather than assuming the expenses of having a car.

daily routine of planning, organizing, and preparing meals, but this skill must be mastered for individuals to achieve an adult level of independence. Similarly, the ability to maintain clothing and a clean living area will be expected as part of adult daily functions. Most adolescents assist with some housework, but do not assume the responsibility for planning or assuring that the work is done. Young adults living with their parents are less likely to do household tasks than are those living on their own. Although there has been some shift away from this, women of all ages do the bulk of household tasks (U.S. Department of Labor, 2013). Household tasks include food preparation and clean-up, household cleaning, laundry, and lawn and garden care. Culture, socioeconomic status, gender expectations, and personal values will all influence what household tasks young adults value and master.

Caring for Household Objects

This category of function includes maintaining and repairing personal belongings and devices that people need in their everyday activities. This includes both interior and exterior maintenance, repair, and decoration. As individuals move into adult roles and lifestyles, they need to learn to care for and repair clothing, appliances, and household processes such as plumbing and ventilation. Culture, socioeconomic status, gender expectations, and personal values will influence the caring for household objects in much the same way that they influence the performance of household tasks. Personal finances and living situations will make this category of skills quite varied. Individuals living in rented apartments may gain skill in communicating with their landlord about needed repairs, and people with lower incomes may need to gain skills in areas that their wealthier peers may omit, such as learning to repair clothing. Also included in this category is the communication with and supervision of others hired to assist with the care of the household.

Sometimes young people learn these skills from their families, and sometimes they learn them from personal experience. When people rent an apartment, the landlord usually requires a substantial "security deposit" to protect against damage to the apartment. Renters who do not care for their living space may find the cost of renting prohibitive, whereas those who have rented and left an apartment in good condition may have an advantage in finding a new apartment.

Assisting Others

This activity includes all of the aspects of assisting household members and others with their learning, communicating, self-care, and movement within the house or outside. This could be the care of partners, children, or any other person of significance to individuals. In early adulthood, individuals express their connections to others by being concerned about the well-being of others. During this stage of life, many people choose to have children. Although the act of becoming a parent is biological, the assumption of the social role of parent is both a complex occupation and a major life event. **Parenting** is the conscious decision to promote and support the physical, emotional, social, and intellectual development of a child from infancy to adulthood. Like most adult occupations, the occupation of parenting changes with the passage of time and with the growing experiences of the parent in question. Parenting is an example of an occupation that is mutually engaged in by two or more people. At a minimum, it incorporates the dynamic interrelationship between a parent and a child. In many instances, the occupation of parent may include several people, both other adults and other children. Parenting is a **co-occupation**, an occupation that is mutually engaged in. Many adult occupations are co-occupations, involving two or more people who are active in building a shared meaning and have a shared goal in the performance of either necessary or chosen occupations.

RELATIONSHIPS

Relationships are interpersonal connections that require skills to build and maintain. In this section, we will consider the actions and tasks required for basic and complex interactions with people in a contextually and socially appropriate manner. Relationships may take many forms. In this discussion, we will consider formal relationships, informal relationships, family relationships, intimate relationships, and romantic relationships.

Formal Relationships

The structure of the family and the educational system offer maturing people opportunities to interact and build relationships with teachers, coaches, religious leaders, and many other people in positions of authority. By early adulthood,

TABLE 16-2   Top Five Civility Traits All Employees Need to Succeed

1. Become aware of communication strengths and limitations and then use that knowledge to build better interactions. Most incivility occurs due to differences in communication and learning styles.

2. Use technology wisely. No one is more important than the person with whom you are speaking. Just because it rings, you don't have to answer it. Just because it alerts you that you have a message, you don't have to read it immediately. Be willing to turn it off so you aren't tempted to be distracted by it.

3. Be on time. When you show up late, you are communicating that what you were doing is more important. When we consistently turn up late, people feel disrespected.

4. Take responsibility for mistakes, apologize, and offer solutions. Say "please," "thank you," "you're welcome," and "I'm sorry." There is strength in admitting mistakes and even more strength in offering solutions.

5. Be IN the moment. Whether you're in a meeting, a one-on-one conversation, or a webinar, show consideration and respect to whoever is speaking and other participants. You have to give it if you want to get it.

Adapted from Stanyon, D. (2012). Top Five Civility Traits All Employees Need to Succeed. Retrieved from http://www.emilypost.com/on-the-job /workplace-relationships/906-top-five-civility-traits-all-employees-need-to-succeed.

people must master the ability to interact with others in a contextually and socially appropriate manner that includes showing consideration and esteem when appropriate.

A **formal relationship** is an association based on employment or social interactions between two parties who are linked because of a mutual affiliation or goal. Often these relationships are with people in positions of authority, but they may also be with subordinates and equals.

Creating and maintaining formal relationships is one of the most important new demands in early adulthood. Through formal relationships, people build social networks that can be invaluable in finding desired housing, employment, and recreational opportunities. Young people who have been heavily involved in electronic communications may undervalue the importance of etiquette in adult life. Stanyon (2012) lists "civility traits" needed for the workplace that heavily emphasize communication skills and manners. These are listed in **Table 16-2**.

In early adulthood, the ability to recognize and conform to both implicit and explicit rules for behavior in formal relationship will be an important predictor of success in entering the workforce and engaging productively within communities. For the net generation who has grown up texting and "tweeting," a whole new standard for electronic communications in formal relationships must be learned. For example, emails at work should be grammatically correct, free of spelling errors, and free of abbreviations. The widespread growth in social networking services that allow individuals to construct a public profile and build a list of connections (other users that they select) leads to a blurring between public and private relationships (Whitfield, 2013). The public profiles, which include lists of "friends" and a permanent record of activities and interactions, on social networking sites are an increasing source of concern

for employers. Not only must young adults learn to never say in an email anything you wouldn't say to someone's face, and that cute emoticons do not make up for rudeness in workplace communications, they must learn that their "profile" on the web can negatively impact them in the workplace.

Informal Social Relationships

Relatively little has been studied about informal social relationships in early adulthood. The most prevalent informal social group for this age is the group of friends. It was noted that in adolescence, friends were a source of affirmation and acceptance. Friends influence decision making and provide support in times of stress. Friends continue to offer these resources in early adulthood (Berk, 2010). Especially for those from middle or higher socioeconomic backgrounds, the postponement of marriage and childbearing allows for an extended period of personal exploration and identity development. Where earlier generations moved quickly into marriage partnerships, peer friendships have taken the forefront as social supports for today's emerging adults. Settersten and Ray (2010) remind their readers that television reflects the times. A couple of generations ago, *Father Knows Best* and later *All in the Family* provided a model for successful young adults. Today, television shows depicting young adults are centered on ensembles of friends. Shows like *Sex in the City, The Big Bang Theory,* and *How I Met Your Mother* all characterize modern emerging adults and the importance of friendships. Christakis and Fowler (2009) find that the size of our social network and our position in it are more influential and predictive of success than race, class, gender, or education.

Many young adult friendships are based on proximity and shared experiences, perhaps a shared college or workplace. These friendships are supportive and cordial, but they may lack true intimacy. With Internet connectivity and the wide array of social networking options, it is easier than ever before to find like-minded people and build relationships virtually. Many young adults have web-based friends that they value as or more highly than their face-to-face friends. Christakis and Fowler (2009) report that it will be "friends of friends" who connect emerging adults to job leads, romantic partners, and career growth.

Social relationships influence health behaviors by instilling a sense of collegiality and concern for others that influences individuals to engage in behaviors accepted in their social groups (Umberson & Karas Montez, 2010). These influences on health may be either positive or negative depending on individuals' social network.

Family Relationships

In many cases, after young people marry or become established in committed relationships, they invest less time in developing a romantic partnership and their relationships with siblings may expand. Siblings who are emotionally close or even emotionally neutral to one another often build stronger relationships during this period. When family experiences have been positive, relationships between adult same-sex siblings offer a bond that includes a shared background and similarity in values and perspectives. Conversely, when the relationship is negative, as in cases where there is a childhood history of parental favoritism, interpersonal competition, and sibling rivalry, sibling bonds may be disrupted and relationships with siblings may be discarded (Berk, 2010).

As recently as 15 years ago, there was an assumption of a clear point in development when young adults "leave home." The combination of changes in educational demands for workforce participation, the delaying of marriage, and economic recession has resulted in dramatic changes in young adults' relationships with their family. This is a transitory life stage in which people may move into and out of romantic and marital relationships, attend college, change schools, enter the labor force, and perhaps also change jobs (Aquilino, 2006). In this developmental period, in addition to gaining autonomy in necessary occupations (such as ADLs and IADLs), young adults also explore many occupations that are new or of interest to them. They chose to explore occupations that bring them pleasure or a sense of personal satisfaction.

Understandably, in the midst of all this change, young adults' relationships with their family of origin is transformed dramatically. Historically, in the stage of emerging adulthood, people would see their parents, their siblings, and their other relatives less frequently than ever before (Hutchison, 2011). Recent studies have shown a reversal

of this trend. Settersten and Ray (2010) report that "one-half of young adults between the ages of 18 and 25 say they see their parents at least once a week. Nearly two-thirds live within an hour of their parents. If they do not see one another, they talk on the phone regularly." Work, romantic attachments, geographic distance, and a desire for independence may all influence the ability to maintain contact with family members. In spite of this, relationships with parents are both important and influential. Aquilino (2006) writes "A secure, affectionate parent–emerging adult bond that extends the balance of connection and separation established in adolescence promotes many aspects of adaptive functioning: favorable self-esteem, identity progress, successful transition to college life, higher academic achievement, more rewarding friendships and romantic ties, and reduced anxiety, depression, loneliness, and drug abuse" (p. 367). During the economic challenges of establishing oneself as an adult, the bond with parents can support the young adults' achievement of independence if they feel secure, supported, and loved within their family of origin.

Boomerang generation is a term applied to young adults that plays on the idea that they "keep coming back." Young people in the emerging adulthood period often choose to cohabitate with their parents after a brief period of living on their own, "boomeranging" back to their place of origin. For many parents, this is unsettling, as it would have been considered a "failure" in an earlier generation. It also may cause tension in some relationships, as all parties will have less privacy and less independence than they had on their own.

Young adults often have active ongoing interactions with their own parent at the same time that they become parents themselves. When young adults accept a role as parent, they experience changes in all aspects of everyday life. The costs of child care and medical care can exceed the financial resources of young people just joining the workforce. Young adults who are parents may have built a large network of friends, but after childbearing, they tend to spend less time with the friends they made earlier and more time with family. This group of young adults is the most likely to "boomerang" for the social support and assistance with expenses that they can find with their own parents.

Even when they maintain their own household, young adults with young children are often drawn back to their family of origin. The challenges of parenting often lead individuals to seek support from others who have shared the experience and who may offer support both emotionally and physically for this adult occupation. As illustrated in **Figure 16-4**, young adults often strengthen relationships with their parents and siblings and take a more active role in family activities such as holiday celebrations and vacations as part of their adult occupational choices.

Young adults who do not have financially stable and supportive parents may be in an especially precarious position. There are concerns about the growing "underclass" of young people who are unable to establish themselves in

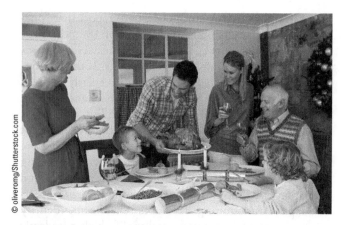

Figure 16-4 When young adults have their own children, they often strengthen ties with their own parents and become more active in family holidays and traditions.

the workforce because of limited education, health access, and employment. This social pattern, emerging in 2012, is expected to result in significant social challenges in the upcoming decade (Draut, 2005).

Intimate Relationships

Identification of and commitment to personal values and goals is the first step toward preparing young adults for intimacy in relationships (Aquilino, 2006). Interestingly, another support to the development of intimacy is skill in behavioral self-regulation (Busch & Hofer, 2012). Self-regulation reflects increased cognitive flexibility and allows people to adjust to societal and situational demands that they encounter on a daily basis (Baumeister & Vohs, 2007).

Eryilmaz and Atak (2009) offer eight aspects of intimacy: physical intimacy, nonverbal communication, self-disclosure, presence, cognitive intimacy, affective intimacy, commitment, and mutuality. Physical intimacy is sharing touch and physical closeness. It can include a range of behaviors from standing in close physical proximity to sexual contact. Intimacy through nonverbal communication is a private communication using gestures, facial expressions, or some other private physical signal. **Self-disclosure** is the intimate act of revealing private information, such as the personal feelings of one person toward another. Presence is the subjective feeling that a person you are intimate with is present in either a physical or nonphysical manner when the person is not actually present. Cognitive intimacy is characterized by feelings of "knowing" the other.

Affective intimacy is the reception and expression of a deep sense of love, caring, compassion, and positive attraction for one another. Commitment is the extent to which partners in a relationship perceive their relationship as ongoing for an indefinite period. Finally, mutuality is the assumption that intimate partners are co-engaged in a common cause. Intimate relationships may be romantic relationships, but successful young adults build intimacy

with friends, siblings, coworkers, and other important people in their life as well.

Romantic Relationships

Romantic love is traditionally considered to lead young adults toward commitment and marriage. **Marriage** is a social union or legal contract between people called spouses that legally identifies kinship and in which committed interpersonal relationships, usually intimate and sexual, are acknowledged. Marriage as a committed interchange between people who share a common goal may also be considered a gateway to the co-occupation of "spouse" or "life partner." At the level of intimacy and romantic relationships, same-sex couples experience much the same pressures and stresses as do heterosexual couples in early adulthood. The primary difference these couples experience that is documented in the literature is less support from their families of origin and a more limited association with their family networks (Hutchison, 2011).

The average age of first marriage in the United States has risen and is 25.5 for women and 27.5 for men (Berk, 2010). Nearly 90 percent of Americans marry at least once. "Marriage is an event of great social and economic significance in most societies. It is a rite of passage that marks the beginning of an individual's separation from the parental unit, even if families continue to be socially and economically interdependent. In many developing countries, marriage represents the union not only of two individuals, but also of two families or kinship groups" (Quisumbing & Hallman, 2006, p. 200).

The decision to marry is influenced by many personal, economic, and social factors. Many young people are influenced by the idea that one "should" get married within a particular age range. Failing to marry within an expected time frame may lead to constant questioning and perhaps even criticism from relatives and peers. Wang and Taylor (2011) note that although marriage and parenthood have traditionally been linked milestones on the journey to adulthood, this is no longer the case. In the United States, the proportion of adults that are married has been declining for several years. Cohn (2011) reports that this trend is most marked in early adulthood, with only 20 percent of 18- to 29-year-olds choosing to marry in 2010, compared with 59 percent in 1960.

Traditional marriages involve a clear division of a husband's and wife's roles. In this type of marriage, the husband's primary responsibility is the maintaining the economic well-being of his family through employment side of the home. In this arrangement, the wife is responsible for managing the household and caring for her husband and children. The traditional wife is not employed outside of the home.

In the 2012 U.S. Census, both the husband and the wife were employed in 53.6 percent of all married households, reflecting a significant move away from traditional marriage roles. In only 21.7 percent of marriages, only the husband worked, and in 7.5 percent of marriages, only the wife worked. In the remaining 16.6 percent of couples, neither partner participated in the workforce. In marriages where both partners work outside the home, household management, child care and leisure activities must be negotiated and shared between partners. In spite of the increasing number of women in the work force, women still have primary responsibility for the maintenance of the home and the welfare of the children in most U.S. families.

Cohabitation is a living arrangement in which two adults who are not legally married are in a sexual relationship and share domestic tasks and responsibilities. For today's young adults, cohabitation is often the first co-residential union formed. Cohabitation reflects a level of commitment to the durability of a relationship, and partnerships of this sort could be considered co-occupations when there are shared goals and a consistent intent to collaborate on the achievement of these goals.

PARENTHOOD

The decision to have a child begins a lifelong relationship. Wang and Taylor (2011) report that today's young adults value parenthood more highly than marriage, and that the two social patterns are increasingly seen as distinct, with more out-of-wedlock childbirths every year. These authors reported that 52 percent of current young adults say that being a good parent is "one of the most important things" in life as compared to only 30 percent who say the same thing about a good marriage.

Especially in early adulthood, people underestimate the impact that having a child will have on their lifestyle. With the onset of parenthood, young adults face new obligations and responsibilities. According to Martinez, Daniels, and Chandra (2012), more than a half of first births occur to women in their 20s, and nearly a third occur to women younger than age 20. For men, about two-thirds of first births occur to those in their 20s, and one out of five first births occur to those aged 30 years and over. For both men and women aged 22 to 44 years, the higher the level of education, the lower the percentage who had a first birth before age 20. Between 2006 and 2010, about 25 percent of women aged 15 to 44 had a first birth before their first marriage.

Clearly, the decision of whether or not to have children is a major one, with an effect at the level of the individual, the child, and society in general. For many couples, the decision to become parents is part of a well-coordinated plan that considers such factors as educational attainment, personal values, biologic and medical conditions, and the couple's readiness to incorporate parenting roles into their current routine. For others, pregnancy with the prospect of parenting is an unplanned and surprising discovery. In either case, the anticipation is both exciting and stressful, and results in a degree of life change that can be difficult to predict. As with other developmental tasks during the transition

LONELINESS

Young adults are at risk for loneliness. With the social pressure to build relationships and marry, the individual who is not following this path may feel isolated. Loneliness is "the unhappiness resulting from a gap between the social relationships we currently have and those we desire" (Berk, 2010, p. 376). Loneliness is, in many ways, a positive motivator for social and identity development. Without the structure of compulsory schooling to bring people in contact with others, loneliness can motivate young people to explore and extend their social relationships. Although extreme loneliness is associated with depression and anxiety, living with mild to moderate loneliness may have positive benefits such as offering time for personal reflection to help individuals understand themselves better, and learning to strike a balance between gratifying relationships with others and contentment within ourselves (Berk, 2010).

MAJOR LIFE AREAS

One of the most important factors impacting the current generation of young adults is the change in the economy. Relatively few jobs that involve a skilled or unskilled labor force, such as manufacturing, mining, construction, mechanical, and other types of physical work, are available. These jobs have historically offered a living wage and benefits for people who did not earn a college education. Today, there are unskilled jobs in the service industry as salespeople and in food service, but these jobs often do not offer health benefits or assure a living wage.

As they face these challenges, young adults bring a willingness to take risks and to creatively combine their skills to meet the changing social, civic and employment environment.

EDUCATION

Settersten and Ray (2010) start their book, *Not Quite Adults*, with the sentence, "Higher education is the most important first step on the road to adulthood." This quote illustrates the primacy of education in emerging adulthood. These authors also remark that, "It is a little-known fact today, but only one-fourth of young adults between ages twenty-five and thirty-four have a bachelor's degree, in a world in which nearly half of all jobs require a degree of some sort." Virtually all of the jobs that pay a decent wage require a degree or certificate.

Not only that, but in many fields, the academic credentials required for entry into the profession are rising. This trend has been true in both occupational and physical therapy professions. Today's higher-wage jobs are both in shorter supply and require more lengthy, specialized training that was not true in earlier generations. This makes education, whether it is technical, vocational, or college-based, required to compete in the workplace (Settersten & Ray, 2010).

Participation in vocational and college education programs require self-regulation and personal discipline, as well as financial resources. Many young people, especially those from lower-income or working-class families, do not gain the skills in high school that they will need to succeed in college. For these individuals, the path toward gaining credentials for employment may be very long and may involve remedial coursework to bring their skills up to a college level.

Young people whose parents had a college education and those who come from more affluent families have an advantage in pursuing advanced education. These individuals are more likely to have financial resources (such as their parents), they are more likely to have been encouraged to perform well in high school (and thus be college-ready), and they are more likely to receive good advice and emotional support from their extended families. Issues associated with access to, support during, and strategies for maintaining an adequate level of academic performance are all central concerns during early adulthood. Individuals with disabilities or special learning needs may be left behind in the competitive academic and workplace environments that young people face today.

WORK AND EMPLOYMENT

Braveman and Page (2012) comment that "in one form or another, most of us will spend much of our adult lives working" (p. 3). Work is an area of occupation that serves many functions throughout adulthood. Work provides a source of income, but it also offers a daily routine and an opportunity to interact and extend our social networks. For many adults, work provides access to better health care and child care options. In many instances, even recreational and leisure opportunities are associated with work.

A common ideal in early adulthood is to find work that is meaningful and personally satisfying. Young adult choices about work at this age are closely tied to their sense of personal identity. Beginning in adolescence, young people engage in a long period of vocational choice. This vocational choice and the subsequent vocational exploration period guide educational choices in early adulthood. This process results in the development of an occupational identity. Braveman and Page (2012) define **occupational identity** as the subjective sense of capacity and effectiveness for participation in a chosen task. Occupational identity encompasses those things that people find interesting and satisfying to

do, the roles and relationships that are sustained through participation, and a sense of comfort and familiarity with the routines associated with the chosen life path. Vocational choice ideally reflects occupational identity.

As young adults explore vocations through actual work experiences, they face the everyday constraints like travel, availability of jobs in their geographical area, transportation, and the need for child care. This reality factor offers constraints to the pursuit of "dream jobs." An emotional factor to vocational choice relates to the individuals, and to their feeling about what is (or is not) acceptable in a workplace. This may be as simple as "I could never work at a desk job" or "I absolutely cannot deal with blood," or it may be a more subtle issue about authority and power relations. In many entry-level service jobs, workers are told not only what to wear and when to arrive, but many personal things like jewelry, hair color, perfume, and posture may be criticized and regulated. When individuals feel strongly about personal expression, they may balk at this level of supervisory control. Finally, individual values will be central in the identification of a vocational path that individuals have enough commitment to that they can withstand the pressures of education and supervision.

The first time academics looked at and theorized about vocational choice was in the 1950s. As the workplace and social expectations have changed, many of the early vocational theories are little used today. Eli Ginzberg and associates (1951) proposed their **developmental theory of vocational choice**. This theory states that the process of occupational choice follows a developmental progression that begins in childhood and spans into the early adult years. The childhood years are marked by fantasizing about career options that tend to reflect those professions that are familiar, glamorous, or exciting to the children. During this fantasy period, people are likely to express a desire to one day become a teacher, doctor, athlete, or superhero. It typically lasts until approximately age 11 or 12, at which time more realistic thinking about one's eventual career begins.

Decision making within the tentative period, according to Ginzberg, is marked by tentative consideration of one's personal skills, capacities, and values. The seemingly endless opportunities that characterized the fantasy period begin to meet the realities of what career one might be suited for. This tentative period is said to begin around the ages of 13 and 14 years and progresses to late adolescence, with an increasing level of awareness of factors that may pose restrictions on available career options. These considerations include economic realities and various potential personal and environmental barriers.

Following the period of realistic career exploration during late adolescence, young adults move to an experimentation period within the chosen career category. Ginzberg and associates view the selection of career category as a process whereby information is collected and various options consistent with one's personality are investigated. Ultimately,

TABLE 16-3 Theories of Vocational Development Compared

	Ginzberg (Developmental)	Super (Self-Concept)
Childhood developmental period	*Fantasy period*, when career preferences reflect glamorous, exciting careers that bear little relation to eventual career choice.	Ideas about the self formed (self-concept).
Perspectives on adolescence	*Tentative period* of evaluating capacities and values during early period; *realistic exploration* in later period that considers economic and practical realities.	Continued development of vocational self-concept; growing clarity about the self and ideas about the self crystallize.
Early adulthood	Experimentation within career category following exploration process.	Particular occupations specified between ages 18 and 21; implementation of career decisions occurs between 21 and 24; vocational choices stabilize from 25 to 35.

in this model, crystallization of vocational choice occurs whereby a single occupation is selected from within a career category, such as choosing to be a nurse following a period of considering a career in health care.

The work of Donald Super (1984) is closely related to that of Ginzberg, and is compared with the stages of Ginzberg and colleagues in **Table 16-3**. Super, like Ginzberg describes career development as an ongoing, continuous, process extending the lifespan. He proposes that the career development process reflects the interaction of people's abilities, personality traits, and self-concepts with the demands and skill required for specific careers. Both Ginzberg and Super present career development as an orderly path to a single career. Both of these theories have been criticized as not reflecting vocational choice experience of today's young adults. The main criticism is that. both are stage theories and are linear. This assumes that the vocational path is singular and does not account for interruptions or changes in the vocational path. Also, neither theory considers contextual factors such as gender, family influences, socioeconomic status, or culture.

If you carefully consider Ginzberg's and Super's theories of vocational development, you can see that they assume vocational and career development to be a linear process. This linear path toward a career does continue to exist for many young adults, but most experience more diverse paths and timetables for career development. The models Ginzberg and Super propose are **continuous career path models**, from completion of formal education to retirement. This continuous career path is much less common in real life than it once was. Young adults today change jobs frequently. Some of the job change is related to being employed in temporary positions as they pursue advanced training. Another factor is that younger workers are often the segment of the workforce most likely to be impacted by social or economic trends. In the U.S. economic recession that extended into 2010, the hardest hit were young men who had less than a high school education and young black

women. The Bureau of Labor Statistics (2012) reported that "the percentage of employed young men with less than a high school diploma dropped almost 12 percentage points from December 2007 to June 2009, and the percentage of employed black women dropped more than 10 percentage points during the same period" (p. 2).

Discontinuous career paths, paths interrupted or deferred by child rearing, need for additional education, disability, or trauma are increasingly the norm (Berk, 2010). Grote and Raeder (2009) note that many employers have restructured hiring to allow flexibility in employment that would better handle demands in current economic and societal environments. These organizational changes include allowing for work being done from home, open time arrangements (for example, flextime), and variable pay (for example, pay for performance). Although these changes have been good for many people, they have also increased the use of contingent labor. Many young adults will find that they must take several part-time jobs rather than one full-time job. This employment pattern may limit their access to employment benefits (health insurance, retirement benefits, and so on) and upward mobility within their chosen vocation.

With increasing workplace demands for extensive and specialized training, and the great availability of young workers, the transition to the U.S. workforce today is more challenging than it has been since the Great Depression in the 1930s. Even before the economic recession, many young adults sought to gain any employment, including employment outside of their field of interest. In one study that followed 1,200 young people for seven years after they finished their schooling, only 20 percent were working in a field consistent with their greatest interest at any given point in time (Athanasou, 2002).

In spite of the near-equivalent participation of young adult men and women entering the workforce, most women work in lower-paying, female-dominated occupations. This trend is, at least in part, because the female-dominated professions have traditionally offered greater access to flexibility and family-friendly benefits (Glauber, 2011). People of either gender with higher levels of education are more likely to be able to find desirable flexible employment than those who are working in unskilled or service industry positions.

Settersten and Ray (2010) comment that, even of those who do not have young families, many in this generation of young people are committed to the idea of work-life balance. **Work-life balance** is a lifestyle choice in which the person sets priorities about the relative value of career and career ambitions and family, relationship, and leisure pursuits. Morganstern (2008) says that **work-life balance** "is not about the amount of time you spend working vs. not-working. It's more about how you spend your time working and relaxing, recognizing that what you do in one fuels your energy for the other." Today's young adults are less likely to allow themselves to be defined by their work than the previous generation. They are also less likely to see work as preeminent, taking precedence over self-care, family, and leisure. This means that young people are less likely to stay in jobs that require long working hours and that are very high-pressure/high-stakes jobs. Employers have complained that today's young adults are lazy and have a poor work ethic. Another perspective may be that young adults today have a higher expectation for preserving their own health and well-being than employers saw in earlier generations (Settersten & Ray, 2010).

Workplace flexibility has been slowly increasing, but tends to increase only in an effort to retain valued employees. In 1985, 12.4 percent of employed men and women worked a flexible schedule, whereas by 2004, 27.5 percent worked a flexible schedule (U.S. Department of Labor, 2005). This reflects a very modest increase when compared to the social and technological changes in the 20 years separating the two sets of statistics.

IMMIGRATION AND WORK

The already challenging labor market facing young adults is most accessible to well-educated young adults with mainstream middle-class values and experiences. Immigrants and children of immigrants are disadvantaged in this competitive market. Batalova and Fix (2011) report that "Youth and young adults from immigrant families today represent one in four people in the United States between the ages of 16 and 26—up from one in five just 15 years ago. This population will assume a greater role as the U.S. workforce ages, and how it fares in the classroom and in the workplace is of signal importance not just for these individuals but for the vibrancy of the overall U.S. economy and local communities" (p. 1).

This group of young adults will have a profound impact on society as they move into adult life roles.

Although many of the mainstream institutions that provide employment opportunities are not open to the undocumented, these young people have had access to the public school system are educated as well as any typical American high school graduate. For the undocumented children of immigrants, avenues into adulthood (jobs or postsecondary education) after public school are severely constrained, because of the lack of employment options and because the undocumented are denied access to most publicly funded work programs. Because undocumented immigrants are ineligible for most college financial aid programs, they also face enormous barriers to higher education (Flanagan & Levine, 2010). In spite of this, longitudinal studies show impressive gains in educational achievement each generation after immigration in all immigrant groups. Additionally, women of all immigrant generations and ethnicities have better educational outcomes than their male counterparts (Batalova & Fix, 2011). In spite of these gains, Settersten and Ray (2010) identified people of immigrant and minority background as at high risk for poor educational preparation and poor financial resources to help them build the skills needed to compete in the workplace.

SUPPORTED EMPLOYMENT

Supported employment is an approach to helping people with disabilities participate in the competitive labor market, helping them find meaningful jobs and providing ongoing support from a team of professionals. Supported employment was first described in the amendments to Rehabilitation Act of 1973. In this document, supported employment means "competitive work in integrated work settings, or employment in integrated work settings in which individuals are working toward competitive work, consistent with the strengths, resources, priorities, concerns, abilities, capabilities, interests, and informed choice of the individuals, for individuals with the most significant disabilities for whom competitive employment has not traditionally occurred; or for whom competitive employment has been interrupted or intermittent as a result of a significant disability." Supported employment is an approach to help individuals with developmental and mental health conditions gain skills and thus gain entry into the workforce. It provides assistance such as job coaches, job development, job retention, transportation, assistive technology, specialized job training, and individually tailored supervision. Supported employment often refers to both the development of employment opportunities and ongoing support for those individuals to maintain employment. Both occupational and physical therapists may work in supported employment settings, and may work with individuals who would benefit from their services in their efforts to enter the adult workforce.

COMMUNITY, SOCIAL, AND CIVIC LIFE

This section is about the actions and tasks required to engage in organized social life outside the family, in community, social and civic areas of life. It is in this age group that people become fully independent in their choices about civic engagement. Young adults' tasks of leaving their family of origin, marriage, and parenthood are more discontinuous now with young people cohabitating, divorcing, returning to their parents' home, and postponing parenthood. Many traditionally young adult tasks have been extended into the middle adult years, and will be discussed in depth in the next chapter.

PARENTING

Engaging in community social life through parenting groups, parent-teacher associations, and as coaches and supporters of youth activities are common community activities of young adult parents.

Many young adults first enter into community, social and civic life in their role as parents. Engaging in activities with and in support of their children, young adults begin to relates to themselves as a member of the community at large.

In the ICF framework, parenting demands are distributed through many aspects of activities and participation, including the "general tasks and demand" area of handling stress and other psychological demands.

Child care is a significant issue for young adult parents and community supports for parents can be a significant aspect for community engagement in early adulthood. Without many high-wage employment options, most young couples must both work and must be able to afford and access child care while they work. **Figure 16-5** shows the diversity of child care arrangements that parents of preschoolers commonly use. Laughlin (2013) report that children under 5 years old were more likely to be cared for by a relative (42 percent) than by a nonrelative (33 percent), and 12 percent of children in the study were regularly cared for by both. In this study, she also noted that 39 percent of preschoolers had no regular child care arrangement.

Although both employed and nonemployed parents make similar choices in types of child care, children with employed mothers spent about 15 hours more in child care than children with nonemployed mothers.

The cost of child care and the lack of access to quality care limit employment options for low-income families. These families are likely to have no regular child care arrangement to provide care. Similarly, families of children with disabilities may be unable to find appropriate child care options and may then be limited in their ability to seek employment.

Child Care Arrangements of Working Mothers 15 to 44 Years of Age with at Least One Child Under 13 Years of Age:

	2002[1]	2006–2010[2]
Child cares for self, Head Start, or other arrangement	4.0%	4.5%
Kindergarten or school	6.9%	13.9%
Family day care	3.8%	4.1%
Child's brother or sister	5.6%	6.0%
Other parent or stepparent	7.3%	9.8%
Before or after school care	10.0%	11.6%
Nonrelative	16.7%	13.4%
Day care center or preschool	22.6%	23.0%
Grandparent or other relative	35.1%	40.3%

Note: Percentages add to more than 100 because more than one response was allowed.

Figure 16-5   Child Care Arrangements.

Source: Centers for Disease Control and Prevention, Vital and Health Statistics, Series 23, Number 25 (DHHS Publication No. (PHS) 2006-1977

RECREATION AND LEISURE

As was noted earlier, there is a recent trend for young adults to spend less time at work, and more time in valued activity with family or friends. This shared time can be face-to-face or through some electronic media. Although this is a growing pattern, young adults do often work long hours and use their leisure time resting and regrouping rather than in organized leisure pursuits. In childhood and in late adulthood, people have the most time and options for recreation and leisure. In early adulthood, recreation and leisure are usually linked to the educational and work settings in which individuals are involved. Extramural sports teams and fitness programs are available at most colleges. For young adults who are working, leisure time often consists of meeting friends for a drink after work or watching a movie at home in the evening.

Returning to the opening case, DeAndre had been very athletic and involved in his church prior to his injury. At this time, he does not engage in any social or leisure activities other than watching TV and playing *World of Warcraft*. Although it may be some time before DeAndre is physically able to return to sports, finding social outlets in the community or through the Internet can help him begin to rebuild his social life.

Adults who choose leisure activities that involve the commitment to participate in a group endeavor, such as participation in a sports team or a musical group, are choosing to engage in leisure co-occupations. Co-occupations such as these can be highly rewarding and can be protective against the loneliness some young adults experience.

RELIGION AND SPIRITUALITY

Among the many aspects of identity development that occur in early adulthood, one of the important things that individuals do is explore and refine their belief systems (Hutchison, 2011). Many young adults change their faith practices in this period of life. A foundation of this is individuals' personal spirituality. **Spirituality** is belief in an inner path that gives meaning, purpose, and direction to life and life choices. Spiritual practices, including meditation, prayer, and contemplation, are intended to develop individuals' inner life. Spirituality "manifests itself through one's ethical obligations and behavioral commitments to values and ideologies" (Hutchison, 2011, p. 284). **Religiosity,** on the other hand, represents attitudes and behaviors that connect individuals to specific organized faith practices.

Table 16-4 summarizes the findings of Smith (2009) from the reports of the National Study of Youth and Religion. This study was done on individuals between 18 and 23 years of age, and so does not capture the entire period of early adulthood. The Pew Research Center Report (2010) had similar findings. They report that Americans between the ages 18 to 29 are considerably less religious

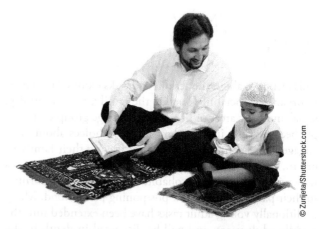

Figure 16-6   Although religiosity is relatively low in many young adults, those with children often return to faith practices and share those with their children.

than older Americans. Fewer young adults belong to any particular faith, and they are less likely to be affiliated with an organized faith than their parents' generations were when they were young.

There is evidence that religious beliefs often grow with age, even in the young adulthood period. Young adults with children will often return to organized religion as their children grow, and share their beliefs with growing children. **Figure 16-6** shows a young father teaching Muslim worship activities in Ramadan holy month to his son. The benefits of religious affiliations include rich social resources with a strong sense of ethics. Idler (2008) notes that core beliefs of all of the world's religious traditions include a concern for others less fortunate and the deliberate turning of attention away from ourselves.

TABLE 16-4   National Study on Youth and Religion (NSYR) Findings on Young Adult Spirituality
Fifteen percent are *committed traditionalists* who "embrace a strong religious faith, whose beliefs they can reasonably well articulate and which they actively practice" (p. 166).
Thirty percent are *selective adherents* who adhere to aspects of their religious tradition that they consider important and drop other aspects or simply ignore certain topics (p. 167).
Fifteen percent are *spiritually open,* not personally very committed to a religious faith but receptive to and interested in some spiritual topics or activities (p. 167).
Twenty-five percent are *religiously indifferent* or what other research identifies as "Nones." They simply don't care about religion or spirituality; they don't oppose it or argue about it and even listen. They are neither for it nor against it. (p. 168)
Five percent are *religiously disconnected* and have "little or no exposure to . . . religious people, ideas, or organizations. They are neither interested in nor opposed to religion" (p. 168). They don't have enough information to have an opinion about religion.
Ten percent are *irreligious* or skeptics about religion in general and specific faiths. These are the people who "make critical arguments against religion generally, rejecting the idea of personal faith" (p. 168).
Pew Research Center, A Pew Forum on Religion & Public Life Report; Religion Among the Millennials, February 2010

Because DeAndre had previously been active in his church, reestablishing his link to the faith community could be a valuable tool to help him cope with his impairments and the traumatic events he has recently experienced. Spirituality has been found to be a support during stressful life events and has been emotionally supportive in facing illness and family problems. Many health benefits have also been associated with religion, including greater length of life and better recovery time from operations and depression (Koenig, 2008). Although it remains unclear whether it is faith that is central to the health benefits or the social support safety net and the general optimism that is often associated with people of strongly religious views, the overall value of the affiliation makes it important for health professionals to recognize and address within the comfort levels of their clients.

POLITICAL LIFE AND CITIZENSHIP

Settersten and Ray (2010) state that "over the last four decades, young adults have retreated from 'civic engagement' of every kind, whether reading newspapers, attending club meetings, joining formal groups, working on community projects, voting, joining unions, or joining religious groups." There has been much speculation about what has fueled this trend. One finding, especially among young adults in the 30- to 40-year age bracket is disillusionment in political systems and general distrust that the government works toward their own needs and interests.

According to family life cycle theory, stable patterns of civic engagement will usually emerge when individuals have settled into adult roles, such as steady jobs, marriage, and parenting, that build up their stake in community affairs (Flanagan & Levine, 2010). For many young adults, civic involvement tends to be episodic, perhaps influenced by the workplace or through family activities they are drawn into by their children. Although early adulthood is a low point for most adults in civic engagement, it is the period in which lasting viewpoints and political identities are often formed.

The younger people in the early adulthood cohort, the "emerging adults," have a more positive viewpoint than their slightly older peers. As seen in the youth activism in both the 2008 and the 2012 U.S. elections, young adults are looking to the government as a solution to social problems. True to themselves and their social world, emerging adults are using social networking to support causes, get involved, and to create interest in issues they find compelling (Settersten & Ray, 2010). Among this group, the frequency and amount of time spent in volunteer activities is higher today than it was during the 1970s and 1980s. Flanagan and Levine (2010) report that young adults today are more likely than their contemporary elders to engage in global activism, to use the Internet for political information, and to engage in lifestyle and consumer politics.

SUMMARY

A successful transition from adolescence to adulthood is marked by the ability to make repeated, major, life-altering decisions without the life experiences necessary for complex problem solving. Although many young people leave high school believing themselves to be immune to the risks of unsuccessful careers, failed marriages, career dissatisfaction, and serious health consequences, young adults face all of these trials. With the competitive employment market, the oversupply of unskilled workers, and the economic recession, young people are taking longer to settle into traditional adult roles. The exploration and mastery of new occupations, both necessary and chosen, are central to the development of people's occupational identity and patterns of participation that extend through adulthood. The manner by which people approach and manage the tasks of early adulthood are influenced by the experiences of childhood and adolescence, and by the social and economic resources that young people bring with them into early adulthood. People from underprivileged backgrounds, such as low-income families or families of undocumented immigrants, are at far greater risk for failure in early adulthood. Individuals with disabilities also have difficulty competing in the field of remunerative employment and civic engagement.

Although young adults are generally viewed as healthy, it is important to remember that many young adults are returning veterans with both disabilities and mental health problems that may benefit from ongoing therapy. The increasing survivorship of infants with disabilities leads to a subsequent increase in young adults with chronic, lifelong impairments. As health care consumers, young adults are often consumers of both adult care and care for their dependent children. In this age group, quality of life is impacted not only by one's own health, but also by the access to and adequacy of health care services for dependent children. As health care providers, we may need to become politically active ourselves to ensure that young adult clients can receive the therapy services they need for both themselves and their children.

CASE 1

DeAndre...Continued

DeAndre has been working with both an OT and PT to help him regain function. He has a home exercise program to help with his walking and his physical endurance. The OT has been helping him learn to adjust to his visual problems and has helped him with little tricks to keep him on task in his daily activities. He has added several "apps" to his smartphone that remind him when it is time to exercise and to take his medications. He has started learning to cook, and through doing this, he is able to help his parents. DeAndre has found that the VA will transport him to the local support group, and through this group he is able to talk about his experiences with others who will understand what he went through.

Although it is likely that DeAndre will make an excellent physical recovery, his more difficult impairments are the social and emotional ones. With the support of his family, his church, and the VA, he is likely to redefine himself and start a new adult path that will let him be independent and successful.

Guiding Questions

Some questions to consider:

1. PTSD has been mentioned in several instances, including DeAndre's combat-related PTSD. People living with PTSD may have difficulty adhering to therapy expectations. Look up PTSD symptoms and list three challenges that you think would limit people as they try to return to their daily occupations.
2. DeAndre is in the time of life where many people find romantic partners and in which sexuality is a central feature of the relationship. If DeAndre confided in you and expressed concerns about his impairment and his ability to function sexually, what would you do? Look in your professional practice guidelines to learn what your profession could do to support DeAndre.

CASE 2

Daniela

Daniela loves to exercise, golf, and watch the Pittsburgh Steelers on television. "This is the year for the Steelers," she says, smiling. She really means it. Daniela has a mild intellectual disability. She finished school at age 18, able to work productively but unable to read above a second-grade level. Now 27, Daniela lives with her parents. Since finishing high school, she has worked at a major grocery chain bagging groceries 20 hours a week. Recently, Daniela talked to her mother and said that she "didn't want to be a bagger when she turned 50." She said that she got too tired and people were sometimes very rude to her in the grocery store. Daniela went to the local rehabilitation center for a functional capacity evaluation. She had good strength and range of motion with good endurance. She was independent in ADL tasks and could do many IADL tasks with minimal prompting. Daniela worked with a physical

Continues

Case 2   *Continued*

therapist, an occupational therapist, and a job coach. With these supports, it was noted that Daniela had difficulty holding instruction and multiple step sequences in her mind, but was able to manage well if they were written down for her. She learned to use a voice recorder to keep lists and reminders for herself. Daniela had no difficulty applying the knowledge gained through practice of tasks and was able to learn new tasks with time and repetition.

She wanted a job where she had more responsibility and variety, and less contact with "customers." A local business was willing to work with her to build a supported employment arrangement. Daniela now works five mornings a week at Mike's Market, a specialty meat and deli market where she stocks the shelves and cleans and helps prepare food. She is paid minimum wage and is a valued employee in this small business.

With her improved job status and her parents' support, Daniela was able to move into a group home with three housemates, one without disabilities. When living at home, Daniela had continued to see herself as the "child" and expected her parents to make decisions for her. Now Daniela is gaining self-confidence and making decisions for herself. She has been spending time with her housemates and has become interested in dancing. Daniela has learned the city bus independently so that she can get from work to the mall and to dance classes. A local agency organizes activities for people with disabilities and has a monthly pizza and movie night. This has become the highlight of Daniela's month.

When Daniela's younger sister Claudia came home from college, she was startled by the change in Daniela. Now that she is in the group home, her life is much more like that of other young adults, and she has developed friendships as well as gained skills to help her advocate for herself.

Guiding Questions

Some questions to consider:

1. Depression is common in young adults with intellectual and developmental disorders because of the combination of life challenges they face, including prolonged dependency, lack of friendships, and social isolation. What aspect of Daniela's new lifestyle do you think will contribute the most to her life satisfaction? Why?
2. What other things do you think you, as a health professional, could recommend to build healthy routines for Daniela that would help her remain healthy both mentally and physically?

Speaking of
Labels

COLLEEN ANDERSON, PARENT OF A YOUNG MAN
WITH AUTISM AND DEVELOPMENTAL DELAY

When Kenny was a baby, getting a diagnosis that explained why he was developing differently seemed very important to me. When I was told he had cerebral palsy, I thought, "Now I know what I'm dealing with." Then, years later, a doctor did an MRI and found no brain damage, so Kenny could no longer have the diagnosis of cerebral palsy but was diagnosed with autism and developmental delay. The school district checked his IQ and said he was profoundly mentally impaired, all because they had no way to test a child who was nonverbal. The labels changed, but it was all still my Kenny.

Continues

Speaking of   Continued

Kenny is 22 now. He walks with a walker and communicates with gestures and one or two words and phrases, and on occasion you will even get sentences out of him. Kenny's personality and humor shine through all the labels. Kenny may have major impairments, but he still perceives himself as a young adult ready for the challenges of new people and places. He was unhappy in the rush and crush of the large local high school, and was homeschooled all of those years. Although he qualified for school-based services until the age of 21, at 18, he announced that he was "all done," and we started the next phase of his life.

Kenny has been a volunteer worker at the local Center for Excellence in Disabilities since he finished school. At "work," Kenny met many new people and challenges. His ability to communicate increased more in the first few months than it had for years in special education, because now he had a real need to communicate. He learns more in the real setting than in some "pretend" setting. Since then, he has continued to gain skills that no one ever expected a "profoundly impaired" person to gain.

In many ways, Kenny is a very typical 22-year-old. He has a job, loves to spend time with young women, teases and flirts, and fights with his mother. Kenny is also Uncle Kenny, a role that has become a central focus of his life. As a parent, I would like to encourage student therapists to look for the person behind the label, and to offer support with community transitions so that more people like Kenny can find a productive niche when they have finished school. Remember, labels are not the person.

REFERENCES

Aimone, J. B., Wiles, J., & Gage, F. H. (2006). Potential role for adult neurogenesis in the encoding of time in new memories. *Nature Neuroscience, 9,* 723–727.

American Occupational Therapy Association (AOTA). (2014). *Occupational therapy practice framework: Domain and process* (3rd ed.). Bethesda, MD: AOTA Press.

Aquilino, W. (2006). Family relationships and support systems in emerging adulthood. In J. J. Arnett & J. L. Tanner (Eds.). *Emerging adults in America: Coming of age in the 21st century* (pp. 193–217). Washington, DC: American Psychological Association.

Arnett, J. (2000). Emerging adulthood: A theory of development from the late teens through the twenties. *American Psychologist, 55*(5), 469–480.

Arnett, J. (2007). Emerging adulthood: What is it, and what is it good for? *Child Development Perspectives, 1,* 68–73.

Athanasou, J. (2002). Vocational pathways in the early part of a career: An Australian study. *The Career Development Quarterly, 1,* 78–86.

Baldwin, C. L., & Ash, I. K. (2011). Impact of sensory acuity on auditory working memory span in young and older adults. *Psychology and Aging, 26*(1), 85–91.

Bar-Shalita, T., Vatine, J., Parush, S., Deutsch, L., & Seltzer, Z. (2012). Psychophysical correlates in adults with sensory modulation disorder. *Disability & Rehabilitation, 34*(11), 943–950.

Batalova, J., & Fix, M. (2011). *Up for grabs: The gains and prospects of first- and second-generation young adults.* Washington, DC: Migration Policy Institute.

Baumeister, R. F., & Vohs, K. D. (2007). Self-regulation, ego depletion, and motivation. *Social and Personality Psychology Compass, 1,* 1–14.

Baumeister, R. F., & Bushman, B. J. (2011). *Social psychology and human nature* (2nd ed.). San Francisco, CA: Cengage.

Becker, S. (2005). A computational principle for hippocampal learning and neurogenesis. *Hippocampus, 15,* 722–38.

Berk, L. (2010). *Exploring lifespan development* (2nd ed.). Upper Saddle River, NJ Prentice Hall.

Braveman, B., & Page, J. (2011). *Work: Promoting participation & productivity through occupational therapy.* Philadelphia, PA: F.A. Davis.

Busch, H., & Hofer, J. (2012). Self-regulation and milestones of adult development: Intimacy and generativity. *Developmental Psychology, 48*(1), 282–293.

Carlson, D. L., Lennox Kail, B., Lynch, J. L., & Dreher, M. (2014). The Affordable Care Act, Dependent Health Insurance Coverage, and Young Adults' Health. *Sociological Inquiry, 84*(2), 191-209. doi:10.1111/soin.12036

Christakis, N., & Fowler, J. (2009). *Connected: How your friends' friends' friends affect everything you think, feel, and do.* Boston, MA: Back Bay Books.

Christiansen, C., and Townsend, E. (2010). *Introduction to occupation: The art and science of living* (2nd ed.). New Jersey: Pearson.

Cohn, D. (2011). Marriage rate declines and marriage age rises. *Pew Research: Social and Demographic Trends.* Retrieved from http://www.pewsocialtrends.org/2011/12/14/marriage-rate-declines-and-marriage-age-rises/

Copen, C., Daniels, K., Vespa, J., & Mosher, W. (2012). First marriages in the United States: Data from the 2006–2010 National Survey of Family Growth. *National Health Statistics Report*, 49. Retrieved from http://www.cdc.gov/nchs/data/nhsr/nhsr049.pdf

Davis, B., Dutzik, T., & Baxandall, P. (2012). *Transportation and the new generation: Why young people are driving less and what it means for transportation policy*. Frontier Group and U.S. PIRG Education Fund. Retrieved from http://www.uspirg.org/reports/usp/transportation-and-new-generation

Draut, T. (2005). *Strapped: Why America's 20- and 30- somethings can't get ahead*. New York: Doubleday.

Eryilmaz, A., & Atak, H. (2009). Ready or not? Markers of starting romantic intimacy at emerging adulthood: The Turkish experience. *International Journal of Social Sciences, 4*(1), 31–38.

Feldman, R. (2010). *Development across the life span* (6th ed.). Prentice Hall.

Flanagan, C., & Levine, P. (2010). Civic engagement and the transition to adulthood. *The Future of Children, 20,* 159–179.

Flegal, K., Carroll, M., Kit, B., & Ogden, C. (2012). Prevalence of obesity and trends in the distribution of body mass index among US adults, 1999–2010. *JAMA, 307*(5), 491–497.

Ginzberg, E., Ginsberg, S., Axelrad, S., & Herma, J. (1951). *Occupational choice: An approach to a general theory*. New York: Columbia University Press.

Glauber, R. (2011). LIMITED ACCESS: Gender, occupational composition, and flexible work scheduling. *The Sociological Quarterly, 52,* 472–494.

Goldberg, J., Hayes, W., & Huntley, J. (2004). *Understanding health disparities*. Health Policy Institute of Ohio.

Grote, G., & Raeder, S. (2009). Careers and identity in flexible working: Do flexible identities fare better? *Human Relations, 62*(2), 219–244.

Hutchison, E. (2011) *Dimensions of human behavior: The changing life course* (4th ed.). Thousand Oaks, CA: Sage Publications.

Idler, E. (2008). The psychological and physical benefits of spiritual/religious practices. *Spirituality in Higher Education Newsletter, 4,* 1.

Kempermann, G., Wiskott, L., & Gage, F. (2004). Functional significance of adult neurogenesis. *Current Opinions in Neurobiology, 14,* 186–191.

Koenig, H. G. (2008). *Medicine, religion and health: Where science and spirituality meet*. West Conshohocken, PA: Templeton Foundation Press.

Laughlin, L. (2013). *Who's minding the kids? Child care arrangements: Spring 2011*. Household Economics, U.S. Census Bureau. Retrieved from https://www.census.gov/hhes/childcare/

Li, Y., Baldassi, M., Johnson, E. J., & Weber, E. U. (2013). Complementary cognitive capabilities, economic decision making, and aging. *Psychology and Aging, 28*(3), 595–613.

Martinez, G., Daniels, K., & Chandra, A. (2012). Fertility of men and women aged 15–44 years in the United States: National Survey of Family Growth, 2006–2010. *National Health Statistics Reports, 51.*

Mayo Foundation for Medical Education and Research. (2014). Drug addiction risk factors. Retrieved from http://www.mayoclinic.org/diseases-conditions/drug-addiction/basics/risk-factors/con-20020970

Millman, J. (2014). Wonkblog: Young adults signing up at higher rates off Obamacare exchanges. *The Washington Post*, March 25, 2014. Retrieved from http://www.washingtonpost.com/blogs/wonkblog/wp/2014/03/25/young-adults-signing-up-at-higher-rates-off-obamacare-exchanges/

Morganstern, J. (2008). Work-life balance: A new definition. *Bloomberg Business Week,* July 11. Retrieved from http://www.businessweek.com/business_at_work/time_management/archives/2008/07/work-life_balan.html

National Institute on Drug Abuse. (2010). *Drugs, brains, and behavior: The science of addiction*. NIH Publication number 10-5605. Retrieved from http://www.drugabuse.gov/publications/science-addiction

Ogden, C., Carroll, M., Kit, B., & Flegal, K. (2012). *Prevalence of obesity in the United States, 2009–2010*. NCHS Data Brief No. 82. Retrieved from http://www.cdc.gov/nchs/data/databriefs/db82.pdf

Payne, V. G., & Isaacs, L. D. (2012). *Human motor development: A lifespan approach* (8th ed.). New York: McGraw Hill.

Pew Research Center Report. (2010). *Religion in the millennial generation*. Forum on Religion and Public Life. Retrieved from http://pewresearch.org/pubs/1494/millennials-less-religious-in-practice-but-beliefs-quite-traditional

Quisumbing, A., & Hallman, K. (2006). Marriage in transition: Evidence on age, education, and assets from six developing countries (Chapter 7). In C. Lloyd, J., N. Stromquist, & B. Cohen (Eds.), *The changing transitions to adulthood in developing countries: Selected studies*. Washington, DC: The National Academies Press.

Rehabilitation Act of 1973, 29 U.S.C. §§ 701-796l, Pub. L. No. 93-112.

Saloumi, C. C., & Plourde, H. H. (2010). Differences in psychological correlates of excess weight between adolescents and young adults in Canada. *Psychology, Health & Medicine, 15*(3), 314–325.

Schaie, K., & Willis, S. (2000). Chapter 10: A stage theory of adult cognitive development revisited. In R. Rubenstein, M. Moss, & M. Kleban (Eds.), *The many dimensions of aging* (pp. 175–193). New York, NY: Springer Publishing Company.

Settersten, R., & Ray, B. (2010). *Not quite adults: Why 20-somethings are choosing a slower path to adulthood, and why it's good for everyone*. London, England Bantam Press.

Shore, N. (2012). Millenials: The new American dreamers. HLNTV.com, Cable News Network. Retrieved from http://www.hlntv.com/article/2012/11/14/nick-shore-mtv-gen-y-millennial-making-america

Smith, C. (2009). *Souls in transition: The religious and spiritual lives of emerging adults*. Oxford University Press.

Stanyon, D. (2012). *Top five civility traits all employees need to succeed*. Retrieved from http://www.emilypost.com/on-the-job/workplace-relationships/906-top-five-civility-traits-all-employees-need-to-succeed

Steinberg, L. (2012). What the brain says about maturity. *New York Times*. Retrieved from http://www.nytimes.com/roomfordebate/2012/05/28/do-we-need-to-redefine-adulthood/adulthood-what-the-brain-says-about-maturity

Substance Abuse and Mental Health Services Administration (SAMSHA). (2011). *Results from the 2010 National Survey on Drug Use and Health: Summary of national findings*. NSDUH Series H-41, HHS Publication No. (SMA) 11-4658. Rockville, MD: Substance Abuse and Mental Health Services Administration.

Super, D. (1984). Career and life development. In D. Brown & L. Brooks (Eds.), *Career choice and development.* San Francisco: Jossey-Bass.

United States Bureau of Labor Statistics. (2012). Young adult employment in the recent recession. *Issues in Labor Statistics.* Retrieved from http://www.bls.gov/opub/ils/pdf/opbils91.pdf

U.S. Department of Labor (2013). *Table A-1. Time spent in detailed primary activities, and percent of the civilian population engaging in each detailed activity category, averages per day by sex.* Retrieved from http://www.bls.gov/tus/tables.htm.

U.S. Department of Labor. (2005). *Workers on flexible and shift schedules.* Washington, DC: U.S. Department of Labor.

Umberson, D., & Karas Montez, J. (2010). Social relationships and health: A flashpoint for health policy. *Journal of Health & Social Behavior, 51*(1), S54–S66.

Wang, W., & Taylor, P. (2011). For millennials, parenthood trumps marriage. *Pew Research and Social Demographic Trends.* Retrieved from http://www.pewsocialtrends.org/2011/03/09/for-millennials-parenthood-trumps-marriage/

Whitfield, B. N. (2013). Social media @ work: #policyneeded. *Arkansas Law Review (1968–Present), 66*(3), 843–878.

Wiskott, L., Rasch, M. J., & Kempermann, G. (2006). A functional hypothesis for adult hippocampal neurogenesis: Avoidance of catastrophic interference in the dentate gyrus. *Hippocampus, 16,* 329–343.

World Health Organization. (2001). *ICF: International classification of functioning and disability.* Geneva, Switzerland: World Health Organization.

CHAPTER 17

Middle Adulthood

Anne Cronin, PhD, OTR/L,
Associate Professor, Division of
Occupational Therapy,
West Virginia University,
Morgantown, West Virginia

Objectives

Upon completion of this chapter, readers should be able to:

- Describe the physiological changes and health challenges that are common in middle adulthood;

- Describe the difference between cohort and developmental effects in studies of cognitive abilities in middle adulthood;

- Identify the age-related changes in vision and hearing that begin in middle adulthood;

- Explain why considering aging adults in terms of "three types of age" help us gain insight into the diversity and multifactorial aspects of aging;

- Recognize the role of locus of control, stress and coping abilities throughout adulthood and the potential impacts of these on health;

- Identify socioeconomic factors and their influence on occupation, occupational roles, occupational balance, and occupational performance in adulthood;

- Explain why the increasing trends toward multigenerational households are a significant consideration in understanding performance and function in middle adulthood;

- Identify trends in participation in leisure, community, and civic activities for the midlife adult; and

- Discuss occupational deprivation and its potential impact in adult participation and activity performance.

Key Terms

absolute threshold

adaptive coping

aerobic capacity

aging-associated disease

arthritis

atherosclerosis

biological age

bone remodeling

cancer

chronic stressor

civic engagement

cognitive appraisal

deceleration stage

diabetes mellitus

difference threshold

establishment stage

exploration stage

flexibility

home establishment and
    management

hypertension

kinkeeper

maintenance stage

metabolic equivalent unit (MET)

occupational balance

occupational deprivation

osteoarthritis

osteoporosis

palliative coping

presbycusis

presbyopia

psychological age

role strain

sandwich generation

sarcopenia

sensorineural hearing loss

sexual interest

social age

stress hardiness

type 2 diabetes

visual accommodation

CASE 1

Sandy

Sandy is a 52-year-old woman who was diagnosed with multiple sclerosis (MS) when she was 22. She has been in the acute care hospital due to an exacerbation of her condition, and has just been discharged to home and home health therapy. She lives with her spouse, her daughter, and her two granddaughters in a two-story house. Sandy is a homemaker, and for the last two years has provided day care for her granddaughters (ages 5 and 7). On a typical day, she is up at 6 a.m. to get the kids up and ready to meet the school bus. After the kids leave, she typically takes a nap, then does a light workout, followed by whatever chores or housework is needed. When the girls come home from school, she supervises their play and prepares an evening meal for the family. Sandy's daughter works as a beautician and often works evenings, and on those days Sandy's husband John helps her clean up and then helps care for the girls while Sandy rests.

Since her discharge from the hospital, Sandy has not been able to keep up with her old routine. Her husband, John, is very supportive and has taken time off work to care for the girls while Sandy was in the

Continues

Case 1 *Continued*

hospital. Sandy's daughter is divorced and does not get regular child support payments. She does not earn vacation time in her work at the beauty parlor and is afraid to take off too much time because she might lose clientele (and thus lose income). Sandy knows that she needs to cut back on her child care responsibilities to regain her health. But she is reluctant to do this because of the problems it will cause for her daughter.

Physical and occupational therapists come to the home to provide outpatient therapy for Sandy. Sandy has numbness and weakness in both arms, and when tired she has tremors in her hands and an unsteady gait. She tires easily, and her symptoms become worse when she is tired. Sandy and her therapists are working on ways she can conserve her energy and simplify the household tasks that she does so that she is able to do all that needs to be done in a regular day.

Continues on page 399

INTRODUCTION

"As people grow older . . . variability among similarly aged individuals increases over the life course" (Settersten & Mayer, 1997, p. 239). Increasingly, as we consider adults, the specific chronological ages assigned to the chapter become less reliable and less meaningful. Middle adulthood is traditionally associated with adults who are established in their adult roles. Adult roles include having started a family, persisting in a career, and becoming engaged in civic and community activities. For the most part, middle adulthood encompasses the issues of people between the chronological ages of 40 and 65. Yet, due to the combination of the postponement of childbearing and marriage in early adulthood and advances in life expectancy in late adulthood, the period of family caregiving responsibilities has extended. The central developmental tasks associated with this period include learning to express love through more than sexual contacts, to be proud of accomplishments, to maintain a standard of living, and to adjust to the physiological changes of middle age.

In the remainder of this text, we will consider *three types of age:* biological age, psychological age, and social age. **Biological age** relates to the condition of individuals' organ and body systems. People who have been active and exercised regularly are likely to have a "younger" cardiovascular system than chronologically younger people with a more sedentary lifestyle. **Psychological age** refers to individuals' ability to adapt, solve problems, and cope with life events. For example, a person may be 90 years old and physically frail, but mentally active and interested in life events. Finally, **social age** refers to habits, beliefs, and attitudes. Young adults may have had to take on the role of supporting a family while still in their teens, and may have struggled socially and economically, so that they have taken on

the cautious, conservative behavior of much older people. The life events experienced in adulthood do not occur in the same sequencing or with the same timing for any two people. For this reason, readers should consider people first before age as they consider both their developmental needs and their personal challenges.

As with early adulthood, many descriptive names are applied to people in middle adulthood. The two most common are "the sandwich generation" and "generation X." The baby boomers, the generation of Americans who were born in the "baby boom" following World War II (roughly between 1944 and 1964), includes individuals in both middle adulthood and late adulthood. Generation X is the generation born after the post–World War II baby boom ended, and makes up much of the remainder of individuals in middle adulthood. Much of the literature on adult development divides this period of midlife into "early" and "late," respecting the differing historical and personal experiences of the "boomers" and "generation X."

Middle adulthood is often a period in which individuals experience conflicts between the demands of their life roles and occupations. Some common conflicts in this age group are work-lifestyle conflicts and conflicts between caregiving demands. The term **sandwich generation** was coined to describe the conflicts associated with caregiving. The "sandwich" refers to middle-aged adults caught between providing support or caregiving to both older and younger cohorts in the population. Now with the boomerang generation bringing their own children along, midlife adults may have four generations sharing the same home. **Figure 17-1** illustrates the pressures of the sandwich generation.

Today, adults in the middle years make up about a third of the U.S. population (Hutchison, 2011). **Figure 17-2** illustrates the changing age demographics in the United States today. These demographics are important to consider

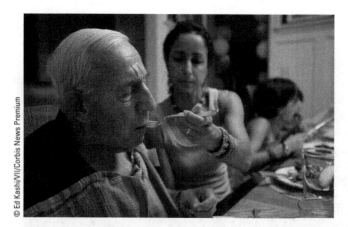

Figure 17-1   Caring for a frail older person can dramatically change family dynamics and add both emotional and physical pressure in middle adulthood.

as the largest middle-age cohort ever moves into late adulthood, and relatively few young adults will be moving into middle age to fill their shoes.

The Pew Research Center calls the baby boomers the "gloomiest generation." They report that boomers "are more downbeat about their lives than are adults who are younger or older" (Pew Research Center, 2008). In this survey, boomers give their overall quality of life a lower rating than adults in other generations, and they are likely to worry that their incomes won't keep up with inflation—this despite the fact that boomers enjoy the highest incomes of any

age group. How much of this negativity is associated with the extended caregiving strain, and how much is associated with the economic recession is impossible to determine, but it seems reasonable to assume middle adulthood's descent from the pinnacle of achievement, financial security, respect, and personal independence that it was in the late twentieth century to the most stressful period in the adult life span would justify the "gloomy" outlook that the researchers found.

As we consider the experiences of midlife adults, we will also consider the concept of occupational balance. **Occupational balance** is defined as the extent to which an individual's pattern of occupation is perceived by that person to be satisfactory, fulfilling, and compatible with that individual's values and goals (Christiansen & Townsend, 2010). As individuals engage in both obligatory and discretionary activities in daily life, they find their lifestyle to be harmonious and cohesive when they have occupational balance.

BODY FUNCTIONS AND STRUCTURES

Middle adulthood, like early adulthood, is for most people a period of good physical and mental performance. Lifestyle and personal expectations often define adults' level of satisfaction with their physical and mental performance. This is the age span that sees menopause in women and the accompanying physical and emotional challenges that

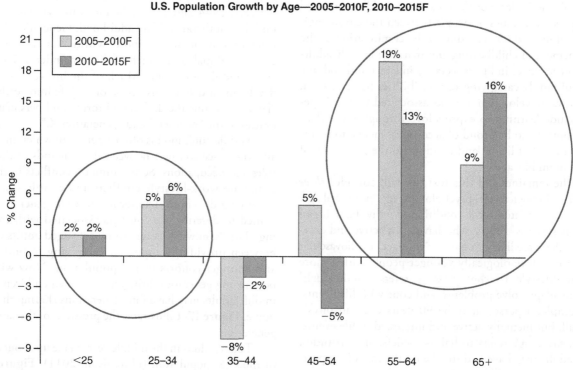

Figure 17-2   Changing Age Demographics in the U.S. Today
Source: U. S. Census Bureau

may occur during this process. While these changes are not a focus of this chapter, they can result in sleeplessness and depression in some women, leaving them at higher risk for other health conditions. Age-related declines in some area of function may emerge toward the end of this period, but for most people they occur gradually and are easy to adapt to.

BRAIN AND NERVOUS SYSTEM

Although neurogenesis does continue into middle age, it is balanced by a gradual shrinkage of the hippocampus, some parts of the cortex, and the cerebellum (Raz, Ghisletta, Rodrigue, Kennedy, & Lindenberger, 2010). Although brain shrinkage has been consistently documented, there are significant individual differences in shrinkage rates, with healthy diet, exercise, and genetics all weighing in as potentially protective against brain tissue loss. These brain changes begin in middle age, but extend through the remainder of the life span. For most people, the changes that occur in the brain and nervous system associated with aging that begin in middle adulthood are not enough to affect the overall function of the individual.

COGNITIVE FUNCTIONS

There is clear evidence that cognitive performance remains stable for most people during middle adulthood (Hutchison, 2011). Although there are changes in cognitive function that are detectable in psychology studies, most individuals do not experience noticeable changes in performance until late middle adulthood or late adulthood. In spite of this, "what people fear the most about aging is not the loss of physical abilities, but rather the loss of cognitive abilities" (Levy, 2011, p. 117). Some biological risk factors are associated with midlife cognitive decline such as hypertension, type 2 diabetes, and high cholesterol. Each of

these conditions is discussed later in this chapter. Protective factors that support persistent high function are education, work, and physical exercise (Willis & Schaie, 2005). In a longitudinal study, Willis and Schaie (2006) found that middle adulthood is a period of peak performance in the mental abilities of inductive reasoning, spatial orientation, vocabulary, and verbal memory. This study identified six mental abilities that changed in the midlife period. These six abilities are listed in **Table 17-1**.

Men reach peak performance on spatial orientation, vocabulary, and verbal memory in their 50s, 10 years earlier than women achieve their peak performance in the same abilities. Women have greater improvements overall in mental abilities in midlife than men do. Both studies by Willis and Schaie (2006) and Deary, Allerhand, and Der (2009) found cohort differences in measures of cognitive abilities and processing speed. In both longitudinal studies, more recent cohorts performed at a higher level than earlier cohorts. There is also evidence that individual differences, including intelligence and health status, contribute significantly to cognition patterns in middle age. The good news is that cognitive decline in middle adulthood is not usually significant, and can be reduced with healthy lifestyle choices and active engagement in cognitively challenging activities.

Several recent studies have shown that with specific training, cognitive abilities—particularly working memory—can improve in middle adulthood. This training requires daily cognitive challenges that include novelty and problem solving, and the effects can impact other cognitive abilities, such as fluid intelligence (Richmond, Morrison, Chein, & Olson, 2011). Websites and game developers have jumped on this research with a variety of "train your brain" games and activities you can subscribe to. Unfortunately, many of these do not meet the standards for novelty of presentation and challenge level to offer the effects reported in the scientific studies.

TABLE 17-1 Changing Mental Abilities in Middle Adulthood	
Mental Ability	**Direction of Change**
Vocabulary: ability to understand ideas expressed in words	↑
Verbal Memory: ability to encode and recall language units	↑
Number: ability to perform simple mathematical computations quickly and accurately	↓
Spatial Orientation: ability to visualize stimuli in two- and three-dimensional space	↑
Inductive Reasoning: ability to recognize and understand patterns in and relationships among variables to solve problems	↑
Perceptual Speed: ability to quickly make discriminations in visual stimuli	↓

Adapted from Hutchison, E. (2011) Dimensions of Human Behavior: The Changing Life Course, 4th edition. Thousand Oaks, CA: Sage Publications. p. 327

Another effective tool for retaining cognitive abilities and preventing age-related physical decline is to maintain cardiovascular fitness. Reis et al. (2013) found that good cardiovascular health in young adulthood supported cognitive function in midlife and beyond. Fitness as a lifestyle choice in middle adulthood supports healthy aging and continued active engagement in valued occupations and occupational roles.

SENSORY FUNCTIONS

Sensory organ function, sensory processing, and sensory perception all are negatively impacted by age. With peak function in early adulthood, middle-aged adults may begin to notice changes, especially in vision and hearing. For most people, these changes are small and gradual, and therefore easily accommodated. Although sensory function changes occur in middle adulthood, significant impairments usually do not emerge until late adulthood.

Vision

Visual functioning is stable through early and much of middle adulthood. Normal age-related changes begin approximately at the age of 50, (Payne & Isaacs, 2012). The term **absolute threshold** is used in neuroscience to indicate the smallest detectable level of a stimulus. With vision, this refers to the smallest amount of light required to see an object. As the eyes change, individuals may need more light to read, and they may have more difficulty seeing at night. The **difference threshold** is the smallest change in stimulation that people can detect. By improving lighting and choosing materials that offer greater visual contrast, change is absolute, and difference thresholds in vision are easily accommodated for in middle adulthood (Hayslip, Patrick, & Panek, 2011).

Changes in vision occurring with age include decreased lens transparency, a decrease in the amount of light contacting the eye, and a decrease in the number of macular neurons by approximately half from the ages of 20 to 80 years old. **Visual accommodation** is the process during which the eyes adjust their focus, whether to near or far objects, to gain visual clarity. The process of visual accommodation becomes less effective with aging, secondary to deterioration of ciliary muscle action. Ciliary movement is necessary for changing the curvature of the lens. This diminished ability to accommodate results in **presbyopia**, an age-related decline in the eyes' ability to focus on near objects. The physiological process of presbyopia is illustrated in **Figure 17-3**.

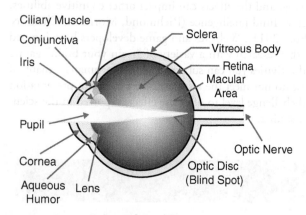

Schematic View of the
Normal Human Eye

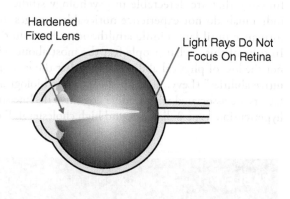

Schematic View of Eye
with Hardened, Fixed Lens

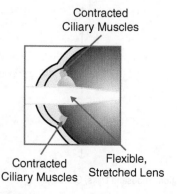

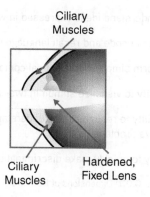

Figure 17-3 Ocular Changes Resulting in Presbyopia

Individuals between the ages of 40 and 50 will usually need some form of visual correction (WebMD, 2012). In this period, many people begin to use reading glasses or change existing visual correctors (eyeglasses or contact lenses) to include a bifocal feature to enhance near focusing.

Hearing

As with vision, the absolute threshold for the lowest level sound that can be heard increases with age. In addition, beginning as early as age 30, an increasing difficulty hearing high-frequency sounds begins to develop. This most common of form of age-related hearing loss is called **presbycusis** For most people in middle adulthood, this change is very slow and not noticeable until after the age of 60 (Kidd Iii & Bao, 2012).

Another more limiting type of hearing loss may also develop in middle adulthood. The type of hearing loss that results from prolonged exposure to very loud noise is **sensorineural hearing loss.** Sensorineural hearing loss is due to poor cochlear hair cell function. The cochlear hair cells may be damaged due to environmental exposure, such as a loud workplace without hearing protection. Sensorineural hearing loss affects individuals' sensitivity to sound, speech comprehension, and maintenance of equilibrium (Bonder & Bello-Haas, 2008).

Many industries now require workers to wear ear protection to prevent sensorineural hearing loss, but this has not always been the case. In addition, some young people fail to use ear protection that is recommended, believing that they will not be impacted by the exposure. Sensorineural hearing loss can also occur with frequent exposure to loud music or to having headphones set to high volumes for a long period. **Figure 17-4** shows a carpenter using recommended hearing protection as he uses loud power tools. Although hearing protection may be required in the workplace, household or recreational activities that involve exposure to loud noises are not regulated and not considered by individuals to be of concern.

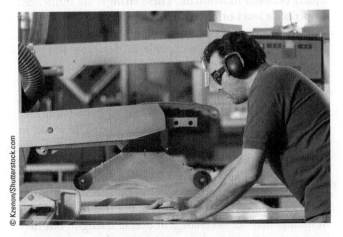

Figure 17-4 Power tools are common offenders as causes of hearing impairment. In many trades, power tool users are required to have hearing protection.

PHYSICAL FUNCTIONS

As a result of access to improved advances in medicine and in preventative health care, individuals today can expect to live well into old age, barring any physical trauma or illness. According to the National Vital Statistics Reports, the average life expectancy for a baby born in the United States was 76.3 years for males and 81.1 years for females (Hoyert & Xu, 2012). Longer life expectancy will lead to a greater percentage of people experiencing the normal age-related physiologic changes in the musculoskeletal system that occurs as one progresses from young through middle adulthood and finally into late adulthood. There is strong evidence that physical activity and healthy lifestyles in middle age can lead to less physical decline later in life (Chang et al., 2013).

Musculoskeletal System

Skeletal maturity is reached in early adulthood when the bones (and spine) finished growing, and the skeletal system reached its maximal, or peak, bone mass. Throughout the life span, a process of *bone remodeling* occurs. **Bone remodeling** is the dynamic balance between the absorption of bone tissue (osteoclastic functions) and simultaneous deposition of new bone (osteoblastic functions). Through early adulthood and much of middle adulthood, osteoblastic and osteoclastic functions are in a state of equilibrium (Payne & Isaacs, 2012). However, for many people, after age 35, bone loss will begin to exceed bone formation. **Figure 17-5** illustrates the changes in bony tissue resulting from aging.

Osteoporosis occurs when the body fails to form enough new bone, when too much old bone is reabsorbed by the body, or both. Osteoporosis is a multifactorial metabolic bone disease with genetic and environmental causes (Hammond, Chapman, & Barr, 2011). Osteoporosis is the most common type of bone disease in this age group. The leading causes of osteoporosis are a drop in estrogen in women at the time of menopause and a drop in testosterone in men. Women over age 50 and men over age 70 have a higher risk for osteoporosis (A.D.A.M. Medical Encyclopedia, 2010). *Osteopenia* is a less severe, early stage of what may develop into osteoporosis. Sandy, from the case at the start of this chapter, is at risk for osteoporosis because of her chronic medical condition. Multiple sclerosis is a progressive condition in which the body's immune system damages the myelin sheath on the peripheral nerves. Because Sandy has been so involved in child care, she has not been able to get the type of weight-bearing exercises that could help keep her bones healthy.

Arthritis is a disease condition involving the inflammation of one or more joints. Normal joint surfaces are covered with a smooth layer of cartilage. Cartilage is a type of connective tissue that is capable of withstanding mechanical stress and compressive loads that serves as a shock absorber, providing a surface for the sliding and rolling between joints. When cartilage undergoes a mechanical load or compressive

Normal

Osteoporosis

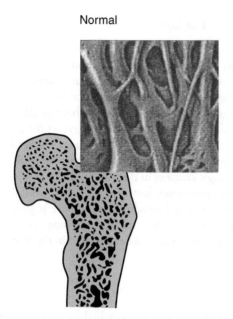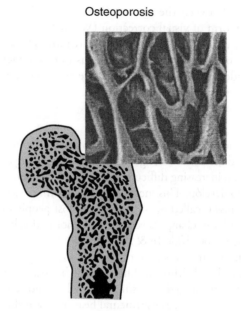

Figure 17-5   Changes in Bone Structure with Osteoporosis

force, fluid and nutrients are pushed out. Conversely, as the cartilage is unloaded, fluid and nutrients flow back into the matrix. This process is essential for adequate lubrication and nutrition of the cartilage. With aging, this process is disrupted and often results in dehydration, poor nutrition, and increased degradation of weight-bearing surfaces (Cech & Martin, 2011). When, the cartilage between bones is worn thin, the bones rub against each other, causing stiffness, pain and loss of joint movement. This condition is called **osteoarthritis** results. Osteoarthritis (OA) is an age-related form of arthritis and most commonly affects joints in the hands, knees, hips and spine. **Figure 17-6** compares a normal knee joint to one with osteoarthritis.

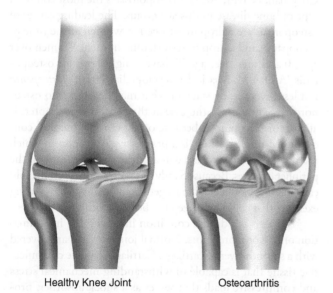

Healthy Knee Joint   Osteoarthritis

Figure 17-6   Osteoarthritis often develops in the knees, the hips, and in the spine.

Osteoarthritis (OA), the most common form of arthritis, and is associated with risk factors, such as overweight/obesity, history of joint injury, and age. The risk factors for osteoarthritis are listed in **Table 17-2**.

MUSCULOSKELETAL CHANGES

Several alterations in musculoskeletal physiology begin between 30 and 40 years of age. Body mass index (BMI) measures reflect a steady increase for most people through adulthood (Payne & Isaacs, 2012). Americans' BMIs begin to rise in adulthood, peaking in the 55 to 59 age group at an average of 28.5 (Gallup Well-Being, 2012). During middle adulthood, lean body mass and bone density begin to decrease, but degree and rate of loss vary widely between individuals. These changes are influenced by people's level of physical activity, genetics, and other lifestyle factors (such as smoking or drinking). Strength training in particular is capable of delaying and even avoiding some of the natural deterioration seen in aging muscles (Payne & Isaacs, 2012).

Muscle force production begins to show a slight decline beginning between the years of 40 to 65 (Williams, Higgins, & Lewek, 2002). These age-related decreases in strength are attributed to several factors. One such factor is a decline in the total number of skeletal muscle fibers according to size and type, called **sarcopenia** (Payne & Isaacs, 2012). Sarcopenia tends to specifically affect the Type II (fast twitch) muscle fibers the most. For this reason, adults in midlife may see no change in overall strength, but may begin to see change in the speed of muscular contractions.

With changes in muscle/fat ratios and changes in activity level, decreasing flexibility is also common in midlife adults.

TABLE 17-2 Risk Factors for Osteoarthritis

Genetics There are likely genetic variations that can contribute to the cause of arthritis, although these are not yet well understood.

Age Cartilage becomes more brittle with age and has less of a capacity to repair itself. As people grow older, they are more likely to develop arthritis.

Weight Because joint damage is partly dependent on the load the joint has to support, excess body weight can lead to arthritis.

Previous Injury Joint damage can cause irregularities in the normal smooth joint surface. Previous major injuries can be part of the cause of arthritis.

Occupational Hazards Workers in some high-demand jobs such as assembly line workers and heavy construction are more prone to develop arthritis.

Some High-Level Sports Sports participation can lead to joint injury and subsequent arthritis. However, the benefits of activity likely outweigh any risk of arthritis.

Illness or Infection People who experience a joint infection (septic joint), multiple episodes of gout, or other medical conditions, can develop arthritis

Adapted from Cluett, J. (2011). What causes Arthritis? About.com Guide. Retrieved from http://orthopedics.about.com/od/arthritis/f/arthritiscauses.htm

Flexibility, in this context, refers to the range of motion available to joints during functional activity. Flexibility allows the performance of everyday tasks such as bending over to pet the dog, tying your shoes, stepping out of the shower, and traversing up and down stairs. As with other physiological functions, without continued practice, flexibility decreases with age. Payne and Isaacs (2012) note that decreases in flexibility are usually very gradual up to the age of 49, and then significant drops in flexibility occur for both genders. Individuals such as those pictured in **Figure 17-7**, who participate in fitness activities such as yoga, may maintain their flexibility well into late adulthood.

CARDIOVASCULAR FITNESS

Aerobic capacity is the maximal amount of physiologic work that individuals can do as measured by oxygen consumption. Aerobic capacity is greatly affected by age- and disease-related processes. The measure of aerobic capacity is often expressed as a **metabolic equivalent unit (MET)**. One MET is equal to approximately the body's utilization of 3.5 ml of oxygen per kilogram of body weight per minute (ml O_2/kg/min). One MET is the average energy cost of just resting. Walking 2 miles per hour requires 2.5 METs. If a person's maximum functional capacity is only 5 METs, that person will have to use 50 percent of his functional capacity just to walk at this pace.

Aerobic capacity is a common measure of cardiovascular fitness. Cardiovascular fitness serves as a protective factor against the changes in BMI, sarcopenia, and osteoporosis that typically manifest in middle age. Although studies are not conclusive, "it appears that fitness and physical activity more strongly influence the cardiovascular system in older men

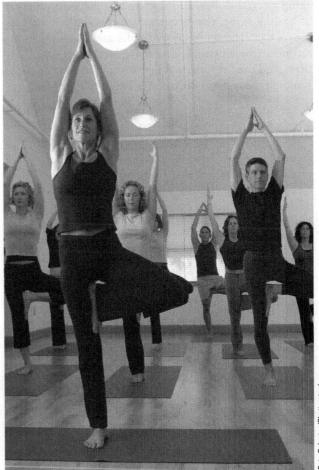

Figure 17-7 Yoga not only supports fitness and flexibility, it also protects against the development of balance problems later in life.

© Pete Saloutos/Shutterstock.com

versus women . . . [T]he growing body of evidence regarding chronic disease risk and physical activity/inactivity in men and women also indicates that physical activity plays a less effective role, and physical inactivity a more substantive role, in modulating certain chronic disease risks in women" (Parker, Kalasky, & Proctor, 2010, p. 244). This means that although cardiovascular fitness serves to slow the aging process and slow the onset of age-related diseases, the overall positive effects of cardiovascular fitness are greater for men than they are for women.

HEALTH RISKS IN MIDDLE ADULTHOOD

Health during middle age is typically good to excellent. Both male and female fertility declines with advancing age, and women will experience menopause, which ends natural fertility, in their late 40s or early 50s. Many changes in health begin in middle adulthood. These changes may be subclinical (too small to be noticed without medical testing), but over time may develop into more significant problems. These small changes may be the beginning of an **aging-associated disease**. These are true diseases, not a part of healthy aging, that occur with increasing frequency as people age. The aging-associated diseases discussed in this section are hypertension, cardiovascular disease, type 2 diabetes, and cancer. Osteoarthritis, one of the most common health problems, was discussed earlier in this chapter.

HYPERTENSION

Hypertension is commonly called high blood pressure. Blood pressure is the force of blood pushing against the walls of arteries as it flows through them. In hypertension, the force of the blood is increased and over time contributes to many health problems. Many people have hypertension without knowing it. Hypertension is a leading risk factor for heart disease and stroke. Left uncontrolled, hypertension can also lead to kidney disease and vision problems. Adults with hypertension are more likely to have other chronic conditions than those without hypertension, including a higher incidence of cognitive impairments in late adulthood (Taylor et al., 2013). Several risk factors are associated with hypertension. These are African American heritage, obesity, frequent stress or anxiety, high alcohol consumption, high levels of salt in the diet, family history of high blood pressure, diabetes, and smoking (U.S. Library of Medicine, 2014).

CARDIOVASCULAR DISEASE

Cardiovascular diseases are diseases of the heart and blood vessels. Most cardiovascular diseases are related to a process called atherosclerosis. **Atherosclerosis** is a condition that develops when a substance called plaque builds up in the walls of the arteries (American Heart Association, 2014). Atherosclerosis narrows the arteries, making it harder for blood to flow through, potentially leading to heart attack or stroke.

Cardiovascular disease includes a number of conditions affecting the structures or function of the heart. These include coronary artery disease (narrowing of the arteries), heart attack, abnormal heart rhythms (arrhythmias), congestive heart failure, heart valve disease, and vascular disease (blood vessel disease). Cardiovascular disease is one of the leading causes of morbidity and mortality in both middle and late adulthood (WebMD, 2014).

DIABETES MELLITUS

Diabetes mellitus, or simply diabetes, is a group of metabolic diseases in which people have high blood sugar, either because the body does not produce enough insulin, or because cells do not respond to the insulin that is produced. **Type 2 diabetes**, once known as adult-onset diabetes, is the most common form of diabetes. Type 2 diabetes results from insulin resistance, a condition in which cells fail to use insulin properly, sometimes combined with an absolute insulin deficiency (U.S. National Library of Medicine, 2013). Obesity and lifestyle factors significantly impact the development of this condition. Type 2 diabetes is more common in African Americans, Latinos, Native Americans, Asian Americans, Native Hawaiians, and other Pacific Islanders. In type 2 diabetes, the body's fat, liver, and muscle cells do not respond correctly to insulin. This is called insulin resistance. As a result, blood sugar does not get into these cells to be stored for energy and high levels of sugar build up in the blood resulting in *hyperglycemia*. Type 2 diabetes usually occurs slowly over time, and can be delayed or controlled with lifestyle changes.

CANCER

Cancer is the uncontrolled growth of abnormal cells in the body. Cancerous cells are also called malignant cells (U.S. National Library of Medicine, 2012). There are many different kinds of cancer. Cancer can develop in almost any organ or tissue, such as the lung, colon, breast, skin, bones, or nerve tissue. The likelihood that an individual will develop cancer increases with age. Among adults aged 40 through 64, 4 percent of men and 6 percent of women have been diagnosed with cancer at some point in time (Pfizer Foundation, 2005). Issues related to cancer treatment and survivorship in middle adulthood center around the fact that those individuals are usually employed and may find it difficult to balance work and family demands with managing illness. Although the disease itself is frightening, one of the more challenging aspects of cancer is managing the disruption that occurs in everyday life. Meadors (2011) reports that "when someone is diagnosed with cancer, regardless of the type, the diagnosis can evoke a great deal of worry and fear throughout the family. The uncertainty regarding the type of cancer, prognosis, and treatment options can be overwhelming for patients and family members. In fact, partners and family members often exhibit more distress than the cancer patient. This distress may be a result of losing control, feeling hopeless, financial difficulties, and anticipatory loss that are often associated with a cancer diagnosis. While cancer can have a substantial impact on physical health, there are also varying degrees of psychological and social implications that result from being diagnosed and treated for cancer."

ACTIVITIES AND PARTICIPATION

Middle adulthood is typically a period during which individuals demonstrate competence in a diverse array of activity demands, occupations, and roles. In middle adulthood, the range of functional abilities is broad. The ICF category of "activities and participation" includes all aspects of adult occupation. Decline in function in any of these areas during midlife would be a nonnormative pattern.

Roles are culturally determined guidelines, a set of rights, duties, expectations, norms, and behaviors that people have to face and fulfill (Hindin, 2007). By middle adulthood, individuals have developed many roles, both formal and informal. People may have also modified or rejected socially prescribed patterns of role performance to meet their personal lifestyle and social preferences. Some of the critical roles commonly managed in middle adulthood are child, parent, spouse, friend, citizen, worker, mentor, and grandparent. If you reflect back to the discussion in Chapter 16 on co-occupations, you will note that many of the roles listed involve intentional collaborative relationships with others that serve as co-occupations. Each role adds meaningful occupations, but each role can also add stress. **Role strain** (also called role overload) is the feeling of anxiety and tensions that arise when there is a conflict in the demands of roles, when individuals do not agree with the assessment of others concerning their performance in their role, or from accepting roles that are beyond an individual's capacity (Hayslip, Patrick, & Panek, 2011). Role strain is a particular form of occupational imbalance, because individuals experience distress due to excessive demands and their perception that they have an insufficient capacity to meet those role demands.

Role strains include ongoing problems that arise from social roles, particularly family relationships. Role strains, such as caregiving, peak in midlife when one in five provides some degree of caregiving (Scott, Whitehead, Bergeman, & Pitzer, 2013). The sense of having too much to do in a normal amount of time is a common source of role strain in midlife.

Sandy, the woman with multiple sclerosis that was presented earlier in this chapter is suffering from role strain. She has been functioning as a wife, mother, homemaker, grandmother, and child care provider. The exacerbation of her illness has added the role of patient, and the patient role interferes with her other valued roles.

HANDLING STRESS AND OTHER PSYCHOLOGICAL DEMANDS

When perceived stress and coping resources were examined as predictors of life satisfaction among three age groups, it was found that the youngest adults (18 to 40) experienced the highest levels of stress as compared to the older age groups, 41 to 65 years and 66 years and older (Hamarat, Thompson, Zabrucky, Steele, & Matheny, 2001). In addition, older adults experienced highest satisfaction with life. This is in accordance with other research that has found no significant differences in coping resources among middle-aged (45 to 64), young-old (65 to 74), and oldest-old (75 and older) age groups. The idea of a midlife crisis, or of midlife being an especially stressful life stage is not supported by the data (Hamarat, Thompson, Steele, Matheny, & Simons, 2002). In middle age there will be some people who face major changes in life focus, perhaps away from childrearing to more community participation, or away from a competitive focus in the workplace to more time for recreations or leisure. People who have difficulty adapting to these changes may experience a period of "midlife crisis" or "empty nest syndrome", but these reactions do not occur inevitably or to the majority of persons in midlife.

While the typical young adult is faced with many acute stresses. In middle age the stresses are more likely to be ongoing, chronic problems, such as those associated with caregiving or financial well-being.

In Schaie and Willis's stages of cognitive development, people in middle adulthood typically experience the *responsible stage* described in Chapter 16. The responsible stage is associated with the establishment of a family, and complex cognitive skills are required as responsibilities for others are acquired on the job and in the community. People who assume leadership positions—whether in family, community, or career paths—may also move into the *executive stage*. Schaie and Willis note that not all adults move into the executive stage; they must have the opportunities to gain and practice leadership skills to function at the executive level.

Self-efficacy is the belief that you can succeed in a specific area of your life. Most adults maintain their overall sense of self-efficacy as they age. *Locus of control* is how much control the person feels that he or she has over a situation. The person who believes they control over what happens, are considered to have an internal locus of control. If a person believes that they have no control over what happens and that external variables are to blame, they are described as having an external locus of control. In middle and later adulthood, some seem to have a diminishing belief that they have control over life events, and the individual's locus of control becomes more external (Schaie & Willis, 2011). Having an internal locus of control is associated with positive health behaviors because people believe that they can make a difference. A central developmental accomplishment in this age group is having a positive sense of accomplishment. The sense that you have done well in important life tasks can be protective against the growing experience that there are things you cannot control. There is evidence that an age-related decline in perceived control toward and external locus of control may have a negative impact on health and well-being. In aging, "a lowered sense of control may have affective, behavioral, motivational, and psychological effects, including greater levels of stress and anxiety, lower levels of effort, and persistence and strategy use, as well as less frequent engagement in memory tasks or physical activities" (Schaie & Willis, 2011, p. 181). Locus of control is useful because it helps us understand the variability in people's response to stress. People with a more internalized locus of control tend to feel less stress and have fewer health problems associated with chronic stress.

Stress is the internal sense that one's resources to cope with demands will soon be depleted. As described earlier in this text, stress may have damaging effects on an individual's health, if the individual's ability to cope with the stress is ineffective. Commonly observed stress reactions are mental exhaustion, depression, anxiety, memory problems, somatic symptoms, and sleep-related disturbances (Kulmala et al., 2013). Stress increases heart rate and blood pressure, increasing the risk for cardiovascular diseases. With aging, many of the acute stressors that were experienced in early adulthood decrease. This is because the daily interactions of people in middle adulthood, established in their jobs and families, become more predictable, and middle adults will choose to avoid situations that are stressful. Unfortunately, those stresses that are experienced are more likely to be chronic and more likely to negatively impact health. These midlife stressors, including health, workplace, and caregiver stresses, are long lasting and often seen as outside of individuals' control, contributing to the externalized locus of control described earlier. Kulmala and colleagues (2013) reported that between 14 and 23 percent of their midlife-aged sample had chronic stress symptoms.

Chronic stressors include enduring problems, conflicts, and threats that people face in their everyday lives that persist over time (Scott et al., 2013). Chronic stressors may result from actual pressures on individuals, and from the emotional distress caused by concern about people in their social network. An example of a social network stressor would be the economic strain that an adult child experiences in "boomeranging" back home. Another network stressor could be the sense of loss experienced by an middle adult's parent who loses cherished friends to old age. Middle adulthood is a time of relative personal stability with workplace and network stresses. Loneliness, poor health, and financial difficulties can be a source of chronic stress for some individuals. Scott and colleagues (2013) found that significant stressors in midlife rarely occur in isolation, and that most people were experiencing a proliferation of stressors that cascaded into chronic distress rather than having a series of discrete stressful events. **Stress hardiness** is a mindset exhibited by individuals that makes them resistant to the negative impacts of stressful circumstances and events. Hardiness is due to a combination of people's interpretation of the stresses, the degree to which they feel in control of the stresses, and their stressor reactivity.

People who are stress-hardy have learned how to think through stressful situations and respond to them differently. Planning and enacting specific strategies to restore occupational balance is a positive response to chronic stress and contributes to stress hardiness. Lifestyle balance was described by Christiansen and Townsend (2010) as "a pattern of occupations resulting in reduced stress and improved well-being" (p. 240).

In middle adulthood, health and family challenges require thought and planning. Efforts to build and maintain lifestyle balance require careful consideration and planning. In this age group, many people have gained experience and skill in cognitive appraisal. **Cognitive appraisal** is a process of trusting individuals' personal interpretation of an event or illness in determining their emotional reaction. Cognitive appraisal is a strategy taught as a tool to address stress and mental health challenges and to support positive coping. Lazarus and Folkman (1984) identify two forms of coping based on cognitive appraisal that individuals of all ages frequently use. This model is illustrated in **Figure 17-8**. The first—*problem-focused* or **adaptive coping**—focuses on the problem by attempting to solve a problem, master the situation, or expand resources to deal with a situation. It is primarily used as a coping mechanism when individuals feel that they have a realistic chance to effect change. Changing careers or quitting a stressful job in midlife are good examples of problem-focused coping in middle-aged adults.

The second form of coping is **palliative coping**. Palliative coping focuses on strategies to help the person feel better through the management of the emotional response to a stressful situation. People tend to use this type of emotion-focused coping when they feel that they can do nothing to change a stressful condition (Lazarus & Folkman, 1984). The use of substances such as alcohol and cigarettes as a distraction from marital problems arising from difficulties balancing work and family is a good example of emotion-focused coping in individuals who are in middle age.

It is evident that the stressors encountered in middle adulthood can have a negative effect not only on the health of these individuals, but also on the relationships that they have with significant others, such as spouses, children, and colleagues at work. Finding positive and effective coping strategies is especially important and salient for this group of individuals. Research indicates that positively biased appraisals of negative experiences that are relatively uncontrollable are associated with better mental health over time (O'Mara, McNulty, & Karney, 2011).

SELF-CARE

Adult self-care demands are the most extensive of those at any point in the life span. In addition to competence in the ADL and IADL tasks described earlier in this text, adults need skill in home management, community mobility, financial management, health management and maintenance, meal preparation and cleanup, safety precautions and emergency responses, shopping, child rearing, and care of others.

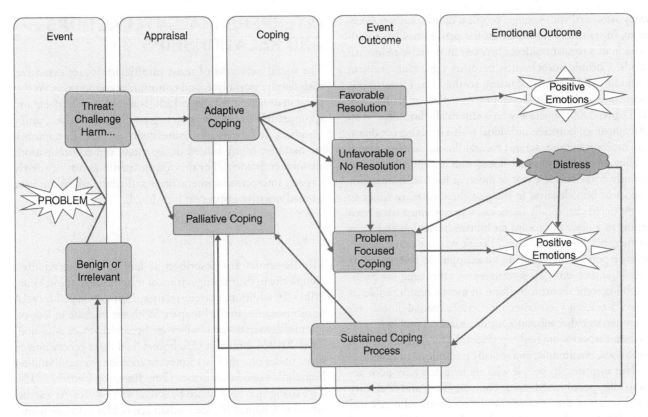

Figure 17-8 Adaptive coping is a problem-solving approach used to effect change. When this approach does not resolve a problem, distress results and moves individuals into a sustained cycle of stress and coping.

Although adults have been refining self-care and process skills since childhood, adults are expected to have effective process skills, including knowledge of the task and the tools for that task. Adults should be able to choose the right tools before initiating a task without hesitation. The tool may be a computer, a forklift, or a pencil sharpener, depending on the task and the challenges offered by it. Occupationally competent adults know what task objects are needed for different activities that make up the day. They have the knowledge to use the tools and materials that they have chosen for different tasks according to their intended purpose in a safe manner.

Adults are more independent in their work and self-care activities than are children or adolescents, and they are expected to be goal-directed in all activities and to see them through to completion. Adults typically complete familiar tasks without asking questions and are aware of the need to seek information when a task exceeds their skill level.

DOMESTIC LIFE

In early adulthood, most people begin to build a home for themselves by acquiring a place to live, food, clothing and other necessities, as well as skills in household cleaning and repairing, caring for personal and other household objects, and assisting others. The American Occupational Therapy Association (2014) describes instrumental activities of daily living (IADLs) as "activities to support daily life within the home and com-

munity that often require more complex interactions than self-care used in ADL" (p. 42). IADLs are of central importance in middle age. Some examples of IADLs are care of others (including selecting and supervising caregivers); child rearing; financial management; and home establishment and management. **Home establishment and management** is a central focus of this age group and maintaining a standard of living is one of the central developmental tasks of this period. Home establishment and management involves "obtaining and maintaining personal and household possessions and environment (e.g., home, yard, garden, appliances, vehicles), including maintaining and repairing personal possessions (clothing and household items) and knowing how to seek help or whom to contact" (American Occupational Therapy Association, 2014, p. 43). Of most middle-class Americans, midlife adults are most likely to be established in a secure housing arrangement. Poverty and poor economic conditions can limit the ability of some adults in the establishment of a home. In the earlier discussion of "boomerang kids," there was an assumption that middle adult parents could provide support for their children. In cases when there is not a secure housing arrangement, or where financial resources are limited, the inability to offer aid to children or parents may be a significant additional stress for midlife adults.

Homelessness

Homelessness can occur at any point in the life span, and is not a uniquely middle adult problem. The type of homelessness usually associated with younger people is called *transitory homelessness*. In transitory homelessness the person may have periods without a regular residence between more stable residential periods. Chronic homelessness becomes a growing problem in middle adulthood. According to the U.S. Department of Housing and Urban Development definition of *homeless* (HUD.gov, 2009), a person who is chronically homeless "is an unaccompanied homeless individual with a disabling condition (e.g., substance abuse, serious mental illness, developmental disability, or chronic physical illness) who has either been continuously homeless for a year or more, or has had at least four episodes of homelessness in the past three years. In order to be considered chronically homeless, a person must have been sleeping in a place not meant for human habitation and/or in an emergency homeless shelter." People who are homeless frequently report health problems; for example, 38 percent report alcohol use problems, 26 percent report other drug use problems, 39 percent report some form of mental health problems (20 to 25 percent meet criteria for serious mental illness), 66 percent report either substance use or behavioral problems, and 29 percent report acute health problems including HIV/AIDS, tuberculosis, pneumonia, and sexually transmitted diseases.

Not surprisingly, people who are homeless have poor access to all types of health care. Thomas, Gray, and McGinty (2011) reviewed the literature on the occupational needs and goals of people who experience homelessness. Four areas of needs were identified: employment and education, money management, coping skills, and leisure skills. These authors reported that extreme poverty resulting from lack of employment, or from alcohol and drug abuse that resulted in little experience with or understanding of banking and budgeting. Skills in the areas of stress management, anger management, and assertiveness were also identified as a need. Finally, there was a need to enhance employment opportunities through setting and meeting work or education goals.

Occupational Deprivation

Occupational deprivation, the inability to engage in valued occupations as a result of an external circumstance, was first described in Chapter 4. Using the example of homelessness, the ability to make meals or build family bedtime routines, although highly valued occupations, may not be possible for a young mother who is living in a homeless shelter. Occupational deprivation may occur secondary to homelessness, chronic poverty, natural disasters, or in any other situation in which individuals lose the capacity to structure their own time and daily life tasks. The best-described example of this is the limitation of occupational choices and activities that are available to individuals incarcerated in prisons due to criminal behavior (Brown & Stoffel, 2011). Occupational deprivation, when it persists, can lead to diminished ability to perform daily activities, reduced self-efficacy, and a loss of occupational identity that may negatively impact individuals as they face future lifestyle and participation decisions.

INTERPERSONAL INTERACTIONS AND RELATIONSHIPS

The social networks of most midlife adults are extensive, with family, workplace, and community connections. At this point in development, typical adults are able to effectively and appropriately interact with strangers, friends, relatives, family members, and lovers in a contextually and socially appropriate manner. Many valued occupations and co-occupations are inherently social. For this reason, anything that negatively impacts interpersonal interactions and relationships can have a broad negative impact on individuals.

Relationships with Family

Middle adults are described as having "unprecedented complexity in their configuration of relationships" (Hutchison, 2011). In addition, current relationships are shaped by relationships earlier in the life span. With the increase in longevity, multigenerational families are becoming more common. As of 2010, 4.4 million U.S. homes held three generations or more under one roof, a 15 percent increase from 3.8 million households two years earlier (Pew Research Center, 2010). This change has been fueled by several social forces. As was discussed in Chapter 16, the median age of first marriage is later than ever before, and thus there are more unmarried 20-somethings in the population who continue to live in their childhood home. The immigration of Latin Americans and Asians has also resulted in more multigenerational family households.

Divorce

Marriage and divorce happen throughout adulthood. Chapter 16 included an in-depth discussion of the institution of marriage, and this discussion is equally applicable to the midlife and older adult. Similarly, the discussion of divorce presented here is equally applicable to other adult age groups. In Western cultures, more than 90 percent of people marry by the end of the midlife period. About 25% of first marriages end in divorce. The divorce rate for subsequent marriages is above 50% (Centers for Disease Control and Prevention, 2011). Most people marry with the expectation that the marriage will be lasting and divorce is both undesired and often unanticipated. The dissolution of a marriage is a painful and disruptive experience for an entire family. Hayslip, Patrick, and Panek (2011) state that in divorces, at least one of the partners leaves with a deep sense of failure and rejection. In addition, both parties have losses in personal finances, social networks, social roles, self-concept, and material possessions. Divorce is especially common in middle adulthood, because, as Hayslip, Patrick, and Panek (2011) remark, "Mid-life may be a time of pruning the unsatisfactory relationships from our social network" (p. 99). Divorce is also responsible for an increase in the number of blended families today, and an increase in the number of families headed by a single parent.

Blended Families

In 2011, 29 of 1,000 divorced or widowed Americans remarried (Jayson, 2013). Increasingly, though, divorced or widowed people are choosing to cohabitate rather than remarry. As a result of both remarriage and cohabitation, there is an increasing number of blended families in the United States. A *blended family* is a family that includes children of a previous marriage of one spouse or both. Parental roles are often harder to negotiate when they are stepparent/stepchild relationships. Building positive stepchild relationships in blended families can be an enormous challenge for a parent (Hayslip, Patrick, & Panek, 2011).

Kinship

Though one's family of origin is a given, not actively chosen, there is an element of choice regarding which kin ties are honored. Research findings show that these choices are guided by, among other factors, kinship norms. For example, the strongest kinship obligation is normally toward children, followed by that toward parents. Kinship relationships do not exist in isolation. They form a network of bonds of varying intensity across time and across members.

Siblings who had a close relationship in childhood tend to be close in middle and late adulthood. For most adults, feelings of closeness with siblings increases with age and patterns of conflict between siblings dissipates with age. Research has shown that the decision to provide help and companionship to parents is structured by kin network expectations about what siblings will do. Those who have a sibling who is emotionally closer or lives nearer to the parent are less inclined to step in and help (Hayslip, Patrick, & Panek, 2011).

Beyond sibling connections, with all of the changes in patterns of family formation and dissolution, what is a kin relationship today? Do the family ties of nonmarried cohabitees fall into the category of kin? What about the complexities introduced by divorce, remarriage, and the formation of stepfamilies? Finally, there are the "chosen families" of gays and lesbians that often include former spouses, friends, children from heterosexual marriages, and children acquired through adoption or the use of birth technologies, which are personally constructed rather than governed by rules of blood and marriage. In this context, kinship is a close connection recognized by the individuals in question that is marked by biological, legal and/or social ties. Kinship networks include persons who are chosen by mutual interests or affection. Family members may be excluded from a kinship network and non-family members may be included based on the choices of the members of the kinship group.

In multigenerational families and extended kinship groups, midlife adults often serve as kinkeepers. **Kinkeepers** are family members who work at keeping in touch with family members or keeping family members in touch with one another (Rosenthal, 2013). Specific family members, often women, fulfill the role of keeping others informed about what is happening in the family, organizing get-togethers, and encouraging direct interactions. Kinkeeping serves to facilitate access of members of the kin network to one another.

Relationships with Spouse or Partner

With the high incidence of divorce, remarriage, and cohabitation it is difficult to characterize midlife partnerships. People in midlife now often have more egalitarian relationships than those seen in earlier generations. Looking at diversity patterns in midlife partnerships, the least egalitarian relationships are the traditional heterosexual couples with children. African American and GLBT couples were found to engage in more role sharing than white married couples (Hutchison, 2011).

Although most adults remain sexually active throughout middle adulthood, sexuality is no longer the central focus of relationships that it was in early adulthood. One of the significant developmental tasks of this period is to learn to express love through more than sexual contacts. In midlife people begin to face their own limitations in terms of family, career, and health. Age-related physical changes may make some people feel vulnerable and less desirable. This awareness often occurs at a time in a relationship when the couple is no longer so intensely focused on each other. Because sexuality is associated with a sense of attractiveness and desirability, some people will go to great lengths to reassert their sexuality in middle adulthood. One result of this is the trend toward increasing marital infidelity during midlife. Other results may be spending money on plastic surgery or designer clothes to regain a sense of youthfulness. When midlife partnerships are "out of sync," with each partner having differing standards for behavior and appearance, marital discord is likely to follow.

Intimate Relationships

Sexual interest is defined by Hayslip, Patrick, and Panek (2011) as "primarily a psychological experience that pertains to a person's desire to engage in sexual behavior" (p. 41). Sexual interest is distinct from sexual activity, the act of actually engaging in sexual behaviors. From puberty and throughout adult life, sexual interests exceed sexual activities. Lindau and colleagues (2007) report that the frequency of sexual activity did not decrease substantially with increasing age through 74 years. These researchers also found that the likelihood of being sexually active was positively associated with self-reported health.

Although sexual interest remains fairly stable across adulthood, the level of sexual activity begins to decline for some people. Many factors influence this, including the quality of the intimate relationship, and the physical and mental health of both individuals. Some health conditions common to middle adulthood have been found to be associated with decreased sexual activity. These are cardiovascular disease, arthritis, cancer, and depression. Overall, in both middle age and later adulthood, sexual satisfaction is highly correlated with measures of quality of life (Penhollow, Young, & Denny, 2009).

Relationships with Children

Midlife parents may be parenting children of any age in today's society of postponed pregnancies and treatments for infertility. The boomerang generation, described in Chapter 16, results in a phenomenon called *prolonged parenting* for midlife parents. When the young adult returns to live in the family home, the midlife parent continues and sometimes extends his or her parental roles. Rather than having an "empty nest" associated with a diminishing of direct parental responsibilities, some midlife parents find that they continue to parent as their children boomerang back. Most midlife parents today did not anticipate the extended role as parent, including the care for their "boomerang children" and grandchildren that is rapidly becoming the norm. For many midlife parents, this extended role is a source of distress. Supporting children in the transition to adulthood is an important developmental role for midlife parents. In the case of "boomerang children" the midlife adult may feel a sense of failure. This is further compounded when the adult children have problems such as chronic disease, emotional problems, or substance abuse problems. In these cases, the midlife parents' sense of well-being is often lowered (Hutchison, 2011).

There have also been changes in societal expectations of parents. Even if the midlife adult is parenting young children, studies indicate that more than in earlier generations, the "lifestyles of baby-boom parents revolve around their children" (Blieszner & Roberto, 2006, p. 270). Parents expect to orchestrate the lives of young children to assure that they have the best possible experiences on which to build their adult life. Rather than sending children out to play on their own in the neighborhood, playdates are arranged and potential friends screened and chosen by parents. For some parents, this pattern of directing their child's life extends far beyond early childhood. That some midlife parents are so enmeshed in the life of their children reflects both the high value they place on their parental role and also potentially the difficulty they have in relinquishing control as their children mature and need to build their own organizational skills and interpersonal skills. A negative description of parents that has emerged in the popular press is the label "helicopter parent." A *helicopter parent* is a parent who "hovers" or pays extremely close attention to a child's experiences and problems, particularly at educational institutions, well beyond the age at which children are able to bear the responsibility for their own behavior and performance.

Stepparenting

The stepparent role is more difficult and less clearly defined than the parent role. Being a stepmother is more difficult than being a stepfather, primarily because stepmothers often are expected to assume primary responsibility for child care. In cases where a family includes both stepchildren and biological children, the role strain on the mother is often

great. Some children may resist the changes associated with "blending" a family and this resistance is greater if the breakup of their family of origin is fairly recent. Not surprisingly, stepmothers report higher levels of stress and greater dissatisfaction with their role than do stepfathers. Stepparents may also be involved in all of the challenges faced by other parents such as boomerang children, extended child care, and extended financial support of adult children.

Grandparenting

Some people become grandparents in their 30s and 40s, whereas others do not become grandparents until their 70s or 80s. For this reason, it is hard to characterize the grandparent role for all age groups. In this discussion, we will focus on middle adults as grandparents. The roles grandparents play within the family group varies widely, but some common grandparent functions are to serve as a safety net and mediator in times of crisis, to share news of the family to all family members in the role of kinkeeper, and many grandparents serve a family historians. Grandparenting is an increasingly important societal and occupational role, with the increase in multigenerational households and the increase in life expectancy. The grandparent/grandchild relationship may now extend more than 20 years.

For many families, grandparents serve as sort of family historians and teach the grandchildren ethnic traditions, culture, history, and sometimes even language that reflects their heritage. Both race and ethnicity are influences on the grandparent role. For example, studies have shown that African American grandparents had almost twice the involvement with their grandchildren that Caucasian grandparents had (Hayslip, Patrick, & Panek, 2011). The age of the grandchildren and the age of the grandparents are both significant factors in shaping the relationship as well.

Grandmothers in particular are increasingly taking on important roles as child care providers. Zauszniewski and colleagues (2014) stated that "more than 1.7 million grandmothers provided basic care (food, shelter, and clothing) for their grandchildren, 40 percent of whom lived in the grandmothers' households. They also found that almost 70 percent of the grandmothers were between the ages of 30 and 59, and therefore likely to be in the workforce while providing care to their grandchildren" (p. 42).

Relationships with Caregivers

Caregiving demands are greater in middle adulthood than they have ever been before. Pew Research Center (2005) reports that 50 percent of all boomers were raising one or more young children while also providing primary financial support to one or more adult children. The challenge of assuming the role of caretaker of one's children, spouse, and aging parent in addition to facing one's own life crises can take a toll on marriage and relationships between a caretaker and children and between a caretaker and parents. "Thirty percent of U.S.

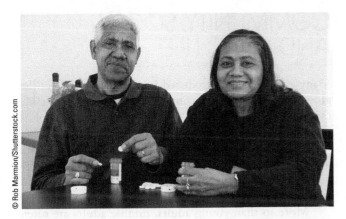

Figure 17-9 Both older parents and their midlife children may have difficulty adjusting roles as a child assumes caregiving responsibilities.

adults help a loved one with personal needs or household chores, managing finances, arranging for outside services, or visiting regularly to see how they are doing. Most are caring for an adult, such as a parent or spouse, but a small group cares for a child living with a disability or long-term health issue" (Pew Internet and American Life Project, 2012). Support and interactions with aging parents can be rewarding, but also may place children in the position of supervising basic parental ADLs, like medication management, such as pictured in **Figure 17-9**.

More women than men are caregivers: An estimated 66 percent of caregivers are female, and the average age of a female caregiver is 48 (Family Caregiver Alliance, 2012). Consistent with the changing social and gender roles seen in the generation X population, the balance in the younger cohort shifts close to equal participation (47 percent of caregivers are male), while among the 50+ recipients, it tips to females (32 percent male, 68 percent female). Not surprisingly, caregivers have far less time to perform their own personal tasks. The services that they provide are not only physical, but are time-consuming and may be emotionally draining. The Family Caregiver Alliance (2012) reports that caregivers reported that they spend an estimated 13 hours per month researching care services or information on disease, coordinating physician visits, or managing financial matters.

Midlife caregivers are likely to be juggling a caregiving role while also working. Of working caregivers, 69 percent report having to rearrange their work schedule, decrease their hours, or take an unpaid leave to meet their caregiving responsibilities (Family Caregiver Alliance, 2012). Compromises made by caregivers include turning down promotions at work, choosing early retirement, and even giving up working entirely. Associated with these compromises, caregivers suffer loss of wages, health insurance and other job benefits, retirement savings or investments, and Social Security benefits (Family Caregiver Alliance, 2012). These losses can have serious impacts as midlife caregivers age. Culture and personal lifestyle choices play a role in influencing whether providing care to aging parents is experienced as a gain or a loss. Even in cultures that value caregiving in multigenerational families, long-term intensive caregiving

relations often have negative effects on the caregivers due to chronic stress and role strain (Hutchison, 2011).

Relationships with Friends

Although familial relationships seem to hold greater values for many people in midlife, friendships remain important. Friendships seem to serve as protective influences against the many stresses experienced in middle adulthood. Friendships are especially important for midlife individuals with low or no family support. In particular, the "chosen families" of gay and lesbian midlife adults are a group of enduring friends that provide both care and support to each other (McGoldrick, 2005).

MAJOR LIFE AREAS

For many, middle age is a stable time in which individuals are negotiating familiar ground as they manage their educational and employment-related occupations. Educational pursuits may occur within the scope of the individuals' employment, or they may be explorations into areas of interest that were put aside in early adulthood. For many people, this is a period of economic self-sufficiency. Most midlife adults have an interest in ensuring their economic security as they approach retirement age.

WORK

Traditionally, the establishment and progression of a career begins in the middle 20s, with individuals progressing in their mid-30s up the career ladder (Super, 1985). As introduced in Chapter 16, Super's theory is one of the most influential theories of adult career development. This theory relies on the concept of career stages based on clusters of distinctive attitudes, motivations, and behaviors that arise in sequence over the span of career development. In an expansion of his original theory, Super proposes that the career stages bear no invariant relationship to chronological age, and that the psychological changes achieved by passing successfully through a given stage are not necessarily permanent (Super, 1990).

Super's theory proposes four stages of adult career development: (1) exploration, (2) establishment, (3) maintenance, and (4) disengagement. The timing of transitions between career stages is a function of individuals' personality and life circumstances, not their chronological age. The decision to return to higher education after a period of employment, to dabble in widely varied career options, or to delay career entry until the completion of child rearing may lengthen the time it takes to pass through the exploration stage, with consequent delays in completion of each of the subsequent stages (Super, 1990).

The **exploration stage** is the period during which people begin to specify and implement a career choice. Different roles are tried and various employment options are explored. The second of Super's adult stages is the **establishment stage**.

This stage occurs when a suitable field is selected and efforts are made to secure a long-term place in the chosen career. Super's third adult stage, known as the **maintenance stage**, is distinguished by the maintenance of prestige, authority, and responsibility. This stage is characterized by constancy: (1) *holding on* (stagnating or plateauing), or (2) *keeping up* (updating or enriching). Continuity, stress, safety, and stability tend to be the standard. Today, there is much job mobility among middle-aged workers, and workers in midlife might be functioning in any of the early stages on the career development ladder if they have had to change careers or workplaces. Women, more than men, may have periods of job disruption, where they have withdrawn from the workforce because of caregiving responsibilities (Braveman & Page, 2012).

Work-role attachment is defined as the "degree to which individuals' commitment to their work-role influences their desire to remain a member of the workforce" (Adams, Prescher, Beehr, & Lepisto, 2002, p. 126). According to this theory, workers who have a high degree of job involvement value their role within their particular job; workers who strongly identify with their company are characterized as committed to their organizations, whereas workers who have a high degree of professional attachment value their role as an active member in a particular profession (Adams et al., 2002).

When individuals have a strong work-role attachment, that valued occupational role may serve as a positive, protective influence on midlife adults facing chronic stressors and occupational imbalance due to these stressors. Some individuals find their work role alienating. These individuals are more vulnerable to experience work-lifestyle conflicts and role strain. Adults in midlife who do not have a strong work-role attachment tend to look toward retirement as a time of release and of being empowered (Drentea, 2002). Work-role attachment variables such as job involvement, organizational commitment, and career commitment served as predictors of intention to retire in a sample of men and women ranging in age from 45 to 77 years.

Super's **deceleration stage** is the adult life stage where people begin to prepare for retirement and begin to engage more in leisure activities than they have since adolescence. Super (1985) noted that by their late 50s, most workers begin to distance themselves emotionally and physically from their workplace. This timeline may be somewhat delayed in contemporary American culture, where the average age of retirement has risen steadily from 57 to 61 (Harter & Agrawal, 2014). In the current group reaching retirement ages, Harter and Agrawal note that "Nearly half (49%) of boomers still working say they don't expect to retire until they are 66 or older, including one in 10 who predict they will never retire" (2014). Gupta and Sabata (2012) remark that in addition to the tangible financial benefits, work results in intangible benefits for older workers, including the ability to be productive contributors to their community and to society. Work also organizes the day into work and nonwork (or personal) time and imposes daily routines. For many people, work provides opportunities to cultivate relationships and extend social connections.

COMMUNITY, SOCIAL, AND CIVIC LIFE

Many of the topics introduced in this chapter reflect the growing participation in community, social, and civic life that often occurs in middle adulthood. Increasing involvement in the community activities of older children, whether they be sports, theater, or musical events, not only gives midlife adults an opportunity to visit with others, but for many also offers opportunities to volunteer, teach, and mentor young people other than their own relatives.

More so than young adults, midlife adults are often widely engaged in an organized social life outside the family, in community, social, and civic areas of life. This pattern of social engagement grows throughout middle adulthood and into the period of retirement and late adulthood. It is only when individuals' health begins to decline that adults will again narrow the scope of their social engagements to a limited set of friends and family.

COMMUNITY LIFE

Engagement in voluntary activities and associations contributes to society in many ways. Voluntary association participation generally peaks in middle age as work and family responsibilities spur social engagement. In 2011, the highest rate of volunteering was among people between the ages of 35 and 44 (31.8 percent reported volunteerism) followed by a 28.1 percent volunteerism rate in those aged 55 to 64 (Burr, Tavares, & Mutchler, 2011). Adults in midlife are active in religious organizations, union halls, political parties, and groups that support valued sectors within their community such as youth sports or adult literacy (Yunqing & Ferraro, 2006). Volunteerism is a way to build social integration. *Social integration* was described by Yunqing and Ferraro (2006) as social embeddedness of individuals, typically due to multiple social roles. Active engagement and social integration "promotes social support, social interactions, and other psychosocial resources that enhance resilience in the face of disease" (p. 499). Volunteering benefits midlife adults in that it has been shown to improve personal well-being over time, with improvements in aspects of well-being and reducing depression (Herrera et al., 2011).

Veterans as a subgroup are more likely than their peers to work with their neighbors to fix community problems (10.5 percent versus 7.8 percent), to exchange favors with their neighbors (63.4 percent versus 56.9 percent), and to have voted in the 2008 election (70.9 percent versus 56.8 percent). In addition, people who have access to the internet in their homes and people who use the Internet wherever they have the opportunity are more likely to get involved in almost every type of activity studied by the Corporation for National and Community Service (2012). The most

TABLE 17-3	Civic Service in the United States	
Type of Service	**Percent Participation**	**Summary**
Volunteering with an Organization		26.5%
Civic, political, professional, or International	5.4%	
Educational or youth service	26.6%	
Hospital or other health	8.3%	
Religious	35.6%	
Social or community service	13.8%	
Sport, hobby, cultural, or arts	3.5%	
Other	6.9%	
Working with Neighbors to Fix Community Problem		7.9%
Attending Public Meeting		9.3%
Fundraise or sell items to raise money	26.6%	
Collect, prepare, distribute, or serve food	23.5%	
Engage in general labor or transportation	20.5%	
Tutor or teach	19.0%	

Adapted from Corporation for National and Community Service (2010). Civic Life in America: key finding on the civic health of the nation. Retrieved from http://www.nationalservice.gov/pdf/factsheet_cha.pdf.

frequently engaged-in types of community service are listed in **Table 17-3**. Although religious participation was addressed earlier in this chapter, it is worthwhile to note that it is also considered to be a form of civic engagement.

RECREATION AND LEISURE

Leisure activities are important in maintaining quality of life in adulthood. Adults engage in leisure activities because they enjoy them, not because they need to be done or because they offer social advantages. Leisure, like play, is intrinsically motivated. Participation in leisure activities enhances health and well-being and can be an important tool in restoring occupational balance for adults in midlife. Leisure can enhance cognitive function, can reduce bone loss, improve balance, and extend the adults' social network. Herrera and colleagues (2011) report that leisure activities provide positive support to individuals' emotional and mental health. Leisure activities such as handcrafts, computing, art, music, and social games help reduce social isolation, provide mental stimulation, or offer physical activity that reduces health risk factors.

Freysinger (1995), based on interviews with 54 middle-aged men, categorized leisure as either self-oriented or other-oriented. She explains, "Through these two types of leisure, adults try to balance social expectations and individual needs, and in doing so adapt to the developmental concerns

and issues of middle adulthood" (Freysinger, 1995, p. 71). Leisure can be seen as *agency,* an outlet from the roles of work and family, and as *affiliation,* a way of sharing oneself with others.

Through affiliation, some middle-aged individuals will find pleasure in sharing activities or spending time with family or friends. For individuals who seek this form of leisure activity, leisure is a way of gaining or maintaining closeness with family and friends. In some instances, affiliation with family serves as a way to interact and share in the development of one's children. This is done by serving as a positive role model for learning for the children. In some ways, leisure appears to parallel changes that occur in the family life cycle. Between the ages of 30 and 44, leisure activities tend to be centered on the home and family. After the age of 45, when children are becoming more independent, the focus of leisure activities may expand to reflect this freedom from responsibility (Hayslip, Patrick, & Panek, 2011).

For some people, health may limit participation in the more action-oriented activities that they preferred as young adults. In middle adulthood, people begin to anticipate retirement and consider leisure activities that they can continue into later adulthood. These may be small changes, such as serving as the coach to an office softball team, rather than playing shortstop. It could also mean exploring a long postponed interest such as art or music. Enrolling in adult education courses, joining dinner clubs, and going on travel

TABLE 17-4 Compiled Research Findings on Midlife and Older Adults and Religion
Religion and associated activities are common among older adults (9 of 10 older adults rate religion important in their lives).
Many people use their faith practices to help them cope with stress throughout adulthood.
Most older people report that religion helps them cope or adapt with losses or difficulties.
African American black women are more religious than African American black men and all Caucasians.
People do not necessarily become more religious as they age.
Religious participation offers a social support network that becomes more important with aging.

tours are all ways that people explore leisure options as they move through middle adulthood.

RELIGION AND SPIRITUALITY

Patterns of religious participation during midlife are highly variable and subject to change in response to life experiences. For example, temporary increases in religious activity are documented as increasing during child rearing, and reductions in religious participation tend to follow divorce or declines in health. In light of the complexity of the data, and the presence of contradictory data from subsets of the population, McCullough and colleagues (2005) suggest that "the search for a single trajectory of religious development over the adult life course may be misguided because several trajectories can hypothetically exist in any population" (p. 78). Although life-stage specific patterns do not hold true, longitudinal studies do offer some interesting insights into faith and religiosity. People who are highly religious relative to their peers tend to stay highly religious relative to their peers, while at the same time, the intensity of individuals' religiousness can increase, decrease, or even increase and then decrease over the adult life course (McCullough, Enders, Brion, and Jain, 2005).

Although religiosity does not have a predictable development progression, it does remain important to the majority of adults in midlife. **Table 17-4** lists some of the findings of diverse studies on the perceived value of participation in organized religion in adulthood.

POLITICAL LIFE AND CITIZENSHIP

During middle adulthood, people often become more civically engaged. **Civic engagement** is defined by an individual's interest with the improvement of community programs, and taking actions to respond to political and public affairs (Kaskie, Imhof, Cavanaugh, & Culp, 2008). The reasons listed by Binstock (2006) for the increases in civic engagement that begin in middle age are that older people are more likely to pay attention to the news, they are more directly impacted (with issues of Social Security and Medicare), and they have greater identification with political parties.

Civic engagement can include very simple things such as taking an interest with issues of public concern, participating in activities such as joining a neighborhood association, assisting a frail elder in the neighborhood, or attending a community concert.

Some middle adults have an increased interest in the political process, and people may become more active in local as well as national politics through working to increase voter registration, contributing to and working in political campaigns, contacting public officials, and serving on local public advisory boards.

SUMMARY

The years from young adulthood into middle adulthood are complex and characterized by changes occurring in many facets of individuals' lives. These transformations occur as part of a normal developmental process that brings change in the physiology, motor, and sensory systems. Transformation also extends into the many roles assumed by individuals during these years. As demonstrated in this chapter, navigation through the various transformations can be difficult for young or middle-aged adults, but these transformations can also be seen as opportunities to discover or rediscover oneself through exercise, sport, and leisure activities. The concept of occupational balance becomes especially important in this developmental period as individuals face complex chronic stressors and role demands. Adults in midlife commonly use participation in leisure and in civic activities as common tools to help them maintain a meaningful and productive lifestyle.

CASE 1

Sandy...Continued

At this time, Sandy continues to be a fall risk and is easily overfatigued. She is using a standard walker for support during ambulation. She uses the walker well, but can only ambulate for about 5 minutes before she needs to rest. An OT and PT are involved to help Sandy return to her homemaker role and to help her develop some short-term plans for kitchen and bathroom modifications to reduce fatigue while performing her daily routine. They are also interested in helping her return to her child care role at a modified level so that she can continue this valued role as well as maintain her own health needs.

Guiding Questions

Some questions to consider:

1. What kinds of home reorganization can you think of that would help Sandy limit the amount she needed to walk as she cared for the girls?
2. How might you enlist the girls to help Sandy so that Sandy gets the exercise she needs?
3. Sandy has been so busy that she no longer engages in cross-stitch and the other craft activities she enjoys. Do you think it would be important for you as a therapist to encourage her participation in leisure activities? Why?

CASE 2

Kaamil

Kaamil is a 54-year-old man hospitalized for an open depressed skull fracture secondary to a motor vehicle accident with subarachnoid hemorrhage. Kaamil is currently dependent in most areas of self-care. He is unable to dress or walk without maximal assist. Prior to his accident, Kaamil had been independent in all ADLs and IADLs. He worked with maintenance at a local long-term care facility (6 a.m. to 3 p.m.) five days a week and he has provided most of the income for the family. He enjoys outdoor activities, including attending his son's sports events, gardening, and playing cards with his friends.

Kaamil is motivated to get better and to return home with his wife Bakula and their children. Bakula had been working about 15 hours a week doing bookkeeping for a local business. Since his hospitalization she has taken on another job and now works 30 hours per week. Kaamil is worried about the stress this places on her as she also maintains the household and cares for the children. They live in an apartment with their 15-year-old daughter and a 12-year-old son. The goals Kaamil set for himself are to be able to "take care of self," "move around better," "use right hand," "get back to work," and "get back to driving." On initial assessment, Kaamil's difficulties with problem solving, memory, and safety awareness exaggerated the limitation caused by his physical impairments.

Continues

Case 2 *Continued*

Kaamil is able to use his left arm independently and is not able to use his right arm to offer even minimal assistance in bilateral tasks. He has decreased awareness of the right body side, and no active movement in the right upper extremity. He was right handed and is no longer able to write.

Bakula has been very attentive and helpful in the hospital, but is concerned about how Kaamil will manage at home. She has been encouraged by the neurologists that much return of function can be expected. An OT and PT need to help Kaamil prepare for his discharge to home. Because the couple needs some income, Bakula would like it if Kaamil could be safely home alone during the day, and help with the supervision of the children before and after school. Kaamil's mother is coming from India to stay with the family during his recuperation. This will provide some much-needed assistance, but will also create more financial problems for the family.

Guiding Questions

Some questions to consider:

1. Search the Internet to discover what kind of cognitive problems Kaamil might be dealing with. How might these complicate your therapy with him?
2. One of Kaamil's goals is to return to driving. Do you think this is a realistic goal? Why?
3. At this time, Kaamil has lost several important life roles. He can no longer interact with any family member in the way that he used to, he can no longer work at his job, and he has become dependent on others for most daily tasks. How do you think you might support him in regaining valued roles as part of your therapy plan?

Speaking of
Adulthood: The High Points and Challenges

ANN CHESTER, PhD HEALTH SCIENCES EDUCATION
PROFESSIONAL, DAUGHTER, WIFE, AND MOTHER

Christmas vacation? That's when you "work so much you look forward to going back to the office to rest up." When people ask me how my Christmas holidays were this year, I could say they are just a reflection of my life: *complex*. For my family of five, the week of Christmas was decorating, shopping, cooking, wrapping, sending off packages of gifts, and more wrapping. But, turns out, getting ready for Christmas was the easy part. I have always looked forward to the time after Christmas to relax and catch up. Not this year. This year, without thinking about what we were doing, my husband, Jim, and I gave our 16-year-old daughter a room makeover. That translates to spending two solid days buying supplies, taping the edges, and painting trim and walls all over again (even though we just did this two years ago). That's the "benefit" of having a daughter interested in interior design who has been inspired by a number of design shows on TV. She chose some unlikely color combination that you'd swear wouldn't work in a room with cedar walls and ceiling. Kelly green on one plaster wall with a window, sky blue on the other plaster wall with the door, and yellow trim on the window. After the painting was finished, we hung her very own photos of flowers (she's so talented) and a couple of neat posters in nice frames. We even put a picture light underneath one big poster over her window to accent it. I must say, the girl has a different eye from mine, but it all worked. When we were done, Jim and I were exhausted, but we love facilitating our kids' achievements: Isn't that what being a foundation for your kids is all about?

Continues

Speaking of   *Continued*

After one evening of relaxation, Jim and I got the bright idea of paying some attention to ourselves in an effort to enjoy life longer as healthy, fit, and energetic adults. This meant turning our unused basement recreation room into a workout room, with recumbent bike, weight machine, step- and free-weight space, and the essential couch to sit on to contemplate working out. Taking the lead from our artistic daughter, we painted the room cornflower blue, maize, and cranberry. What a job that was . . . still is. It isn't completely done. We had only a day to spend on it. It looks a lot better, though, than it did before. Just getting rid of the holes in the wall and scuff marks from boys playing table tennis and throwing footballs—and occasionally one another—up against and through the drywall. A day for ourselves, that's not too extravagant, is it?

Then we went to my parents' home for New Year's. My parents are both 81 years old and in pretty good health. My sister and her two teenagers joined us from Tennessee. What was supposed to be a relaxing few days playing bridge with our elderly parents turned into a marathon home-moving affair. This involved moving our even more elderly (92) unmarried and childless aunt from independent living to assisted living. This couldn't have been done by my parents, because we're talking a major mess and heavy lifting. Ohhh, myyyy!! It couldn't have been done by the children; they just wouldn't have known how to do what we did. We had a day and a half to move many years of accumulated possessions from a three-room apartment to a single room—quarters less than half the size. My sister and I and my husband and all five of our wonderful children pitched in. Yep, my aunt is now in "assisted living" and happy. She cannot find anything, but, then, she couldn't remember where she put stuff before we moved it, so that's not much different. In the move from the old apartment, we found food in the strangest places. We found gallons of gin, bourbon, scotch, white wine from 1958, and tiny little bottles from airlines from who knows what year (people must give the elderly liquor, because I know she didn't buy it. She couldn't carry a cup of coffee, much less a gallon of liquor). We found bills in even stranger places. We found 5,000 pipe cleaners bent up to make cat toys all over the floor. We found inches of dust and kitty litter and coffee spills from one end of the apartment to the other. But we did it! She's moved. She was smiling when we left—till she can't find her favorite coffee cup.

I'm exhausted and mentally overwhelmed with the thought of aging at the moment. My aunt is 43 years older than I am. I came back home from "vacation" and exercised in my newly painted beautiful basement workout space to try to make sure I can continue to live life the way I want to. If I can make it through these years of being responsible for myself (which is hard enough) with a full-time job, plus my children and my parents' generation—I hope to be climbing mountains when I'm 92!

Speaking of
Life in the Middle

TRACY J. HOUGH, COTA/L, OCCUPATIONAL THERAPY
ASSISTANT AND STUDENT IN MOT PROGRAM

In my postcollege adult years, I had many typical experiences, including moving, setting up a household, learning to balance my family demands, and keeping space in my life to play.

Now as I look at the young adult students around me, I can still remember the enthusiasm and idealistic expectations from that time. Enthusiasm, however, is not necessarily limited to youth: In the middle years, enthusiasm merged

Continues

Speaking of *Continued*

with the experiences of life can create an exciting environment; it affords you the opportunity to continue the quest for satisfaction while tempering the limitations of idealistic expectations.

Prior to my work experience and reeducation as a certified occupational therapy assistant, I spent my early years in a corporate environment as a manufacturer representative for three different companies over an 18-year span. The life and work experiences there provided me with many of the life skills necessary to succeed in many work environments, including OT, and now also carry over to my education while enrolled as a master's of occupational therapy (MOT) student. Much of what you learn and develop early on in your professional career transfers to new opportunities, perhaps in a different format, but the skills, qualities, and characteristics remain. These skills—maturity, work ethic, focus, determination—all transition well into career changes.

Each year, I lecture to a graduating occupational therapy assistant (OTA) class on marketing yourself in an OT environment. What I tell these new grads, many of whom have life experiences, is to use those life experiences and these skills, as skills that translate into OT. Interpersonal skills, time management skills, organizational skills, teamwork, persistence, determination—the "soft skills" learned in life's roles—are skills that carry you through and separate the ordinary OT from the exemplary OT.

The enthusiasm gained from entering a new work environment, as a midlife career change, provides the spark so often needed for middle-aged workers. The so-called burnout can be avoided because the environment and the job-specific "hard skills" are new but the unrealistic expectation of the work environment is tempered.

In my experience, when reentering the workforce at 40 with a new career, I was able to bring a renewed zest for work through my new career and combine it with my life knowledge and experience. I entered the workforce armed with much enthusiasm, eager to practice my new craft. On the other hand, I, from many years of work experience, was able to understand that change does not happen immediately. I also was able to understand that not everything that I would do as a COTA would save the world. That concept and belief was for the youth, the inexperienced. That concept, however, is vital to young adults because it is part of their development. Idealism is something that fades with maturity but is also something that should never be forgotten. It is the remembrance of that idealism that continues to fire the soul each day, why you continue to persevere. Maturity does not eradicate idealism entirely, but tempers it, channels it, and makes it a memory of how you would like things to be.

REFERENCES

A.D.A.M. Medical Encyclopedia (2010). Osteoporosis. Retrieved from http://www.ncbi.nlm.nih.gov/pubmedhealth/PMH0001400/

Adams, G. A., Prescher, J., Beehr, T. A., & Lepisto, L. (2002). Applying work-role attachment theory to retirement decision-making. *International Journal of Aging and Human Development, 54,* 125–137.

American Heart Association (2014). *What is cardiovascular disease (heart disease)?* Retrieved from http://www.heart.org/HEARTORG /Caregiver/Resources/WhatisCardiovascularDisease/What-is -Cardiovascular-Disease_UCM_301852_Article.jsp

American Occupational Therapy Association. (2014). *Occupational therapy practice framework: Domain and process* (3rd ed.). Bethesda, MD: AOTA Press.

Binstock, R. H. (2006). Older people and political engagement: From avid voters to "cooled-out marks." *Generations, 30*(4), 24–30.

Blieszner, R., & Roberto, K. (2006). Perspectives in close relationships among baby boomers. In S. Whitbourne & S. Willis (Eds.), *The baby boomers grow up: Contemporary perspectives on midlife* (pp. 261–281). Mahwah, NJ: Lawrence Erlbaum.

Bonder, B., & Bello-Haas, V. (2008). *Functional performance in older adults* (3rd ed.). Philadelphia: F.A. Davis.

Braveman, B., & Page, J. (2011). *Work: Promoting participation & productivity through occupational therapy.* Philadelphia, PA: F. A. Davis.

Brown, C., & Stoeffel, V. (eds.) (2011). *Occupational therapy in mental health: A vision for participation.* Philadelphia, PA: F. A. Davis.

Burr, J. A., Tavares, J., & Mutchler, J. E. (2011). Volunteering and hypertension risk in later life. *Journal Of Aging & Health, 23*(1), 24–51.

Cech, D. J., & Martin, S. (2011). *Functional movement development across the lifespan* (3nd ed.). Philadelphia: W.B. Saunders.

Centers for Disease Control and Prevention (2011). *FastStats: Marriage and Divorce.* Retrieved from http://www.cdc.gov/nchs/fastats/marriage-divorce.htm.

Chang, M., Saczynski, J. S., Snaedal, J., Bjornsson, S., Einarsson, B., Garcia, M., & . . . Jonsson, P. V. (2013). Midlife physical activity preserves lower extremity function in older adults: Age gene/environment susceptibility-Reykjavik study. *Journal of the American Geriatrics Society, 61*(2), 237–242.

Christiansen, C., and Townsend, E. (2010). *Introduction to occupation: The art and science of living* (2nd ed.). New Jersey: Pearson.

Cluett, J. (2011). *What causes arthritis? About.com Guide.* Retrieved from http://orthopedics.about.com/od/arthritis/f/arthritiscauses.htm

Corporation for National and Community Service. (2010). *Civic life in America: Key finding on the civic health of the nation.* Retrieved from http://www.nationalservice.gov/pdf/factsheet_cha.pdf

Deary, I. J., Allerhand, M., & Der, G. (2009). Smarter in middle age, faster in old age: A cross-lagged panel analysis of reaction time and cognitive ability over 13 years in the west of Scotland Twenty-07 Study. *Psychology & Aging, 24*(1), 40–47.

Drentea, P. (2002). Retirement and mental health. *Journal of Aging and Health, 14,* 167–194.

Family Caregiver Alliance. (2012). *Selected caregiver statistics.* Retrieved from http://caregiver.org/selected-caregiver-statistics

Freysinger, V. J. (1995). The dialectics of leisure and development for women and men in midlife: An interpretive study. *Journal of Leisure Research, 27,* 61–84.

Gallup Well-Being. (2012). *In U.S., being middle-aged most linked to having higher BMI.* Retrieved from http://www.gallup.com/poll/156440/middle-aged-linked-having-higher-bmi.aspx

Gupta, J., & Sabata, D. (2012). Older workers: Maintaining a worker role and returning to the workplace. In B. Braveman & J. Page (Eds.), *Work: Promoting participation and productivity through occupational therapy* (Chapter 8; pp. 172–197). Philadelphia, PA: FA Davis.

Hamarat, E., Thompson, D., Steele, D., Matheny, K., & Simons, C. (2002). Age differences in coping resources and satisfaction with life among middle-aged, young-old, and oldest-old adults. *Journal of Genetic Psychology, 163,* 360–367.

Hamarat, E., Thompson, D., Zabrucky, K. M., Steele, D., & Matheny, K. B. (2001). Perceived stress and coping resource availability as predictors of life satisfaction in young, middle-aged, and older adults. *Experimental Aging Research, 27,* 181–196.

Hammond, G., Chapman, G., & Barr, S. (2011). Healthy midlife Canadian women: How bone health is considered in their food choice systems. *Journal of Human Nutrition & Dietetics, 24*(1), 61–67.

Harter, J., & Agrawal, S. (2014). Many baby boomers reluctant to retire: Engaged, financially struggling boomers more likely to work longer. *Gallup Economy.* Retrieved from http://www.gallup.com/poll/166952/baby-boomers-reluctant-retire.aspx

Hayslip, B., Patrick, J., & Panek, P. (2011). *Adult development and aging* (5th ed.). Malabar, FL: Krieger Publishing Company.

Herrera, A. P., Meeks, T. W., Dawes, S. E., Hernandez, D. M., Thompson, W. K., Sommerfeld, D. H., & . . . Jeste, D. V. (2011). Emotional and cognitive health correlates of leisure activities in older Latino and Caucasian women. *Psychology, Health & Medicine, 16*(6), 661–674.

Hindin, Micelle J. (2007). Role theory. In George Ritzer (Ed.), *The Blackwell encyclopedia of sociology* (pp. 3959–3962). Hoboken, NJ: Blackwell Publishing.

Hoyert, D., & Xu, J. (2012). Deaths: Preliminary data for 2011. *National Vital Statistics Reports, 61*(6), 1–52.

HUD.gov. (2009). A clearer national perspective on homelessness. *Research Works, 6.* Retrieved from http://www.huduser.org/portal/periodicals/ResearchWorks/decjan_09/RW_vol6num1t3.html

Hutchison, E. (2011) *Dimensions of human behavior: The changing life course* (4th ed.). Thousand Oaks, CA: Sage Publications.

Jayson, S. (2013). Remarriage rate declining as more opt for cohabitation. *USA Today.* Retrieved from http://www.usatoday.com/story/news/nation/2013/09/12/remarriage-rates-divorce/2783187/

Kaskie, B., Imhof, S., Cavanaugh, J., & Culp, K. (2008). Civic engagement as a retirement role for aging Americans. *Gerontologist, 48*(3), 368–377.

Kidd Iii, A., & Bao, J. (2012). Recent advances in the study of age-related hearing loss: A mini-review. *Gerontology, 58*(6), 490–496.

Kulmala, J., von Bonsdorff, M. B., Stenholm, S., Törmäkangas, T., von Bonsdorff, M. E., Nygård, C., & . . . Rantanen, T. (2013). Perceived stress symptoms in midlife predict disability in old age: A 28-year prospective cohort study. *Journals Of Gerontology Series A: Biological Sciences & Medical Sciences, 68*(8), 984–991.

Lazarus, R. S., & Folkman, S. (1984). *Stress, appraisal, and coping.* New York: Springer.

Levy, L. (2011). Cognitive aging. In N. Katz (Ed.), *Cognition, occupation and participation across the life span* (3rd ed.; Chapter 7, pp. 117–141). Bethesda, MD: AOTA Press.

Lindau, S., Schumm, L., Laumann, E., Levinson, W., O'Muircheartaigh, C., & Waite, L. (2007). A study of sexuality and health among older adults in the United States. *New England Journal of Medicine, 357*(8), 762–774.

McCullough, M., Enders, C., Brion, S., & Jain, A. (2005) The varieties of religious development in adulthood: A longitudinal investigation of religion and rational choice. *Journal of Personality and Social Psychology, 89,* 78–89.

McGoldrick, M. (2005). Becoming a couple. In B. Carter & M. McGoldrick (Eds.), *The expanded family life cycle: Individual, family, and social perspectives* (3rd ed.; pp. 231–248). Boston: Allyn & Bacon.

Meadors, P. (2011). *Adult cancer.* American Association for Marriage and Family Therapy. Retrieved from http://www.aamft.org/imis15/Content/Consumer_Updates/Adult_Cancer.aspx

O'Mara, E. M., McNulty, J. K., & Karney, B. R. (2011). Positively biased appraisals in everyday life: When do they benefit mental health and when do they harm it? *Journal of Personality & Social Psychology, 101*(3), 415–432.

Parker, B. A., Kalasky, M. J., & Proctor, D. N. (2010). Evidence for sex differences in cardiovascular aging and adaptive responses to physical activity. *European Journal Of Applied Physiology, 110*(2), 235–246.

Payne, V., & Isaacs, L. (2012). *Human motor development: A lifespan approach* (8th ed.). New York, NY: McGraw Hill.

Penhollow, T., Young, M., & Denny, G. (2009). Predictors of quality of life, sexual intercourse, and sexual satisfaction among active older adults. *American Journal of Health Education, 40*(1), 14–22.

Pew Internet and American Life Project. (2012). *Family caregivers online.* Retrieved from http://pewinternet.org/Press-Releases /2012/Family-Caregivers-Online.aspx

Pew Research Center (2005). Baby boomers: From the Age of Aquarius to the Age of Responsibility. Washington, DC: Pew Social and Demographic Trends. Retrieved from http://www .pewsocialtrends.org/2005/12/08/baby-boomers-from-the-age -of-aquarius-to-the-age-of-responsibility/?loc=interstitialskip

Pew Research Center (2008). *Inside the middle class: Bad times hit the good life.* Washington, DC: Pew Social and Demographic Trends. Retrieved from http://www.pewsocialtrends.org /files/2010/10/MC-Middle-class-report1.pdf

Pew Research Center. (2010). *The return of the multigenerational family household.* Washington, DC: Pew Social and Demographic Trends. Retrieved from http://www.pewsocialtrends.org /files/2010/10/752-multi-generational-families.pdf

Pfizer Foundation. (2005). *Pfizer facts: The burden of cancer in American adults.* Pfizer U.S. Pharmaceuticals. Retrieved from http:// www.pfizer.com/files/products/The_Burden_of_Cancer_in _American_Adults.pdf

Raz, N., Ghisletta, P., Rodrigue, K. M., Kennedy, K. M., & Lindenberger, U. (2010). Trajectories of brain aging in middle-aged and older adults: Regional and individual differences. *Neuroimage, 51*(2), 501–511.

Reis, J., Loria, C., Launer, L., Sidney, S., Liu, K., R, & . . . Yaffe, K. (2013). Cardiovascular health through young adulthood and cognitive functioning in midlife. *Annals of Neurology, 73*(2), 170–179.

Richmond, L. L., Morrison, A. B., Chein, J. M., & Olson, I. R. (2011). Working memory training and transfer in older adults. *Psychology & Aging, 26*(4), 813–822.

Rosenthal, C. (2013). Kinkeeping. In H. Reis & S. Sprecher (Eds.), *Encyclopedia of human relationships.* Retrieved from http:// knowledge.sagepub.com/view/humanrelationships/n305.xml

Schaie, K. W., & Willis, S. L. (eds.). (2011). *Handbook of the psychology of aging.* San Diego, CA., Elsevier

Schaie & Willis, 2011, p. 181, Handbook of the Psychology of Aging. Academic Press.

Scott, S. B., Whitehead, B. R., Bergeman, C. S., & Pitzer, L. (2013). Combinations of stressors in midlife: Examining role and domain stressors using regression trees and random forests. *Journals of Gerontology Series B: Psychological Sciences & Social Sciences, 68*(3), 464–475.

Settersten, J. A., & Mayer, K. (1997). The measurement of age, age structuring, and the life course. *Annual Review of Sociology, 23*(1), 233.

Super, D. E. (1985). Coming of age in Middletown: Careers in the making. *American Psychologist, 40,* 405–414.

Super, D. E. (1990). A life span, life-space approach to career development. In D. Brown, & L. Brooks (Eds.), *Career choice and development* (2nd ed.). San Francisco: Jossey–Bass.

Taylor, C., Tillin, T., Chaturvedi, N., Dewey, M., Ferri, C. P., Hughes, A., & . . . Stewart, R. (2013). Midlife hypertensive status and cognitive function 20 years later: The Southall and Brent revisited study. *Journal of the American Geriatrics Society, 61*(9), 1489–1498.

Thomas, Y., Gray, M., & McGinty, S. (2011) A systematic review of occupational therapy interventions with homeless people. *Occupational Therapy in Health Care, 25,* 77–90.

U.S. National Library of Medicine. (2012). A.D.A.M. medical encyclopedia: *Cancer.* Retrieved from http://www.ncbi.nlm.nih.gov /pubmedhealth/PMH0002267/

U.S. National Library of Medicine. (2014). Medline Plus: High Blood Pressure. Retrieved from http://www.nlm.nih.gov/medlineplus /ency/article/000468.htm

U.S. National Library of Medicine. (2013). A.D.A.M. medical encyclopedia: Type 2 diabetes. Retrieved from http://www.ncbi .nlm.nih.gov/pubmedhealth/PMH0001356/

WebMD. (2012). *Presbyopia and your eyes.* Retrieved from http:// www.webmd.com/eye-health/eye-health-presbyopia-eyes

WebMD. (2014). *Heart and cardiovascular diseases.* Retrieved from http:// www.webmd.com/heart-disease/guide/diseases-cardiovascular

Williams, G. N., Higgins, M. J., & Lewek, M. D. (2002). Aging skeletal muscle: Physiologic changes and the effects of training. *Physical Therapy, 82,* 62–68.

Willis, S., & Schaie, K. (2005). Cognitive trajectories in midlife and cognitive functioning in old age. In S. Willis & M. Martin (Eds.), *Middle adulthood: A lifespan perspective* (pp. 243–275). Thousand Oaks, CA: Sage Publications.

Willis, S., & Schaie, K. (2006). Cognitive functioning in the baby boomers: Longitudinal and cohort effects. In S. Whitbourne & S. Willis (Eds.), *The baby boomers grow up: Contemporary perspectives on midlife* (pp. 205–234). Mahwah, NJ: Lawrence Erlbaum.

Yunqing, L., & Ferraro, K. F. (2006). Volunteering in middle and later life: Is health a benefit, barrier, or both? *Social Forces, 85*(1), 497–519.

Zauszniewski, J. A., Musil, C. M., Burant, C. J., & Au, T. (2014). Resourcefulness training for grandmothers: Preliminary evidence of effectiveness. *Research in Nursing & Health, 37*(1), 42–52.

CHAPTER 18

Late Adulthood

Anne Cronin, PhD, OTR/L,
Associate Professor, Division of
Occupational Therapy,
West Virginia University,
Morgantown, West Virginia
with contributions from

Pamela Reynolds, PT, EdD,
Associate Professor, Gannon University,
Erie, Pennsylvania

Objectives

Upon completion of this chapter, readers should be able to:

- Describe the two major categories of aging theories, and relate these to the changes in function described in the chapter;

- Recognize normal and usual neurological and cognitive characteristics of aging, including changes in orientation, attention, memory, and learning;

- Identify the functional implications of age-related changes in vision, hearing, balance, taste, smell, and somesthesia;

- Describe the cardiovascular, pulmonary, and changes in aerobic capacity associated with aging, and offer examples of changes in function caused by these alterations;

- Describe the psychosocial characteristics of aging, including education and socioeconomic factors, family roles, social support networks, leisure activities, work, retirement, and community roles;

- Explain the value of the updated four-factor successful aging model to inform decision making and enhance quality of life for older persons with health challenges; and

- Describe aspects of human occupation in the aging population including occupational transitions and occupational balance.

Key Terms

age-associated memory
   impairment (AAMI)

benign senescent forgetfulness (BSF)

bridge employment

continuing care retirement
   community

coronary heart disease

dynamic visual acuity

environmental modifications

fast twitch (type II) muscle fibers

fear of falling (FOF)

gray power

Hayflick limit

keeper of the meaning

kyphosis

leisure competence

medication reconciliation

medication toxicity

naturally occurring retirement
   communities (NORCs)

occupational transition

orthostatic hypotension

presbyastasis

programmed aging theories

random error theories (stochastic)

rule of thirds

senescence

slow twitch (type I) muscles fibers

somesthesia

successful aging model

useful field of view (USOV)

Vaillant, George

CASE 1

Linda

Linda is an 83-year-old woman who was admitted to the rehabilitation hospital following a right cerebral vascular accident (CVA) with left weakness. Upon admission, Linda was identified as a fall risk and requires assistance in both ADLs and IADLs. At this time, Linda walks independently with a "toe drag" on the left, and is walking throughout the facility using a standard walker. Increased muscle tightness was noted throughout the left upper extremity.

On initial assessment, Linda could feed and groom herself, given setup. She needs minimum assistance in transfers and moderate assistance in bathing. She uses her right hand for most tasks, and will use the left arm as a gross assist in some activities. Her left shoulder and elbow are weak, with muscles scoring in the "fair" grade of strength.

Linda has an impaired awareness of light touch on her left body side and she has left visual inattention. Linda is interested in participating more in dressing and cooking tasks, but requires prompting to stay on task and to follow a schedule for task completion.

Goals Linda set for herself in rehabilitation include: "walk like I used to," "use left hand when I need to," and "pain control." Linda's husband Bob has visited her daily while she was hospitalized, but has not wanted her discharged to home because he did not feel competent to care for her. Both Bob and Linda will need a lot of support as she transitions back to living in her home.

Continues on page 428

INTRODUCTION

In the 2010 U.S. Census, 16.2 percent of the population was made up of people aged 62 and over (U.S. Census Bureau, 2011). In recent years, the U.S. population has grown at a faster rate in the older ages than in the younger ages. This increase in the number of older adults offers some challenges and many opportunities. Most of our best and most reliable information about normative aging and development is gained through longitudinal studies. It has only been fairly recently that longitudinal studies were available to describe the period of late adulthood, the period of life spanning between 65 and 80 that many psychologists call "the young old." This "young old" group will be the focus of this chapter. Although any discussion of aging must include a discussion of age-associated disease, poor health does not have to be an inevitable consequence of aging (CDC, 2012a).

Another group, the adults over 80, is the fastest-growing segment of the American population. Their growth rate is twice that of those 65 and over and almost four times that of the total population. The U.S. Census Bureau projects that the population age 85 and over could grow from 5.5 million in 2010 to 19 million by 2050 (AgingStats.gov, 2012). This group of the "old old" has distinctive developmental changes and health-related issues. This is also a group that is less well understood, because as a cohort, they are relatively new. Very few studies guide our understanding of healthy aging in the "old old" segment of the population.

It has been estimated that by the year 2030, Americans over 65 will make up 20 percent of the population (U.S. Census Bureau, 2011). We will again refer to the distinctions between the three types of age listed in Chapter 17: biological age, social age, and psychologic age. A consideration of the three types of age is important because adults over 64 years of age are more varied in their performance skills and their daily functions than any other age group. Some of this variance can be best understood in terms of the three types of age. In this chapter, some common chronic health problems will be discussed, but our focus will be on healthy aging and supports to healthy aging.

THE BIOLOGY OF AGING

Senescence is the term used to describe the process of biological aging. Although a decline in many body processes is documented during aging, there is much heterogeneity in age-related decline. Older adults of the same chronologic age may reflect broad differences in biologic age in demonstrating "physical function that ranges from the physically elite to the physically dependent and disabled" (Shumway-Cook & Woollacott, 2012, p. 223). The study of the process of aging as a biologic process has led to many theories that attempt to explain age-related changes. Increasingly scientific data is replacing theory in the understanding of biologic aging, but theories of the aging process continue to guide research in this area. In this chapter, we will focus on the two most prominent categories of biological theories of senescence.

Programmed aging theories are those theories of aging that state that life expectancy is predetermined with cells programmed to divide a certain number of times. Functional changes in the cells cause aging of the cells. In this conception, aging is based on an internal built-in genetic "clock" and follows a preset biological timetable. This group of theories reports that the DNA cannot duplicate itself indefinitely, and as we age, the replication of cells slows. One of the first

to propose this approach, Dr. Leonard Hayflick, was honored by later scientists who named this slowing of cell replication the "Hayflick limit" (Austad, 2009).

This group of DNA-based programmed aging theories has three subcategories: (1) *programmed longevity*, theorizing that aging is the result of a sequential switching on and off of certain genes, with senescence being defined as the time when age-associated deficits are manifested; (2) *endocrine theory*, proposing that biological clocks act through hormones to control the pace of aging; and (3) *immunological theory*, which proposes that the immune system is programmed to decline over time, which leads to an increased vulnerability to infectious disease and thus aging and death (Jin, 2010).

The random error theories (also called the stochastic theories) consist of several specific theories based on the effects of random events occurring over time and include free radical generation, gradual wear and tear, mutation over time, and differences in metabolic rate. Some of the best known of these are: (1) *wear and tear theory*, an older theory that posits that cells wear out from repeated use, slowly killing themselves and then the body; (2) *somatic mutation theory*, based on the concept that (random) chromosomal changes occur as a result of miscoding, translation errors, chemical reactions, irradiation, and replication of errors, causing changes in the genetic sequence and slowly reducing cell viability; (3) *cross-linking theory*, suggesting that an accumulation of cross-linked proteins damages cells and tissues, slowing down bodily processes and resulting in aging; and (4) *free radicals theory*, which proposes that superoxide and other free radicals cause damage to the macromolecular components of cells, and the accumulated damage causes cells and eventually organs to stop functioning.

Scientific evidence supports and sometimes refutes aspects of all of the theories presented in this chapter. Most of these theories were developed in 1950s or 1960s, and they have served to provide research questions and directions for many years now. This group of theories, although helpful in directing scientific research, results in a fairly pessimistic view of aging, because the premise is that functional loss is inevitable and invariant. This may lead people and therapists to have self-limiting perceptions, and accept suboptimal functioning as they age (Shumway-Cook & Woollacott, 2012).

A different approach to aging, the approach most often used by rehabilitation professionals, uses a model of health and well-being, rather than a model of illness and degeneration. Successful aging models emphasize the importance of adaptation and emotional well-being in successful aging. For most senior citizens, subjective quality of life is more important than the absence of disease and other objective measures relating to physical and mental health. The original successful aging model is shown in **Figure 18-1**.

Rowe and Kahn (1998) suggested that because physical function is decreasing for elders, prevention of disease and keeping physically healthy is an important factor of successful aging. These authors presented an integrative perspective of successful aging that incorporated three main factors: avoidance of disease and disability, maintenance of cognitive capacity, and active

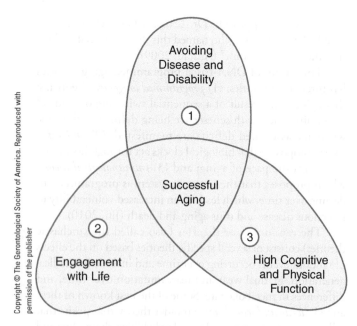

Figure 18-1 Interdependent Relationship among Components of Successful Aging

engagement in life. This model has had broad influence across health care fields and it the reason the focus of many health promotion campaigns aimed at older adults is on physical fitness. More recently, Montross and colleagues (2006) found that 92 percent of the elderly people in their study claimed they are aging successfully, though many of them claimed to have chronic disease and disability. Supporting this, Reichstadt and colleagues (2007) found that older adults place greater emphasis on psychosocial factors as being key to successful aging, with less emphasis on longevity and absence of disease. Chaves and colleagues (2009) add another perspective in their study, which found that successful agers participated in 1.5 times more leisure activities than did normal agers. While physical fitness and continued engagement in physical activities contributes to successful aging, mental health, social support, and leisure participation also have significant impacts on quality of life in late adulthood. Lee, Lan, and Yen (2011) surveyed older adults considering this new information and found that the top three conditions perceived to be related to successful aging were having good health (68%), psychological health, (48%), and involvement in social activities (36%). From this finding Lee and colleagues proposed an updated four factor model of successful aging. Added to the original three factors described by Rowe and Kahn, is a expanded fourth factor, participation in leisure activities.

BODY FUNCTIONS AND STRUCTURES

In late adulthood, age-related declines in function become noticeable. Many changes in both body functions and body structures occur during this period. About 20 years ago, a "**rule of thirds**" was being widely promoted in the study of aging. In this conception, aging is considered a combination of three things: (1) normal age-related changes plus, (2) the effects of disuse, and (3) the effects of age-related diseases. With this *rule of thirds*, an increased focus on fitness emerged that continues to be central to contemporary views on successful aging. This model suggests that at least a third of age-related changes can be prevented through exercise and lifestyle changes. Although this model has recently been considered overly negative as a model of quality of life, the original premises about activity and prevention continue to be sound.

BRAIN AND NERVOUS SYSTEM

The aging brain remains plastic in that individuals can purposely continue to gain or retain complex skills. As mature adults, aging people may have reached their biologic capacity for brain growth, but they can continue to channel their resources or energies into valued skills and activity competence.

A number of changes in the brain and CNS occur as part of the aging process. Chapter 14 provided a link between emerging metacognitive functions and the maturation of the prefrontal cortex. In late adulthood, we see some reversals of this process. Sowell, Thompson, and Toga (2004) note that there is a decrease in gray matter volume between middle adulthood and old age. The most extensive decreases in gray matter density occur over dorsal, frontal, and parietal lobes. The parietal lobe integrates information from the sensory modalities, particularly determining spatial sense and navigation skills. As we look in more detail into age-related changes in motor functions, we will see the functional impact of decreased parietal lobe function.

The brain loses neurons in the aging process, which is a factor in age-related cognitive decline. However, the cognitive changes associated with senescence are not linked to a significant loss of neurons; rather, there is a loss of neuronal elements, including changes in the branching of axons and in the number or size of synaptic contacts (Kumar & Foster, 2007). Aging is associated with a shift in the timing or level of transmission through neural structures. Both PET and fMRI studies show that older adults activated more and different brain areas than younger adults. One explanation for this is that age-related overactivation indicates compensatory processing. Older adults could be using additional brain regions to implement the same cognitive strategies as young adults (Reuter-Lorenz & Park, 2010). The normally aging brain has lower blood flow and gets less efficient at recruiting different areas into operations. Associated with this decreased blood flow, older people often experience declines in verbal fluency, and have to work harder at executive functions. In addition, older people often have more difficulty recovering from physical and emotional stress and returning to pre-stress levels.

In addition to changes in the cerebral cortex, a loss of Purkinje fibers from the cerebellum may influence control of posture and balance, locomotion, movement sequencing, repetitive and alternating movements, and smooth eye movements (Guccione, Wong, & Avers, 2011).

Overall, the volume of cortical white matter and myelin decreases (Sullivan & Pfefferbaum, 2006). As noted earlier in the text, myelin is important for the rapid, accurate, and effective transmission of neural signals. The compromise of the myelinated structures contributes to the slowing of psychomotor speed, increased processing time required for complex information, and transmission of motor responses via the corticospinal and peripheral neural pathways (Guccione, Wong, & Avers, 2011).

COGNITIVE FUNCTIONS

Changes in cognitive function occur in late adulthood. Although there are tremendous individual differences in the type and rate of cognitive change, there are some trends in cognitive performance for healthy individuals in the period. Recall the mental functions described in the ICF. Global mental functions including consciousness functions, orientation functions, intellectual functions, global psychosocial functions, temperament and personality functions, energy and drive functions, and sleep functions tend to remain intact. For example, although increasing disorientation is a stereotype of aging, studies suggest that orientation does not decline as part of the normal aging process. Benton, Eslinger, and Damasio (1981) found that 92 percent of normal elderly adults (65 to 84 years) presented with perfect or near-perfect orientation.

The area in which most change is noted is in the area of specific mental functions. Gradual changes often begin in late middle age. These changes are in attention functions, memory functions, and psychomotor functions.

Attention

Many influences on attention must be considered in the older population. Functional attention requires both good working memory and inhibitory control. Performance differences in working memory between younger and older adults are generally minimal on simple tasks. Imaging studies of item recognition, however, reveal pronounced activation differences, despite age-equivalent recognition accuracy, especially in regions of the prefrontal cortex. Older adults recruit more of the prefrontal cortex as compared with younger adults in working memory tasks. This pattern of prefrontal overactivation suggests that older adults are engaging additional "executive" resources to support short-term memory maintenance (Reuter-Lorenz & Park, 2010).

Inhibitory Control

In older adults, the excitatory or activational aspects of attention are preserved, but brain imaging has documented specific inhibitory impairment. Older adults are more vulnerable than young adults to interference from distrac-

tors during tasks requiring attention (Gazzaley, Cooney, Rissman, & D'Esposito, 2005). Recent studies suggest that sustained attention shows no decline with age, remaining relatively stable through the seventh decade of life (Carrier, Cheyne, Solman, & Smilek, 2010).

Related to inhibitory control is mind wandering. Mind wandering is a shift of attention away from a primary task toward personal thoughts and memories (Jackson & Balota, 2012). Again, although the stereotype suggests that mind wandering will be greater in the older population, this has not been seen in research studies. Older adults have similar or reduced rates of mind wandering when compared to younger adults. What is greater in the older adults is post-error slowing. This means that when they detect that they have made an error, they slow their response speed much more than young adults do. Jackson and Balota (2012) state that post-error slowing can be attributed to the process of redirecting attention to the primary task after an error is detected. These researchers suggest that this pattern shows that older adults have a decreased ability to reengage the task set after the set has been lost, leading to the error.

The case of Linda that opens this chapter presents aging in the face of a disease process. Because Linda has had a CVA, the age-related cognitive changes in attention and inhibitory control may be greatly worsened. Also associated with problems in inhibitory control are problems with emotional regulation. The trauma of the CVA, followed by hospitalization and rehabilitation, would be distressing for anyone. When this distress is compounded by cognitive changes, you may notice that an individual has lability of emotion or flattening of affect. Efforts to help Linda recover and to return to her prior lifestyle and achieve occupational balance must offer support for these cognitive changes as well as support for her physical challenges.

Processing Speed

Neural processing speed deficits with age are associated with diminished white matter volume and white matter integrity. Different cognitive measures (for example, processing speed, episodic memory, working memory, inhibition, and attention) have been associated with different localized regions or networks of white matter decline (Kennedy & Raz, 2009). Research has consistently shown that the abilities to manipulate (that is, processing speed) and retain (that is, memory) acquired information exhibit steady decline over the life span, with a marked decline after about 60 to 70 years of age (Henninger, Madden, & Huettel, 2010).

MEMORY FUNCTIONS

Memory changes associated with normal aging do not reflect a pattern of general decline, rather there are some specific aspects of memory that tend to decline first. These in episodic memory (what did I eat for lunch?), source memory (who told me that?), and what psychologist call flashbulb memory (where were you on Sept. 11, 2001?) (American Psychological Association, 2014). Poor memory in older adults stems, in part, from deficient encoding and decoding. During memory tasks, older adults often show weaker activation in regions of the medial temporal lobe (including the hippocampus and parahippocampus), but increased activation in prefrontal regions compared with younger adults. Interference, such as distractions, blocks encoding and slowed processing can make information retrieval more difficult. When specific encoding instructions are provided in a structured way or through practice, improvements in functional memory can result (Reuter-Lorenz & Park, 2010).

Age-associated memory impairment (AAMI) is a clinical state that involves complaints of memory impairment with everyday activities and is a very modest loss of memory function in healthy people aged 50 and older. In contrast, **benign senescent forgetfulness (BSF)** is a term associated with healthy individuals who experience brief transitory episodes of cognitive decline. It is attributed more to inattentiveness and distractions than to the actual aging process. BSF is not severe enough to interfere with daily activities.

PSYCHOMOTOR FUNCTIONS

There is a pronounced slowing in psychomotor processing speed with aging. Rodríguez-Aranda and Jakobsen (2011) noted that healthy elderly adults are slower to initiate and produce speech. Age-related deficits in motor coordination are noted in other psychomotor patterns as temporal impairments in movements that are reflected in difficulties with bimanual tasks such as synchronized tapping. Similarly, in tests of reaction time and balance (discussed later in this chapter), older adults' performance is far inferior to that of young adults.

SENSORY FUNCTIONS

Sensory changes can have a profound functional impact in late adulthood. The changes vary in type, timing and degree in all people, but these changes are a part of the normal aging process and are experienced to some degree by most people. For example, based on findings from the National Health and Nutrition Examination Survey, one out of six people in late adulthood has impaired vision; one out of four has impaired hearing; one out of four has loss of feeling in the feet; and three out of four have abnormal postural balance testing (Dillon, Gu, Hoffman, & Ko, 2010).

Vision

The prevalence of self-reported vision impairment increases with age. Among people age 65 and older, more than 21 percent report some form of vision impairment (Dillon et al., 2010). *Presbyopia,* the most common visual problem among older adults, was presented in Chapter 17.

Presbyopia does not reflect a disease state; it is simply a normal aspect of aging. Additional age-related changes in visual function emerge in late adulthood.

Because of the physical changes in the eye, older people have greater difficulty with visual acuity when there is low contrast between the stimulus and the background and in the presence of glare. These changes may require some accommodations in everyday life, such as providing more light and making print and other objects larger and more distinct.

Dynamic visual acuity is the ability to accurately identify a moving target. This can be the ability to perceive objects accurately while actively moving the head. Or the person's head can be stable and the object can be moving. An example of this would be the ability to read a street sign while in a moving car. The more quickly the object is moving, the greater the problem for the older person. This can be a significant problem for older people who drive a car.

The **useful field of view (UFOV)** (Ball, Wadley, & Edwards, 2002) is the visual area over which information can be extracted at a brief glance without eye or head movements. With age, people notice the size of the UFOV decreases, reflecting reduced attentional resources, and less ability to ignore distracting information (Cosman, Lees, Lee, Rizzo, & Vecera, 2012). UFOV performance is correlated with a number of important real-world functions, including risk of an automobile crash (Wood, Chaparro, Lacherez, & Hickson, 2012). UFOV and overall driving safety can be assessed and improved by using clinic- and computer-based simulations and cognitive training programs (Bedard, Parkkari, Weaver, Riendeau, & Dahlquist, 2010).

Color vision also changes with aging. This is due in part to the yellowing of the lens of the eye and in part because the cells in the retina that are responsible for normal color vision decline in sensitivity as we age. The result is that colors become less bright and the contrast between different colors becomes less noticeable. Aging also causes a normal loss of peripheral vision, with the size of our visual field decreasing by approximately one to three degrees per decade of life. For people in their 80s, the peripheral visual field loss is about 20 to 30 degrees. This loss of visual field increases the risk for automobile accidents. Several common eye diseases also become more common in late adulthood. These are described in **Table 18-1**. The most common causes of age-related visual disorders in the elderly are presbyopia, cataracts, age-related macular degeneration, primary open-angle glaucoma, and diabetic retinopathy (Loh & Ogle, 2004).

In Linda's case, it is reported that she has left visual inattention. Visual inattention is a condition experienced by people who have had a CVA that results in an inability to attend to part of their visual field. Because of her left visual inattention, Linda appears to be unaware of her left arm. In Linda's case, this inattention is compounded by decreased sensation on the left side. This means that her brain is getting less information about her left limbs, and it will make it harder for her to relearn their use. Educating both Linda and her husband on the impact of inattention on daily function will be important for

TABLE 18-1 Vision and Aging Eye Problems

Age	Eye Problems	Solutions
50s	Presbyopia becomes more advanced. Risks increase for cataracts, glaucoma, and macular degeneration.	Multiple eyewear solutions might be needed for presbyopia. Risk of dry eye increases for women after menopause.
60s	Risks increase for cataracts, glaucoma, and macular degeneration. Ability to see in low lighting decreases.	Use brighter lights for reading. Allow more time to adjust to changing light conditions.
70s and 80s	Most people in this age group already have or will develop cataracts. Color vision declines, and visual fields begin to narrow.	Cataract surgery is the only option for correcting cataracts. Explore eyewear or lens options for increasing contrast vision.

both occupational and physical therapists. Lack of limb awareness can make her a fall risk and a safety risk in the kitchen.

Hearing

Hearing loss is a common problem in older adults. It can be caused by exposure to loud noises, aging, some types of disease, and heredity. Hearing is a complex sense that involves both the ear's ability to detect sounds and the brain's ability to interpret those sounds. Older people may report no difficulty with hearing because the loss is very gradual or because they are very sensitive about admitting the loss. Functional limitations caused by hearing loss include difficulty participating in conversations, hearing the telephone, hearing verbal instructions, and hearing traffic noises.

The factors that determine how much hearing loss will negatively affect a person's quality of life include the degree of the hearing loss, the pattern of hearing loss across different frequencies, whether one or both ears is affected, the ability to recognize speech sounds, a history of exposures to loud noise and environmental or drug-related toxins that are harmful to hearing, and the age of the person. The ability to hear decreases dramatically enough after age 65 to compromise performance on many daily activities. The incidence of hearing loss is 23 percent in people over 65 years of age. Older people may report no difficulty because the loss is very gradual or because they are very sensitive about admitting the loss. Functional limitations may occur in participating in conversations, hearing the telephone, hearing verbal instructions, and hearing traffic noises.

With advances in technology, hearing aids are improving. Four basic styles of hearing aids are currently recommended. The basic styles of hearing aids include behind-the-ear (BTE), in-the-ear (ITE), in-the-canal (ITC), and intra-canal (CIC). The style of hearing aid describes where and how the hearing aid fits the ear. The different levels of technology are described as conventional (analog), improved (analog/programmable instruments), and advanced (fully digital programmable). Even the best hearing aids cannot bring damaged hearing back to normal. New technology, however, has made a significant difference in the way these devices compensate for hearing loss. One of the main problems with traditional hearing aids is that they amplify all sounds, both loud and soft. The result is often confusion and frustration for hearing aid users. The newest, most sophisticated hearing aids can be adjusted to compensate for some of the natural patterns of hearing loss, and provide greater flexibility and clarity in difficult listening environments. Approximately 70 percent of older Americans with hearing loss in at least one ear could potentially benefit from using a hearing aid, but do not use one (Dillon et al., 2010).

Balance

One of the leading health concerns for people over 60 is falling. The ability to maintain balance depends on information that the brain receives from three different sources—the eyes, the muscles and joints, and the vestibular organs in the inner ears. All three of these sources send information in the form of nerve impulses from sensory receptors, special nerve endings, to your brain. Changes in vision that might impact balance have already been introduced. Anatomical studies have shown that the number of nerve cells in the vestibular system grows smaller with age, beginning at about age 55. The loss becomes more severe as age progresses.

Although the sense of balance is built on information from three sensory systems, Shumway-Cook and Woollacott (2012) describe the vestibular system as "an absolute reference system with which the other systems (visual and somatosensory) may be compared and calibrated" (p. 236). With declining vestibular system function, the CNS will have greater difficulty dealing with conflicting information coming from the visual and somatosensory systems. This is believed to contribute to the sense of unsteadiness that some older people report, a condition known as **presbyastasis**. Presbyastasis is an impairment of the vestibular function associated with aging. This condition is common, with a third of those aged 65 to 75 reporting that balance problems adversely affect their quality of life (Dillon et al., 2010). Presbyastasis is often noted clinically as a tendency toward a broad-based gait, staggering, and unsteadiness on turns.

Presbyastasis can lead to individuals developing a **fear of falling (FOF)**. Many older adults are afraid of falling and the fear becomes more common as people age. FOF can cause older people to avoid activities such as walking, shopping, or taking part in social activities. FOF is commonly reported among older adults and is associated with poorer health status and functional decline. Recommended interventions for FOF include education, environmental safety considerations, discussion of risk-taking behaviors, assertiveness training, and improving physical fitness (Legters, 2002).

Taste and Smell

The chemical senses of taste and smell become less acute with age, and saliva flow decreases (Hayslip, Patrick, & Panek, 2011). *Hyposmia* is the decreased sensitivity to smell that occurs in the olfactory system, and *hypogeuia* is the decreased sensitivity to taste that occurs in the gustatory system. Decreased perception of both taste and smell may make food less appealing and lead to poor nutrition. It may also place older people at risk for failing to recognize (1) food that may be spoiled or (2) toxic gases such as cooking or heating fuels, because they cannot detect these warning cues. To compensate for these dampened senses, food choices should highlight appearance and texture for their appeal, and the social aspect of mealtime should be emphasized.

Somesthesia

Somesthesia is the faculty of bodily perception, including information from all of the sensory systems associated with the body. This includes sensitivity to touch, vibration, temperature, kinesthesia, proprioception, and pain. With aging, people experience a decline in each of the senses contributing to somesthesia. The functional result of these changes includes a decline in fine touch and in pressure/vibration sensation. With this loss of information from the body sensory organs, individuals rely more on other sensory systems, such as vision. In addition, there are delays in muscle response to perturbations, resulting in delayed equilibrium and protective responses (Shumway-Cook & Woollacott, 2012).

PHYSICAL FUNCTIONS

The progressive increase in body fat accompanied by a decrease in lean body mass that begins earlier in adulthood continues into late adulthood. In addition, the total body water content of the body also decreases with age, which is exhibited intracellularly as either dehydration of cells or a decrease in cell mass when hydration is adequate. Dehydration is a frequent problem in the elderly, especially during exercise (Guccione, Wong, & Avers, 2011).

Musculoskeletal System

The degeneration of the articular joint surfaces leading to osteoarthritis and progressive demineralization of bones, resulting in osteoporosis, was discussed in Chapter 17.

Osteoporosis is a medical condition in which the bones become brittle and fragile from loss of tissue. Some of the biggest changes to osteoporosis occur in the vertebral bones of the spine and in the long bones of the arms and legs. The vertebrae lose some of their mineral content, making each bone thinner. Because of this the spinal column becomes curved and compressed. The joints become stiffer and less flexible. Osteoporosis is a major public health problem that has both a medical and economic impact around the world. Fractures caused by either osteoporosis can lead to chronic pain, disability, and even death. In the United States each year, broken bones due to low bone mass or osteoporosis cause more than 432,000 hospital admissions, almost 2.5 million medical office visits, and about 180,000 nursing home admissions (National Osteoporosis Foundation, 2012).

Physical inactivity is only one of the many factors contributing to pathogenesis of osteoporosis but it is one of the one that is easiest to change. During normal activity or exercise, three forces act on the bone: gravity, weight bearing, and the pulling forces of the muscle on the bone. Bone loss occurs when physical activity levels and weight bearing are decreased. Physical activity increases remineralization of the bone tissue in people who exercise (Guccione, Wong, & Avers, 2011).

Range of Motion

Decreased range of motion and loss of spinal flexibility contribute to postural changes commonly noted in the elderly. Spinal flexibility shows the greatest decline of any joints with aging, with up to 50 percent less extensor flexibility by age 85. This loss of spinal flexibility results in a pattern of postural changes that includes a displacement of the center of body mass to the rear, and a forward head position, resulting in a posture of **kyphosis**. Kyphosis is illustrated in **Figure 18-2**. When kyphosis is severe, people may develop a secondary lordosis to help regain the overall alignment of the body. *Lordosis,* as described in Chapter 10, is part of the normal alignment of the trunk. When individuals have a kyhpotic posture, the lordosis becomes more extreme as an abnormal forward curvature of the spine in the lumbar region. Kyphosis may result in functional impairments such as impaired balance, slower walking, difficulty with stair climbing, a shorter functional reach, and decreased ADL performance. Other potential range of motion changes include declines in ankle flexibility (by 50 percent in women and 35 percent in men) and reduction in cervical rotation in the neck. In addition, osteoarthritis and pain may limit the functional range of motion of any joint (Shumway-Cook & Woollacott, 2012).

efficient at using oxygen to generate more fuel for continuous, extended muscle contractions over a long time, and **fast twitch (type II) muscle fibers**, which use anaerobic metabolism to create fuel, making them much better at generating short bursts of strength or speed than slow fibers. However, fast twitch fibers fatigue more quickly. Fast twitch fibers generally produce the same amount of force per contraction as slow fibers, but they get their name because they are able to fire more rapidly. The size and number of type I (slow) fibers does not change substantially with age. However, the type II (fast) fibers undergo selective atrophy resulting in sarcopenia (Shumway-Cook & Woollacott, 2012).

The muscle fiber is one part of the motor unit, pictured in **Figure 18-3**. Another significant component is the motor neuron. The number of motor neurons also decreases with age. Some of the "orphaned" muscle fibers do become reinnervated by a remaining motor neuron through collateral sprouting. The result of this is that, with aging, some motor units become larger. In a seemingly contradictory pattern, motor units become larger (hypertrophy) whereas the overall proportion of muscle mass is diminished (sarcopenia).

The potential functional impact of these changes is a decline in muscle strength, changes in postural alignment, impairments in balance, impairments in gait, and a decrease in the maximal speed of movement (Bonder & Bello-Haas, 2009). Strength training has been found to be an effective tool to slow the impact of aging on muscles (Hurley, Hanson, & Sheaff, 2011). Strength training interventions have two major categories: endurance training and strength training. *Endurance training* refers to exercise directed at improving stamina (the duration that a person can maintain strenuous activity) and aerobic capacity, whereas *strength training* refers to exercise directed at improving the maximum force-generating capacity of muscle.

Table 18-2 summarizes the age-related physiologic attributes, their functional significance, and effects of exercise training on that attribute.

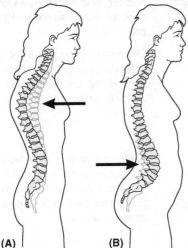

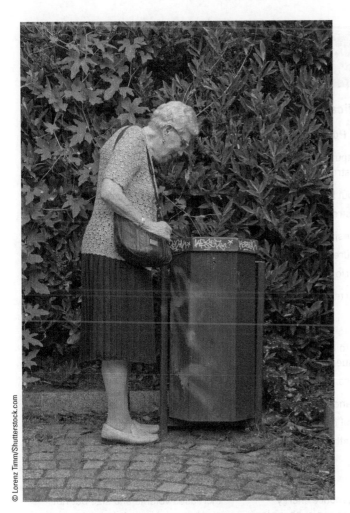

Figure 18-2 Kyphosis is the extreme curvature of the upper back. A. Kyphosis. B. Lordosis.

Musculoskeletal Changes

Skeletal muscle is made up of bundles of individual muscle fibers. These muscle fibers can be broken down into two main types: **slow twitch (type I) muscles fibers**, which are more

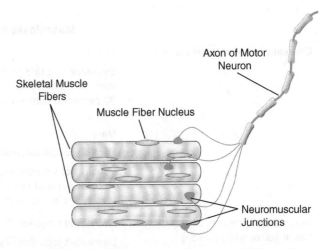

Figure 18-3 The skeletal motor unit consists of both type I and type II fibers, as well as the neuromuscular junction and the motor neuron.

TABLE 18-2   Age-Related Physiologic Attribute, Functional Significance, and Effect of Exercise on Change

Age-Related Change	Functional Significance	Effect of Exercise and Activity
Cardiovascular and Pulmonary System		
Decreases of 2 to 4 bpm resting heart rate.	Decreased cardiac output—if not accompanied by increase in stroke volume.	Does not seem to have any effect.
Decreased cardiac heart muscle and heart volume.	Decreased cardiac output by 25 to 30 percent. Decreased maximum stroke volume.	Delays and diminishes decline.
Decreased elasticity of blood vessels.	Increased peripheral resistance. Increased blood pressure. Increased cardiac afterload.	Slows decline and improves cardiovascular proficiency.
Increased systolic blood pressure (10 to 40 mm Hg); increased diastolic blood pressure (5 to 10 mm Hg).	Increased risk of hypertension, AMI, and CVA.	Upon initial onset, elderly persons show a greater decrease in hypertension with exercise training.
Decreased capillary/muscle fiber ratio.	Decreased blood flow to muscle beds and related connective tissue. Delayed healing process.	Delays and diminishes decline. Ratio can actually increase with exercise training.
Decrease of 40 to 50 percent vital capacity. Increase of 30-50 percent residual capacity.	Increased lung compliance. Decreased elastic recoil of lungs. SOB (shortness of breath).	Exercise training may delay or limit these changes. However, in the absence of disease, these changes are compensated for by the respiratory system's large reserve capacity.
Decreased size and number of mitochondria.	Decreased potential to produce energy required for any muscular and/or physiologic work.	Increased volume and size but not number, which contributes to meeting need for increased metabolic energy production.
Decrease of 20 to 30 percent functional work capacity.	Decline in ability to perform ADLs and IADLs; average 5 to 7 METs average 2.5 METs.	Exercise training slows decrease of work capacity and aids in maintaining functional skills and ability to participate in recreational activities.
Musculoskeletal System		
Decreased bone mineral content.	Women: Decrease of 2 to 3 percent/yr from menopause to 5 years after menopause = 30 percent on bone mineral loss by age 70. Men: Decrease of 0.4 percent/yr beginning at age 50. Usually not a problem until age 80. Increased risk of bone fracture, especially vertebral, hip, and wrist fractures.	Exercise is beneficial in decreasing the amount of bone mineral loss, and resistive exercises have been shown to increase bone mineral density in some instances.
Increased stiffness of connective tissue surrounding joints.	Decreased flexibility 20 to 30 percent. Decreased joint stability and mobility.	Improved flexibility and mobility.

Continues

TABLE 18-2   Age-Related Physiologic Attribute, Functional Significance, and Effect of Exercise on Change   *(continued)*

Age-Related Change	Functional Significance	Effect of Exercise and Activity
Decreased cartilage water content.	Decreased nutritional fluid exchange in cartilage, leading to increased degenerative joint changes. Loss of height in spine and increased risk of vertebral compression fractures and kyphosis.	Provides increased nutritional fluid exchange for cartilage. Spinal extension exercises can decrease risk of vertebral compression fractures and may help to prevent deformity.
Neuromuscular System		
Decrease of 25 to 40 percent muscle mass.	Decreased lower extremity musculature > upper extremity. Decreased distal musculature > proximal. Type II (FT) > Type I (SO). Loss of strength and endurance.	Increased strength and endurance. Muscle hypertrophy occurs with resistive exercise training, but is unlikely with only aerobic exercise training.
Decrease of 10 to 15 percent nerve conduction velocity.	Changes in threshold for action potential. Increased refractory period. Widening of the synaptic cleft Functional denervation.	Exercise training increases the proficiency of motor unit recruitment for movement.
Decreased "psychomotor speed".	Decreased reaction time. Loss of balance and coordination. Increased risk of falls.	Exercise delays decline and preserve functional reaction time for activities such as crossing a street.
Metabolic		
Decrease of 15 percent basal metabolic rate.	Decreased physical activity. Loss in muscle mass accounts for age-associated decrease in BMR. Fewer calories are required to supply energy, but nutritional requirements are unchanged.	Slows decline of BMR. Exercise training with adequate intensity will decrease accumulation of internal fat deposits.
Decreased lean body mass.	Diminished strength leads to compromise of ability to perform ADLs/IADLs; increased chance of falls.	Resistive exercise training can increase muscle mass; strengthening muscle of LE has been shown to decrease fall risks.
Increased fat mass. Decreased glucose tolerance and insulin responsiveness.	Increased risk for chronic disorder (atherosclerosis, hypercholesterolemia, hypertension).	Aerobic exercise with adequate intensity can decrease fat mass. Aerobic exercise improves glucose tolerance.
Decrease of 30 to 50 percent renal function.	Slower clearing of metabolic waste products. Increased risk of drug toxicity and electrolyte imbalance.	Exercise can improve clearing of metabolic waste products.
Decreased total body water.	May present increased risk when exercising.	Adequate hydration is necessary during exercise; however, exercise has not been shown to alter age-related decreases in total body water content.

CARDIOVASCULAR AND PULMONARY SYSTEMS

Cardiovascular health risks, including poor fitness and hypertension, were introduced in Chapter 17 of this text. The changes that began in midlife continue through late adulthood. The heart has a natural pacemaker system (the sinoatrial [SA] node) that controls the heartbeat. The SA node also loses some of its cells. In some people, these changes may result in a slightly slower heart rate. In addition, a slight increase in the size of the heart, especially the left ventricle, is not uncommon. The heart wall thickens, so the amount of blood that the chamber can hold may actually decrease despite the increased overall heart size. These changes cause the ECG of normal, healthy older people to be slightly different than the ECG of healthy younger adults.

Blood Vessel Changes

Atherosclerosis, described in chapter 17, is a disease of the arteries characterized by the deposition of plaques of fatty material on their inner walls. Over time, these plaques can block the arteries and more serious cardiovascular problems. Baroreceptors are pressure-sensitive receptors in the blood vessels which initiate changes in blood volume to help maintain a fairly constant blood pressure when a person changes positions or activities. The baroreceptors become less sensitive with aging. This may explain why many older people have **orthostatic hypotension,** a condition in which the blood pressure falls when they go from lying or sitting to standing. This causes dizziness because less blood flows to the brain. Orthostatic hypotension due to increasing autonomic dysfunction is more frequently seen in the elderly and can contribute to age-related vulnerable states of health (Barantke et al., 2008).

Another blood vessel change is that the main artery from the heart (the aorta) becomes thicker, stiffer, and less flexible. This is probably related to changes in the connective tissue of the blood vessel wall. This makes the blood pressure higher and makes the heart work harder, which may lead to thickening of the heart muscle. The other arteries also thicken and stiffen. **Blood pressure** is the pressure of the blood in the circulatory system. It is measured because it is closely related to the force and rate of the heartbeat and the diameter and elasticity of the arterial walls. About 65 percent of Americans aged 60 or older have high blood pressure (U.S. Department of Health and Human Services, 2012). People in late adulthood may be less able to tolerate increased aerobic demands. Physical exertion is the most common way to increase heart workload. Heart workload may also be increased by some medications, emotional stress, illness, and injuries. **Figure 18-4** shows an older man shoveling snow. Engaging in occasional activities, like

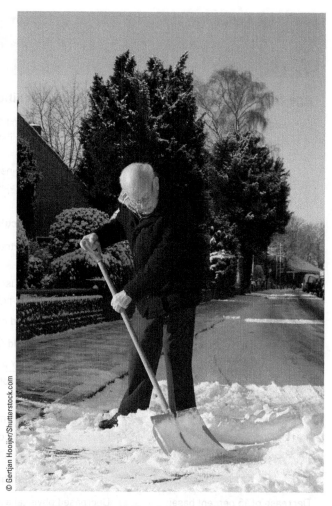

© Gertjan Hooijer/Shutterstock.com

Figure 18-4 In late adulthood, the physical exertion of shoveling snow may challenge the cardiovascular system by exceeding its effective workload.

shoveling snow, that put a heavy workload on the cardiovascular system may result in distress, discomfort, or more serious complications.

INTEGUMENTARY SYSTEM

The skin changes undeniably as it ages. The epidermis thins and flattens, making it more susceptible to shearing stresses, which can lead to blisters and skin tears. The dermis also atrophies and has diminished vascularity. There is a loss of collagen, and the loss of tissue support for the remaining capillaries results in an increased tendency to bruise (senile purpura). Lentigos (flat pigmented age spots) increase with exposure to the sun. The number and size of oil and sweat glands decreases as well, resulting in less sweat production. Older skin does not stay as moist or as well lubricated as younger skin and may need extra attention in personal hygiene activities (Hutchison, 2011). These changes are illustrated in **Figure 18-5**.

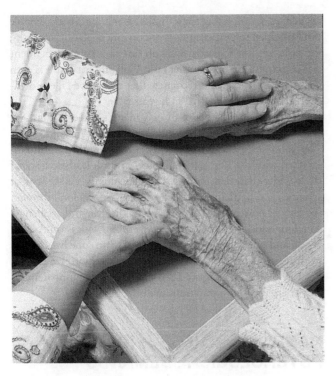

Figure 18-5 Changes in skin are common to aging.

HEALTH RISKS IN LATE ADULTHOOD

Cardiovascular conditions, when left untreated or unresolved, often lead to heart disease. Heart disease is the leading cause of death in the United States. The precursors to heart disease, poor cardiovascular fitness, hypertension, atherosclerosis, and hypercholesterolemia, usually begin in middle adulthood, with problems persisting into late adulthood. Over 30 percent of men and 20 percent of women between 65 and 74 years of age have some form of heart disease (CDC, 2012b).

A prevalent cardiovascular disease associated with age is coronary heart disease. **Coronary heart disease (CHD)** is caused by a narrowing of the coronary arteries, which results in a decreased supply of blood and oxygen to the heart. CHD includes myocardial infarction, commonly referred to as a heart attack, and angina pectoris, or chest pain. "Adults with heart disease are much more likely to have difficulties with activities of daily living, or ADLs, such as bathing, dressing, eating, using the toilet, walking, and getting into and out of bed. Difficulties are most common among older age groups. Among those with coronary heart disease, about one-third of those age 51 to 61 and about half of those age 70 and older have difficulty with one or more ADL" (National Academy on an Aging Society, 2000a).

Table 18-3 presents the top five reported chronic health conditions in people over age 64 in the United States. The top four of these were presented in Chapter 17.

Almost a quarter of people aged 65 or over will have been diagnosed with cancer by 2040, one study finds (Russell, 2012). The most common types of cancer in the elderly are prostate, breast, and lung cancer. In addition to new instances of cancers, many cancer survivors with ongoing health and functional impairments are moving into late adulthood.

Depression (also called a depressive mood disorder and first described in Chapter 14) is an illness that involves the body, mood, and thoughts and that affects the way people eat, sleep, and feel. Depression affects more than 6.5 million of the 35 million Americans aged 65 years or older (National Alliance on Mental Health, 2009). Depression in the elderly is also frequently confused with the effects of multiple illnesses and the medicines used to treat them. The symptoms of depression include loss of interest in activities that were once interesting or enjoyable, including sex; loss of appetite, with weight change; loss of emotional expression (flat affect); a persistently sad, anxious, or empty mood; feelings of hopelessness, pessimism, guilt, worthlessness, or helplessness; and social withdrawal. Also, older people with depression report unusual fatigue, low

TABLE 18-3	Chronic Health Conditions in Late Adulthood	
Common Name	**Medical Name**	**% of Population Reporting the Condition**
High blood pressure	Hypertension	58.4%
High cholesterol	Hypercholesterolemia	48.6%
Diabetes	Type 2 Diabetes	22.6%
Cancer	Carcinoma	19.2%
Depression	Depressive mood disorder	15.7%

Adapted from Gallup-Healthways Well-Being Index (2012). Key Chronic Diseases Decline in the Unites States, Retrieved from http://www.gallup.com/poll/152108/key-chronic-diseases-decline.aspx

energy level, and a feeling of being slowed down. They may have insomnia, and trouble concentrating, remembering, or making decisions. Older people with depression often do not seek help, as they and their families assume that the changes in their everyday functioning are associated with aging rather than a disease process.

Depression doubles elderly people's risk of cardiac diseases and increases their risk of death from illness. At the same time, depression reduces elderly people's ability to rehabilitate. Studies of nursing home patients with physical illnesses have shown that the presence of depression substantially increases the likelihood of death from those illnesses. Depression also has been associated with increased risk of death following a heart attack. The National Institute of Mental Health considers depression in people age 65 and older to be a major public health problem (MedicineNet.com, 2012).

Older adults who practice healthy behaviors, take advantage of clinical preventive services, and continue to engage with family and friends are more likely to remain healthy, live independently, and incur fewer health-related costs. An essential component to keeping older adults healthy is preventing chronic diseases and reducing associated complications. The practice of occupational therapy and physical therapy in services to the well elderly reflects the growing needs of this segment of the population. With education and activity support, many older people can remain healthy well into their 80s.

ACTIVITIES AND PARTICIPATION

With the new longitudinal information on aging, there is much more optimism about this stage of life than ever before. In his book, *Aging Well*, **George Vaillant** (2002) identifies six "adult life tasks" that must be successfully accomplished for people to mature as adults. These are not stages; they are more like challenges. Completing these "tasks" is not automatic. People can be helped to purposefully work on any or all of these tasks; the tasks are not hierarchical, with one task being dependent on the acquisition of an earlier task. Vaillant says that it is even possible for people who recognize that they have failed to address a task to work on that task years later.

Table 18-4 presents all six of Vaillant's tasks. The task we will focus on here is the late-adult "keeper of the meaning" task. The **keeper of the meaning** teaches and shares the traditions of the past with the next generations. This task leads to a social circle wider than that produced by generativity. As we look at activities and participation in late adulthood, we look through the lens of positive adaptation, mental health, and resiliency. The foundation of the *keeper of the meaning* task is on conservation and preservation of the culture in which one lives and its institutions. Through activities and participation, we can see this role played out. **Figure 18-6** shows proud grandparents as they share their faith traditions with their grandson.

HANDLING STRESS AND OTHER PSYCHOLOGICAL DEMANDS

One of Vaillant's (2002) important findings was that in the absence of brain disease, mental health improves with age. Although stressors remain, the overall number and seriousness of these stressors tend to diminish in late adulthood. Defensive coping mechanisms have been a focus of Vaillant's studies for many years. Vaillant (2011) described *mature defenses* as strategies that maximize gratification and allow relatively more conscious awareness of feelings, ideas, and their consequences. Some examples of mature defense strategies in response to psychological demands are altruism, suppression, and humor. As noted earlier in this chapter, although this period of life does not tend to be more stressful than earlier periods, the older adult may have more difficulty recovering from the stressful experience than a younger person would.

TABLE 18-4 Vaillant's The Six Adult Life Tasks

1. The adolescent must evolve an identity that allows one to become separate from parents.

2. Then the young adult should develop intimacy, which permits one to become reciprocally, and not narcissistically, involved with a partner.

3. The middle adult achieves career consolidation. Mastery of this task permits the adult to find a career that is both valuable to society and as valuable to one as she once found play.

4. Later in middle adulthood comes the task of generativity, building a broader social circle through which one manifests care for the next generation.

5. In late adulthood the task is to become a "keeper of the meaning," that allows one to link the past to the future.

6. In very late adulthood, the task is to achieve a sense of peace and unity with respect both to one's own life and to the whole world.

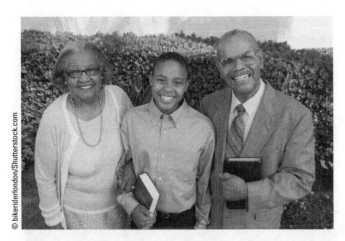

Figure 18-6   Sharing faith practices with a younger generation is a way to serve as a "keeper of the meaning."

SELF-CARE

In the absence of disease or disability, most older adults retain their independence in ADLs well past the age of 80. These ADLs may be done differently, or assistive devices may be used to compensate for age-related changes, but there is no loss of independence. For example, bathroom adaptations are common adaptations to assist older people with washing themselves. Hand-held showerheads and grab bars allow older people to compensate for loss of balance and mobility in bathing. Providing good lighting in the bathroom area also allows for improved care for skin, teeth, hair, and fingernails.

Toileting accommodations may be needed for women in particular who have urinary urgency (urge incontinence), or stress incontinence. Adhesive pads, much like the pads used to control menstrual flow in younger women, are now available for women with occasional incontinence. For people with poor balance, grab bars or side rails can be placed near the toilet for support. For people with osteoarthritis or other orthopedic problems, raising the height of the toilet seat may reduce strain on their joints and may make getting off of the toilet more manageable.

Balance may also be a limiting factor in dressing and undressing. People may choose to be seated for more of the dressing process, and may choose clothing with elastic waists that are easier to manage with one hand. For some people, footwear poses a particular problem. The use of slip-on shoes, although convenient, may also present a fall risk. Long-handled shoehorns and supportive shoes are recommended for people who have balance or orthopedic problems.

Most people in late adulthood take some type of medications or nutritional supplements. To be effective in the management of medications, individuals must have a basic understanding of what the medication offers them, they must be physically able to access the medication, and they must remember to take the medications on the prescribed schedule. Pill organizers with the days of the week and a.m./p.m.

designations are easily available to help with this. If asked, most pharmacies will provide large print labels and containers that are easier to open for storing medications.

Older adults are the largest users of prescription medication (Marek & Antle, 2008). As people age, their bodies are slower to metabolize both medications and food supplements. This change in metabolism causes an extension in the period during which the drug is active in the body. A complication of this is medication (or drug) toxicity. **Medication toxicity** occurs when people accumulate too much of a drug in their bloodstream, leading to adverse effects within the body. Approximately 30 percent of hospital admissions of older adults are drug related, with more than 11 percent attributed to medication nonadherence and 10 to 17 percent related to adverse drug reactions (Marek & Antle, 2008). There are two important components to managing medication toxicity. The first of these is increasing overall hydrations, and the second is *medication reconciliation.*

Medication reconciliation is the process of comparing a patient's medication orders to all of the medications that the patient has been taking. This reconciliation is done to avoid medication errors such as omissions, duplications, dosing errors, or drug interactions. Medication reconciliation is typically managed by a primary care physician or nurse, but is a process in which other health care providers may be involved. Community-based older adults may keep stores of old medications from earlier conditions, and they may confuse these with their current medications, or they may self-prescribe medications using these older medications (Marek & Antle, 2008). In addition to managing medications, older people need to pay attention to remaining hydrated, and may need to put the day's fluids in a special cup, so that they can keep track of how much they drink.

There are complex issues associated with adherence to recommended medication protocols. For adults who do not drive, not filling or refilling prescriptions is a common cause for medication nonadherence. Few pharmacies provide a delivery service, and most will not even allow older people to call in their credit card information ahead of time so that others can pick up the medicines for them. A current focus of national legislation is the rising costs of medications, as inability to afford medication is another common reason for nonadherence to recommended medication regimes. Management of medications may need special attention and planning for older adults, especially for those living alone.

Another important consideration is that rates of substance abuse are higher in people currently in their 50s than in previous generations (Neergaard, 2012). Neergaard (2012) reports that at least 5.6 million to 8 million Americans age 65 and older have a mental health condition or substance abuse disorder. As the number of seniors in the population grows, this number of older people needing mental health support will also grow. Adding in a proportionally higher number of people with substance abuse problems in the baby boom generation, this proportion of older people needing mental health support may nearly triple. Neergaard (2012) reflects that all health workers who see older patients need some training to recognize the signs of geriatric mental health problems and provide at least basic care. All of the adaptations to ADL tasks described earlier are considered environmental modifications. **Environmental modifications** are internal and external physical adaptations to the home, which are supportive in ensuring the health, welfare, and safety of older adults. **Table 18-5** presents several types of common environmental modifications. These types of adaptations are usually minor,

and often are already available in the community if individuals are able to identify and express their needs to pharmacists, therapists, and other health and wellness professionals.

DOMESTIC LIFE

Late adulthood is a period of occupational transition. An **occupational transition** is a "major change in the occupational repertoire of a person in which one or several occupations change,

---

TABLE 18-5 Common Environmental Modifications

Vision Impairments

Use enlarged text, and the use of electronic devices such as e-readers that allow for customization of text presentation.

Use large face clocks, watches, calendars, and playing cards.

Preprogram commonly used phone numbers and have a simple high-contrast display on telephones.

Improve illumination in work areas, using indirect lighting and motion-activated night lights.

Reduce distracting visual glare with antiglare screen protectors on cell phones and other electronic devices, and avoid glossy paints and glossy flooring. Encourage the use of sunglasses when outside.

Hearing

Use sound amplifiers on telephones and other electronic devices.

When background noise is a distracter, acoustical ceiling tile and carpeting can reduce interior noises. Exterior noise can be reduced through insulated doors and windows, and the use of landscaping to absorb traffic sounds.

Smoke alarms that offer flashing as well as sound alerts are also recommended.

Balance

Keep floor surfaces free of obstacles, including throw rugs and extension cords.

Add handrails and grab bars. Good places are at doorways that require stepping up or down to go through, and the shower or bathtub where people must step over a threshold or walk on a potentially wet surface.

When possible, use nonslip tile in all areas of the home and workplace.

Arrange the home so that unstable furniture and towel racks are outside of the major traffic patterns, so they will not be considered sources of support when people feel unsteady.

Use wider, shallower steps (4 inches as opposed to 8 inches), and keep step heights consistent within any set of stairs.

Memory

Be sure that smoke alarms are installed properly and are close to potential problem areas such as the kitchen.

Use clocks whose faces offer the day of the week as well as the time.

Use timers or the schedule prompts available through many cell phone apps to remember times for medications and appointments.

Within individuals' financial ability, replace appliances for those with alarms or auto shut-offs. Many coffee pots, curling irons, and stovetops are available with this option. For those with higher financial resources, there are refrigerators that buzz if the door is left open too long and home alarm systems that alert you when doors and windows are not properly closed.

Pill organizers can be left in a conspicuous area, like the kitchen table, to prompt medication use and to serve as a reminder as to whether the day's medications have already been taken.

disappear, and/or are replaced with others" (Christiansen & Townsend, 2010, p. 212). For example, workplace demands typically decrease or disappear in this developmental period, and ordinary ADL and IADL activities gain importance. These tasks often become harder to perform and may take up an increasing proportion of older adults' day. In late adulthood, many people first need environmental modifications to their homes and workplaces. Some simple modifications, like rearranging storage in cabinets, closets, and storage areas to make the most used items most accessible, can greatly improve people's ability to perform tasks independently. Common home modifications used with well elderly are the installation of handrails and grab bars both inside and outside of the house, the widening of doorways for greater ease of access, and a variety of bathroom and kitchen modifications, additions, or adjustments to allow accessibility or improved ability to manage water faucet controls and work surfaces.

For many people, shopping for necessities involves driving an automobile. Limitations in vision, reaction times, mobility, and coordination will all impact the safety with which older people can drive. Drivers over the age of 65 are often more conservative drivers, but they are also more likely than younger ones to be involved in multivehicle crashes, particularly at intersections. "After the age of 75, the risk of driver fatality increases sharply, because older drivers are more vulnerable to both crash-related injury and death. Three behavioral factors in particular may contribute to these statistics: poor judgment in making left-hand turns; drifting within the traffic lane; and decreased ability to change behavior in response to an unexpected or rapidly changing situation" (SmartMotorist.com, 2012). National initiatives such as *CarFit* (AARP & AAA, 2012), an educational program that offers older adults the opportunity to check how well their personal vehicles "fit" them offer much-needed help in supporting the continued safe participation of older people who need to drive to remain independent in their homes.

Housing

As older adults face changes in employment, family demands, and health, they often begin to think about future housing arrangements. Currently, more than 95 percent of older people in the United States live in community settings, and 77 percent own their own homes. Of the older adults living in the community, 81 percent live in single-family dwellings (Bonder & Bello-Haas, 2009). Although we hear much about nursing and "care" homes, only a very small proportion of the elderly live in these settings.

The American Association of Retired Persons (AARP) reports that, "Nine out of 10 people age 50 and older say they want to remain in their homes and communities for as long as possible" (2011). The freedom from paid employment demands does create an opportunity to reevaluate their current housing situation. This is a time in which some people plan a move to care for their own aging parents, some people choose to move to be closer to their children, and some people choose to follow their dreams and buy a recreational vehicle for travel or to move to a nicer climate.

Although most people don't discuss strengths and weaknesses of their current home until a crisis, the earlier older adults consider their housing options, the more choices and control they will have over future living arrangements. To remain safely in their current home, older people may need to invest in home modifications to address accessibility issues. The first step in reviewing housing is to consider the home in terms of universal design criteria. *Universal design,* in this context, refers to broad-spectrum strategies to build homes and environments that are accessible to both people without disabilities and people with disabilities. Some essential home design features recommended by AARP for making homes accessible to support aging in place are presented in **Table 18-6.**

For older adults who want to or need to move, the differences between the various types of housing options for older adults can be confusing. Many factors influence

TABLE 18-6 Essential Universal Design Features for Housing
At least one no-step entry into the house.
Entryway doors that are 36 inches wide, interior doors with widths of 34 to 36 inches, and passageways measuring 42 inches wide.
Light controls, electrical outlets, and thermostats that are easily reachable for a person in a seated position.
A three-foot wide corridor free of hazards and steps that connects all rooms on the main floor.
Lever-style door handles and faucets that don't require grasping or twisting to operate.
A bedroom, kitchen, entertainment area and a full bathroom (with plenty of space for maneuverability) on the main floor.
Reinforced bathroom walls that allow for the addition of grab bars.
Adapted from American Association of Retired Persons (AARP) (2011). Home Fit Guide. Retrieved from http://www.aarp.org/home-garden/livable-communities/info-07-2011/aarp-home-fit-guide-aging-in-place.html

which choices are appropriate and available to each person, but of these, the most significant factor is financial. The first choice for many people would be to stay in their current home with modifications done to meet their needs. Home modifications can be expensive, and may end up costing more than the value of the home. For people with the financial resources to buy a home, a good option is a continuing care retirement community.

A **continuing care retirement community** is a planned residential arrangement, usually including apartments and townhouses, that include social, recreational, meal, and housekeeping services for a monthly fee. These communities include a range of housing levels from independent housing through nursing care, so that as more skilled care is needed, individuals can remain within their social community for as long as possible. A retirement community is similar, except that it only offers independent housing, and does not include the options of assisted living or nursing care. Both of these options are expensive and available only to people of higher socioeconomic status.

Naturally occurring retirement communities (NORCs) are areas that were not built as retirement communities, but happen to have a high concentration of older residents. They can be in apartment buildings, neighborhoods, or rural areas. These communities may include people of all ages, not just the elderly. In a NORC, social service agencies partner with residents to provide resources that allow older residents to continue to live independently.

For elders who are no longer independent and rely on their children for support, a common solution is an accessory apartment (also called a grandmother suite), which is an apartment in or attached to a single-family home that includes a private sleeping area, bathroom, and living space. Many times these apartments will also have a kitchen and a separate entrance. An old idea with a new name is called ECHO—*elder cottage housing opportunity* (ECHO), a housing strategy which uses small freestanding, prefabricated dwellings placed near a single-family home. In the past, small trailers or motor homes were used. Now there is a whole ECHO industry. ECHO units can be a fairly affordable housing option when compared to an assisted-living center.

Household Tasks

There are many easily available environmental modification to help people remain independent in valued household tasks. For example, one of the most basic household skills needed for people to be independent in their home is preparing meals. Individuals have differing expectations for themselves in this area. Some people may be content to prepare very little; others may feel strongly that meal preparation is central to their role in the family and their sense of well-being. Some of the most common kitchen modifications are appliances that indicate when they are hot, appliances with automatic off switches, and the use of kitchen timers. Large-print cookbooks are available, and people are increasingly using electronic resources, like Internet-based recipes, to meet special dietary needs. The use of an electronic device for recipes also allows users to adapt the screen to optimize the material to meet their visual needs.

Similar environmental modifications could be applied to doing housework. The maintenance of clear walking pathways within the home, the use of lightweight appliances or robotic appliances for cleaning, and maintaining a good level of lighting within the home will all support the performance of housework. Because some types of housework, such as disposing of garbage and laundering clothing, may involve going outside the house, handrails and other outdoor safety features may be needed. Some people will consider maintaining the outdoor area around their home part of routine housekeeping tasks. When a task is potentially strenuous, such as shoveling snow, older people may need to break the task into smaller parts and take frequent breaks to avoid overtaxing their cardiovascular system. One of the most common types of support for older people that family members and members of the community provide is help with the more strenuous of household management tasks.

Basic competence in self-care is a life role often overlooked by younger, more able people, but becomes a significant concern as individuals age. The ability to care for one's self is a source of personal dignity and contributes to a sense of well-being. The ICF lists "caring for others" as a domestic task. Many older people are involved in caregiving, either full- or part-time. They may provide care to a spouse, a sibling, an adult child, or a grandchild.

INTERPERSONAL INTERACTIONS AND RELATIONSHIPS

In Chapter 2, when we introduced the *life course model* as a framework for human development, we focused on the importance of transitions. We have discussed transitions throughout all of the age spans, but many of these transitions, such as going to school, leaving home, and having children, have included an extended period of time. They have included time to consider the transition, experience the transition, and then to adapt and move forward. In late adulthood, some transitions continue in this manner; the decision to retire and the choice of whether to remain in the current home or to relocate are often changes considered over the long term. Both of these are examples of occupational transitions that involve the exit from one pattern of occupational behaviors and the acceptance of new occupations and occupational behaviors.

However, these considered and planned-for occupational transitions are only a small part of the transitions most people experience in late adulthood. For many people, abrupt transitions cluster in late adulthood. Abrupt transitions often are the result of an injury or serious illness, such as Linda's CVA. This incident triggered a move from her home, the enforced dependency of the hospital and rehabilitation setting, and then a transition back to her own home with many new physical and cognitive impairments. Although his health was not impaired, Linda's husband Bob has experienced a related cluster of transitions. Bob's role of spouse became extended into primary caregiver and nursing assistant for Linda in the hospital. He has had to serve as Linda's advocate with the health care team, and in his own home he has had to take on cooking and homemaking roles. As Linda adjusts to her impairments and slowly recovers, Bob and Linda will experience changes in their interpersonal interactions and their relationship.

These abrupt transitions typically begin in an intense, often medically focused, period of treatment and recovery. The lifestyle changes that are required to accommodate the individual's change in health or physical abilities unfold slowly as the person regains (or fails to regain) skills and faces the changes in lifestyle and corresponding occupational transitions that result. Abrupt transitions are often more challenging for such individuals and their family, because they are sudden and may limit the pursuit of desired and planned-for retirement activities.

Relationships with Family

Nearly 80 percent of older adults are parents of living children, most of whom are middle-aged. Most of these people report that their adult children are often in touch, even when they live far from each other. Positive bonds with adult children reduce the negative impact of physical impairments and other losses (such as death of a spouse) on psychological well-being. Historically, aging parents and adult children have provided each other with occasional and modest forms of help. This pattern may be changing for today's elders. Older adults who own their own home are now more likely to be providers than recipients of help. This balance shifts toward the adult children as providers of support, but well into late adulthood, elders give more than they receive, especially in financial support (Grundy, 2005). Many grandparents (and some great-grandparents) provide child care or housing for the younger adults in their families as well.

Although it is clear that multigenerational family relationships benefit all parties, the greatest pattern of support is from an elder parent to younger family members as long as the parent remains healthy. Later in life, older adults increasingly look to their children for emotional support as their social network begins to shrink. While older parents enjoy social and emotional support from their children, it is only with the onset of physical limitations that older parents will usually welcome assistance with housework and errands. Most Americans in late adulthood value their independence and tend not to seek their children's assistance unless there is a pressing need. Older parents may also express annoyance when their adult children are overprotective or insist on helping when they have not been invited (Berk, 2010).

A newer trend is in social networking use by older people to keep up with their extended families. Although young adults may object to their parents and grandparents "lurking," the use of social networking has allowed older people to keep up more easily with the people they love but rarely see. "More than 20 percent of grandparents over 60 have a social media presence and most of those who do are on Facebook" (Warman, 2011). One of the most common reasons older people gave for social networking was that younger people in their families encouraged them.

Relationship with Spouse or Partner

Even with the high U.S. divorce rate, one in every four or five first marriages is expected to last at least 50 years (Berk, 2010). The significance of the marital or partner relationship increases in late adulthood. Trudel and colleagues (2008) note that after retirement, older people organize their life primarily around the house and their partner or spouse. With this change, their social network shrinks down to the people in their immediate vicinity. This is a mixed blessing, as the marital satisfaction in retirees tends to reflect the level of marital satisfaction prior to retirement. If the relationship was positive, the postretirement period may be very rewarding for the committed couple. If a spousal relation is already experiencing certain difficulties, these difficulties are likely to be amplified after retirement (Trudel, Villeneuve, Anderson, & Pilon, 2008).

Older partners tend to feel greater acceptance, and find marital life a source of support against stressors (Smith & Moen, 2004). Rabin and Rahav (1995) note that looser adherence to stereotypes of traditional gender roles (that is, housewife and breadwinner) proves another positive factor fostering greater marital satisfaction after retirement. Additionally, couples who maintain an interest in sex and opt for an active sex life in late adulthood report a higher quality of life and higher scores on assessments of marital satisfaction (Trudel et al., 2008).

As older couples spend more time together, interpersonal characteristics, such as sense of humor, can become factors in relationship satisfaction. Trudel and colleagues (2008) included sense of humor as a positive influence on both health and marital satisfaction. Playful interactions, such as the one pictured in **Figure 18-7**, help build stronger and more positive bonds between older couples.

Widowhood

Death of a spouse is considered one of the most difficult and disruptive transitions within the entire life course (Hutchison, 2011). Widowhood also results in significant occupational transitions for a surviving spouse. Widows may need to take on household roles that are unfamiliar or uncomfortable for them. Spouses who have been a caregiver through a long illness will experience a loss of an important role and may have difficulty organizing their daily routines without caregiving to provide structure. Social support and assistance with the required occupational transitions can greatly relieve the stress faced by the newly bereaved.

Social contact during the earlier stages of bereavement tends to be focused on adult children and provides an important source of emotional support (Isherwood, King, &

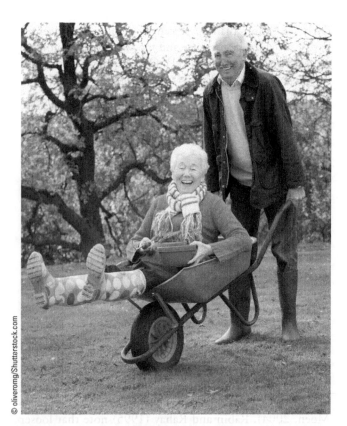

© oliveromg/Shutterstock.com

Figure 18-7 Laughter and a sense of humor help build positive social interactions and strengthen partnerships after retirement.

often provides them with a more stable source of care than that which is available in the community. Musil and colleagues (2013) focused their study on the impact of caregiving on grandmothers. These researchers found that those grandmothers raising grandchildren reported more stress and less reward than age peers, or than grandmothers without child-rearing responsibilities. Other worrisome patterns found were that grandmothers raising grandchildren reported the worst self-rated health and most depression among age peers.

As occupational and physical therapists, these findings are important. We may be providing health care support to either the grandparent or the grandchild. We need to carefully consider any exercise programs or other therapy routines that we may ask the grandparent to implement. In addition, we must be protective of the safety and health of both parties in all of our dealings with them.

Relationships with Friends

Friendship patterns in late adulthood are similar in pattern and structure to those in middle adulthood. The only significant change in later-life friendships is that with retirement, most people find their social network shrinking, and they have less casual contact with new people and casual friends in their everyday routines. This is particularly true for married couples who tend to rely heavily on each other as they move into their retirement years. As noted previously in the discussion on widowhood, after the immediate bereavement period, widows and widowers often rebuild friendships and social networks. People who are divorced or never married tend to maintain the same friendship patterns that they had in middle adulthood.

Luszcz, 2012). Later in the process people gradually let other friends and acquaintances offer support and social contact.

As noted earlier, older partners often become closer and have a smaller social network than they maintained when they were younger. Longitudinal studies report that after the immediate bereavement period, when social contact is focused on children, participation in social activities during widowhood was shown to increase each year after bereavement, reaching a peak at 5.8 years. Isherwood, King, and Luszcz (2012) report that "high levels of social engagement during widowhood may not only assist individuals in successfully overcoming the challenges of spousal bereavement, but may also enhance healthy aging" (p. 227).

MAJOR LIFE AREAS

There are changing patterns of participation in major life areas in late adulthood. Although work remains important for many, it becomes less of a focus for people in this age group. Educational pursuits are more likely to be motivated by personal interests than by career advancement or work-related skills. Many people retire from paid employment in late adulthood and may face economic challenges. Recreation and leisure take a more prominent role in the daily life of older adults.

Grandparenting

"In the United States, there are 4.1 million households of grandparents living with grandchildren and 34% have no parents in the home; of the latter, 38.5% of grandparents have been responsible for grandchildren for 5 or more years and 23% for less than 1 year" (Musil et al., 2011 p. 86). This trend reflects both the economic challenges younger adults face and a strong sense of filial responsibility among family members. In most cases, the care of grandchildren is done by grandmothers, in part reflecting the greater longevity of women, and in part reflecting traditional gender roles. This relationship seems to have no ill effect on grandchildren, and

WORK

The median age at exit for paid work is estimated for the 2005–2010 period as 61.6 years of age for men and 62 years of age for women (Gendell, 2008). These statistics are simplistic though, and do not offer a complete picture of work participation in late adulthood. People retire either because they have the financial resources to manage, or because they are forced to by workplace policies. People in higher socioeconomic levels are more likely to retire early, and people at lower socioeconomic levels tend to retire later.

In addition, there is a widespread trend of workforce re-entry, in which retirees leave long-term full-time employment with retirement benefits, but return to the workplace part-time to maintain their lifestyle. Changes in the economic climate over the past two decades have resulted in a lowering of both Social Security and employer-supported retirement benefits. As it becomes increasingly difficult for many workers to accumulate sufficient resources to maintain their standard of living in retirement, there has also been a significant rise in longevity. This means that workers need to prepare for a retirement that could last 25 years or more (Gendell, 2008).

More people in late adulthood are employed than ever before, and there are many more patterns of work and retirement than ever before. Some people are involved in phased retirement programs in their workplace that allow them to decrease the amount of time worked over a span of 5 to 15 years. Phased retirement allows workers to keep the health and financial benefits of employment with less strenuous work demands.

Many older workers who change jobs, and especially those who change careers, "downshift" into part-time work that involves less stress and responsibility and more flexible work schedules than their previous jobs. Many older job changers end up working for themselves. These new careers pay less per hour and are less likely to offer benefits. They also tend to have less social standing than the former jobs held by older workers who make these transitions. Most older job changers say they enjoy their new jobs more than say they enjoyed in their former positions, despite the fact that the new jobs do not pay as well and are less likely to offer benefits such as health insurance (Johnson, Kawachi, & Lewis, 2009, p. viii).

Bridge employment is any paid work after individuals retire or start receiving a pension (Hayslip, Patrick, & Panek, 2011). *Career bridge employment* refers to working within your established career field under different conditions, a different employer, different work hours, and so on. An example of this would be an occupational therapist who specialized in pediatrics and retires from a large children's hospital. He wants to continue his work, but in a more leisurely and more rewarding manner. The retired occupational therapist gains bridge employment in a home health agency providing home therapy care to infants with chronic illness. This allows him to earn money, have more time to pursue leisure interests, and engage in a career he values. The age of such retirees, their nonwork interests, the desire to make use of their skills, and the desire to earn more money are all significant predictors of employees wanting to engage in career bridge employment instead of full retirement (von Bonsdorff, Shultz, Leskinen, & Tansky, 2009).

Noncareer bridge employment is working outside of your career field after retirement. An example of this might be a retired bank manager who wants to earn some money, but no longer wants to work in an office setting. This person might choose a more physical job, such as working in child care or as a cook.

Re-careering is career change at older ages. In a 2009 study, 27 percent of workers employed full-time at age 51 to 55 changed occupations by age 65 to 69 (Johnson, Kawachi, & Lewis, 2009). Re-careering is more common among workers with lower levels of formal education. These people may no longer be able to physically manage their prior workplace, and may seek education to gain credentials that qualify them to work in a new field. **Figure 18-8** shows an older man who has sought training as a surveyor, a career that allows him to work flexible hours with only mild to moderate physical labor.

Although many older people retire and then return to the workforce in some form of bridge employment or through re-careering, a significant proportion of older workers actually do retire. For those individuals who have been able to amass adequate resources to finance a retirement, the first postretirement year is described as the *liberation stage*. In the liberation stage, retirees enjoy the freedom away from the grind of work. Braveman and Page (2012) comment that this liberation stage "is a short-lived period, and then retirees spend the next 2 to 15 years trying to reorient themselves to their postwork lives" (p. 180).

The United States is a work-oriented society, and for many people, work is central to people's mental and physical health. The loss of the worker role, even in planned retirement, may result in stress and a decreased sense of well-being. Retirement impacts many aspects of people's

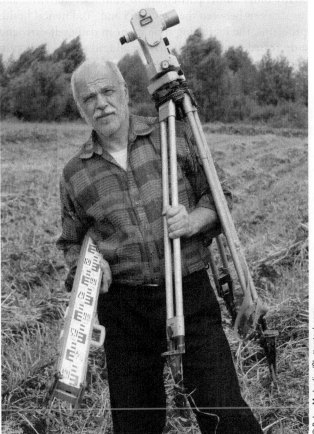

Figure 18-8 Older adults often continue to work in many fields, and some seek additional training to work in skilled, less physically strenuous careers.

lives, and some of the impacts are unanticipated. The loss of identity, social networks, material wealth, and even a structure to the day may leave retired workers disillusioned and ready to consider a return to the workforce or an investment in volunteer, unpaid labor (Braveman & Page, 2012).

COMMUNITY, SOCIAL, AND CIVIC LIFE

Throughout the literature on quality of life in late adulthood, there are a couple of constant themes. Physical fitness and social engagement consistently support a sense of well-being and serve to protect against stress, cardiovascular decline, and depression. Personality remains fairly stable throughout adult life, and those people who were socially engaged in middle adulthood are likely to remain engaged as they move through late adulthood. People without spouses and without children are the least likely to be engaged with the community at any point in the adult life cycle (Berk, 2010).

COMMUNITY LIFE

Many older adults participate in voluntary activities and associations between the ages of 65 and 70. Physical health problems, the increasing time spent in daily self-care, and a decreased comfort with driving all lead to a reduction in participation as volunteers over time. Those people who were highly involved as volunteers earlier in adulthood are likely to remain active as long as they are able. There are opportunities to volunteer in social, community, and service programs, but most require that older people be able to drive. Some organizations, such as senior centers, offer volunteer and social activities under one roof to help address the transportation limitations of older people.

Many older people take on caregiving roles in late adulthood. For some, caregiving is a community service. One well-established program in the United States is the *Senior Corps* program. Senior Corps is a program of the Corporation for National and Community Service, an independent federal agency created to connect older adults with people and organizations that need their skills. One senior corps program, the *Foster Grandparent Program,* connects volunteers with children and young people with exceptional needs. The *Senior Companion Program* brings together volunteers with adults in their communities who have difficulty with the simple tasks of day-to-day living. Volunteer companions help out on a personal level by assisting with shopping and light chores, interacting with doctors, or just making a friendly visit.

In addition to formalized organizational volunteer activities, older people may provide child care to grandchildren or support a spouse with disabilities. Older adults who are friends or neighbors may call each other frequently and share skills and resources. One person might be comfortable driving while another might have been a hairdresser before she retired. As a team, the two may visit friends who are "shut in" and deliver the local news and haircuts. These same two women may need help in their own homes with other things, so this becomes a time of simultaneous caregiving and care receiving.

Recreation and Leisure

Janke, Davey, and Kleiber (2006) report a significant causal relationship between health measures and leisure activity. In spite of this, Americans have a mixed view of leisure. The United States is a work-focused country that is proud of its Protestant work ethic. From early childhood, Americans are socialized to be working and contributing members of society. For this reason, many people find it difficult to retire, and they find it difficult to engage in leisure activities. With folk wisdom relaying that "Idleness is the beginning of all vices," many older people seek activities in which they are needed (like child care) in preference to activities that they enjoy. Berk (2010) comments that, "after a 'honeymoon period' of trying out new options, many new retirees find that interests and skills do not develop suddenly. Instead, meaningful leisure and community service pursuits are usually formed earlier and sustained or expanded during retirement" (p. 496). Braveman and Page (2012) describe a **leisure competence** as the understanding of what leisure activities are meaningful and rewarding for you as an individual. They describe the acquisition of leisure competence as a process. People who are strongly work-focused may enter late adulthood without considering or exploring leisure options. Other people will enter this stage of life with clear interests that are within their capability to pursue. A leisure interest may be something like playing duplicate bridge that you started playing when you went to college, and have played occasionally throughout adulthood. You may enter late adulthood with a goal of becoming a "life master" in bridge. Sometimes people enter late adulthood hoping to indulge in a long deferred goal, such as traveling or learning to play a musical instrument. For this group of people, organized groups like the Road Scholar program build travel and educational programs that allow people to both pursue a passion and socialize with others.

There are many forms of leisure activity, but leisure-time physical activity has received special attention from gerontologists because of its profound health benefits. Janke, Davey, and Kleiber (2006) found that women's involvement in leisure activities declined over time whereas men's involvement stayed relatively stable until their mid-80s. The Centers for Disease Control recommends light to moderate exercise of at least 30 minutes each day for people in late adulthood. The benefits of this exercise include improved cognitive function, improved health, and an improved sense of well-being. However, despite all public health education efforts, only 29 percent of adults aged 65 and older participate in leisure-time physical activity. In fact, approximately 58 percent of people in this age cohort are totally sedentary (Dergance et al., 2003)!

When Dergance and colleagues sought to understand the low physical activity engagement in late adulthood, they found that elders reported that older people are expected to be sedentary, and they were self-conscious and did not want to stand out. Additionally, most community-based exercise programs tend to focus on high-intensity exercise that is either not enjoyable or manageable for many elders. "The findings of this study are that self-consciousness and lack of time, knowledge, companionship, and facilities are prevalent barriers" (2003, p. 865).

There is a profound health need for senior activity programs that are appealing and adaptable to the needs of an aging population. Perhaps as the current generation in middle adulthood move into the retirement years, older people will be more open to the traditional gym facility and workout model, as adults in midlife now have been exposed to this most of their lives. The group currently in late adulthood predated the "fitness craze" of the 70s and 80s and may find today's high-tech exercise gyms very intimidating.

RELIGION AND SPIRITUALITY

As with the other life areas, there is little change in religious beliefs or levels of spirituality between middle and late adulthood. Because many of the present cohort of elderly were religious in their youth, a large percentage of them will retain their religious interest. Many people in late adulthood attach great value to religious beliefs and behaviors, and religious practices are one of the most commonly emphasized in their role as *keepers of meaning*. Of Americans age 65 and older, 72 percent say that religion is very important in their lives, the most value any age group places on religion (Newport, 2006). Over half of U.S. elders attend religious services or other events weekly, nearly two-thirds watch religious TV programs, and about one-fourth pray at least three times a day (Princeton Research Center for the Study of American Religion, 1999). Older adults indicate that religion is important to them and helps them cope with or adapt to losses or difficulties.

Religious involvement is also associated with an improved perception of physical and psychological well-being. In addition, both organized and informal religious participation predicted longer survival, after family background, health, social, and psychological factors known to affect mortality were controlled (Helm & Hays, 2000; Strawbridge, Shema, Cohen, & Kaplan, 2001).

POLITICAL LIFE AND CITIZENSHIP

Since the 1980s, the American Association of Retired Persons (AARP) has been a lead organization in promoting the political power of older Americans. People in late adulthood control 30 percent of the nation's wealth and are the biggest contributors to congressional and presidential campaigns. Voting is valued in both middle and late adulthood, and 72 percent of older

adults in the United States vote (AARP, 2012). Many organizations, including the AARP, have developed powerful political influence through their political action committees. These groups hire lobbyists to represent the issues and concerns of their members. Because of these powerful political lobbies, the term gray power was coined in the 1980s to describe the organized influence elderly people as a group exert, especially for social or political purposes or ends.

Although younger people may list the Internet as their primary source of political information, and older people rely more on television, in 2012, there was only a seven-percentage-point spread separating 18- to 24-year-olds and 55- to 64-year-olds in Internet use for political information. In another age-related trend, older adults tend to rely more on the issues important to them to guide their vote than to ally strongly with any political party (AARP, 2012).

The biggest hindrance to political participation for elders is the problem of transportation and their own health. The ongoing issue of transportation brought up several times in this chapter impacts the life of the elderly in myriad ways. In recent years, many states within the United States have allowed "early voting." Although there is still a single designated election day in a designated period, registered voters can opt to cast their votes early, usually about two to four weeks before the official Election Day. This has been a great advantage for the elderly, as it allows them more time and flexibility to arrange transportation. As illustrated in **Figure 18-9**, older volunteers are

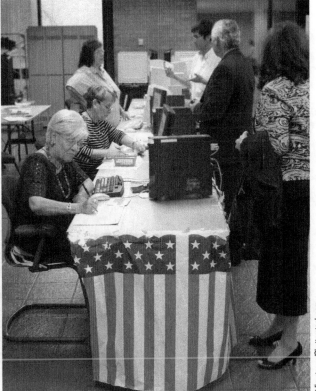

Figure 18-9 Civic responsibility leads older adults to volunteer more in the political process and to vote more regularly than young citizens.

often involved in manning polling places, as well as voting and campaigning for causes of interest to them.

Although much of this discussion has centered on the AARP, many of the groups to which older adults belong also participate in politics. The high religious participation of elders is an example of participation in a group that then influences (and organizes) the political actions of elders. Because they are such a large, well-funded, and active part of American civic life, people in late adulthood have a profound impact on American politics.

SUMMARY

In the span between 65 and 85 years of age, older people tend to think of their health in relatively positive terms. In spite of this, many older adults report that they have at least one physical impairment (visual, hearing, or orthopedic problems or cataracts) or chronic health problem (heart disease, hypertension, emphysema, chronic bronchitis, diabetes, or arthritis). From late adulthood on, chronic diseases predominate, and they increasingly predominate as individuals' age increases. Most older adults accept these conditions gracefully as problems to be dealt with, but not a focus of their lives.

Even with chronic conditions or functional limitations, most older adults see themselves as healthy and satisfied with their lives. Older adults have a profound impact on society. They are central to the support of younger generations, pass down values and traditions, are actively engaged in both paid and volunteer work, and are the age cohort most engaged in civic participation (Hayslip, Patrick, & Panek, 2011).

It is likely that in the future we will see older people active in the community and remaining in paid employment for longer. It is also likely that more people will be living alone and will need support in home modifications and more community-based social and recreational activities. Churches, libraries, and local parks departments will all thrive if they build programs to serve this vibrant older cohort of society.

Recent data suggest that, beyond a certain age, living longer involves a decline in function, an increase in chronic health conditions, and an increasing incidence in disability. So, as health care professionals, we need to focus on what we can do to push back chronic illness and disability so that people will live their lives as independently as possible.

CASE 1

Linda... Continued

Linda lives with her husband Bob in a one-story home that has two steps (with no handrail) to enter the house. At home she now has a walker, a lift chair, a shower chair, and grab bars in the bathroom. Linda is unable to dress herself, requiring Bob to assist with both upper-body and lower-body dressing. Linda has home health therapy support and is highly motivated to improve. Because her ADL activities and her therapy activities take most of her day, both she and Bob have had little ability to socialize or maintain their relationships in the community.

Guiding Questions

Some questions to consider:

1. It is common that older people with illness or disability become more isolated from their community. Look in your own community for senior centers or senior support services. Can you find some leisure or recreation activities that Bob and Linda might participate in during Linda's recovery?
2. Look at the discussion of home modification that can help support healthy aging. Some of these could be beneficial to Linda and Bob. List some that you think would be good ideas, and why you chose them.

CASE 2

Charles

Charles has chronic obstructive pulmonary disease (COPD) and is an 80-year-old widower living in the first floor of a two-family house that he owns. Chantelle, his daughter, lives on the second floor with her daughter and two young children, his great grandchildren. Charles had a recent hospitalization due to an upper-respiratory infection and now, during even light activity, his oxygen saturation drops below 90 percent. Charles is very anxious and is afraid of getting out of breath with any activity. He has a very rigid routine and does not like to deviate from it. He says that he does not want to go into a nursing home or assisted living facility. Charles is proud that Chantelle and her family have benefitted from his rental apartment and feels that letting them use it at cost contributes to the well-being of all of them.

Charles receives intermittent oxygen therapy during the day and wears an oxygen mask at night, both of which he can manage on his own. He can transfer independently in and out of bed, and he spends his day in one chair in the living room. He has difficulty with any sustained activity. For example, he is able to take showers, but is so exhausted afterward that he has to rest for an hour.

Chantelle helps with the groceries, laundry, and light homemaking tasks. Charles spends his day watching TV and reading newspapers. Occasionally friends from his church stop by. He says that his greatest love is for his "grands". He used to go up and visit them often, but now does not because the stairs are too difficult for him to manage.

His goals are to be able to shower, shave, and dress without getting fatigued. In addition, he would like to regain the ability to go up the 12 stairs needed to visit his daughter, his granddaughter and the great grandchildren. This is especially important to him because his granddaughter's fifth birthday is in a month, and she has asked him to come to her party.

Charles has resigned himself to needing oxygen for the rest of his life, and says that he is comfortable enough at home. He won't go out in public because he feels people are staring at him, and because of the oxygen tank, he needs help getting around. Charles used to be active in his church community and enjoyed playing banjo and jamming with local folk musicians. He has discouraged church members from visiting because he to not want to be a focus of their pity. He is now alone much of the time. He feels that he still has things to contribute, and he wants to do more for his family, but mostly he just feels lonely and depressed.

Guiding Questions

Some questions to consider:

1. Charles will need to learn to pace his days so that periods of activity are alternated with periods of rest. If he conserves his energy in this way, he may be able to work on building up his physical activity over time. What modifications to his routine can you think of that would help him complete his ADLs with less fatigue?
2. Charles is at risk for developing depression. What can you think of that might help support Charles emotionally?

Speaking of
The Simple Things

BARBARA HAASE, MHS, OTH, BCN OCCUPATIONAL THERAPIST
RICHARD HAASE, MA REHABILITATION COUNSELOR

She was dying. She, her husband of 39 years, and her family all knew it, yet they at times denied it. She had been well taken care of at the hospital, by many of the same nurses she had trained there. Now she was home, for her final days, to die.

Her caregivers through hospice were good at their jobs. They came every day to give her a bed bath, to provide supplementary feedings, to adjust the morphine, and to provide support to her and her family. There were good days and bad—those days when she reminisced through pictures of happier times and those when she lived for the next push on her morphine drip. There were quiet times, storytelling, and many tears.

It is the simple things, at times like this that mean so much. What do you do for a person who is dying, especially when it is your mother? My mother lived a full and active life. She raised three kids and was beginning to enjoy grandchildren. She was a registered nurse professionally. Her life was beautiful, and she handled dying with grace and without fear. The greatest gift I gave her during these last days, in addition to just being with her, was arranging for hospice to bring in a shower seat so she had a shower. What a joy this was for her.

As an occupational therapist, I have met and worked with people of all ages, from all walks of life, and at different stages of their lives. The study of aging and cognition were part of my master's specialization. I have gained considerable experience with the clinical aspects of aging. Sometimes, as a therapist, I feel better using a new technology because this may be what the consumer wants, or a sophisticated research protocol, because it reflects my own clinical talents. But, as my mother reminded me, it is not high tech or research that are important. In reality, the simple things, the daily life activities, are the most important.

REFERENCES

AgingStats.gov. (2012). *Population.* Retrieved from http://www.agingstats.gov/Main_Site/Data/2012_Documents/Population.aspx

American Association of Retired Persons (AARP) and American Automobile Association (AAA). (2010). *Carfit: Helping mature drivers find their safest fit.* Retrieved from http://www.car-fit.org/

American Association of Retired Persons (AARP). (2011). *Home fit guide.* Retrieved from http://www.aarp.org/livable-communities/info-2014/aarp-home-fit-guide-aging-in-place.html

American Association of Retired Persons (AARP). (2012). *Politics and society: The power of the 50+ voter.* Retrieved from http://www.aarp.org/politics-society/

American Psychological Association, (2014). *Memory changes in older adults.* Retrieved from http://www.apa.org/research/action/memory-changes.aspx.

Austad, S. (2009). Comparative biology of aging. *Journal of Gerontology and Biological Science Medicine, 64,* 199–201.

Ball, K., Wadley, V., & Edwards. J. (2002). Advances in technology used to assess and retrain older drivers. *Gerontechnology, 1,* 251–261.

Barantke, M., Krauss, T., Ortak, J., Lieb, W., Reppel, M., Burgdorf, C., & . . . Bonnemeier, H. (2008). Effects of gender and aging on differential autonomic responses to orthostatic maneuvers. *Journal of Cardiovascular Electrophysiology, 19*(12), 1296–1303.

Bedard, M., Parkkari, M., Weaver, B., Riendeau, J., & Dahlquist, M. (2010). Assessment of driving performance using a simulator protocol: Validity and reproducibility. *American Journal of Occupational Therapy, 64,* 336–340.

Benton, A., Eslinger, P., & Damasio, A. (1981). Normative observations on neuropsychological test performances in old age. *Journal of Clinical Neuropsychology, 3,* 33–42.

Berk, L. (2010). *Exploring lifespan development* (2nd ed.). Upper Saddle River, NJ: Prentice Hall.

Bonder, B., & Bello-Haas, V. (2009). *Functional performance in older adults* (3rd ed.). Philadelphia: F.A. Davis.

Braveman, B., & Page, J. (2011). *Work: Promoting participation & productivity through occupational therapy.* Philadelphia, PA: F.A. Davis.

Carrier, J., Cheyne, A., Solman, G., & Smilek, D. (2010). Age trends for failures of sustained attention. *Psychology and Aging, 25,* 569–574.

Centers for Disease Control and Prevention. (2012a). *Chronic disease prevention and health promotion—Healthy aging.* Retrieved from http://www.cdc.gov/chronicdisease/resources/publications/AAG/aging.htm

Centers for Disease Control and Prevention. (2012b). *Selected measures of disability and health status among adults 65 years of age and over, by urbanization level and selected characteristics: United States, average annual, 2002–2004 through 2008–2010* (Table 58, p. 1 of 5). Retrieved from http://www.cdc.gov/nchs/data/hus/hus11.pdf#058

Chaves, M. L., Camozzato, A. L., Eizirik, C. L., & Kaye, J. (2009). Predictors of normal and successful aging among urban-dwelling elderly Brazilians. *Journal of Gerontology Series B: Psychological Science & Social Science, 64,* 597–602.

Christiansen, C., & Townsend, E. (2010). *Introduction to occupation: The art and science of living* (2nd ed.). New Jersey: Pearson.

Cosman, J., Lees, M., Lee, J., Rizzo, M., & Vecera, S. (2012). Visual search for features and conjunctions following declines in the useful field of view. *Experimental Aging Research, 38,* 411–421.

Craik, F., & Salthouse, T. (2007). *The handbook of aging and cognition* (3rd ed.). Taylor and Francis, Inc.

Dergance, J. M., Calmbach, W. L., Dhanda, R., Miles, T. P., Hazuda, H. P., & Mouton, C. P. (2003). Barriers to and benefits of leisure time physical activity in the elderly: Differences across cultures. *Journal of the American Geriatrics Society, 51*(6), 863–868.

Dillon, C., Gu, Q., Hoffman, H., & Ko, C. (2010) *Vision, hearing, balance, and sensory impairment in Americans aged 70 years and over: United States, 1999–2006.* NCHS data brief, no 31. Hyattsville, MD: National Center for Health Statistics.

Gallup Well-Being. (2012). Key chronic diseases decline in the United States. Retrieved from http://www.gallup.com/poll/152108/key-chronic-diseases-decline.aspx

Gazzaley, A., Cooney, J., Rissman, J., & D'Esposito, M. (2005). Top-down suppression deficit underlies working memory impairment in normal aging. *Nature Neuroscience, 8,* 1298–1300.

Gendell, M. (2008). Older workers: Increasing their labor force participation and hours of work. *Monthly Labor Review,* 41–54.

Grundy, E. (2005). Reciprocity in relationships: Socioeconomic and health influences on intergenerational exchanges between third age parents and their adult children in Great Britain. *British Journal of Sociology, 56,* 233–255.

Guccione, A., Wong, R., & Avers, D. (2011). *Geriatric physical therapy* (3rd ed.). Philadelphia: Mosby.

Hayflick, L. (1974). Cytogerontology. In *Theoretical aspects of aging,* edited by M Rockstein (pp. 83–103). New York, Academic Press.

Hayslip, B., Patrick, J., & Panek, P. (2011). *Adult development and aging* (5th ed.). Malabar, FL: Krieger Publishing Company.

Helm, H., & Hays, J. (2000). Does private religious activity prolong survival? A six-year follow-up study of 3,851 older adults. *Journals of Gerontology Series A: Biological Sciences & Medical Sciences, 55A,* pp. M400–M405.

Henninger, D. E., Madden, D. J., & Huettel, S. A. (2010). Processing speed and memory mediate age-related differences in decision making. *Psychology and Aging, 25*(2), 262–270.

Hurley, B. F., Hanson, E. D., & Sheaff, A. K. (2011). Strength training as a countermeasure to aging muscle and chronic disease. *Sports Medicine, 41*(4), 289–306.

Hutchison, E. (2011) *Dimensions of human behavior: The changing life course* (4th ed.). Thousand Oaks, CA: Sage Publications.

Isherwood, L., King, D., & Luszcz, M. (2012). A longitudinal analysis of social engagement in late-life widowhood. *International Journal of Aging and Human Development, 74,* 211–229.

Jackson, J. D., & Balota, D. A. (2012). Mind-wandering in younger and older adults: Converging evidence from the sustained attention to response task and reading for comprehension. *Psychology and Aging, 27*(1), 106–119.

Janke, M., Davey, A., & Kleiber, D. (2006). Modeling change in older adults' leisure activities. *Leisure Sciences, 28*(3), 285–303.

Jin, K. (2010). Modern biological theories of aging. *Aging and Disease, 1,* 72–74.

Johnson, R., Kawachi, J., & Lewis, E. (2009). *Older workers on the move: Recareering in later life.* AARP Public Policy Institute. Retrieved from http://www.urban.org/uploadedpdf/1001272_olderworksonthemove.pdf

Kennedy, K. M., & Raz, N. (2009). Aging white matter and cognition: Differential effects of regional variations in diffusion properties on memory, executive functions, and speed. *Neuropsychologia, 47,* 916–927.

Kumar, A., & Foster, T. (2007). *Neurophysiology of old neurons and synapses* (serial online). Ipswich, MA: MEDLINE.

Lee, P., Lan, W., & Yen, T. (2011). Aging successfully: A four-factor model. *Educational Gerontology, 37*(3), 210–227.

Legters, K. (2002). Fear of falling. *Physical Therapy, 82*(3), 264–272.

Loh, K.Y., & Ogle, J. (2004). Age-related visual impairment in the elderly. *Medical Journal of Malaysia, 59,* 562–568.

Marek, K., & Antle, L. (2008). Medication management of the community-dwelling older adult. In R. Hughes (Ed.), *Patient safety and quality: An evidence-based handbook for nurses* (Chapter 18). Rockville (MD): Agency for Healthcare Research and Quality.

MedicineNet.com. (2012). *Depression in the elderly.* Retrieved from http://www.medicinenet.com/depression_in_the_elderly/article.htm

Montross, L. P., Depp, C., Daly, J., Reichstadt, J., Golshan, S., Moore, D., & Jeste, D. V. (2006). Correlates of self-rated successful aging among community-dwelling older adults. *American Journal of Geriatric Psychiatry, 14,* 43–51.

Musil, C. M., Gordon, N. L., Warner, C. B., Zauszniewski, J. A., Standing, T., & Wykle, M. (2011). Grandmothers and caregiving to grandchildren: Continuity, change, and outcomes over 24 months. *Gerontologist, 51*(1), 86–100.

Musil, C. M., Jeanblanc, A. B., Burant, C. J., Zauszniewski, J. A., & Warner, C. B. (2013). Longitudinal analysis of resourcefulness, family strain, and depressive symptoms in grandmother caregivers. *Nursing Outlook, 61*(4), 225–234.

National Academy on an Aging Society. (2000a). Heart disease, a disabling yet preventable condition. Challenges for the 21st century: Chronic and disabling conditions, 3. Retrieved from http://www.agingsociety.org/agingsociety/pdf/heart.pdf

National Alliance on Mental Health. (2009). *Depression in older persons fact sheet.* Retrieved from http://www.nami.org/Template.cfm?Section=By_Illness&template=/ContentManagement/ContentDisplay.cfm&ContentID=7515

National Osteoporosis Foundation. (2012). *OVERVIEW: Clinician's guide to the prevention and treatment of osteoporosis.* Retrieved from http://nof.org/files/nof/public/content/file/344/upload/159.pdf /

Neergaard, L. (2012). Report: Too little mental health care for seniors. *USA Today,* July 11, 2012. Retrieved from http://usatoday30.usatoday.com/news/health/story/2012-07-10/aging-mental-health/56132426/1

Newport, F. (2006). Religion most important to blacks, women, and older Americans: Self-reported importance of religion decreases with education. *Gallup News Service,* November 6, 2006.

Princeton Research Center for the Study of American Religion. (1999). *Religion in America.* Princeton, NJ: Princeton University Press.

Rabin, C., & Rahav, G. (1995). Difference and similarities between younger and older marriages across cultures: A comparison of American and Israeli retired non-distressed marriages. *American Journal of Family Therapy, 23,* 237–249.

Reichstadt, J., Depp, C. A., Palinkas, L. A., Folsom, D. P., & Jeste, D. V. (2007). Building blocks of successful aging: A focus group study of older adults' perceived contributors to successful aging. *American Journal of Geriatrics, 15,* 194–201.

Reuter-Lorenz, P. A., & Park, D. C. (2010). Human neuroscience and the aging mind: A new look at old problems. *Journal of Gerontology: Psychological Sciences, 65B*(4), 405–415.

Rodríguez-Aranda, C., & Jakobsen, M. (2011). Differential contribution of cognitive and psychomotor functions to the age-related slowing of speech production. *Journal of the International Neuropsychological Society, 17*(5), 807–821.

Rowe, J. W., & Kahn, R. L. (1998). *Successful aging.* New York: Dell.

Russell, P. (2012). *Cancer rates among the elderly set to triple.* Boots-WebMD. Retrieved from http://www.webmd.boots.com/cancer/news/20120820/cancer-cases-among-elderly-set-to-triple

Shumway-Cook, A., & Woollacott, M. (2012). *Motor control: Translating research into clinical practice* (4th ed.). Philadelphia PA: Lippincott Williams & Wilkins.

SmartMotorist.com. (2012). *Older drivers, elderly drivers, seniors at the wheel.* Retrieved from http://www.smartmotorist.com/traffic-and-safety-guideline/older-drivers-elderly-driving-seniors-at-the-wheel.html

Smith, D. B., & Moen, P. (2004). Retirement satisfaction for retirees and their spouses: Do gender and the retirement decision-making process matter? *Journal of Family Issues, 25,* 262–285.

Sowell, E., Thompson, P., & Toga, A. (2004). Mapping changes in the human cortex throughout the span of life. *Neuroscientist, 10,* 372–392.

Strawbridge, W., Shema, S., Cohen, R., & Kaplan, G., (2001). Religious attendance increases survival by improving and maintaining good health behaviors, mental health, and social relationships. *Annals of Behavioral Medicine, 23,* 68–75.

Sullivan, E. V., & Pfefferbaum, A. (2006). Diffusion tensor imaging and aging. *Neuroscience and Biobehavioral Reviews, 30,* 749–761.

Trudel, G., Villeneuve, V., Anderson, A., & Pilon, G. (2008). Sexual and marital aspects of old age: An update. *Sexual & Relationship Therapy, 23*(2), 161–169.

U.S. Census Bureau. (2011). Age and sex composition, 2010. *2010 Census Briefs.* Retrieved from https://www.census.gov/population/age/publications/

U.S. Department of Health and Human Services. (2012). *Who is at risk for high blood pressure?* National Heart, Lung, and Blood Institute. Retrieved from http://www.nhlbi.nih.gov/health/health-topics/topics/hbp/atrisk.html

Vaillant, G. (2002). *Aging well: Surprising guideposts to a happier life from the landmark Harvard study of adult development.* New York, NY: Hachette Digital, Inc.

Vaillant, G. (2011). Involuntary coping mechanisms: A psychodynamic perspective. *Dialogues in Clinical Neuroscience, 13,* 366–370.

von Bonsdorff, M., Shultz, K., Leskinen, E., & Tansky, J. (2009). The choice between retirement and bridge employment: A continuity theory and life course perspective. *International Journal of Aging & Human Development, 69,* 79–100.

Warman, M. (2011). "One in seven" grandparents on Facebook. *The Telegraph,* June 22, 2011. Retrieved from http://www.telegraph.co.uk/technology/facebook/8589986/One-in-seven-grandparents-on-Facebook.html

Wood, J., Chaparro, A., Lacherez, P., & Hickson, L. (2012). Useful field of view predicts driving in the presence of distracters. *Optometry and Vision Science, 89,* 373–381.

CHAPTER 19

Family and Disablement in Adulthood

Anne Cronin, PhD, OTR/L,
Associate Professor, Division of
Occupational Therapy,
West Virginia University,
Morgantown, West Virginia
and

Garth Graebe, OTR/L,
Assistant Professor, Division of
Occupational Therapy,
West Virginia University,
Morgantown, West Virginia

Objectives

Upon completion of this chapter, readers should be able to:

- Identify common physically and mentally disabling conditions in early, middle, late, and very late adulthood;

- Identify the risks and issues concerning domestic violence and abuse experienced by adults with disabilities;

- Discuss the importance of considering when the disability happened, whether the disability is visible or invisible, whether the condition is physical or mental, and the gender and cultural milieu of the person;

- Offer examples of ways in which disability impacts participation in major life activities such as education, relationships, and workforce participation;

- Define self-determination and self-advocacy in adult life roles and in their roles in the disability rights movement in the support of disabilities with cognitive and mental disabilities; and

- Explain the unique challenges, including those of housing and paid employment, faced by people with disabilities and by their families.

- Describe the common residential options for adults with disabilities who cannot care for themselves.

433

Key Terms

Alzheimer's disease (AD)

chronic obstructive pulmonary
   disease (COPD)

congestive heart failure

developmental niche

disability fraud

disability rights movement

domestic violence

elder abuse

essential tremor

group home

homebound

hospice

integrated employment

low back pain

neglect

nursing home

ocular cataract

Parkinson's disease (PD)

rheumatoid arthritis (RA)

self-advocacy

self-determination

sheltered workshop

subsyndromal depression

traumatic brain injury

vascular dementia

welfare

INTRODUCTION

Throughout this chapter, we will explore disablement and disability in adulthood introducing the basic issues in the experience of people with both congenital and acquired conditions. Because average people will spend 55 to 65 years as adults, the information will be presented separately for the period of early/middle adulthood and the period of late/very late adulthood. The World Health Organization (WHO) reports that "about 15% of the world's population lives with some form of disability, of whom 2–4% experience significant difficulties in functioning" (WHO/WB, 2011, p. 7). As the proportion of older people within the population increases, so too does the number of people with disabilities. The Centers for Disease Control (2012) reports 7 out of 10 deaths among Americans each year are from chronic diseases. Their findings indicate that in 2005, 133 million Americans—almost 1 out of every 2 adults—had at least one chronic illness. In this chapter, we will look at some of the contextual factors impacting disability in adulthood.

Some pervasive contextual factors, like poverty and health policy, influence adult occupations and the experience of disability. More specialized contextual factors include disability subcultures, science and technological influences, and social support systems. Some individuals do not expect or achieve independence in typical adult occupations due to disability. This group of adults often lives full active lives with adaptations and external supports. In spite of this, there continues to be a division of understanding between disabled and nondisabled individuals that is reflected in the comment, "although they know themselves to be full participants in the human community, with strengths, desires, foibles, and triumphs common to all people, disabled people are typically viewed as existing outside the boundaries of human experience" (Albrecht, Seelman, & Bury, 2001, p. 365). This view of people with disabilities as distinct from the mainstream is believed to contribute to many of the struggles that will be presented in this chapter. Struggles include victimization, employment discrimination, educational segregation, and environmental barriers. "A tragic victim, after all, is not likely to be considered a strong job candidate, a capable learner, a wise consumer, or an equal citizen of the community.... Sufferers, however noble, are not likely to be welcomed as helpful neighbors, reliable friends, desired lovers, or competent parents or spouses" (Albrecht, Seelman, & Bury, 2001, p. 365).

COMMON CAUSES OF DISABILITY IN ADULTHOOD

Throughout this text, examples of disabling conditions have been offered. There are many possible causes of disability; some of the causes are congenital, such as autism, and some are acquired, such as spinal cord injury. Although it is impossible to cover all possible causes of disability in adulthood, we will look at the most common causes in this chapter, giving particular attention to those conditions that have not received attention in earlier chapters. **Table 19-1** offers the top causes of disability across all adults in the United States. All of the causes of disability listed become more common as people age.

ARTHRITIS

Osteoarthritis was described in Chapter 18. The other major form of arthritis is rheumatoid arthritis, sometimes called rheumatism. **Rheumatoid arthritis (RA)** is a chronic and systemic inflammatory disorder that may affect many tissues and organs, in addition to the joints. RA can be a disabling and painful condition, leading to loss of functioning and mobility. RA can occur at any age, but becomes increasingly common from middle adulthood. Most people with

Rank	Condition	Number (in millions) of the 47.5 Million U.S. Adults with a Disability
1	Osteoarthritis and rheumatoid arthritis	8.6
2	Back or spine problems	7.6
3	Cardiovascular disease	3.0
4	Mental or emotional problem	2.2
5	Lung or respiratory condition	2.2
6	Type 1 and type 2 diabetes	2.0
7	Deafness or hearing problem	1.9
8	Stiffness or deformity of limbs	1.6
9	Blindness or vision problem	1.5
10	Cerebrovascular accident (stroke)	1.1

TABLE 19-1 Top 10 Causes of Disability

Adapted from Centers for Disease Control and Prevention (CDC), (2011). 47.5 Million U.S. Adults Report a Disability; Arthritis Remains Most Common Cause. CDC Features. Retrieved from http://www.cdc.gov/Features/dsAdultDisabilityCauses/

RA experience intermittent bouts of intense disease activity called flares. In a flare, fluid builds up in the joints, causing pain in the joints and inflammation that's systemic—meaning it can occur throughout the body. Flares are inflammatory responses of the capsule around the joints (synovium) secondary to swelling of synovial cells, excess synovial fluid, and the development of fibrous tissue in the synovium. Over time, the disease process often leads to the destruction of articular cartilage and ankylosis (fusion) of the joints. Early diagnosis and aggressive treatment to put the disease into remission is the best means of avoiding joint destruction, organ damage, and disability (Arthritis Foundation, 2012).

LOW BACK PAIN

Common age-related changes to the musculoskeletal system results in decreased spinal flexibility and reduced cushioning in the discs between the vertebrae resulting in back or spine problems. Low back pain is a common musculoskeletal symptom that may be either acute or chronic. It may be caused by a variety of diseases and disorders that affect the lumbar spine. Many back conditions, such as strains, are temporary and resolve over time. Chronic back pain persists beyond three months and includes long-term pain with daily activity. If the spine becomes overly strained or compressed, a disc may rupture or herniate, as shown in **Figure 19-1.**

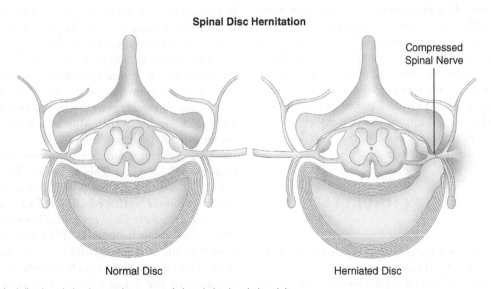

Spinal Disc Hernitation

Compressed Spinal Nerve

Normal Disc   Herniated Disc

Figure 19-1 Spinal disc herniation is a major cause of chronic back pain in adults.

This rupture may compress one of the nerves rooted to the spinal cord causing chronic back pain.

A complication of a ruptured disc is *cauda equina syndrome,* which occurs when disc material is pushed into the spinal canal and compresses the bundle of lumbar and sacral nerve roots. An example of this would be sciatica. *Sciatica* is the term for the condition when a herniated disc presses on the sciatic nerve. This compression causes low back pain combined with pain down one leg. Additional symptoms may include sleep disturbances, morning stiffness, and anxiety. Skeletal irregularities, including scoliosis, kyphosis, and lordosis can produce strain on the vertebrae and supporting muscles, tendons, ligaments, and tissues supported by the spinal column resulting in back pain. Other causes of low back pain include arthritis, osteoporosis, viral infections, and congenital abnormalities in the spine. Scar tissue created when the injured back heals itself does not have the strength or flexibility of normal tissue. Buildup of scar tissue from repeated injuries eventually weakens the back and can lead to more functional limitations.

CARDIOVASCULAR DISEASE

The functional impact of cardiovascular disease is measured through its impact on everyday life. At its mildest, called functional capacity class one, people may be diagnosed with cardiac disease yet have no limitation of physical activity. At this stage ordinary physical activity does not cause undue fatigue, palpitation, dyspnea, or anginal pain. Cardiovascular disease is both chronic, and without treatment, progressive. People with severe cardiac disease, at functional capacity class four, are unable to carry on any physical activity without discomfort. At this level symptoms of heart failure or the anginal syndrome may be present even at rest. If any physical activity is undertaken, discomfort is increased.

There are many types of cardiovascular disease. The most common type of cardiovascular disease, coronary heart disease was described in Chapter 18. Another condition, **congestive heart failure**, is a condition in which the heart works inefficiently and fails to pump enough blood through all the organs within the body. Cardiac rehabilitation programs often focus on persons with coronary artery disease and congestive heart failure. Congestive heart failure is often an end-stage condition experienced by people who have experienced heart disease in the past. This is a progressive condition that results in death.

EMOTIONAL AND BEHAVIORAL CONDITIONS

Although the terms *behavioral health* is increasingly used, adults, as compared to children, are more likely to be labeled as mentally ill. A reason for the increased use of the label behavioral medicine is that the term *mental illness* is stigmatizing and, for this reason, many people do not seek help for mental illness. As with children, the most common behavioral health conditions in adults are anxiety and mood disorders. The anxiety disorders are a spectrum of mental disturbances characterized by anxiety as a central or core symptom. An estimated 28 million people suffer from an anxiety disorder every year. *Panic disorders* and *phobias* are two specific types of anxiety disorders that cause distress both in real time and in worry over recurrence of the trigger event. *Obsessive-compulsive disorder (OCD)* is an anxiety disorder that, in adults, is marked by unwanted, intrusive, persistent thoughts or repetitive behaviors that reflect the patients' anxiety or attempts to control it (Mayo Clinic, 2012).

All of these types of anxiety disorders can be serious problems, and may significantly interfere with valued activities and participation in adult life. Anxiety disorders are believed to contribute to the high rates of alcohol and substance abuse disorders. These substance abuse patterns are described as a form of "self-medication" for individuals with anxiety impairments (NIMH, 2012).

LUNG AND RESPIRATORY CONDITIONS

Chronic respiratory diseases are diseases of the airways and other parts of the lung. Some of the most common are asthma, chronic obstructive pulmonary disease (COPD), lung cancer, cystic fibrosis, sleep apnea and occupational lung diseases. Respiratory diseases affect people of all ages, but like many conditions the impact of the condition often increases in late adulthood. The most common respiratory condition is asthma. There are effective treatments for asthma that can prevent the onset of symptoms and can control symptoms once they occur. **Chronic obstructive pulmonary disease (COPD)** is the occurrence of chronic bronchitis or emphysema, a pair of commonly coexisting diseases of the lungs in which the airways become narrowed. This leads to a limitation of the flow of air to and from the lungs and makes it difficult to breathe. There are two main forms of COPD: chronic bronchitis, which involves a long-term cough with mucus, and, emphysema, which involves destruction of the lungs over time (National Heart, Lung, and Blood Institute, 2012). Most people with COPD have a combination of both conditions.

One of the most common symptoms of COPD is shortness of breath (dyspnea). This condition, like congestive heart failure, reflects an end-stage response to chronic lung problems that cannot be treated using ordinary measures. Over the years, dyspnea tends to get gradually worse and, with this, activity limitations increase. COPD is associated with long-term exposure to noxious particles or gas, most commonly from tobacco smoking, which triggers an inflammatory response in the lungs (Global Initiative for Chronic

Obstructive Lung Disease, 2011). Rehabilitation personnel are often involved in supporting persons with COPD.

THE EXPERIENCE OF ACQUIRED DISABILITY IN EARLY AND MIDDLE ADULTHOOD

Each individual has a unique life story, and disability may become part of the story. So we will begin this section with the story of Stephanie. Stephanie is smart and beautiful. She is 25 years old and is almost finished earning her doctorate in physical therapy. Stephanie lives in Florida, is an avid scuba diver and tennis player, and aspires to work in sports medicine when she finishes her degree. Then Stephanie had a car accident. Now beautiful, smart, young Stephanie has a spinal cord injury (SCI) resulting in paraplegia. Stephanie will be in a wheelchair for the rest of her life. Stephanie, in the start of early adulthood, has lost her self-defined life role. She is still smart and beautiful, but many people see the wheelchair she must use only, and never really see her. She cannot graduate with her class, because of the time she needs for recovery from her injury. Stephanie must come to grips with her many losses, while her peers are moving forward with their lives and living their dreams. Because of the life challenges and social expectations associated with early adulthood, Stephanie's injury is likely to have the most negative impact at this time that it would have at any point in her life.

Now, we will jump 15 years ahead in Stephanie's story. Stephanie has come to accept herself, has finished school, and has developed a niche practice consulting with businesses on accessibility and accessible design. She has many friends, owns her own home, and has learned to pursue scuba and tennis with adaptive devices. Stephanie is, by all accounts, a successful person. She is even inspirational... rising above adversity and all that! But Stephanie still has a disability. Stephanie has now spent 15 years using her arms and shoulders to push her wheelchair, and she is noticing that she gets aches and pains more often now. The prevalence of shoulder pain is significantly greater than normal in the SCI population and increases with time after injury. Because of pain, Stephanie starts to do less overhead reaching, less driving, less wheelchair propulsion, and less housework. She can no longer play tennis. Stephanie is dually disabled, both by her SCI but also by the wear and tear of her everyday life. We could take the story further, and she would continue to have ups and downs. She may marry. She may have children. She may get her life story published! Many things can happen. Some of the things are not as good. Stephanie may get depressed or may develop osteoporosis. Her life story will unfold differently than her college peers. Although she has a disability, factors other than the disability itself will end up defining her quality of life.

Stephanie had a typical developmental experience until the time of her injury. She acquired her disability at a time of peak performance, when her body could recover well, and Stephanie made the most of it. But although Stephanie worked to redefine her self-concept, much of society stopped seeing her as an individual and only saw the wheelchair. Like a person from a disadvantaged minority, Stephanie will have to decide whether to fight the stigma, assumptions, and expectations of people and make them see her, or whether to stay in a safe cocoon of loved ones and avoid the prejudices of others.

Disabilities always impact your self-concept, they always are cumulative, and they always change your view of the world. The time when they occur in the life cycle greatly influences how they change you. If Stephanie had become a paraplegic at age 6, she would have built the disability into emerging self-concept. Disabilities occurring before age 10 more easily are integrated into emerging self-concept and identity formation, and become part of the consideration in planning adult life transitions. Disabilities occurring during late adolescence or young adulthood force a loss of identity (since an identity was already well formed) and a loss of desired life roles. The sense of loss and potential psychological risk is greatest when disabilities are acquired in this period. If the accident had happened late adulthood, it would have been challenging but not as devastating as at earlier life periods. Acquired disabilities are always mediated in their impact on individuals by the life stage and life goals of the individuals.

Before you get too tired of Stephanie, I want to retell her story. This time she does not have a spinal cord injury, but rather she is diagnosed with multiple sclerosis. Multiple sclerosis (MS) is a disease in which the body's immune system destroys the myelin that covers the nerves and causes interference with the communication between the brain and the rest of the body. Multiple sclerosis is a progressive debilitating disease, and there is no cure. Stephanie may need to adapt to her condition by working shorter days, and extending the length of her clinical training, but she will probably still graduate with her class and, unlike our first Stephanie, will be able to work at the job she expected. Stephanie has an invisible disability; the only people who will know about it are those she tells. She does not have the problem of being seen first as a wheelchair, but she has different problems. She gets very tired and cannot work more than six hours a day. She is developing weakness on her left body side that is impacting her ADLs. She cannot continue to play tennis because heat exacerbates her symptoms. When Stephanie in the first scenario dated, there were challenges, but no surprises. What you saw was what you got. She was paralyzed and in a wheelchair, take it or leave it.

For the Stephanie with MS, interpersonal relationships are much more complex. Should she tell her love interests? If she married, could she expect a long happy partnership, or would her condition advance so that she became dependent in all ADLs and IADLs? The wheelchair-bound Stephanie was viewed socially as a paragon of virtue and model of perseverance because she overcame her impairment. The Stephanie coping with MS is the same person, but tired, in pain, and unable to do her work well. She is likely to be seen by her coworkers as a slacker and a whiner, because they cannot see her physical limitations. We will not jump this Stephanie 15 years ahead. . . . You can do that in your imagination. As therapists for people with disabilities, an important part of your job is to look into their future and invest early in interventions that will support them in remaining active and interested in their lives, even if their disability progresses.

The data shows that adults with physical disabilities participate less than people without disabilities in the domains of work and social activities. The barriers that they experience include inaccessible buildings and public transport, as well as social impediments such as stereotyped images (Meulenkamp et al., 2013). So, in review, to support participation for an adult with a disability, the person always comes first. *When* the disability happened is important, because it frames the life challenges that are impacted by the change. Whether the disability is *visible* or *invisible* matters, because it influences the social reaction to how the person's limitations are perceived. Whether the condition is *physical* or *mental* matters, because physical problems are indisputable but we do not always believe in the mental ones. No one questions whether a spinal injury is real, or assumes that they could overcome it if they just demonstrate some personal discipline. Mental disabilities are not always truly recognized as disabilities, and are even less well received socially than Stephanie's multiple sclerosis.

Finally, *culture* matters. Stephanie (with MS) may be quite successful as a stay-at-home mother, pacing herself and resting as needed. If she were from a society that valued at-home pursuits for women, the condition would still be debilitating, but it might be tolerated in a way that would not be in the same culture if she were wheelchair-bound Stephanie rather than Stephanie with MS. Social role expectations including gender roles impact a person's adjustment to disability. If the person is able to continue in desired roles with the condition the impact is less than if there is the loss of valued roles. In providing client-centered care, the rehabilitation professional should help the person regain valued roles as a component of the overall treatment program.

MAJOR LIFE AREAS

Disability has a pervasive impact on the major life areas described in the ICF, education, work and employment, and economic life. Many adult life roles center around these major life areas, and a limited ability to participate can negatively impact adult quality of life. For adults with chronic disabilities, participation in major life areas often involves adaptations and accommodations. When people cannot aspire to independence in the performance of daily occupations, the focus changes to consider how they may control their destiny with as little assistance from others as possible.

The freedom with which individuals "can choose important life and occupational issues such as where to live, what to do with one's time, who to spend time with, and when, where, and how to get help when experiencing a problem" is called **self-determination** (Brown & Stoffel, 2011, p. 788).

EDUCATION

Getting an education as an adult requires financial support and good preparatory education. In Stephanie's story, she was well prepared for education, and if needed, could have changed degrees and studied something more compatible with her physical limitations. There are many young adults who have work and career plans that are not academically based. A young person who did not seek postsecondary education and then acquired a disability may have a far more difficult path than Stephanie. This is the experience of many of the current generation's newly discharged disabled veterans. Tanielian and colleagues (2008) report that of the 2 million veterans seeking to enroll in higher educational institutions, about 20 percent of them will have suffered **traumatic brain injury (TBI)**. TBI is a nondegenerative, noncongenital insult to the brain from an external mechanical force, possibly leading to permanent or temporary impairment of cognitive, physical, and psychosocial functions, with an associated diminished or altered state of consciousness. In current combat conditions, this is a very common condition with potentially long-lasting impacts of participation in daily occupations. About 20 percent of veterans return home with post-traumatic stress disorder (PTSD) or major depression. All three of these conditions common to veterans, traumatic brain injury, post-traumatic stress disorder, and major depression, will impact their ability to participate in all forms of paid work, not just education-dependent jobs.

Cote (2011) discusses the challenges associated with documenting disabilities to qualify for support services, but even with good disabilities documentation, some impairments are not known until veterans engage the learning and thinking requirements in the educational context. The functional impairments associated with TBI, PTSD, and depression include many types of executive function impairments. Executive function impairments such as difficulty with working memory, organizing, and planning are particularly limiting in higher education and challenging to deal with without one-to-one support.

Access to educational opportunities for adults is influenced by financial resources, the quality of individuals' foundational education, their intrinsic abilities, social policy, and the individuals' interests and motivations. In the United States, there is legislation that assures people with disabilities access to a free public education through age 21. There are supports for education beyond this, but in most cases, the opportunities are more limited and based on people's ability to make satisfactory progress in a chosen field of study.

Increasingly self-paced courses are available with Internet access. This offers options for motivated persons to pursue education at their own pace and in their own home. Part of the rehabilitation specialists role may be to help identify the adaptations and modification that the person needs to interface effectively with web-based learning platforms.

People with low self-expectations or negative experiences earlier in educational settings may not seek further education as adults. Because education has a significant impact on opportunities for work and employment, as well as a resource for social and civic engagement, this decision can have a lasting and profound impact on adult lifestyles.

WORK AND EMPLOYMENT

As noted in earlier chapters, participation in paid work has an important role in facilitating adult role development and social participation. Pitts (2011) also notes that there is a link between engagement in work and individual health, especially mental health. In addition to the financial benefits of paid work, this important occupation also helps individuals by imposing a time structure on their day, helps offer definition to personal social status and identity, and enforces activity, often in a social context, rather than allowing individuals to become isolated and solitary (Pitts, 2011). In July of 2012, 70 percent of working-age adults without disabilities participated in the labor force. In the same time period, only 20.7 percent of people with disabilities were in the workforce (U.S. Department of Labor, 2012). Offering more insight into this gap, the U.S. Senate Committee on Health, Education, Labor, and Pensions (2012b) reported that:

- There is no evidence that employment outcomes for people with disabilities as a whole have improved since 1990, and participation rates have been persistently lower than for people without disabilities. In June 2012, just 32.1 percent of working-age people with disabilities were participating in the labor force, compared with 77.7 percent of those without disabilities.

- Between July 2008 and December 2010, workers with disabilities left the labor force at a rate five times greater than workers without a disability—2.1 percent of the nondisability workforce, versus 10.4 percent of the disability workforce, left the labor force over that period.

- Individuals with disabilities also experience a disproportionate level of poverty because of their low employment participation and earnings rates, their underemployment, and the low levels of federal disability cash benefits. In 2010, the poverty rate for working-age adults with disabilities in the United States was 27.3 percent. The poverty rate

for working-age adults without disabilities was 12.8 percent. (USSCHLP, 2012b)

A corollary to the high unemployment rates among the disabled is the large number of people with disabilities who receive public welfare support. The term welfare encompasses those government programs that provide benefits and economic assistance to no- or low-income Americans. Other terms to describe welfare programs are *government subsidy programs* and *public support*. Welfare programs available in the United States include Medicaid, Supplemental Security Income, food stamps, Housing and Urban Development (HUD) programs, and Medicare. Medicaid is a fee-for-service payment system, and it assists low-income families with medical expenses. Supplemental Security Income (SSI) provides financial support to people with disabilities based on financial need. Finally, Social Security Disability Insurance (SSDI) pays benefits to individuals if they are "insured," meaning that they worked long enough and paid Social Security taxes prior to acquiring the disability. Although intended as a support for people with disabilities, current regulations cause some people to choose not to work for fear of losing these benefits. Workers with disabilities must weigh the benefits of being employed against the possible reduction or loss of welfare benefits. Even when the financial gains of working are adequate to offset these potential losses, the process of qualifying for welfare benefits in the first place is a lengthy and often difficult process. People who have had difficulty maintaining employment in the past may be wary of the possibility of losing their job and then have to go through the qualifying process again (Pitts, 2011). This pattern is seen both in adults and in parents of children with disabilities. In the case of children with disabilities, family income serves as a criterion for levels of welfare support. When children are frequently ill and need ongoing specialized care, parents may have frequent absences from the workplace and have difficulty keeping a job. These parents also may opt out of employment to assure welfare support for their child's care. For this reason, it is common for health care providers to see people who are not highly motivated to enter or return to the workforce. This creates a challenge for clinicians as they work to support full participation in adult life roles for their clients.

There is a widespread social belief that some people pretend to have or exaggerate a medical problem to be declared disabled. Disability fraud is when a person (or a group of people) willingly accepts and collects disability payments when they are not actually disabled. Disability benefits fraud has been a focus of political attention, and the reports of its incidence vary widely.

People working in rehabilitation fields will see the whole gamut of people who seek and receive federal disability support. They will treat people with severe persistent disabilities who may not have adequate support to live safely with their condition. On the same day, they may see a person with a limp, complaining of pain with walking while in the clinic, and then watch that person walk back to the car limp free. Many people that receive welfare payments are legitimately in need of support, but exceptions will abuse the system. Welfare payments can also be a focus of domestic abuse. For example, a disabled person may be kept in a caregiver's home, rather than a more treatment-focused rehabilitation setting, so that the caregiver's family can benefit from the disabled person's welfare payments. People with physical limitations may be more vulnerable to this kind of abuse because they are no longer mobile or independent. When health professionals have reason to believe that welfare fraud is occurring, they are legally and ethically required to report it.

COMMUNITY, SOCIAL, AND CIVIC LIFE

Participation in community, social, and civic life increases through early and middle adulthood for most adults. These increases may be related to family activities, in the contexts of school, religion, and community volunteerism. Participation of this type often occurs as an extension of relationships built in the workplace.

Adults with disabilities have historically faced both social and physical barriers to participation in these areas. Beginning in the 1970s, several disability communities emerged to draw public attention to stigma and to advocate for inclusion and full participation possibilities for people with disabilities (Brown & Stoffel, 2011). Disability rights initiatives and public awareness programs continue to work toward this goal. Some especially influential efforts of this type have focused on media representations of people with disabilities. Initiatives such as the Sprout Film Festival (Sprout, 2014), which focuses on people with intellectual and developmental disabilities, and film reviews by the National Alliance on Mental Illness (NAMI), a consumer advocacy group for people with severe mental illnesses and their families, have led to far more accurate and compassionate depictions of people with disabilities in the media. These types of initiatives can help raise awareness on a societal level that may lead to greater acceptance on an individual level.

COMMUNITY LIFE, RECREATION, AND LEISURE

Disability presents multiple barriers to community volunteerism and leisure participation. For some adults, the acquisition of a disability results in the gradual cessation of previously treasured leisure occupations. Barriers to participation may include decreased capability to perform activities at necessary or desired levels of satisfaction, a myriad of environmental barriers, and discrimination resulting in lack of access to leisure and relationship options, particularly travel and social activities.

Decreased community participation may be due to environmental and transportation barriers as well as

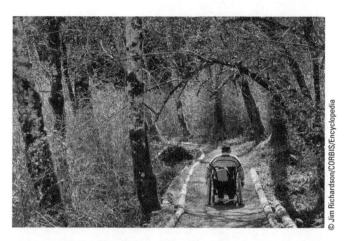

Figure 19-2 This wheelchair-accessible nature trail is coated with crushed rock to make it easier for wheelchair users to traverse.

stigma or discrimination. The energy and amount of effort required by individuals and their caregivers may also result in decreased leisure participation. Current trends toward accessible design and visibility may help, but recreations and leisure interests tend to be highly individualized, and often need individualized solutions. Regardless of the types of barriers to leisure participation, the loss of previously enjoyed activities represents a loss of an important source of identity and coping for individuals with disabilities.

Although many rehabilitation professionals address leisure participation and community reintegration in formal rehabilitation settings, carryover is often limited, and resources for community involvement are sorely lacking. Consumers with disabilities should be encouraged to demand equal access. Some communities are including public recreational sites that use principles of barrier-free design, allowing access to playgrounds, hiking paths, parks, and golf courses (see **Figure 19-2**). These accessible leisure sites are limited and not available in all communities.

As individuals progress through the recovery process, rehabilitation professionals are responsible for being aware of options and resources for addressing the major life task of leisure participation. By attending to leisure needs, individuals with disabilities and their families may experience the opportunity to reduce stress, increase self-confidence and self-esteem, integrate the development of new skills, increase coping skills, affirm their identity, and experience pleasure in the achievement of goals.

In some areas, groups of people with disabilities have worked together to assure access to public transportation. **Figure 19-3** is a historical picture, taken early in the disability rights movement; it shows a public demonstration to help make the needs of people with disabilities evident to the able-bodied mainstream.

As with many things, there are adaptations that can allow people with physical disabilities to participate in many sport and recreational activities, if they can afford to pay for them. The variety and ingenuity of these adaptations can been seen

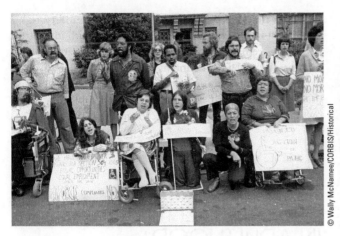

Figure 19-3 This picture, taken in 1977, shows a public demonstration held early in the disability rights movement.

in the Paralympic competitions. The Paralympics are the parallel games to the Olympics, but include only athletes with disabilities. Like the traditional Olympics, the Paralympics have both summer and winter games. In 2012, there were 28 official Paralympic sports. These sports are listed in **Table 19-2**.

These sports are challenging and offer opportunities for competitive sports at elite levels of competition. But they do not meet the needs of more mainstream people with a physical disability. There has been an increased interest in public playground accessibility recently, but less attention has been given to making public parks and museums more accessible for adults with physical limitations. Some communities have Master Gardener programs that support people interested in gardening. These groups may work with community gardens to include raised garden beds and wide pathways to increase access for people in wheelchairs. An enthusiastic gardener working in an accessible community garden is shown in **Figure 19-4**. The Internet has become a growing source of recreational and leisure resources. This new expressive platform permits an opportunity for engagement for many with disabilities. With online gaming, social networking, shopping, selling and blogging all potential recreational and leisure outlets. The Internet also has many

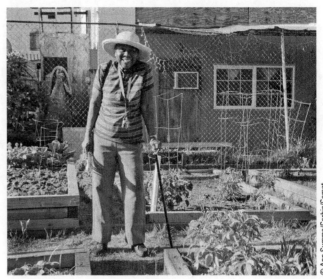

Figure 19-4 A community garden can support accessibility for the elderly and people with physical impairments through providing clear pathways and raised garden beds.

specialized "communities" of people who share experiences or interests. When considering leisure and recreation options, it is important to look broadly at what the person values and help him or her develop a variety of potential leisure and recreational outlets.

Political Life and Citizenship

The **disability rights movement** is an organized political and social action movement to raise public awareness and secure equal opportunities and rights for people with disabilities. In the more than 50 years the movement has been active, significant civil rights legislation has been gained. Some examples of these legislative efforts in the United States are presented in Chapter 21.

This disability rights movement has not been limited to the United States. For people with *physical disabilities,* accessibility and safety are primary issues that this movement works to reform, and the movement has been most

TABLE 19-2	Official Paralympic Sports		
Alpine Skiing	Archery	Athletics	Badminton
Boccie	Cross-country skiing	Equestrian	Football, 5-a-side
Football, 7-a-side	Goal ball	Ice sledge hockey	Judo
Para-canoe	Para-cycling	Para-triathlon	Power lifting
Rowing	Sailing	Shooting	Sitting volleyball
Swimming	Para-table tennis	Wheelchair basketball	Wheelchair curling
Wheelchair dance	Wheelchair fencing	Wheelchair rugby	Wheelchair tennis

effective in this area. There have been noticeable changes in some parts of the world that include the installation of elevators, automatic doors, wide doors and corridors, transit lifts, wheelchair ramps, and curb cuts along sidewalks. **Figure 19-5** shows a commuter train station that has been designed to be accessible to people in wheelchairs.

Advocates for the rights of people with cognitive and mental disabilities have focused mainly on self-determination, self-advocacy, and access to housing where individuals can live independently (Barnartt & Scotch, 2001). Another focus for the disability rights group is access to education and employment. The availability of paid aides in schools and in the home has been one result of this effort. Because people with cognitive and mental disabilities are more vulnerable to abuse and neglect, the disability rights movement has been able to influence broad social institutions, including health care, school, and housing, to identify and recognize the rights of their clients. Some examples of these changes have been a legal requirement for informed consent for treatment, prosecution for failure to maintain the confidentiality of treatment records, and strict supervision in the use of physical and chemical restraints in health care settings.

Self-advocacy, as presented by the disability rights movement, supports that people with disabilities should be able and allowed to speak for themselves, rather than have experts or authority figures determine their fate. This movement promotes that even in the presence of cognitive impairments, individuals are entitled to have control of their own resources

and how they are directed. Although the disability rights movement has made significant gains, people with intellectual disabilities remain among the most vulnerable and isolated members of society. The intent of focusing on self-advocacy is to reduce the isolation of people with disabilities and give them the tools and experience to take greater control over their own lives (Wehmeyer, Bersani, & Gagne, 2000).

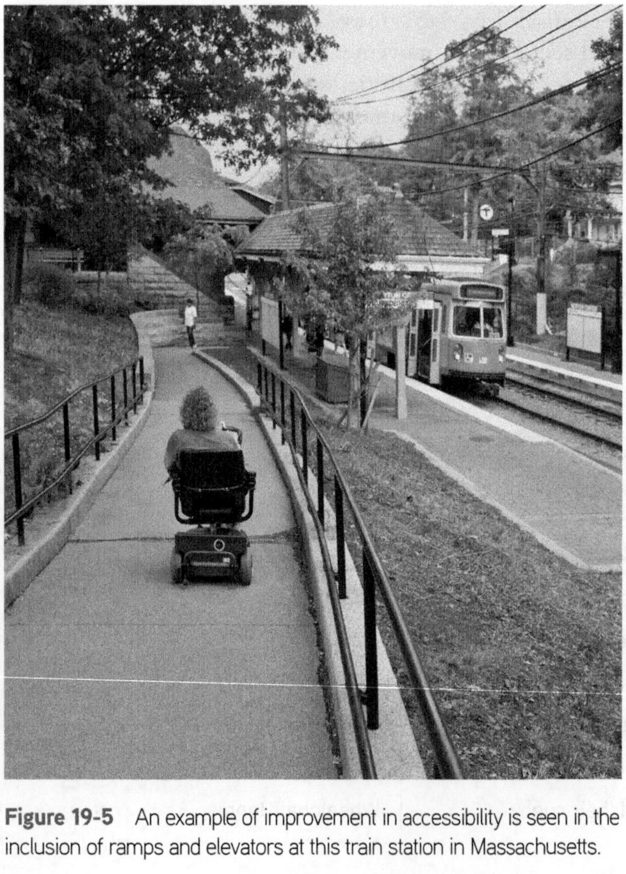

THE EXPERIENCE OF CONGENITAL/ DEVELOPMENTAL DISABILITY IN ADULTHOOD

As we change our focus from people with acquired disabilities to those with congenital conditions, our focus is on people who had a different or atypical developmental trajectory from early childhood. Following the earlier example, this developmental trajectory will be illustrated through a case example.

Rikki, a girl born with a condition called arthrogryposis multiplex congenita (AMC), has profound physical limitations including multiple joint contractures and muscle weakness. Although the disease is nonprogressive, as a child she will experience several painful orthopedic procedures to gain mobility and structural integrity in her skeletal system. Rikki may grow up dependent in most areas of self-care and community mobility. AMC is very rare. There are no large population-based studies on the experiences and impact of growing up with this physically limiting condition that usually leaves cognition intact. As health care providers, we must listen and learn when we meet Rikki in our clinic as an adult. Like Stephanie, who is bound to a wheelchair, Rikki has a highly visible physical limitation and will need special devices and supports to achieve her daily activities. She may be depressed and angry, as Stephanie was, about the isolation and limitations that she experiences because of her condition. Unlike Stephanie, she never knew a different life. Her life of learning, her hopes and expectations were all framed with an awareness of herself as an individual with a physical disability.

Rikki will have access to a free appropriate public school education, but in spite of that, young people like Rikki leave adolescence with low expectations for themselves in terms of education, work, and interpersonal relationships. Higher education and employment levels among individuals with disabilities remain unacceptably low (Carter, Austin, & Trainor, 2012). Working-age people with disabilities participated in the workforce at a rate less than half of that of the general population, and of those that are employed, they are more likely to work only part-time (USSCHELP, 2012a).

In a report from the U.S. Senate Committee on Health, Education, Labor, and Pensions (2012a), it was noted that "despite similar education, those people with disabilities who are working earn less on average than workers without disabilities. In 2010, the median annual

Figure 19-5   An example of improvement in accessibility is seen in the inclusion of ramps and elevators at this train station in Massachusetts.

earnings for workers with disabilities ages 16 and older was $19,500. For workers without disabilities that year the median annual earnings was $29,997. The median earnings for workers with disabilities are less than two-thirds the median wages for workers without disabilities" (p. 9).

So Rikki, now 41, has come to your clinic with jaw and neck pain. She has been working as a medical transcriptionist, using a combination of speech recognition and an infrared optical tracking device to emulate mouse and keyboard access. Rikki lives with her parents and is able to walk and use public transportation; however, between her ADL, medical, and transportation limitations, she has only been able to work 30 hours a week. She is very concerned, because if she has to cut her working hours more, she would be financially better off to stop working and live on federal welfare disability benefits. She does not want to do this because she is able to work, enjoys the challenge and autonomy it offers, and likes being in regular social contact with other people. At this point, Rikki enjoys the prestige of being a "success story," much as Stephanie was, and she does not want to lose this status.

If she chooses to quit her job, she will be financially better off, but much more emotionally and socially challenged. She could choose to continue to work as a "volunteer" and retain the social connections, while receiving disability benefits, but this could be considered disability fraud—if she works at a job she could be paid for, but refuses pay to keep her disability benefits. This is one of the paradoxical situations that adults with disabilities face today. There are not enough alternatives to meet the needs of people who want to work but have limitations that make keeping a traditional job difficult.

In the same report mentioned earlier, it was noted that "In America today, being a person with a disability greatly increases the likelihood of being jobless or underemployed. The likelihood of living in poverty and remaining in poverty for an adult with a disability is significantly greater than it is for a person without a disability. Despite their educational foundation, despite their desire to work, despite their abilities and skills, far too many people with disabilities in our country today are suffering because they have not, in most cases, achieved success in the labor market. Our support programs and the level of benefits often trap people with disabilities in a system that discourages and often punishes their efforts to work, ensnarling them in life-long poverty" (USSCHELP, 2012a, p. 11).

Meulenkamp and colleagues (2013) conducted a three year study considering data from almost 6000 adults with physical disabilities. These authors report that most people wanted to participate more, although how they wanted to participate varied based on individual factors such as age and educational levels. They noted that "when support is needed, it must be tailor-made and fit the specific personal needs, as is also advocated by client-centered rehabilitation approaches" (p. 948). People who work in rehabilitation fields should always be on the front lines of supporting and advocating for people with disabilities. Although Rikki may be able to continue to live with her parents and live on a disability income, the quality of her life will be greatly diminished. The rehabilitation team must be open to exploring and assimilating new assistive technology innovations in creative ways to support the "Rikkis" in our clinical practices. Our role as clinician also extends into an advocacy role for our clients at the community and even national level. Ricardo Pagán (2013) conducted an extensive time-use study of persons with physical disabilities. He found that the increased time needed for self-care, child-care, and household tasks left people with physical disabilities unable to engage in full time employment. His discussion supported the consideration of social policy changes to help people who want to work be more successful in this. He noted that "rehabilitation professionals and others working with disabled people must understand the time constraints, activity patterns, and lifestyle requirements of this group and thus offer a more balanced program through therapy and by increasing the levels of satisfaction in the client therapist relationship" (p. 91).

INTELLECTUAL AND DEVELOPMENTAL DISABILITIES

A special subgroup of people with congenital disabilities are people with intellectual and developmental disabilities (I/DD). More research is available for this subgroup than for others, in part because so many congenital disabilities include differences in cognition and cognitive development. The people in this subgroup have some problems in participation in adult life that are unique to their developmental disabilities.

Health

The life expectancy for people with I/DD is similar to that of the general population, with the mean age at death ranging from the mid-50s (for those with more severe disabilities or Down syndrome) to the early 70s for adults with mild to moderate I/DD (Bittles et al., 2002). The number of adults with I/DD age 60 years and older is projected to nearly double from 641,860 in 2000 to 1.2 million by 2030 (Miniño, Xu, Kochanek, & Tejada-Vera, 2009). Adults with developmental disabilities were significantly more likely to suffer from high blood pressure, cardiovascular disease, arthritis, diabetes, and chronic pain than their typically developing peers (Havercamp, Scandlin, & Roth, 2004).

Complicating this, Havercamp, Scandlin, and Roth (2004) reported that adults with developmental disabilities were even more likely to lead sedentary lifestyles than their typically developing peers. People with I/DD are often segregated from the mainstream of adult life, and continue to rely on their aging parents for assistance, emotional support, and friendship. These people often cannot drive or manage public transportation. Remaining in the family role of "child," they do not build their own social supports or networks outside of their family of origin.

Domestic Life

Some of the difficult challenges that parents of adults with I/DD face are those associated with the tasks listed as "domestic life" in the ICF. The first of these tasks, acquiring a place to live, is often a parental decision rather than the decision of a person with I/DD. In the United States, over 75 percent of adults with I/DD live at home with family caregivers, and over 25 percent of these caregivers are over 60 years or older (Heller & Arnold, 2010).

As parents age, other living arrangements must be considered. The two most common choices in the United States are establishing a sibling as caregiver and placement in a group care home. Group homes are small, residential facilities located within a community and designed to serve people with chronic disabilities. These homes usually have six or fewer occupants and are staffed 24 hours a day by trained caregivers. Group homes allow adults with I/DD to develop skills they need to function in the community, which they may not be able to learn in their family home. Bianco and colleagues (2009) reported that parents of adult children with I/DD took on the responsibility for identifying, anticipating, and planning for services their children would need as they moved into more independent living situations.

A less desirable option for adults with I/DD is a nursing home. The term nursing home is a blanket term for a wide variety of institution-based living arrangement facilities that provides 24-hour supervised care. Nursing homes provide a much-needed service, but are usually designed to provide care for those who are elderly and infirm. Nursing homes are often a poor fit for healthy younger adults with a developmental disability.

The domestic life task of "acquiring goods and services" includes shopping and gathering daily necessities. Adults with I/DD will have the same transportation and access problems described previously. They will also have increased problems of personal safety and may be easy to exploit for money or sexual favors. Martorell and Tsakanikos (2008) report that people with I/DD have a high likelihood of encountering traumatic events throughout their lifetime (such as abandonment by loved ones, abuse, bullying, and harassment). There is a delicate balance between supporting independence and protecting people with intellectual impairments.

INTERPERSONAL INTERACTIONS AND RELATIONSHIPS

The social networks of most adults include family, workplace, and community connections. The interpersonal social networks of adults are important tools to help them cope with change and to serve as a psychological buffer in times of stress (Hayslip, Patrick, & Panek, 2011). Adults with I/DD tend to have very limited social networks and are often dependents within their family. Peer support and friendship is highly valued but difficult to maintain for the adult with I/DD.

Relationships with Family

As noted earlier in this text, parental adaptation to a child's disability is a complex, lifelong process for parents. This process continues as children become adults. For many, the parental role remains unchanged from childhood, with the parent guiding and directing their adult child's daily activities and social interactions. One of the findings that van Ingen and Moore (2010) reported was that parents of adults with I/DD express both pain and emotional distress in moving their adult children out of their house and into another home or institution where professionals provide caregiving . Parents who cannot leave the caregiver role may feel limited in their own growth and opportunities, tied to the constant care of a child who "never grows up." On the other hand, some parents may define their identity in their role as caregiver and may provide more assistance than the individual with I/DD needs. This meets the needs of the parent (needing to be needed), but further infantilizes the adult with I/DD. This is not the experience of all parents, but even those who are content with their caregiving relationship may be isolating their adult child unnecessarily and making the inevitable transition, when the parent is no longer able to provide the needed care, more difficult.

Siblings tend to have long-lasting close relationships with their brother or sister with I/DD, and most are willing to take on a caregiving role (Heller & Arnold, 2010). The most common living arrangement for adults with I/DD is with parents or siblings. This changes when a person with I/DD has challenging behaviors, such as seen in people with mental illness or with a behavioral disorder, or when the caregiving needs are too great. It is hard to care for an adult whose needs are likely to grow rather than diminish over time. This is especially challenging if siblings have children of their own that become more and more independent over time. In these instances, such siblings may be less supportive and less willing to take on a caregiving role. Placement in a residential care facility is often considered in these cases.

Intimate Relationships

Because many people with intellectual impairments never gain academic skills above the most basic level, they are often seen as "childlike," even as adults. Viewing them as perpetual children does them a great disservice. Although people may not gain academic skills, people with I/DD do continue to learn and develop throughout their lives. With maturing bodies and immersed in the culture of their community, adults with I/DD will be interested in romantic and intimate relationships. They will experience hormone surges and sexual attractions in the same way as their age peers. This creates tremendous challenges for both the individuals and their caregivers.

The author of this chapter, once employed in a high school setting, was stopped by a male special educator who was distressed and needed support in both protecting and advocating for an 18-year-old woman with Prader-Willi syndrome. Prader-Willi syndrome affects many aspects of development and is associated with compulsive eating behaviors. The concern of the special educator was that the young woman was enrolled in some classes with typically developing students. She was very social and interested in making friends, but did not understand social boundaries within friendships. Her teacher blurted out, "I can't let her go there by herself. She will do anything for a candy bar!" It was a challenge to support her academic achievement and keep her from being sexually exploited at the same time.

Adults with I/DD can form positive, rewarding romantic and sexual relationships. Like other adults, they tend to choose partners who have similar life experiences and that they meet in their everyday lives. The establishment of romantic relationships, such as the one shown in **Figure 19-6**, is in many ways positive and reflects participation in ordinary adult activities. Many group homes and nursing homes offer conjugal living arrangements for couples.

Abuse and Vulnerability

Although no longer children, people with I/DD are potentially at-risk for sexual, psychological and physical abuse from members of the community much in the same way that children are. **Domestic violence** refers to a pattern of abusive behaviors by one partner against another in an intimate relationship such as marriage, dating, family, or cohabitation. Domestic violence has many forms, including physical aggression or assault, threats, sexual abuse, controlling or domineering behaviors, and intimidation. Adults with I/DD are vulnerable to abuse and are more likely to experience social victimization than any other adult subgroup. Examples of victimization that were reported include money/theft, teasing/persuasion, sexual exploitation, and abuse. This victimization does not seem to directly relate to the level of a person's cognitive functions. Fisher, Moskowitz, and Hodapp (2012) reported that individuals who are higher functioning and thus more aware of vulnerable situations still experience victimization at rates similar to those who are less able to detect risk.

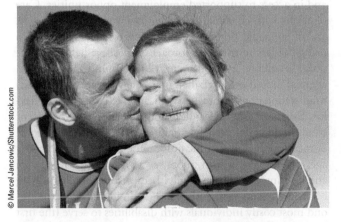

Figure 19-6 Romantic partnerships among people who have intellectual impairments can be rich and fulfilling.

In addition to social victimization, people with developmental disabilities are at an increased risk for becoming victims of sexual abuse. Research has shown that as many as 25 percent of males and 50 percent of females with developmental disabilities experience some form of sexual abuse. The largest group of identified perpetrators of this sexual abuse includes the developmental disability service providers (Bowman, Scotti, & Morris, 2010). This problem is so prevalent that many families endure physical and financial hardship to avoid leaving their adult child in the care of professional service providers.

MAJOR LIFE AREAS

Hayslip, Patrick, and Panek (2011) suggest that all adults seek a developmental niche. A **developmental niche** is an environment in which a person can function optimally. The developmental niche is defined by culture and environment, and is congruent with an individual's skills and abilities. For typically developing adults, a developmental niche might be an employment setting that offers interesting challenges and is consistent with their values and career goals. The establishment of a positive developmental niche for people with I/DD often involves the cooperation of the individuals, their family, potential employers, social service agencies, and community organizations.

Work and Employment

The two most common mechanisms for people with I/DD to engage in remunerative work are through sheltered workshops and integrated employment. A **sheltered workshop** is a facility-based workplace that provides a supportive environment where people with physical or mental challenges can acquire job skills and vocational experience. Activities in workshops tend to be relatively easy to learn and perform. Typically, they involve repetitive tasks such as assembling, packing, woodworking, manufacturing, or sewing, as well as those tasks associated with agriculture (Migliore, Mank, Grossi, & Rogan, 2007). The goals of workshops may vary, ranging from assessment and rehabilitation geared toward transition into the general labor market to long-term placement in the workshops. People with I/DD accept the sheltered workshop model, which offers an alternative to staying at home and an ability to interact with others. The fact that participation in sheltered workshops typically does not lead to engagement in work in the regular workforce is more of a concern for policy makers than for the families and the workers. Most sheltered workshops are independent organizations, and participation in them is voluntary. They are criticized because they do not reflect actual work settings and because all of the workers are people with disabilities. Sheltered workshops in the United States are often private nonprofit enterprises that provide services such as recycling materials into marketable crafts, paper shredding, and food service.

Integrated employment is paid work in the general labor market where the proportion of workers with disabilities does not exceed the natural proportions in the community (unlike sheltered workshops). **Figure 19-7** shows a woman working in an integrated employment position in a local greenhouse that grows ornamental plants. People with I/DD working in integrated employment may work full-time or they may work part-time. Some groups have designated jobs that are only 10 to 15 hours a week, jobs that would not interest typical workers. Wages in integrated employment settings are at least the minimum wage.

"The advantages that integrated employment [have] over sheltered employment include the following: (a) better financial outcomes for people with disabilities, (b) increased opportunities for personal growth for people with disabilities, (c) compliance with the paradigm shift from fitting people into programs to adapting services to people's needs, (d) adherence to the values of social justice in which western democracies claim to have their roots, (e) fulfillment of the preferences of people with disabilities, (f) satisfaction of families' preferences, and (g) greater social integration of people with disabilities" (Migliore et al., 2007, p. 7).

Both sheltered workshops and integrated employment programs are limited in their availability, and in 2010, served only about 20 percent of the adult population with I/DD (Winsor, 2012). In a challenging economic environment with high unemployment, there are fewer options for integrated employment. This is an area of current and growing need as more people with I/DD move into adulthood and are unable to earn a living without additional training and assistance.

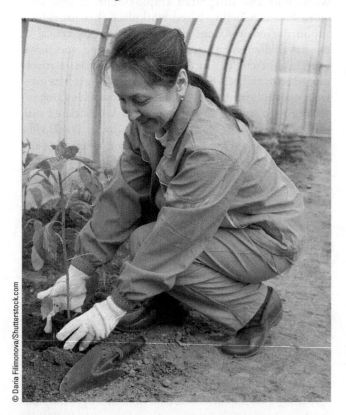

© Daria Filimonova/Shutterstock.com

Figure 19-7 This woman has a disability but is able to contribute positively and is able to earn a wage for her work.

Challenging Behaviors

The most common syndromes associated with developmentally based intellectual disabilities in adults are autism, Down syndrome, fragile X syndrome, and fetal alcohol spectrum disorder (FASD) (The Arc, 2012). The abilities of people with I/DD to regulate behaviors and interact in an adult social environment are key predictors both to employability and to the ability to live in community housing. One of the strongest arguments for inclusive educational environments is the development of these skills.

Challenging behaviors can be part of any condition, but are especially common in people with autism and fetal alcohol syndrome. Currently, the central focus of early childhood treatment of autism is behavioral self-regulation. This is a relatively new trend, and today's adults may not have had intensive behavioral supports early in life, and often have matured with some challenging behaviors. Manente and colleagues (2010) looked at adults with autism, and identified problems of aggression, self-injurious behavior, property destruction, ritualistic behavior, disruption, inappropriate vocalization, and pica (among others). In their review of the literature, these authors found that up to 32 percent of adults with autism demonstrated aggressive behaviors, up to 21 percent demonstrated self-injurious behavior, and up to 19 percent demonstrated patterns of destructive behavior.

The management of these types of challenging behaviors exceeds the abilities of most families, and in fact exceeds the abilities of most nursing homes. This is an extreme problem and one that is growing rapidly as the incidence of autism is greatly increased in the current generation of children and adolescents. Persistent challenging behaviors place adults at risk for high levels of physical restraint, abuse from caregivers/day program staff, and self-inflicted injury (Allen, Lowe, Moore, & Brophy, 2007).

People who did not receive strong behavioral support in childhood and those who need but do not have access to ongoing behavioral support as adults are likely to be excluded from both community integration in daily living arrangements and in access to supported employment opportunities. Care of adults with challenging behaviors is very labor intensive, and often medications are used to limit behaviors rather than using the less restrictive approach of positive behavior supports. Manente and colleagues (2010) found that physical aggression and other challenging behaviors predict the administration of psychotropic medication to control the behavior. Esbensen and colleagues (2009) found that 81 percent of adults and adolescents with autism were taking some form of medication, and that medication use increases with greater age, more severe autism, more severe intellectual handicap, and housing outside the family. Because of these challenging behaviors, adults with autism have been identified as the second most costly individuals with disabilities to serve (the first being people with sensory impairments). Supporting an autistic person financially over their lifetime costs an estimated $3.2 million dollars (Ganz, 2006).

Recreation and Leisure

Adults with I/DD may or may not have physical impairments as well as intellectual impairments. The issues associated with physical impairments will be the same as those described in the category of acquired disability. These are problems of transportation and access. Atypical behaviors and poor socialization may further limit acceptance in group recreational or leisure activities. Adults with high-functioning autism may be physically and intellectually able to play duplicate bridge or ultimate Frisbee, but may not behave socially in ways that are acceptable to the group.

People with intellectual impairments are more likely to have limited interests and not seek out new leisure activities. Social programs for adults with disabilities, particularly those focusing on engagement in the arts, have been very promising in addressing the leisure needs of these individuals, but to date these programs are poorly funded and available only in limited areas.

Religion and Spirituality

Faith communities offer both social support and connections for all adults. This is also true for adults with developmental disabilities. Although challenging behavior patterns are as limiting in this context as they are in others, faith communities often offer a safe and accepting social network for adults with developmental disabilities.

Political Life and Citizenship

Although adults with I/DD are citizens, because of the nature of their limitation, they have not organized as a force in political or civic areas. Family members rehabilitation professionals and other involved adults should advocate for people with these conditions. Several of the most prominent political action groups that advocate for the needs of people with developmental and mental disabilities are listed in **Table 19-3**.

TABLE 19-3 Political Advocacy Groups Supporting People with Developmental and Mental Disabilities	
Organization	**Description of Organizational Mission**
American Association of People with Disabilities http://www.aapd.com	"The American Association of People with Disabilities is the nation's largest cross-disability organization. We promote equal opportunity, economic power, independent living, and political participation for people with disabilities." (www.aapd.com/what-powers-us/aapd-mission.html)
Americans Disabled for Attendant Programs Today (ADAPT) http://www.adapt.org	"ADAPT is a national grass-roots community that organizes disability rights activists to engage in nonviolent direct action, including civil disobedience, to assure the civil and human rights of people with disabilities to live in freedom." (http://www.adapt.org)
The Arc of the United States http://thearc.org	"The Arc promotes and protects the human rights of people with intellectual and developmental disabilities and actively supports their full inclusion and participation in the community throughout their lifetimes." (www.thearc.org/page.aspx?pid=2345)
Bazelon Center for Mental Health Law http://bazelon.org	"The mission of the Judge David L. Bazelon Center for Mental Health Law is to protect and advance the rights of adults and children who have mental disabilities. The Bazelon Center envisions an America where people who have mental illnesses or developmental disabilities exercise their own life choices and have access to the resources that enable them to participate fully in their communities." (http://bazelon.org/Who-We-Are.aspx)
Disability Rights Education and Defense Fund http://www.dredf.org	"The mission of the Disability Rights Education and Defense Fund is to advance the civil and human rights of people with disabilities through legal advocacy, training, education, and public policy and legislative development." (http://www.dredf.org/about/index.shtml)
NAMI: National Alliance on Mental Illness http://www.nami.org	"NAMI, the National Alliance on Mental Illness, is the nation's largest grassroots mental health organization dedicated to building better lives for the millions of Americans affected by mental illness. NAMI advocates for access to services, treatment, supports and research and is steadfast in its commitment to raising awareness and building a community of hope for all those in need." (http://www.nami.org/template.cfm?section= About_NAMI)
National Organization on Disability http://www.nod.org	"The mission of the National Organization on Disability (NOD) is to expand the participation and contribution of America's 54 million men, women, and children with disabilities in all aspects of life. Our current focus is on improving employment prospects for America's 33 million working-aged Americans with disabilities." (http://www.nod.org/about_us/)
TASH http://www.tash.org	"As a leader in disability advocacy for more than 35 years, the mission of TASH is to promote the full inclusion and participation of children and adults with significant disabilities in every aspect of their community, and to eliminate the social injustices that diminish human rights." (http://www.tash.org/about/mission/)

THE EXPERIENCE OF DISABILITY IN LATE ADULTHOOD

Disabilities acquired earlier in life will continue to be prevalent in late adulthood. For this reason, you will see a repetition of many of the disability types described earlier in any description of disability in later life. For example, the age of onset for rheumatoid arthritis is variable. It may occur in early adulthood and continue through late adulthood, or first occur in late adulthood. Statistics show that RA is the most common disease-related cause of acquired disability in middle adulthood. It is also the most common cause of disability in late adulthood, with an increasing incidence in late adulthood. In this discussion of late adulthood, we will consider all forms and developmental patterns of disabilities.

People aged 65 and older report much higher rates of disability (53.9 percent) than people in early adulthood (13.6 percent) (Erickson, Lee, & von Schrader, 2010). The American Community Survey (Erickson, Lee, & von Schrader, 2010) explored the prevalence of functional disability in older people. This survey described the six categories of functional disabilities presented in **Table 19-4**. These disability types are: (1) visual disability—the person is blind or has serious difficulty seeing even when wearing glasses; (2) hearing disability—the person is deaf or has serious difficulty hearing; (3) ambulatory disability— the person has serious difficulty walking or climbing stairs; (4) cognitive disability—this person has serious difficulty concentrating, remembering, or making decisions because of a physical, mental, or emotional condition; (5) self-care disability—the person has difficulty dressing or bathing; and (6) independent living disability—this person has difficulty doing errands alone such as visiting a doctor's office or shopping because of a physical, mental, or emotional condition.

COMMON CAUSES OF FUNCTIONAL LIMITATIONS IN LATE ADULTHOOD

Bonder and Bello-Haas (2009) identify falls as one of the most serious health problems that older people face. Among community-dwelling older people, 28 to 35 percent fall each year. The likelihood and frequency of falls increases with age (Yoshida, 2007). Falls have been identified as a major cause of physical injury, immobility, psychosocial dysfunction, and nursing home placement in the elderly. The risk of falling increases as the frailty of the elder increases. Falls have been associated with visual disorders, neurological disorders, cardiovascular disorders, musculoskeletal disorders, psychological/psychosocial issues, and medications (Bonder & Bello-Haas, 2009). Each of these factors that contribute to the incidence of falls will be discussed briefly.

Visual Disorders

The most common type of visual pathology, impacting about 50 percent of all people between the ages of 65 to 75 years, are ocular cataracts (Loh & Ogle, 2004). An **ocular cataract** is a clouding that develops in the lens of the eye or in its envelope (lens capsule), varying in degree from slight to complete opacity. There are many specific types of cataracts, but the most common are age-related (or senile) cataracts. Early in the development of age-related cataract, individuals may experience nearsightedness, followed by a gradual yellowing and increasing opacity of the lens. Age-related cataracts typically progress slowly, and are highly treatable. Left untreated, cataracts can cause vision loss and eventually blindness.

Age-related macular degeneration (ARMD) is a leading cause of legal blindness among the elderly above 60 years of age, and it presents a global public health crisis (Loh & Ogle, 2004). In this condition, central vision is lost, but peripheral vision almost always remains intact. ARMD is irreversible and is characterized by retinal atrophy, scarring, and hemorrhages in the macula. This condition occurs in about 30 percent of individuals over the age of 75 (Bonder & Bello-Haas, 2009).

Dementia

Dementia is a significant health problem in the elderly, and a significant cause of falls. *Dementia* is a general term describing a deterioration in cognitive functioning that challenges a person's ability to meet the intellectual demands of everyday life. Most dementias are the result of structural brain changes. The most common causes of dementia are

TABLE 19-4	The Prevalence of Functional Disability in Persons Aged 65+	
Vision disability		6.9%
Hearing disability		15.1%
Ambulatory disability		23.8%
Cognitive disability		9.5%
Self-care disability		8.7%
Independent living disability		16.2%

Erickson, W., Lee, C., & von Schrader, S. (2010). Disability Statistics from the 2008 American Community Survey (ACS). Ithaca, NY: Cornell University RehabilitationResearch and Training Center on Disability Demographics and Statistics. Retrieved from www.disabilitystatistics.org

(1) degenerative neurological diseases, such as Alzheimer's disease; (2) vascular disorders; (3) infections that affect the central nervous system, such as HIV; (4) chronic drug use; and (5) depression (Cleveland Clinic, 2012). The dementias associated with degenerative neurological disease and those associated with vascular disorders are the two types most common overall and the types most prevalent in people over 65 years of age.

Alzheimer's disease (AD) is the most prevalent form of progressive dementia among people aged 65 and older. In Alzheimer's disease, brain cells degenerate and die, causing a steady decline in memory and mental function. There are several subtypes of AD, but in general, people with AD usually have a gradual decline in mental functions that eventually results in losses in the ability to maintain employment, and to plan and execute familiar tasks. In the middle to late stages of the disease, communication ability, mood, and personality also may be affected. AD predominantly affects the elderly. AD affects about 3 percent of all people between ages 65 and 74, about 19 percent of those between 75 and 84, and about 47 percent of those over 85 (Naditz, 2003). To date, there are no effective treatments to halt the progression of AD. A class of medications called *cholinesterase inhibitors* has shown positive effects on cognition and ability to complete ADLs in people with AD (Pouryamout, Dams, Wasem, Dodel, & Neumann, 2012). These medications may reduce caregiver burden for a time, but do not impact the overall trajectory of the disease.

Vascular dementia is a general term describing cognitive problems that are caused by brain damage from impaired blood flow to the brain. Cerebrovascular accidents (also called CVA or stroke) are the most common cause of vascular dementia. Vascular dementia also can result from other conditions that damage blood vessels and reduce circulation, such as atherosclerosis. Vascular dementia is the second most common form of dementia after Alzheimer's disease (AD) in older adults (Battistin & Cagnin, 2010). Early detection and accurate diagnosis are important, as vascular dementia is at least partially preventable (American Academy of Neurology, 2007).

Parkinson's disease (PD) is a progressive disorder primarily impacting older adults that effects movement and cognition. PD is characterized by slowed movements (bradykinesia), resting tremor, and postural reflex impairment leading to balance problems. There are medical treatments that are effective at managing the early motor symptoms of the disease. One common type of motor impairment is *essential tremor*. **Essential tremor** is involuntary shaking (tremors), often in the hands. Essential tremors worsen with movement and are aggravated by emotional stress, fatigue, and extremes of temperature. Unlike AD, PD does seem to respond to lifestyle and rehabilitative interventions. In addition, there are some promising new treatments for PD including gene-based therapies, deep brain stimulation to reduce motor symptoms, and stem cell transplants.

Depression

Depression was described in Chapter 18 as a common mental health problem among the elderly. Major depression is seen in about 5 to 10 percent of elders in primary care settings (Lyness, 2012). Much more common than major depression (10 to 25 percent of community-dwelling elders), however, are patterns of clinically meaningful depressive symptoms that do not meet the full diagnostic criteria for depression (Wittchen & Uhmann, 2010). This type of depressive condition is most commonly described as *minor/subsyndromal depression*.

Subsyndromal depression in the elderly, has a functional impact similar to that of a clinically more serious major depression in younger people (Lyness et al., 2006). This type of Late-onset depression in old age has distinctly different risk factors (for example, CVA, PD, or arthritis) than those seen in younger people. In addition, depression in older people is less likely to be associated with sadness or a flattened mood, but is more likely to be associated with sleep disturbance. Rates of depression are highest in those subsets of the elderly population requiring intensive medical attention, including inpatient and residential treatment.

SELF-CARE

Limitations in self-care skills can occur at any age when people experience a disability. The incidence of difficulties with self-care skills increases as people age. In many large-scale census and epidemiological studies, the most frequent definition of disability is as "individuals who require assistance with basic activities of daily living" (Burwell & Jackson, 1994), making ADL performance diagnostic of disability. ADL performance is impacted by sensory impairment, cognitive declines, restricted mobility, decreased flexibility, and reduced strength, all common aspects of aging. Active participation in self-care activities, even if the participation is modified or assisted, supports health, self-esteem, social relationships, and psychological well-being (Brown & Stoffel, 2011).

Self-care impairments are highly individualized and cannot be presented here in more than general terms. An important focus of occupational and physical therapy is in the prevention of further disability. Daniels and colleagues (2011) report that multidisciplinary self-management support, using a mixture of components, is effective in improving clinical outcomes in older people with disabilities. These researchers noted that many older people lack confidence in their capabilities. Many also experience a lack in activities that they enjoy or that give meaning to life. In their study, occupational therapists worked with clients to explore capacities, interests, and satisfaction with meaningful activities. Interventions supported the clients' ability to choose and perform the activities of their choice. Both occupational and physical therapists work with clients to adapt the environment, activities, or skills to enhance performance of ADL and IADL tasks. Interventions may involve retraining strategies for task performance, it may involve the use of assistive technology, or it may involve a functional exercise program to gain needed strength.

DOMESTIC LIFE

Difficulties in acquiring the necessities for daily life will be similar to those described in Chapter 18, although the limitations may be greater. Access to safe, reliable transportation, capability for community mobility, and moderate or better physical endurance will be significant predictors in which of the elderly will be able to maintain independence in this area, and which will need assistance. The categories of performance tasks included in the ICF as domestic life tasks are all likely to be problematic for elderly people with a disability. These include shopping, gathering daily necessities, preparing meals, washing and drying clothes, cleaning the cooking area and utensils, cleaning the living area, using household appliances, and disposing of garbage. This is an area of particular importance to the older adult. Difficulty with the performance of domestic tasks may be reason that the person must move to a residential home. Many occupational roles are associated with activities around the home, difficulties performing these activities may distressing because they reflect a loss of a valued role.

INTERPERSONAL INTERACTIONS AND RELATIONSHIPS

As presented in Chapter 18, there is strong evidence that supportive social networks enhance well-being and health in late adulthood. Disability creates barriers to the development and maintenance of social relationships. Because maintaining these relationships are already issues as a part of healthy aging, older adults with disability are especially vulnerable in this area. The emotional and physical needs of a frail older person can erode even long-standing positive relationships.

Cohen-Mansfield, Shmotkin, and Hazan (2010) studied elders that were homebound. In their studies, they defined being homebound as going out of the house once a week or less. Homebound status isolates people and also restricts access to community, social, and civic life. In this study, it was noted, that even controlling for disability and premorbid mental health conditions, there was a higher level of mental illness in the homebound population. These authors argue that the increased incidence of depression in homebound participants emphasizes the importance of "providing homebound older persons with resources to allow them to get out of the house and calls attention to the need for health and social agencies to address the pain, depressed affect, and general low mental health of those persons" (p. 2362).

Neglect may include the failure to provide sufficient supervision, nourishment, or medical care, or the failure to fulfill other needs for which victims are helpless to provide

for themselves. This term may apply to children, people with I/DD, or to frail older people. Elder abuse is a form of domestic violence. The World Health Organization (2012) defines elder abuse as "a single, or repeated act, or lack of appropriate action, occurring within any relationship where there is an expectation of trust which causes harm or distress to an older person. Elder abuse can take various forms such as physical, psychological or emotional, sexual, and financial abuse. It can also be the result of intentional or unintentional neglect." Abuse may be a single or repeated willful infliction of pain or mental anguish. It can be the willful deprivations of basic needs (Hayslip, Patrick, & Panek, 2011).

Elder abuse is a specific form of domestic violence, and perpetrators of elder abuse can include anyone in a position of trust, control, or authority. Anyone, including a spouse, partner, relative, a friend or neighbor, a volunteer worker, a paid worker, or a member of a faith community can be an abuser. Children and living relatives who have a history of substance abuse or have had other life troubles are of particular concern (Hutchison, 2011). As with other forms of domestic violence, elder abuse can involve physical abuse, emotional abuse, or a combination of the two. *Exploitation* (financial abuse) occurs when a trusted person misuses the older person's income or resources for financial or personal gain. Exploitation may include a broad range of activities including stealing money or possessions, or coercing the older person to legally sign over rights or property. As with child abuse, neglect is also a form of abuse in older adults. Neglect, in the case of the elderly, "is the lack of services necessary to maintain mental and physical health of a disabled person living alone or not able to render self care" (Hayslip, Panek, & Patrick, 2011, p. 111). *Abandonment* is a form of neglect that involves deserting dependent people with the intent to abandon them or leave them unattended at a place for such a time period as may be likely to endanger their health or welfare (Choi & Mayer, 2000). An example of this would be the failure of an adult child who provides support and supervision for an elderly parent to find a caregiver for the period of time he or she plans to be out of town on vacation.

Elder abuse also occurs in care homes and other institutional settings. **Table 19-5** offers some worrying statistics on elder abuse in U.S. nursing homes. "Abusive acts in institutions include physically restraining patients, depriving them of dignity (by for instance leaving them in soiled clothes) and choice over daily affairs, intentionally providing insufficient care (such as allowing them to develop pressure sores), over- and under-medicating and withholding medication from patients; and emotional neglect and abuse" (WHO, 2011).

COMMUNITY, SOCIAL, AND CIVIC LIFE

White and colleagues (2010) discovered that the availability of public parks, walking areas, handicapped parking, and public transportation were features of neighborhoods that

TABLE 19-5	Institutional Abuse of Elders in the United States

Based on a survey of nursing home staff

36 percent witnessed at least one incident of physical abuse of an elderly patient in the previous year.

10 percent committed at least one act of physical abuse toward an elderly patient.

40 percent admitted to psychologically abusing patients.

Adapted from World Health Organization. (2011). Elder maltreatment Fact sheet N°357. Retrieved from http://www.who.int/mediacentre/factsheets/fs357/en/index.html

TABLE 19-6	Where do Older Adults want to Go?
Essential destinations	Bank, physician's office, pharmacy, grocery store, or shopping superstore
Essential to some	Gas station, church, post office, laboratory, etc. in hospital setting
Nonessentials	Restaurants, senior centers, shopping malls, cemeteries, beauty parlor, hospitals, libraries

greatly influenced community leisure participation for older adults with disabilities. Revisiting the concept of visitability introduced in Chapter 7, older people will be more able to accompany others, including grandchildren, in interacting in playgrounds and museums, if those facilities have established a standard of visitability. Many aspects of visitability are relatively simple and inexpensive. For example, placing benches or other seats near children's play areas and at intervals along walking trails greatly improves the usability of these areas for older people with a disability. **Figure 19-8** shows an older couple sitting on a park bench. Older people often limit their excursion out of fear that they will become too tired. Knowledge that there are benches and places to rest can make them much more open to participation in outdoor activities.

Brown and colleagues (2010) studied 19 people over the age of 65 to determine the types of community ambulation people engaged in and the challenges they experienced (see **Table 19-6**). These researchers defined *essential destinations* as locations that were necessary to meet basic needs including food, clothing, money, and health

care needs. The *essential for some* category added locations that would be necessary to meet basic needs for some but not all of the subjects. *Nonessential* were locations that might be considered quality of life enhancers but were not necessary to meet basic needs. Although this study only included a few people in a limited geographical area, it offers insight into the needs and values of elders with physical limitations.

Kono and colleagues (2004) studied older people (mean age of 83.4 years) and the frequency with which they went outside. They found that the functional capacity of all of the elders in their study tended to decrease over time, but "the scores of functional capacity of participants who went outdoors less than once a week at baseline decreased significantly more than the elders who went outdoors more frequently" (p. 277). These researchers conclude that "the frequency of going outdoors among ambulatory frail elders may be a useful and simple indicator of older persons with functional and psychosocial problems and an important predictor of persons at risk for deterioration" (p. 278).

ENVIRONMENTAL CONTEXTS

There are five main ways in which adults receive ADL and IADL supports in the United States. These are adult day service centers, home health agencies, hospices, nursing homes, and residential care communities. About two-thirds of the care provided to adults with disabilities is provided in residential settings (nursing homes and residential care communities) (Harris-Kojetin, Sengupta, Park-Lee, & Valverde, 2013).

The most familiar of these support systems are nursing homes. There are many colloquial names for nursing homes, including *convalescent home, skilled nursing facility (SNF), rest home,* and *old folk's home.* Although many consider a retirement community such as that described in Chapter 18 a desirable living arrangement, a nursing home is often seen as a last resort, and nursing home institutionalization is considered negative. For this reason, much research on how to prevent institutionalization has been conducted. The other services listed previously have less negative connotations, but they are also more expensive for many communities to run and are not universally available, especially to people in rural or remote areas.

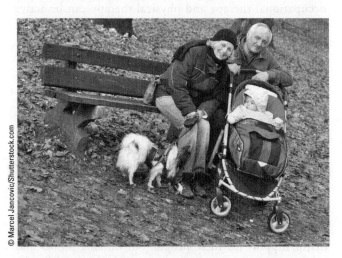

Figure 19-8 This park is "visitable" because it has benches for resting at regular intervals. These grandparents can enjoy the walk without concerns about excessive fatigue.

The risk of needing to have the supports of a nursing home increases with age. Hutchison (2011) reports that only 1.1 percent of older adults between the ages of 65 and 74 reside in nursing homes. Most people in this age range, including most of those with disabilities, live in the community rather than in medical or supervised living settings. Even among adults 85 and older, only 18.25 percent live in nursing homes (Hutchison, 2011). Functional and behavioral impairments are among the most common reasons that older people become institutionalized. Failing health and advancing age are also correlated with institutionalization. Shumway-Cook and Woollacott (2012) reported that the functional physical requirements that are needed for people to remain in community housing are:

- Ability to walk 1,203 feet (366.7 m) to complete an errand in the community

- Gait speed of 1.2 m/s

- Need to carry an average of a 6.7-pound package

- Need to be able to negotiate stairs, curbs, slopes, gravel, grass, uneven pavement

- Need to perform postural transitions—head turns, reaching, looking up, moving backward, and twisting

For people that are unable to continue to function in community housing, whether for physical or cognitive reasons, there are many perceived personal losses. These losses include a loss of control over daily life decisions, a loss of privacy, a loss of relationships, an inability to contribute support to family and friends, and an overall decrease in activity level. Earlier in this chapter, we noted that major depression is seen in about 5 to 10 percent of elders, and subsyndromal depression was seen in 10 to 25 percent of community-dwelling elders. In nursing home residents, major depression was seen in up to 31 percent, and subsyndromal depressive symptoms were seen in up to 75 percent of the population (Choi, Ransom, & Wyllie, 2008).

Choi, Ransom, and Wyllie (2008) report that nursing homes impose environmental and cultural constraints on residents. The constraints may be necessary for health and safety

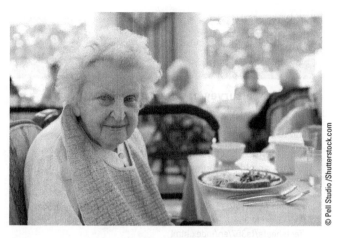

Figure 19-9   Meals in nursing homes may not reflect the preferences and priorities of residents.

reasons, or they may be for the convenience of managing large numbers of people. For example, many nursing homes offer little choice in the food available at mealtimes. In addition, people are expected to sit at a table, wear a bib, and wait patiently for their food to be presented. Food may be ethnically unappealing, people many find a bib infantile, and they may feel degraded in having to sit and wait for assistance while others around them are eating. **Figure 19-9** presents a fairly typical nursing home mealtime arrangement.

Hospice is a specialized type of care for people who are expected to have less than six months to live and who are not seeking a cure for their condition. Hospice care can be provided at home or in a hospice or other freestanding facility, such as a nursing home. The goal of hospice care is to optimize comfort and quality of life. Javier and Montagnini (2011) report that most palliative care patients express a desire to remain physically independent during the course of their disease. Because people in hospice care are highly likely to have physical and emotional challenges, occupational therapy and physical therapy can be active supports in maintaining individuals' highest level of functional ability for as long as possible.

SUMMARY

This chapter has provided an overview of issues associated with disability in its impact on activities and participation in adulthood. This is a broad and diverse topic. Many subjects of particular interest to health care providers were only briefly covered to offer insight into the issue, but will require further study to best understand and address the needs of adults with disabilities. With the improvement in health care and the increasing life span of older people, community and social integration of frail elders will be a growing emphasis in the upcoming years. Increasing public transportation options and building community resources for both household

support and leisure opportunities can help families keep their frail elders in community housing for a longer time.

Another growing social issue will be the care of elderly people with developmental disabilities. Improved health care has extended the life span for many of these people, so that their life span is similar to that of the mainstream adult population. Family caregiving continues to be the major support for these people, but nursing homes and other community care homes are poorly designed for the care of this population. This is of particular concern as the incidence of autism continues to rise. People with autism often have unusual behavior patterns and may not be able to conform to the behavioral expectations in current nursing settings. Many elders with conditions that impact their behavior are faced with physical or chemical restraints when they are placed in institutional care settings. Physical and occupational therapists will have an important role as advocates and as clinicians for both the frail elderly and for aging people with developmental disabilities.

EARLY/MIDDLE ADULT CASE

Mary

Mary is a 40-year-old woman with three children, ages 5, 8, and 10. She was diagnosed with rheumatoid arthritis three years ago. Until recently, she had been managing her symptoms well and has continued to work part-time at a local library, care for her children, and take online courses to work toward a degree in library science. However, after a recent exacerbation of her illness, she has lost more function and now is unable to work or drive. Mary's arthritis causes significant morning stiffness, making it difficult for her to get going in the mornings. Since her children need to catch the school bus at 8:15AM, this is a particular problem for the family. Mary is experiencing increased difficulty with all household activities, especially meal preparation and laundry. Her mother-in-law has been assisting her in these areas on a daily basis. Although Mary appreciates the help from her mother-in-law, their relationship has always been turbulent and conflicted due to personality differences.

To further complicate things, Mary's condition has negatively impacted her intimate relations with her husband. With this and the progressive nature of her condition, Mary feels that she has become a liability to her husband (and she secretly believes her mother-in-law feels the same).

In a typical day she gets up at 7:00 AM, and takes her medicine. She does a short stretching routine then gets the kids going to get ready for school. After the kids leave for school, Mary has her own break-fast. She then rests for about ½ hour and starts doing chores around the house. She works with occasional breaks until about 11:00 AM. After that Mary goes her room to get "fixed up", because she wants to look "presentable" when her mother-in-law comes around noon.

Mary's mother-in-law does the grocery shopping and any of the chores that Mary cannot manage. She also cooks dinner for the family several times a week. Mary knows that she needs the help, but misses cooking and feels "less" of a wife when she cannot feed her family. Miguel, Mary's husband works the early shift and comes home around 1:00 PM. He is tired and goes to bed until about 7 PM when the family shares a meal. He is supportive of Mary and helps when he can, but his work hours make it hard for him to contribute much in the care of the children.

The doctor told Mary that she should exercise regularly to help manage her condition. Mary does not see how this is possible. She has already quit school and work, and still cannot get through the day without outside help. Because she cannot drive, Mary's doctor has recommended therapy services from the home health agency, and although Mary is reluctant, she agrees. Mary does not want to be seen as "handicapped" and "doesn't need anyone else bossing her around".

Guiding Questions

Some questions to consider:

1. Traditional medical approaches to treatment would focus on the physical management of the condition. A "client-centered" approach allows consumers to identify intervention priorities. What would be an advantage of the client-centered approach in Mary's case?
2. Consider Mary's many adult roles that have been interrupted by her arthritis. Mary is most distressed by the limitations in her parenting and homemaking roles. What might be some secondary effects of her inability to conform to her own performance expectations?

OLDER ADULT CASE

Ed

Ed is a 74-year-old widowed male who currently lives alone. He used to run a landscaping business, and enjoyed gardening and doing "handy-man" things around the house and for his neighbors. His wife died nine months ago, and since that time Ed's functional abilities have declined markedly. His two adult children, a son and a daughter, both live over two hours away from him, but each child and their families see him at least once a month. Ed's daughter, Sarah, is a registered nurse and has noticed several concerns in the last two months. She observed that Ed has lost at least 20 pounds and that he frequently has spoiled food in his refrigerator. Ed has also stopped his daily habit of going to the local coffee shop for breakfast with his group of friends. Sarah suspects that Ed is not taking his medications correctly and that he has had several falls, though Ed denies both of these concerns, stating, "I'm fine, really." Ed's son, Sam, has noticed that his father is not attending to the yard work or household chores with his usual interest and skill level. Ed has moderate osteoarthritis, hypertension, low back pain, and a history of a heart attack six years ago. When Ed's wife was living, she motivated him to take care of himself, but now Ed states, "What's the difference?" when prodded by his children to take better care of his health.

The things that are likely to help him function well enough to stay in his home are to have a very structured daily schedule, eat healthy foods, regular exercise and engage in activities that interest him. Ed wants to stay in his own home, and has agreed to ride the senior van to the rehab center twice weekly for an exercise and wellness program run by the rehabilitation department.

Guiding Questions

Some questions to consider:

1. In losing his wife, Ed has also lost many of his interpersonal relationships and many of his valued roles. As his therapist, how could you help him engage with others and build new supportive social relationships?
2. Ed is not interested in cell phones or "apps" to help him manage his health. Think of some low-tech strategies to help Ed remember to eat and to engage in physical activity?

Speaking of
Hanging On to Loved Ones and Home

CORRIE A. MANCINELLI, PT, PhD, CONSULTANT PHYSICAL
THERAPIST TO THE WEST VIRGINIA UNIVERSITY 65+ CLINIC

It is hard to tell a patient that he can no longer safely provide care for his chronically ill wife. This is a true, yet not unique, experience I have had as a therapist.

Mr. A is an 80-year-old gentleman with severe ankylosing spondylitis who sustained a fracture around a total hip replacement. His wife has Parkinson's disease. Mr. A provided care for Mrs. A until the fracture. This acute event

Continues

Speaking of   Continued

interfered with Mr. A's abilities to function in his own home. He was no longer able to care for himself, let alone Mrs. A. They lived in a first-floor apartment with barriers such as thick carpet and a very small bathroom. She spent most of her time in a wheelchair and had a history of falling. He was ambulatory with a rolling walker, but his mobility was markedly limited. He certainly was not able to help her with transfers, bathing, dressing, or meal preparation.

After four months of admissions to acute care hospitals and rehabilitation facilities followed by extensive home health and outpatient rehabilitation, Mr. A recovered enough to provide care for himself, but not for his wife. Mrs. A was no longer a candidate for home health services covered under Medicare because of limited potential to improve. Neither Mr. nor Mrs. A was eligible for daily aid services provided by the local senior center. The only option for care that remained for her was an extended care nursing facility. Mrs. A was willing to accept that she was no longer able to remain at home. She did not want to burden her husband. He, on the other hand, was distraught about not being able to provide for her. He did not want to accept the fact that it was unsafe for both of them to remain in their apartment. He felt as though he was "letting down the love of his life." His core family values were also being disrupted because he was taught from a very young age to take care of all family, no matter how large the task. Mr. A was losing his sense of purpose. He had to rely on his only daughter to visit daily, bathe his wife, cook their meals, and put her to bed. His daughter did this in addition to working full-time and being a mother of two busy teenage boys. She became worn from providing the intensity of care that was needed. In a very short time, Mr. A became aware that the circumstance was emotionally and physically draining for his daughter and unsafe for his wife. He recognized that it was time for Mrs. A to become a resident in an extended care nursing facility. He said, "It is selfish of me to want my wife at home now."

Mr. and Mrs. A celebrated their last evening of being together at home as a couple for 50-plus years. They did so with a mutual respect and a deep love for each other. Mrs. A went to the nursing home the next day. Now Mr. A calls and visits Mrs. A daily. He reports that he feels lonely at times without her but recognizes that she is safer in the nursing home.

Sometimes people are not able to see dangerous home situations because they are not willing to accept disability for themselves or their loved ones. Mr. A was unrealistic about his disablement and ability to provide care for his wife. For health care providers, it is important not only to respect family values and traditions as much as possible, but to also see the dangers that prevail in life circumstances that are unstable because of injury or disease. Mr. A once again has a sense of purpose because he knows that his wife looks forward to his phone calls and visits. He also has learned that he still can provide for her emotional needs, even though he cannot provide for her physical needs. During a recent follow-up phone call, he said to me that his "love for her exceeds his need for her." He didn't realize that he contributed to my understanding of care and support of family just through that statement. I will carry that with me throughout my remaining professional years.

REFERENCES

Albrecht, G., Seelman, K., & Bury, M. (2001). *Handbook of disability studies.* Thousand Oaks, CA: Sage Publications.

Allen, D. G., Lowe, K., Moore, K., & Brophy, S. (2007). Predictors, costs and characteristics of out of area placement for people with intellectual disability and challenging behaviour. *Journal of Intellectual Disability Research, 51,* 409–416.

American Academy of Neurology. (2007). Walking and moderate exercise help prevent dementia. *ScienceDaily.* Retrieved from http://www.sciencedaily.com/releases/2007/12/071219202948.htm

Arthritis Foundation. (2012). *What is rheumatoid arthritis?* Retrieved from http://www.arthritis.org/types-what-is-rheumatoid-arthritis.php

The Arc. (2012). Intellectual disability. Retrieved from http://www.thearc.org/page.aspx?pid=2543

Barnartt, S., & Scotch, R. (2001). *Disability protests: Contentious politics 1970–1999.* Washington, D.C.: Gallaudet University Press.

Battistin, L., & Cagnin, A. (2010). Vascular cognitive disorder. A biological and clinical overview. *Neurochemistry Research, 35,* 1933–1938.

Bianco, M., Garrison-Wade, D. F., Tobin, R., & Lehmann, J. P. (2009). Parents' perceptions of postschool years for young adults with developmental disabilities. *Intellectual & Developmental Disabilities, 47*(3), 186–196.

Bittles, A., Petterson, B., Sullivan, S., Hussain, R., Glasson, E., & Montgomery, P. (2002). The influence of intellectual disability on life expectancy. *The Journals of Gerontology Series A: Biological Science and Medical Science, 57,* 470–472.

Bonder, B., & Bello-Haas, V. (2009). *Functional performance in older adults* (3rd ed.). Philadelphia: F.A. Davis.

Bowman, R. A., Scotti, J. R., & Morris, T. L. (2010). Sexual abuse prevention: A training program for developmental disabilities service providers. *Journal of Child Sexual Abuse, 19*(2), 119–127.

Brown, C., and Stoffel, V. (Eds.) (2011). Occupational therapy in mental health: A vision for participation. Philadelphia: F.A. Davis.

Brown, C., Bradberry, C., Howze, S., Hickman, L., Ray, H., & Peel, C. (2010). Defining community ambulation from the perspective of the older adult. *Journal of Geriatric Physical Therapy, 33,* 56–63.

Burwell, B., & Jackson, B. (1994). *The disabled elderly and their use of long-term care.* U.S. Department of Health and Human Services. Retrieved from http://aspe.hhs.gov/daltcp/reports/diseldes.htm#chap2

Carter, E., Austin, D., & Trainor, A. A. (2012). Predictors of post-school employment outcomes for young adults with severe disabilities. *Journal of Disability Policy Studies, 23*(1), 50–63.

Centers for Disease Control and Prevention (CDC). (2011). 47.5 million U.S. adults report a disability: Arthritis remains most common cause. *CDC Features.* Retrieved from http://www.cdc.gov/Features/dsAdultDisabilityCauses/

Centers for Disease Control and Prevention (CDC). (2012). Chronic diseases are the leading cause of death and disability in the U.S. *Chronic Disease Prevention and Health*

Choi, N. G., & Mayer, J. (2000). Elder abuse, neglect, and exploitation. *Journal of Gerontological Social Work, 33*(4), 5–25.

Choi, N. G., Ransom, S., & Wyllie, R. J. (2008). Depression in older nursing home residents: The influence of nursing home environmental stressors, coping, and acceptance of group and individual therapy. *Aging & Mental Health, 12*(5), 536–547.

Cleveland Clinic. (2012). *Types of dementia.* Retrieved from http://my.clevelandclinic.org/disorders/dementia/hic_types_of_dementia.aspx

Cohen-Mansfield, J., Shmotkin, D., & Hazan, H. (2010). The effect of homebound status on older persons. *Journal of the American Geriatrics Society, 58*(12), 2358–2362.

Cote, F. (2011). Removing barriers to college education for disabled veterans. *Rappaport Briefing* (August 24, 2011). Retrieved from http://rappaportbriefing.net/2011/08/24/removing-barriers-to-college-education-for-disabled-veterans/

Daniels, R., van Rossum, E., Metzelthin, S., Sipers, W., Habets, H., Hobma, S., van den Heuvel, W., & de Witte, L. (2011). A disability prevention programme for community-dwelling frail older persons. *Clinical Rehabilitation, 25*(11), 963–974.

Erickson, W., Lee, C., & von Schrader, S. (2010). *Disability statistics from the 2008 American Community Survey (ACS).* Ithaca, NY: Cornell University Rehabilitation Research and Training Center on Disability Demographics and Statistics. Retrieved from www.disabilitystatistics.org

Esbensen, A. J., Greenberg, J. S., Mailick Seltzer, M., & Aman, M. G. (2009). A longitudinal investigation of psychotropic and non-psychotropic medication use among adolescents and adults with autism spectrum disorders. *Journal of Autism and Developmental Disorders, 39,* 1339–1349.

Fisher, M. H., Moskowitz, A. L., & Hodapp, R. M. (2012). Vulnerability and experiences related to social victimization among individuals with intellectual and developmental disabilities. *Journal of Mental Health Research In Intellectual Disabilities, 5,* 32–48.

Ganz, M. L. (2006). The costs of autism. In S. O. Moldin & J. L. R. Rubenstein (Eds.), *Understanding autism* (pp. 475–502). Boca Raton, FL: CRC Press.

Global Initiative for Chronic Obstructive Lung Disease. (2011). Global strategy for the diagnosis, management, and prevention of chronic obstructive pulmonary disease (rev. 2011). Retrieved from http://www.goldcopd.org/uploads/users/files/GOLD_Report_2011_Feb21.pdf

Guarascio, A., Ray, S., Finch, C., & Self, T. (2013). The clinical and economic burden of chronic obstructive pulmonary disease in the USA. *Clinicoeconomics and Outcomes Research: CEOR, 5235*–5245. doi:10.2147/CEOR.S34321

Harris-Kojetin, L., Sengupta, M., Park-Lee, E., & Valverde, R. (2013). *Long-term care services in the United States: 2013 overview.* Hyattsville, MD: National Center for Health Statistics.

Havercamp, S., Scandlin, D., & Roth, M. (2004). Health disparities among adults with developmental disabilities, adults with other disabilities, and adults not reporting disability in North Carolina. *Public Health Reports, 119,* 418–426.

Hayslip, B., Patrick, J., & Panek, P. (2011). *Adult development and aging* (5th ed.). Malabar, FL: Krieger Publishing Company.

Heller, T., & Arnold, C. (2010). Siblings of adults with developmental disabilities: Psychosocial outcomes, relationships, and future planning. *Journal of Policy & Practice in Intellectual Disabilities, 7,* 16–25.

Hutchison, E. (2011). *Dimensions of human behavior: The changing life course* (4th ed.). Thousand Oaks, CA: Sage Publications.

Javier, N. C., & Montagnini, M. L. (2011). Rehabilitation of the hospice and palliative care patient. *Journal of Palliative Medicine, 14*(5), 638–648.

Kono, A., Rubenstein, L., Kai, I., & Sakato, C. (2004). Frequency of going outdoors: A predictor of functional and psychosocial change among ambulatory frail elders living at home. *Journals of Gerontology Series A: Biological Sciences & Medical Sciences, 59A,* 275–280.

Loh, K., & Ogle, J. (2004). Age related visual impairment in the elderly. *The Medical Journal of Malaysia, 59*(4), 562–568.

Lyness, J. M. (2008). Naturalistic outcomes of minor and subsyndromal depression in older primary care patients. *International Journal of Geriatric Psychiatry, 23*(8), 773–781.

Lyness, J. M., Moonseong, H., Datto, C. J., Have, T., Katz, I. R., Drayer, R., Reynolds, C., Alexopoulos, G., & Bruce, M. L. (2006). Outcomes of minor and subsyndromal depression among elderly patients in primary care settings. *Annals of Internal Medicine, 144*(7), 496–504, W84.

Manente, C., Maraventano, C., LaRue, R., Delmolino, L., & Sloan, D. (2010). Effective behavioral intervention for adults on the autism spectrum: Best practices in functional assessment and treatment development. *The Behavior Analyst Today, 11,* 36–48.

Martorell, A., & Tsakanikos E. (2008). Traumatic experiences and life events in people with intellectual disability. *Current Opinion in Psychiatry, 21,* 445–448.

Mayo Clinic. (2011). *Post-traumatic stress disorder (PTSD).* Retrieved from http://www.mayoclinic.com/health/post-traumatic-stress-disorder/DS00246

Mayo Clinic. (2012). *Anxiety.* Retrieved from http://www.mayoclinic.com/health/anxiety/DS01187

Meulenkamp, T. M., Cardol, M., van der Hoek, L. S., Francke, A. L., & Rijken, M. (2013). Participation of People with Physical Disabilities: Three-Year Trend and Potential for Improvement. *Archives of Physical Medicine & Rehabilitation, 94, 5, 944-950.* doi:10.1016/j.apmr.2012.12.017

Migliore, A., Mank, D., Grossi, T., & Rogan, P. (2007). Integrated employment or sheltered workshops: Preferences of adults with intellectual disabilities, their families, and staff. *Journal Of Vocational Rehabilitation, 26*(1), 5–19.

Miniño, A., Xu, J., Kochanek, K., & Tejada-Vera, B. (2009). Death in the United States, 2007. *NCHS Data Brief, 26.* Retrieved from http://www.cdc.gov/nchs/data/databriefs/db26.htm

Naditz, A. (2003, July). Deeply affected: As the nation ages, Alzheimer's will strike more people close to us. *Contemporary Long-Term Care,* 20–23.

National Heart, Lung, and Blood Institute. (2012). Morbidity and mortality: 2012 chart book on cardiovascular, lung, and blood diseases. Retrieved from http://www.nhlbi.nih.gov/research/reports/2012-mortality-chart-book.htm

National Institute on Mental Health. (NIMH) (2012). *Anxiety disorders.* Retrieved from http://www.nimh.nih.gov/health/topics/anxiety-disorders/index.shtml

Pagán, R. (2013). Time allocation of disabled individuals, *Social Science and Medicine,* 84, 80-93.

Pitts, D. (2011). Work as occupation. In C. Brown & V. Stoffel (Eds.), *Occupational therapy in mental health: A vision for participation* (Chapter 50; pp. 695–710). Philadelphia: F. A. Davis.

Pouryamout, L., Dams, J., Wasem, J., Dodel, R., & Neumann, A. (2012). Economic evaluation of treatment options in patients with Alzheimer's disease: A systematic review of cost-effectiveness analyses. *Drugs, 72*(5), 789–802.

Shumway-Cook, A., & Woollacott, M. (2012). *Motor control: Translating research into clinical practice* (4th ed., pp. 1–20). Baltimore: Lippincott, Williams and Wilkins.

Sprout. (2014). *Sprout: Our mission.* Retrieved from http://gosprout.org/about-us/

Tanielian, T., Jaycox, L., Schell, T., Marshall, G. Burnam, M., Eibner, C., Karney, B., Meredith, L., Ringel, J., & Vaiana, M. (2008). Invisible wounds, mental health and cognitive care needs of America's returning veterans. *Rand Research Brief.* Retrieved from http://www.rand.org/pubs/research_briefs/RB9336.html

U.S. Department of Labor. (2012). Current disability employment statistics, July 2012. Retrieved from http://www.dol.gov/odep/

U.S. Senate Committee on Health, Education, Labor, and Pensions (USSCHELP). (2012a). Unfinished business: Making employment of people with disabilities a national priority. Retrieved from http://harkin.senate.gov/documents/pdf/500469b49b364.pdf

U.S. Senate Committee on Health, Education, Labor, and Pensions (USSCHLP). (2012b). *HELP committee releases report, recommendations on disability employment.* Retrieved from http://www.help.senate.gov/newsroom/press/release/?id=fbf20a90-cad2-4ba8-a236-df6bbc623a8a

van Ingen, D., & Moore, L. (2010). How parents maintain healthy involvement with their adult children: A qualitative study. *Journal of Developmental & Physical Disabilities, 22*(6), 533–547.

White, D. K., Jette, A. M., Felson, D. T., Lavalley, M. P., Lewis, C. E., Torner, J. C., & . . . Keysor, J. J. (2010). Are features of the neighborhood environment associated with disability in older adults? *Disability & Rehabilitation, 32*(8), 639–645.

Winsor, J. (2012). State intellectual and developmental disability agencies' service trends. StateData. *Info Data Note, 38.* Retrieved from http://www.statedata.info/datanotes/datanote.php?article_id=337

Wittchen, H., & Uhmann, S. (2010). The timing of depression: An epidemiological perspective. *Medicographia, 32,* 115–125.

Wehmeyer, M., Bersani, H., & Gagne, R. (2000). Riding the third wave: Self-determination and self-advocacy in the 21st century. *Focus on Autism & Other Developmental Disabilities, 15*(2), 106–115.

World Health Organization. (2011). Elder maltreatment. *Fact Sheet, 357.* Retrieved from http://www.who.int/mediacentre/factsheets/fs357/en/index.html

World Health Organization. (2012). *Elder abuse: What is elder abuse.* Retrieved from http://www.who.int/ageing/projects/elder_abuse/en/

World Health Organization/World Bank (WHO/WB). (2011). *World report on disability.* Geneva, Switzerland: World Health Organization. Retrieved from http://whqlibdoc.who.int/hq/2011/WHO_NMH_VIP_11.01_eng.pdf

Yoshida, S. (2007). *A global report on falls prevention: Epidemiology of falls.* World Health Organisation. Retrieved from http://www.who.int/ageing/projects/1.Epidemiology%20of%20falls%20in%20older%20age.pdf

CHAPTER 20

Wellness, Prevention, and Health Promotion

Ralph Utzman, PT, MPH, PhD,
West Virginia University School of
Medicine, Division of Physical Therapy
and

Anne Cronin, PhD, OTR, FAOTA,
West Virginia University School of
Medicine, Division of Occupational
Therapy

Objectives

Upon completion of this chapter, readers should be able to:

- Explain how health beliefs influence wellness and prevention;

- Discuss the strengths and weaknesses of common measures of health status;

- Describe the disability paradox and the importance of consideration of self-assessed health in addressing the needs of health care clients;

- Provide an example, relevant to your profession, of a population health initiative;

- Define prevention and differentiate the three types of prevention presented in this chapter;

- Differentiate the two health measures, life expectancy and healthy life expectancy, in terms of their impact on individuals and on you as a health professional; and

- Explain the relevance of social cognitive theory and the transtheoretical model to wellness and prevention programs in your profession.

Key Terms

disability paradox

health behavior

health belief model

health promotion

health-related quality
  of life (HRQOL)

Healthy People 2020

incidence

life expectancy

Lifestyle Redesign

morbidity

mortality

National Prevention Strategy

Patient Protection and Affordable
  Care Act (ACA)

population health

prevalence

prevention

prevention programs

primary prevention

secondary prevention

self-assessed health

social cognitive theory

tertiary prevention

transtheoretical model

wellness

INTRODUCTION

The opening chapter of this book introduced readers to the concepts of human health and function. According to the World Health Organization's International Classification of Functioning, Disability and Health (ICF) (2001) presented in Chapter 1, health is determined by a combination of physical, emotional, and social factors over a person's life span. The concept of health is important at both the individual and population levels. Individuals who are healthy in the broadest sense are engaged in life and society. They learn, work, and contribute to their communities through social and economic interaction. This chapter will introduce readers to basic concepts of wellness, prevention, and health promotion, with an emphasis on applying these concepts to populations, as well as individuals.

There is no universally accepted definition of the term *wellness*. **Wellness** is a "condition of good physical, emotional, and mental health,…" (*The American Heritage Medical Dictionary*, 2007), which is similar to the World Health Organization (WHO) definition, but which adds "… especially when maintained by an appropriate diet, exercise, and other lifestyle modifications." Wellness not only is the absence of illness but also includes the motivation to be involved in life, to have a sense of control over one's actions, and to desire interaction and connection with other individuals, and perhaps most prominently, wellness enhances our sense of self-esteem and self-worth. Wellness may also be viewed as a blending of the physical, psychosocial, and spiritual realms. Wellness is a triangulated concept where, if all components work in concert, a positive outcome is achieved.

A second definition important to this chapter is the definition of prevention. **Prevention** is the management of factors that could lead to impairment, disease, or disability so as to maintain and support optimal levels of function and participation. *Life course theory (LCT)* is a conceptual framework to explain health and disease patterns across populations of people over time described in length in Chapter 2. The long-term temporal perspective of LCT allows for a focus on the development of health behaviors and trajectories in development, and has a strong prevention focus for both individuals and populations.

Finally, **health promotion** is the provision of information that makes positive contributions to the health of consumers, whether they are individuals, families, employers, or community groups. Health promotion is also the promotion of healthy ideas and concepts to motivate individuals to adopt healthy behaviors. The World Health Organization's Bangkok Charter for Health Promotion in a Globalized World (WHO, 2005) defines health promotion as "the process of enabling people to increase control over their health and its determinants, and thereby improve their health." This is a broad viewpoint that includes not only education and social marketing focused on changing behavioral risk factors, but also considers the prerequisites of health such as housing, nutrition, and employment.

POPULATION HEALTH AND HEALTHY PEOPLE 2020

Kindig and Stoddart (2003) define **population health** as "the health outcomes of a group of individuals, including the distribution of such outcomes within a group." A population can refer to a group as large as the world's entire population or as small as a group of students in a rural first-grade classroom. The term *population health* is often used synonymously with "community health." Programs to improve or protect the health of populations can be sponsored, designed, and delivered by a wide range of individuals (health providers or teachers, for example) and

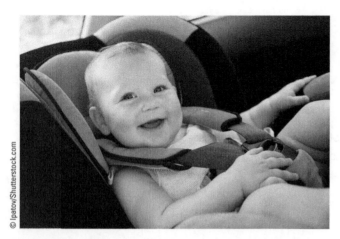

Figure 20-1 Child safety seats are required for infants throughout the United States.

organizations (such as businesses, associations, and governments). One example of a government program to prevent injury is the mandated use of child safety seats, such as the one shown in **Figure 20-1**, for young children traveling in private vehicles. Although child safety seat legislation varies between states in the United States, these policies overall have significantly reduced fatality rates among children 0 to 5 years of age (Houston, Richardson, & Neeley, 2001). This is an issue of interest to health care professionals because some children with disabilities may not be able to sit in a standard child seat, and may need supportive seating in vehicles for much longer than typically developing children. Similarly, some parents with disabilities may not be able to manage a standard child care seat, making it difficult for them to safely transport their child.

Improving population health is important because it helps support successful aging and leads to an improved quality of life for all people. It is also important because the financial costs of many chronic diseases, such as heart disease, diabetes, and cancer, are staggering. For example, the direct medical cost of treating people in the United States with cardiovascular disease was $273 billion in 2010 (Heidenreich et al., 2011). These costs are expected to triple by 2030, when it is projected that over 40 percent of the population will have some form of cardiovascular disease. The indirect costs of cardiovascular disease, which takes into account the loss in productivity that accompanies serious illness, were estimated to be $172 billion in 2010 and are expected to double by 2030 (Heidenreich et al., 2011).

In the United States, the federal government has developed the Healthy People initiative to focus efforts to improve the health of the nation. In 1979, the U.S. Surgeon General published *Healthy People: The Surgeon General's Report on Health Promotion and Disease Prevention* (U.S. Department of Health and Human Services, 2012). The initial report represented the consensus of a broad coalition of federal, state, and local government agencies and numerous national organizations. Every decade since, the

Healthy People document has been revised and updated with new goals for measuring and improving population health. The newest iteration, *Healthy People 2020*, includes almost 600 objectives encompassing 42 different topic areas (U.S. Department of Health and Human Services, 2012). The mission of this initiative includes five major goals: (1) to identify nationwide health improvement priorities; (2) to increase public awareness and understanding of the determinants of health, disease, and disability and the opportunities for progress; (3) to provide measurable objectives and goals that are applicable at the national, state, and local levels; (4) to engage multiple societal sectors to take actions to strengthen policies and improve practices that are driven by the best available evidence and knowledge; and finally, (5) to identify critical research, evaluation, and data collection needs (U.S. Department of Health and Human Services, 2012). A full list of Healthy People 2020 topic areas and objectives can be found at www.healthypeople.gov.

The Healthy People 2020 objectives seek to improve the health of the nation on four categories of health indicators: measures of health status, health-related quality of life, health disparities, and determinants of health (U.S. Department of Health and Human Services, 2012). Each of these four categories will be described briefly to provide greater understanding of health on a population scale.

MEASURES OF HEALTH STATUS

Various epidemiologic statistics are used to measure and describe the health status of populations. These are broadly categorized as measures of mortality and morbidity. **Mortality** refers to the death rate, or the number of people dying during a given period in time. Mortality can be measured for an overall population, or can be measured relative to certain subgroups (for example, infant mortality, discussed earlier in the text) or health conditions (for example, deaths from cancer). **Life expectancy** is a related concept that estimates how long a person is expected to live at a certain point in time. Life expectancy can be estimated from birth or from a specific age. For example, the average life expectancy of a child born in 2009 is 78.5 years, while the average person turning 65 in 2009 can expect to live another 19.2 years (Kochanek, Xu, Murphy, Minino, & Kung, 2011). A newer, important, related concept is healthy life expectancy. *Healthy life expectancy* is the average number of healthy years people can expect to live if age-specific death rates and age-specific morbidity rates remain the same throughout their lifetime. This is an especially useful measure for long-range population-level research and planning, because it provides a "snapshot" of current death and illness patterns that can be used to help us understand the long-range implications of the death and illness rates (U.S. Department of Health and Human Services, 2012).

Measures of **morbidity** reflect the burden of disease in a population. **Incidence** measures the number of new cases of a health condition occurring in a population during a certain period of time. For instance, in 2008, the incidence of cancer in the United States was 462/100,000 (U.S. Cancer Statistics Working Group, 2012), meaning 462 people out of every 100,000 U.S. residents were diagnosed with cancer that year. **Prevalence**, on the other hand, measures the number of people who have a health condition at a particular point in time. As of the end of 2009, the estimated prevalence of HIV in the United States (that is, the number of people living with HIV infection) was 1.1 million (Centers for Disease Control and Prevention, 2012). Like mortality, measures of morbidity can be calculated and reported for various subgroups (age ranges, gender, race/ethnicity, socioeconomic status, and so on). Measuring morbidity and mortality in a population over time allows us to identify and track health problems. This, in turn, allows policy makers to establish goals and priorities for reducing health problems and improving longevity of a population or group. Many of the Healthy People 2020 goals are based on epidemiologic measures. Once these goals and priorities are established, efforts to address the goals can be developed.

Another widely used measure of health status is a self-assessment of health. Self-assessment of health is a measure of how people perceive their health—rating it as excellent, very good, good, fair, or poor. One of the interesting findings presented in Chapter 18 is that many older people with chronic health conditions rate themselves as being in good health. **Self-assessed health** is individuals' perception of their general well-being and quality of life rather than an objective evaluation of disease. This measure is widely used because there is a strong association between poor self-assessed health and other traditional health indicators including morbidity, mortality, and physical disability (Cummings & Jackson, 2008).

A final health status measure used in Healthy People 2020 that is of particular relevance to physical and occupational therapists is called *limitation of activity*. The limitation of activity measure refers to any reported long-term reduction in people's ability to do their usual activities. This health indicator has been especially helpful in improving our understanding of aging. Much of the data about the performance patterns of older adults in activities of daily living and instrumental activities of daily living presented earlier in this text have been gathered by surveys that measure limitation of activity. Limitation of activity measures have been effective in enhancing our understanding of patterns of activity and participation for individuals with both physical and mental health problems (Du Mont & Forte, 2014). People with limitations of activity may also have decreased access to and utilization of health care services.

HEALTH-RELATED QUALITY OF LIFE

Earlier in this text, *quality of life* was defined as a perception of fulfillment both of basic and of complex needs in daily life, leading to life satisfaction. As health professionals, we often focus on quality of life in individuals. Quality of life can also be considered in other contexts. Measures of morbidity and mortality can be seen as measures of quantity of health in a population. Measures of **health-related quality of life (HRQOL)** seek to measure and describe the impact health status has on quality of life in both individuals and groups. Health-related quality of life measures typically include multiple qualitative dimensions, including mental/emotional health, functional status, social support, and socioeconomic status. HRQOL is an especially useful measure because it assesses the positive aspects of a person's life, such as positive emotions and life satisfaction as well as the negative aspects, which are the focus of more traditional health measures. Another advantage to using HRQOL measures is that previous studies have shown significant disparity between self-report and proxy reports of quality of life for individuals with disabilities. Thompson and colleagues (2012) noted that "more than 50 percent of adults with serious and persistent disabilities reported good or excellent HRQOL despite living a daily life that other individuals might regard as less than optimal" (p. 496). This difference noted between self-reported health and assessment of health by others is called the **disability paradox** (Thompson et al., 2012). This paradox emphasizes that individual perceptions of well-being and quality of life are influenced by things other than the absence of disease or disability. As we consider quality of life, it is always important to understand the viewpoint of individuals who are clients and to respond to their perceived needs.

Over the upcoming decade, Healthy People 2020 will monitor HRQOL in the United States through patient-reported outcome measures, well-being measures, and participation measures. One example of a tool used to measure HRQOL is the Short Form (36) Health Survey, or SF-36 (Ware & Sherbourne, 1992). This survey tool and others related to HRQOL are described in greater detail in Chapter 22 of this text. The Healthy People initiative includes objectives related to the evaluation and development of other tools to measure HRQOL on both an individual and a population level.

DETERMINANTS OF HEALTH

Population health is dependent on a number of factors. *Determinants of health*, as described in Healthy People 2020, include diverse influences including biology, genetics, individual behavior, access to health services, and the environment in which people are born, live, learn, play, work, and age (U.S. Department of Health and Human Services, 2012). The Healthy People initiative focuses on five broad determinants of health: biology, social factors, health services, public policy, and personal behavior. **Table 20-1** shows how these determinants relate to various components of the ICF model.

TABLE 20-1	Comparison of Determinants of Health and the ICF Model
Determinants of Health*	**ICF Model**
Biology	Health condition
Social factors	Contextual factors (external)
Health services	Contextual factors (external)
Public policy	Contextual factors (external)
Behavior	Contextual factors (internal)

*US Department of Health and Human Services. (2012). Healthy people. Retrieved October 28, 2012 from http://www.healthypeople .gov/2020/default.aspx

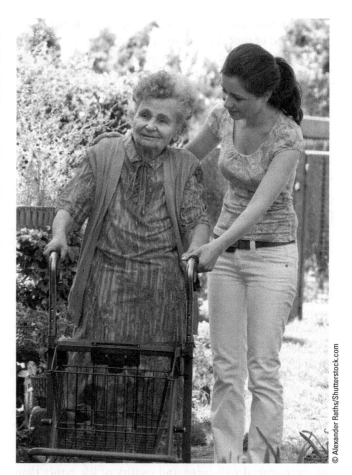

Figure 20-2   In the elderly, outdoor falls are significantly more frequent than indoor falls.

Note that each determinant may influence other determinants, similar to the interaction between the various components of the ICF model. Consider the issue of falls among older adults. One in three adults 65 or older falls each year (Hausdorff, Rios, & Edelberg, 2001), and one in five falls causes serious injury (Stevens, 2006). In 2010, the direct medical cost of falls among older adults in the United States was $30 billion (Stevens, Corso, Finkelstein, & Miller, 2006). Falls among older adults can be caused by a myriad of interrelated factors (Panel on Prevention of Falls in Older Persons, American Geriatrics Society and British Geriatrics Society, 2011). Biologic factors include poor vision, muscle weakness, and impairments in gait and balance. Environmental factors greatly impact fall risks. Outdoor falls are more frequent than indoor falls (57.5 versus 42.5 percent), and bathrooms are the most frequent indoor place for falls (Bergland, Jarnlo, & Laake, 2003). Those most vulnerable to fall are people such as the woman pictured in **Figure 20-2** who has already had a fall, has impaired gait, and osteoporosis.

Social factors include the characteristics of the environment, such as the presence of stairs or other structural barriers, and the availability of social support at home (Panel on Prevention of Falls in Older Persons, American Geriatrics Society and British Geriatrics Society, 2011). Without access to qualify health care, older adults may not receive adequate screening for fall risks. Without such screenings, at-risk seniors will likely not be referred to physical or occupational therapists who can design individualized programs to reduce fall risk. Regular review of medications is also important, as the use of multiple medications has been identified as a risk factor for falls in older people. The costs of caring for older adults following a fall has garnered the attention of policy makers, so now health care providers are encouraged financially by the Medicare system to routinely screen older adults for fall risk. Finally, individuals can influence their own fall risk through their own personal

behaviors. Engaging in regular exercise has been shown to reduce fall risk (Panel on Prevention of Falls in Older Persons, American Geriatrics Society and British Geriatrics Society, 2011).

HEALTH DISPARITIES

Health disparities, as discussed earlier in this text, are differences in health, health services, and health outcomes between population groups or subgroups. Simply stated, some members of the U.S. population are in poorer health than others. Race/ethnicity, gender, disability status, rural versus urban living, and sexual orientation are examples of group characteristics that are often related to health disparities (U.S. Department of Health and Human Services, 2012). For example, African Americans tend to have higher rates of mortality from heart disease than other Americans, yet are less likely to receive lifesaving heart care like bypass surgery, angioplasty, and cardiac rehabilitation (Mead, Cartwright-Smith, Jones, Ramos, & Siegel, 2008). These differences may be due, in part, to socioeconomic and educational differences and variations in access to and utilization of health care. Healthy People 2020 establishes several goals related to better understanding and addressing disparities in our population.

IMPROVING THE HEALTH OF COMMUNITIES

The process for improving the health of a community is similar in many ways to the process rehabilitation therapists use when caring for individual clients. Each therapist performs an examination, works with the clients to devise and prioritize goals, plans and implements therapeutic interventions, and monitors progress and outcomes. **Table 20-2** compares the physical therapy patient/client management model (American Physical Therapy Association, 2003) to the process for community health programs.

In many settings, interprofessional teams collaborate in the provision of community health programs. Community health program development is a process that should begin by identifying community partners and building a coalition of individuals and groups who are also interested in improving community health. Options include individual health care providers, hospitals and other health care organizations, employers, schools, churches, government agencies, and public officials. Partnering with others can help build rapport within the community, reduce duplication, and allow different segments of the community to pool their resources around shared goals. Programs can be very focused, such as aquatic exercise programs for seniors, or more general, such as the provision of screening services at public health fairs. Programs can focus on helping people find useful community resources, they can provide consumer information on a topic such as fall prevention, or they can actually develop a community program for consumers to enroll in such as the aquatic exercise program mentioned earlier.

An interesting approach to the health of communities is an intervention strategy developed in the field of occupational therapy focused on building healthy habits and behaviors. This program, **Lifestyle Redesign**, is an approach to improving health and wellness by preventing and managing chronic conditions through building healthier lifestyles through community-based small groups led by a trained facilitator. This approach was developed through research in Well Elderly studies (Clark & Azen, 1997; Clark et al. 2001). The premise is straightforward and focuses on the process of acquiring health-promoting habits and routines in people's daily life. This small group-based intervention centered on structured group discussion and activities focuses on eight topics: introduction to the power of occupations; aging, health, and occupation; transportation; safety; social relationships; cultural awareness; finances; and an integrative summary. Participants in the Lifestyle Redesign intervention in the Well Elderly studies involved both healthy elders from a culturally diverse group of urban dwellers, and later a group of elders at high risk for developing health disparities. Both research trials documented positive changes in the intervention groups in the areas of enhanced physical health, improved mental health, superior occupational functioning, and increased life satisfaction (Clark & Azen, 1997; Clark et al. 2001).

For wellness and prevention programs such as fall prevention programs and Lifestyle Redesign programs to work, clinicians need to build partnerships in their communities and be client-centered in their interactions. Building partnerships is instrumental in identifying the needs of the community from the community's perspective. Options for gathering data from the community include research surveys, interviewing "key informants" or community leaders, and hosting community forums or focus group interviews. The qualitative information gleaned from this process can be used to clarify and supplement existing quantitative data. Existing data regarding community health can be gathered from a variety of sources, including federal, state, county, and city

---

TABLE 20-2 Physical Therapist Patient-Client Management Model Compared with Community Health Interventions

Patient-Client Management*	Community Health
Examination (including history taking, tests, and measures)	Community needs assessment (including review of existing data, gathering information from the community)
Evaluation, diagnosis, prognosis	Setting goals and priorities
Intervention	Intervention
Reexamination	Monitoring
Outcome (improvements in activities and participation)	Outcome (improvements in morbidity, mortality, etc.)

*Basics of patient/client management. Guide to Physical Therapist Practice (revised 2nd edition) (2003). Alexandria, VA: American Physical Therapy Association.

agencies. The Centers for Disease Control and Prevention, part of the U.S. Department of Health and Human Services, works with state and county governments to monitor birth rates, mortality, and morbidity from a variety of acute and chronic diseases. This information is available to the public at www.cdc.gov/DataStatistics/. Most state governments also provide websites that report public health data; many states provide county-level data as well. Another good source for existing public health data is the Kaiser Family Foundation's website www.statehealthfacts.org. This site allows users to compare states and the nation on numerous indicators of morbidity, mortality, and socioeconomic indicators.

Once the health needs of a community have been identified, priorities and objectives can be developed. Objectives are clear, measurable statements of the intent of a program. For example, objectives may state the intent to increase the number of people having a certain screening test, or to reduce the incidence or prevalence of a disease among a population. Objectives should be measurable, clearly related to health problems identified, and communicated to the public. The objectives will help clearly identify intervention strategies and form the basis for program evaluation.

Community programs such as fall prevention and Lifestyle Redesign reflect traditional physical and occupational service provision models, focusing on a direct interaction between clients and "expert" therapists. In these examples, an intervention is offered to an individual, or a small group of individuals, often over an extended period of time. An example of a community-focused health initiative using a different model is the CarFit initiative described in Chapter 18. CarFit was developed by the American Society on Aging in collaboration with AARP, American Occupational Therapy Association, and AAA (AARP & AAA, 2010). The CarFit model is to sponsor a community event, or to join an existing

community event (such as a health fair). A CarFit event is usually two to four hours, is advertised in advanced, and is open to all people in the community. The CarFit program focuses on the effective use of the safety features in each individual's vehicle. People attending a CarFit event drive their car through a series of stations in which their access to and use of the car's safety features is reviewed. Although the focus of CarFit is safety, its larger aim is to provide a supportive setting to open up the discussion of driving safety and alternatives for aging drivers. This is a model of health promotion, providing education to support healthy behaviors. It addresses a growing societal concern, and involves collaboration between professional and consumer-center organizations at a national level.

COMMUNITY HEALTH INTERVENTIONS

Programs to improve the health of populations are generally referred to as **prevention programs**. Prevention programs can address one or more determinants of health (see **Table 20-3**). Prevention programs can also be classified as primary, secondary, or tertiary, depending on the timing of the intervention with respect to the health condition in question (see **Figure 20-3**).

Primary prevention involves efforts designed to protect people from acquiring an illness or injury. Immunization from infectious diseases is a classic example of primary prevention that addresses biologic health risks. Vaccines are made from materials extracted from infectious organisms (or from an organism that is similar to the infectious organism). Vaccines are then introduced into the body, and antibodies are formed by people's immune system.

TABLE 20-3 Examples of Community Health Interventions by Determinants of Health	
Determinant of Health*	**Example**
Biology	Immunizations
	Mammograms
Social factors	Improving transportation
	Reducing exposure to environmental hazards
Health services	Increasing access to health care services
	Improving quality of care
Public policy	Laws that restrict the sale of tobacco to minors
	Laws that penalize unsafe driving behaviors (texting while driving)
Health behaviors	Programs to educate people about safety, healthy diet, or physical activity

*US Department of Health and Human Services. (2012). Healthy people. Retrieved October 28, 2012 from http://www.healthypeople.gov/2020/default.aspx

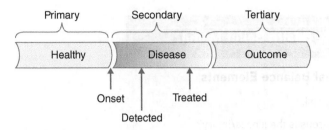

Figure 20-3 Levels of Prevention

When vaccinated people are later exposed to the infectious organism, their immune system is then able to mount a defensive response to the infection. Vaccines are typically harmless, but may produce allergic reactions or mild side effects in a small percentage of people. In the United States, vaccinations for diseases such as polio and measles are required for school-aged children, whereas influenza and pneumococcus vaccines are recommended for older adults.

Other common primary prevention interventions target health behaviors or public policy. Educational programs designed to raise public awareness about brain injury and to increase the use of bicycle helmets are examples of behavioral interventions. Laws making it difficult for children and teens to access tobacco products are examples of policy initiatives geared toward primary prevention. A primary prevention program discussed in Chapter 7 of this text is the *universal design* movement. The principles of universal design emphasize removing or limiting obstacles before they are experienced as obstacles through planning and conscientious design.

Secondary prevention refers to efforts to reduce the duration, severity, and sequelae of an illness or a disability. For many health conditions, people can be asymptomatic in early stages. Examples of such conditions include cancers, some infectious diseases like HIV, and chronic illnesses like hypertension, diabetes, and heart disease. The longer these illnesses go undetected and untreated, the more serious the consequences related to health status, quality of life, and cost. Therefore, secondary prevention efforts are often aimed at developing measures for early detection and intervention. Examples include mammograms to screen for breast cancer, regular blood pressure monitoring, blood tests for high cholesterol, and so on. Screenings can occur in a variety of situations, including regular visits to health care providers, health fairs, and other community events. For screening to be effective, screening tools must be accurate, inexpensive, and readily available, and lead to effective intervention to treat the health conditions. In physical and occupational therapy, secondary prevention could include balance screenings and useful field of view screenings at local health fairs.

Tertiary prevention refers to the rehabilitation, adaption, and accommodation that occur after an illness or injury. Rehabilitation professionals are frequently considered instrumental to this level of prevention. Tertiary prevention can take the form of a custom-made

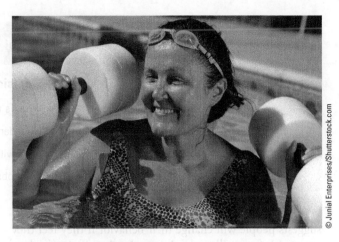

Figure 20-4 Aquatic exercises are a fun and healthy form of exercise for people with arthritis.

orthotic that helps people maintain range of motion, or it can be more general such as a water aerobics class tailored to the needs of people with arthritis, such as the one pictured in **Figure 20-4**. Because physical and occupational therapists focus on returning people to active participation in their life roles, these professions have a unique perspective and skill sets to address population health across all levels of prevention and wellness.

WELLNESS AND HEALTH BEHAVIORS

Wellness not only is the absence of illness but also includes the motivation to be involved in life, to have a sense of control over one's actions, and to desire interaction and connection with other individuals, and, perhaps most prominently, wellness enhances our sense of self-esteem and self-worth. Wellness may also be viewed as a blending of the physical, psychosocial, and spiritual realms. Wellness is a triangulated concept where, if all components work in concert, a positive outcome is achieved.

A **health behavior** is an action taken by individuals that results in supporting health and preventing illness. Some common health behaviors are exercising regularly, eating a balanced diet, and maintaining regular sleep habits. Both the ICF model and Healthy People initiative recognize the impact of personal behavior on health and function. Several theories of health behaviors can be useful when planning prevention strategies for individuals and populations. A brief review of three of these theories follows.

HEALTH BELIEF MODEL

The **health belief model (HBM)** was developed by Rosenstock to study utilization of preventive health services (Rosenstock, Strecher, & Becker, 1988). The model

TABLE 20-4 Components of the Health Belief Model

Component	Decisional Balance Elements
Perceived susceptibility	What is my risk?
Perceived severity	How dangerous is the illness/injury?
Perceived benefits	How will the new behavior improve my life?
Perceived barriers	What obstacles will I face? What is the cost?

suggests people will change their behavior if they feel they are at risk for an illness or injury that is sufficiently dangerous to warrant action. Before deciding to adopt a new behavior, people will weigh the barriers and benefits of the change in behavior; the "decisional balance" must favor the benefits before the person will act. **Table 20-4** summarizes the HBM.

A common intervention to reduce fall risk in older adults is to assess the clients' home environment. A focus of this assessment is to reduce potential environmental hazards like throw rugs and clutter, and enhance problem areas by adding handrails, night lights, and other adaptive equipment (Panel on Prevention of Falls in Older Persons, American Geriatrics Society and British Geriatrics Society, 2011). In a study of 178 older adults at risk for falls, Cumming et al. (2001) concluded that many older adults do not believe home modifications can reduce their risk of falls. This belief has a negative impact on adherence to recommendations by occupational therapists to do so. According to the HBM, older clients will not make home modifications unless they believe the benefits of making these changes (reducing fall risk) outweigh the perceived barriers (cost, inconvenience, and so on).

SOCIAL COGNITIVE THEORY

Social cognitive theory (SCT) was adapted from social learning theory by psychologist Albert Bandura, and has been applied to various health-related personal behaviors. This theory suggests that people acquire skills and perform new behaviors by enacting them, being reinforced for performance, and observing others. SCT suggests that behavior influences, and is influenced by, personal and environmental factors (Basen-Engquist et al., 2013). Some important concepts are implied by this relationship. The concept of "self-efficacy" refers to the degree of confidence people have in their ability to successfully adopt a behavior. Building self-efficacy involves careful attention to all three elements of the SCT model. Strategies include observational learning, building mastery, managing stress, and verbal encouragement/persuasion (Glanz, Rimer, & Lewis, 2002).

People learn by observing their social and physical environments. If a client observes someone execute a

behavior successfully, especially if the client identifies with the actor as a role model, the client is more likely to attempt the observed behavior. Building mastery can be accomplished through careful instruction that helps clients break down complex behaviors into manageable parts. Emotional stress often accompanies adopting new habits; in some cases, clients may also experience physical discomfort (for example, muscular soreness from a new exercise routine). Rehabilitation therapists can help clients manage this stress and discomfort through instruction, counseling, verbal encouragement, and persuasion. The young boy in **Figure 20-5** has demonstrated mastery of his asthma

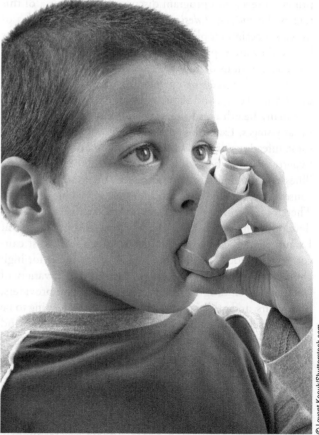

© Levent Konuk/Shutterstock.com

Figure 20-5 The skill and confidence to manage his asthma is an important health behavior for this child.

medication regime. This health behavior is more complex than what a typical child his age has to manage. Through instruction, support, and praise, he has gained this much-needed health behavior.

An example of a program to increase self-efficacy in older adults at risk of falls is *A Matter of Balance*. The program was developed in Europe (Tennstedt et al., 1998) and has been adapted for use in the United States with grant funding by the U.S. Administration on Aging (Healy, Peng, Haynes, McMahon, & Gross, 2008). The program focuses on building seniors' confidence that they can control their fall risk and their fear of falling through increasing physical activity and making environmental modifications.

TRANSTHEORETICAL MODEL

The **transtheoretical model** was developed by James Prochaska and is widely used for a variety of health behaviors (Prochaska et al., 1994). It is often referred to as the "stage of change" model because of its core component. The stage of change concept suggests people adopt new health behaviors in a series of stages: precontemplation, contemplation, preparation, action, and maintenance. In precontemplation, people are not considering changing. In contemplation, they are thinking about changing, but have not yet taken concrete action. In the preparation phase, people are taking preliminary steps to adopt the new behavior. This might include seeking information, buying equipment, or making an appointment with a health care provider. In the action phase, people are actively engaging in the new behavior. After they have sustained the behavior for an extended period (for example, six months), they are considered to be in the maintenance phase (Prochaska et al., 1994).

To assist clients in moving from one stage to the next, rehabilitation therapists employ strategies that are matched to the people's current stage of change. These strategies incorporate the concepts of self-efficacy from SCT and decisional balance from the HBM (Prochaska et al., 1994). For example, for a client in the precontemplation stage, interventions should focus on raising awareness of the problem and the benefits of adopting the new behavior. In later stages, interventions should focus on building self-efficacy, overcoming barriers, and avoiding relapse. Lambert and colleagues (2001) describe a three-session community program designed to encourage older adults to make environmental and personal changes to reduce fall risks. The authors recommended using stage-matched interventions as a way to enhance adherence to recommendations for home environment modifications.

Together with the health belief model and social cognitive theory, the transtheoretical model acknowledges that changing human health behavior is not as simple as just "educating" people to make healthy choices. Health behaviors, like health itself, are dependent on the interaction of various intrinsic and extrinsic factors. To improve the health of the U.S. population, a broad, coordinated approach is necessary.

HEALTH POLICY, PREVENTION, AND THE FUTURE

The **Patient Protection and Affordable Care Act of 2010 (ACA)** represents the most significant regulatory change to the U.S. health care system since the passage of Medicare and Medicaid in 1965.. Additional reforms are aimed at improving health care outcomes and streamlining the delivery of health care. This health care reform law, designed under the auspices of President Barack Obama, includes extensive funding for population health and prevention initiatives. According to the CDC (2014), about half of all adults have one or more chronic health conditions. One of four adults has two or more chronic health conditions. In fact, 7 out of 10 American deaths are the result of chronic diseases, heart disease, and cancer—together accounting for nearly 48 percent of all deaths (CDC, 2014). These diseases account for three-fourths of the money spent on health care in the United States. A 2009 report (Trust for America's Health, 2009) concluded that spending $10 per person on prevention would save $2.8 billion per year in 1 to 2 years, $16.5 billion per year in 5 years, and $18.5 billion per year in 10 to 20 years.

The ACA emphasizes prevention and public health through establishment of national prevention priorities, stimulation of prevention initiatives, reduction of barriers to preventive services, and provision of substantial new funding for public health interventions and infrastructure (Shaw, Asomugha, Conway, & Rein, 2014). President Obama appointed a national council comprised of 17 heads of federal administrative agencies to oversee this sweeping initiative (National Prevention Council, 2011a). The council released its **National Prevention Strategy** in June 2011. This strategy, summarized by **Figure 20-6**, identifies four "strategic directions" and seven "strategic priorities" for improving population health and reducing health care costs (National Prevention Council, 2011b).

The funds from this initiative will be used to expand and sustain public health programs across the nation. In addition, the ACA requires Medicare and other insurers to expand their coverage of health screenings and other preventive services. A notable feature of the ACA and the resulting *National Prevention Strategy* is the recognition that human health, development, and function are important and interrelated in a life course viewpoint, consistent with that introduced in Chapter 2. The National Prevention Strategy builds on the fact that lifelong health starts at birth and continues throughout all stages of life. Prevention begins with planning and having a healthy pregnancy, develops into good eating and fitness habits in childhood,

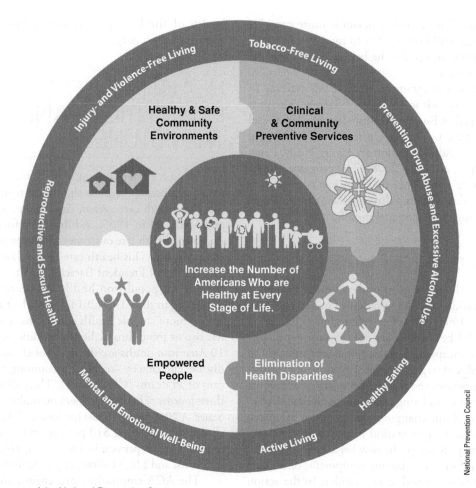

Figure 20-6 Summary of the National Prevention Strategy

is supported by preventive services at all stages of life, and promotes the ability to remain active, independent, and involved in one's community as we age. Students who are healthy and fit come to school ready to learn; employees who are free from mental and physical conditions take fewer sick days, are more productive, and help strengthen the economy; and older adults who remain physically and mentally active are more likely to live independently (National Prevention Council, 2011b, p. 5).

SUMMARY

Although as therapists, we often think about disease and disability as the focus of our efforts, but there is strong evidence that we will be able to make an important impact with people who have no identified problems in helping them make life and activity changes that can support continued health and enhanced quality of life. Wellness and prevention programs, such as the fall prevention and Lifestyle Design programs described in this chapter, serve to support community health and have been proven to be not only beneficial to the participants, but are cost effective as well.

The ACA mandates that new private insurance plans and states with expanded Medicaid programs provide, without cost to consumers, a set of clinical preventive services that have been recommended by a coalition of government public health advocacy groups. The U.S. federal government estimated in early 2013 that this new mandated coverage for private plans provided 71 million additional people with access to preventive services without cost sharing (Shaw, Asomugha, Conway, & Rein, 2014).

Wellness and prevention approaches can be designed for any age, regional, or health risk group. Increasingly, both occupational and physical therapists have been combining traditional client intervention practices with programs aimed at people in the community that are not "patients," but rather are concerned people interested in preventing disease and disability. This is an important, sometimes overlooked area of both clinical practice and social responsibility for today's health practitioners.

CASE 1

Xavier

Xavier is a 26-year-old male with a diagnosis of a mood disorder, major depression, and an above-knee, right leg amputation. Xavier served in the army, and during his second duty tour, lost his left leg from mid-thigh down. Now discharged from the military, Xavier uses a high-tech microprocessor-controlled C-leg, leg prosthesis, and a cane to help him walk. He has been slow to develop confidence with this device. In addition to the challenges of learning to use the prosthetic limb, he has some impairment in attention and working memory attributed to the depression. This results in difficulty persisting at tasks, monitoring his own performance, and in distractibility during task performance.

Xavier has been living with his mother and has not been employed since his medical discharge from the army. At this time, Xavier is able to manage all of his ADLs independently. He helps with the housework, but is unable to manage laundry and heavy cleaning. He is independent in meal preparation, managing money, and computer use. He needs moderate assistance with shopping and has difficulty managing public transportation. His mother says that he is a help around the house, but wants to see him "get back out in the world." Although he has recovered from his injuries, Xavier reports his health as fair.

Prior to his injury Xavier loved basketball and hunting. He has not contacted his old basketball buddies since his discharge and has no leisure activities except for cooking and online gaming. Xavier says that he is ready now. He does not want any more therapy; he wants a life. He wants to hang with friends, play sports, and learn to drive with his prosthesis.

Guiding Questions

Some questions to consider:

1. Considering the development path of a typical young adult, what types of health-promoting behaviors would be developmentally appropriate for Xavier?
2. Xavier has several limitations of activity, including most daily life activities such as education, work, and leisure. What kinds of supports do you think would help Xavier return to these adult life roles?

Speaking of
Wellness and Child Mental Health

ANNE CRONIN, PhD, OTR/L, FAOTA,
PEDIATRIC OCCUPATIONAL THERAPIST

I have followed the advances in public health in my profession closely and have been proud of the positive impact of such broad-based programs as fall prevention, Lifestyle Redesign, and CarFit. These are excellent and important initiatives aimed at adults. As a pediatric therapist, I had always felt that most of my wellness and prevention efforts should be focused on

Continues

Speaking of Continued

the parents of my clients rather than on the children themselves. Then I heard Susan Bazyk, PhD, OTR/L, FAOTA, speak on her grant-funded project "Every Moment Counts: Promoting Mental Health Throughout the Day" (Bazyk, 2011).

This project is a multilevel public health approach to school mental health implemented within the classroom, during lunch, recess, and after-school activities. At the broadest level, the program offers school-wide developmentally appropriate information aimed to promote positive behavior and mental health. This includes social and emotional learning activities embedded in everyday school activities. It also involves a school-wide positive behavioral support framework and includes specific teaching to help students develop and maintain positive mental health. This broad, bottom-of-the-pyramid set of strategies focuses on emphasizing individuals' strength and promoting a positive emotional school climate.

At the next level, the middle of the pyramid, strategies are geared toward students at risk of behavioral and mental health problems due to various situational stressors such as disabilities, overweight/obesity, poverty, trauma/abuse, and so on. Children at this level are generally not identified as having mental health problems but struggle with subclinical challenges that may be resolved with early intervention. Some of the additional prevention and emotional support strategies added for this group of students include education on bully prevention and on promoting and sustaining friendships. Participation in enjoyable extracurricular activities can also support positive mental health. In addition to targeted interventions, students at Level 2 also benefit from universal mental health promotion efforts.

Finally, at the top of the pyramid are the students with identified mental health/behavioral health challenges. At this level, the school-based interventions are individualized and more intensive than the services provided at the lower levels. Level-3 interventions included a comprehensive, integrated continuum of mental health and related services and supports. This approach emphasized youth empowerment and provides opportunities for youths to be decision-making partners in their own care. An additional focus in this group is on reclaiming mental health. Helping build and reinforce a sense of happiness despite chronic illness or disability.

I think that Dr. Bazyk's message is important. First, do not forget the importance of mental health. We think a lot about physical health, but mental health is equally important to maintaining a high quality of life. Second, sometimes we need to bring the whole community into the project, rather than trying to do it all ourselves. And finally, children can and should be active participants in wellness and prevention activities.

REFERENCES

American Association of Retired Persons (AARP) and American Automobile Association (AAA). (2010). *Carfit: Helping mature drivers find their safest fit.* Retrieved from http://www.car-fit.org/

The American Heritage Medical Dictionary. (2007). Wellness. Boston, MA: Houghton Mifflin Co.

American Physical Therapy Association. (2003) Basics of patient /client management. *Guide to Physical Therapist Practice* (rev. 2nd ed.). Alexandria, VA: American Physical Therapy Association.

Basen-Enquist, K., Carmack, C. L., Li, Y., Brown, J., Jhingran, A., Hughes, D. C., & . . . Waters, A. (2013). Social-cognitive theory predictors of exercise behavior in endometrial cancer survivors. *Health Psychology, 32*(11), 1137–1148.

Bazyk, S. (Ed.). (2011). *Mental health promotion, prevention, and intervention for children and youth: A guiding framework for occupational therapy.* Bethesda, MD: American Occupational Therapy Association, Inc.

Bergland, A., Jarnlo, G. B., & Laake, K. (2003). Predictors of falls in the elderly by location. *Aging and Clinical Experimental Research, 15,* 43–50.

Centers for Disease Control and Prevention (CDC). (2012). Monitoring selected national HIV prevention and care objectives by using HIV surveillance data—United states and 6 U.S. dependent areas—2010. *HIV Surveillance Supplemental Report 2012, 17*(3, part A), October 28, 2012.

Centers for Disease Control and Prevention (CDC). (2014). Chronic diseases and health promotion. Retrieved from http://www.cdc.gov/chronicdisease/overview/

Clark, F., & Azen, S. P. (1997). Occupational therapy for independent-living older adults. *JAMA: Journal of the American Medical Association, 278*(16), 1321.

Clark, F., Azen, S. P., Carlson, M., et al. (2001). Embedding health-promoting changes into the daily lives of independent-living older adults: Long-term follow-up of occupational therapy intervention. *Journal of the Gerontology Series B: Psychological Sciences and Social Sciences, 56,* 60e3.

Cummings, J., & Jackson, P. (2008). Race, gender, and SES disparities in self-assessed health, 1974–2004. *Research on Aging, 30,* 137–168.

Cumming, R. G., Thomas, M., Szonyi, G., Frampton, G., Salkeld, G., & Clemson, L. (2001). Adherence to occupational therapist recommendations for home modifications for falls prevention. *The American Journal of Occupational Therapy, 55*(6), 641–648.

Du Mont, J., & Forte, T. (2014). Intimate partner violence among women with mental health-related activity limitations: A Canadian population based study. *BMC Public Health, 14*(1), 1–16.

Glanz, K., Rimer, B. K., & Lewis, F. M. (2002). *Health behavior and health education: Theory, research and practice.* San Francisco, CA: Wiley & Sons.

Hausdorff, J. M., Rios, D. A., & Edelberg, H. K. (2001). Gait variability and fall risk in community-living older adults: A 1-year prospective study. *Archives of Physical Medicine and Rehabilitation, 82*(8), 1050–1056.

Healy, T. C., Peng, C., Haynes, P., McMahon, E., & Gross, L. (2008). Feasibility and effectiveness of translating A Matter of Balance into a volunteer lay leader model. *Journal of Applied Gerontology, 27*(1), 34–51.

Heidenreich, P. A., Trogdon, J. G., Khavjou, O. A., Butler, J., Dracup, K., Ezekowitz, M. D., ... Council on Cardiovascular Surgery and Anesthesia, and Interdisciplinary Council on Quality of Care and Outcomes Research. (2011). Forecasting the future of cardiovascular disease in the united states: A policy statement from the American heart association. *Circulation, 123*(8), 933–944.

Houston, D., Richardson, L., & Neeley, G. (2001). The effectiveness of child safety seat laws in the fifty states. *Policy Studies Review, 18,* 163–184.

Kindig, D., & Stoddart, G. (2003). What is population health? *American Journal of Public Health, 93*(3), 380–383.

Kochanek, M. A., Xu, J., Murphy, S. L., Minino, A. M., & Kung, H. (2011). Deaths: Final data for 2009. *National Vital Statistics Report,* 60, 3. Hyattsville, MD: National Center for Health Statistics.

Lambert, C., Sterbenz, D. E., Womack, L. T., Zarrinkhameh, L. T., & Newton, R. A. (2001). Adherence to a fall prevention program among community dwelling older adults. *Physical & Occupational Therapy in Geriatrics, 18*(3), 27–43.

Mead, H., Cartwright-Smith, L., Jones, K., Ramos, C., & Siegel, B. (2008). *Racial and ethnic disparities in U.S. health care: A chart book.* Retrieved from http://www.commonwealthfund.org/usr _doc/Mead_racialethnicdisparities_chartbook_1111.pdf

National Prevention Council. (2011a). *2011 Annual status report.* Washington, DC: U.S. Department of Health and Human Services, Office of the Surgeon General.

National Prevention Council. (2011b). *National prevention strategy.* Washington, DC: U.S. Department of Health and Human Services, Office of the Surgeon General.

Panel on Prevention of Falls in Older Persons, American Geriatrics Society and British Geriatrics Society. (2011). Summary of the updated American Geriatrics Society/British Geriatrics Society clinical practice guideline for prevention of falls in older persons. *Journal of the American Geriatrics Society, 59*(1), 148–157.

Prochaska, J. O., Velicer, W. F., Rossi, J. S., Goldstein, M. G., Marcus, B. H., Rakowski, W., Fiore, C., ... Rossi, S. R. (1994). Stages of change and decisional balance for 12 problem behaviors. *Health Psychology, 13*(1), 39–46.

Rosenstock, I., Strecher, V., & Becker, M. (1988). Social learning theory and the health belief model. *Health Education & Behavior, 15*(2), 175–183.

Shaw, F., Asomugha, C., Conway, P., & Rein, A. (2014). The Patient Protection and Affordable Care Act: Opportunities for prevention and public health. *Lancet, 384*(9937), 75–82. doi:10.1016 /S0140-6736(14)60259-2

Stevens, J. A. (2006). Fatalities and injuries from falls among older adults—united states, 1993–2003 and 2001–2005. *Morbidity and Mortality Weekly Report, 55,* 45.

Stevens, J. A., Corso, P. S., Finkelstein, E. A., & Miller, T. R. (2006). The costs of fatal and non-fatal falls among older adults. *Injury Prevention: Journal of the International Society for Child and Adolescent Injury Prevention, 12*(5), 290–295.

Tennstedt, S., Howland, J., Lachman, M., Peterson, E., Kasten, L., & Jette, A. (1998). A randomized, controlled trial of a group intervention to reduce fear of falling and associated activity restriction in older adults. *The Journals of Gerontology. Series B, Psychological Sciences and Social Sciences, 53*(6), P384–P392.

Thompson, W. W., Zack, M. M., Krahn, G. L., Andresen, E. M., & Barile, J. P. (2012). Health-related quality of life among older adults with and without functional limitations. *American Journal of Public Health, 102*(3), 496–502.

Trust for America's Health. (2009). Prevention for a healthier America: Investments in disease prevention yield significant savings, stronger communities. Retrieved from http://healthyamericans.org/reports /prevention08/Prevention08.pdf

U.S. Cancer Statistics Working Group. (2012). United States cancer statistics: 1999–2008 incidence and mortality web-based report. Retrieved from http://www.cdc.gov/uscs

U.S. Department of Health and Human Services. (2012). Healthy people. Retrieved from http://www.healthypeople.gov/2020 /default.aspx

Ware, J. E., Jr., & Sherbourne, C. D. (1992). The MOS 36-item short-form health survey (SF-36): Conceptual framework and item selection. *Medical Care, 30*(6), 473–483.

World Health Organization. (2001). *ICF: International classification of functioning, disability and health.* Geneva, Switzerland: World Health Organization.

World Health Organization (WHO). (2005). *The Bangkok charter for health promotion in a globalized world.* Geneva, Switzerland: World Health Organization.

PART 3

Special Topics
in Human
Development
and Performance

CHAPTER 21

Public Policy and Health Care

Barbara L. Kornblau, JD, OT/L, FAOTA, DMASPE, ABDA CCM, CDMS, CPE,
Coalition for Disability Health Equity, Arlington, Virginia, & Florida A & M University, Tallahassee, Florida
and

Anne Cronin, PhD, OTR/L,
Associate Professor, Division of Occupational Therapy, West Virginia University, Morgantown, West Virginia

Objectives

Upon completion of this chapter, readers should be able to:

- Discuss the intent of the United Nations' *Convention on the Rights of Persons with Disabilities* and the potential impact of the *World Report on Disabilities* for health care professionals;

- Explain the difference between antidiscrimination legislation and specific entitlement programs, and offer the strengths and weakness of these two approaches to public policy;

- Describe how the medical model of disability affects policy, as contrasted with how the social model of disability affects policy;

- Reflect on the Health Insurance Portability and Accountability Act of 1996 (HIPAA) as it impacts clinical communications of all types;

- Identify the role of health professionals in public policy advocacy;

- Explain three ways in which public policy can have an impact on clinical practice; and

- Discuss the concept of social justice and how it might relate to political advocacy.

Key Terms

Americans with Disabilities
    Act (ADA)

assistive technology device

essential health benefits

habilitation services

Health Insurance Portability
    and Accountability Act of 1996
    (HIPAA)

ICD-10 (the International Statistical
    Classification of Diseases and
    Related Health Problems)

Individuals with Disabilities
    Education Act (IDEA)

interagency agreements

lobbying

Medicaid

Medicare

Patient Protection and Affordable
    Care Act (PPACA)

political action committee (PAC)

political advocacy

post-acute care bundling

public policy doctrine

Rehabilitation Act of 1973

rehabilitation services

Social Security Disability
    Insurance (SSDI)

Supplemental Security Income (SSI)

telehealth

United Nations Convention on
    the Rights of Persons with
    Disabilities

World Report on Disability

INTRODUCTION

Why is public policy important to health care professionals? The ICF (World Health Organization, 2001) reflects the importance of public policy at local, national, and international levels in its discussion of environmental contexts. Public policy is a broad category that includes legislation as well as policies within social institutions. Earlier in the text, we introduced legislative issues as influential at differing points in the life span. For example, in the United States, the legislation known as Individuals with Disabilities Act (IDEA) provides taxpayer-supported and free therapy services to families of children with identified disabilities, and those at risk for disability under the age of 3. As you have learned, the nervous system is the most plastic, and the opportunity for optimizing function is greatest at these early ages. For this reason,

this legislation serves as a powerful and important asset for families. Another example is provided in the discussion of environmental contexts for function, which included a long discussion of the driver's license legislation, and reflected on its impact for both adolescents and the elderly.

Because much of what the ICF describes as aspects of services, systems, and policies provides the foundation for societal practices and expectations, we often overlook the importance of these influences. For this reason, we will open this chapter with a summary of the ICF descriptors of services, systems, and policies presented in **Table 21-1**. Many of the examples of policies and legislation offered in **Table 21-1** will be discussed in greater detail later in this chapter. The important message is that the scope of this chapter is broad and encompasses issues of social justice for those we serve, as well as more specific issues related to health care professionals.

TABLE 21-1   Services, Systems, and Policies

Category of Services, Systems, and Policies	Descriptor	U.S. Policy Example
For the Production of Consumer Goods	Regulates and approves the medical devices and products consumed or used by people.	The Food and Drug Administration (FDA) protects and promotes public health through the regulation and oversight of certain food safety, prescription and over-the-counter pharmaceuticals, vaccines, medical devices, and other consumer-related products (21 U.S.C. Chapter 9).
Architecture and Construction	Sets national accessibility standards for the design of buildings, public and private.	The Architectural Barriers Act of 1968 requires that facilities designed, built, altered, or leased with funds supplied by the U.S. government meet uniform standards for the design, construction, and alteration of buildings so that people with disabilities can readily access and use the facilities (42 U.S.C. § 4151 et seq.).

Continues

TABLE 21-1   Services, Systems, and Policies   *(continued)*

Category of Services, Systems, and Policies	Descriptor	U.S. Policy Example
Open Space Planning	The planning, design, development, and maintenance of public lands and private lands in the rural, suburban, and urban context that are open to the public.	The Americans with Disabilities Act requires that no individual may be discriminated against on the basis of disability with regard to the full and equal enjoyment of the goods, services, facilities, or accommodations of any place of public accommodation, such as parks and outdoor recreational spaces, including privately owned recreational spaces that are open to the public (Pub. L. No. 101-336).
Housing	Describes policies for the provision of shelters, dwellings, or lodging for people.	The Fair Housing Act protects the buyer/renter of a dwelling from seller/landlord discrimination. Its primary prohibition makes it unlawful to refuse to sell, rent to, or negotiate with any person because a person has a disability. Landlords must make accommodations to their policies and procedures to allow access to enjoyment of the premises and allow tenants to make needed reasonable accommodations to the premises at their own expense (42 U.S.C. § 3601 et seq.).
Utilities	Policies for publicly provided utilities, such as water, fuel, electricity, sanitation, public transportation, and essential services.	The Clean Water Act established the goals of eliminating releases of high amounts of toxic substances into water, eliminating additional water pollution and ensuring that surface waters would meet standards necessary for human sports and recreation (Pub. L. No. 100-4).
Communication	Policies for the transmission and exchange of information.	The Telecommunications Act of 1996 updated earlier legislation to include the Internet in broadcasting and spectrum allotment (Pub. L. No. 104-104).
Transportation	Enabling people or goods to move or be moved from one location to another.	The Americans with Disabilities Act prohibits disability discrimination by all public entities at the local (that is, school district, municipal, city, county) and state level.
Civil Protection	Aimed at safeguarding people and property.	The Federal Emergency Management Agency (FEMA) coordinates the response to a disaster that has occurred when the governor of a state declares a state of emergency and formally requests aid.
Legal Governance	The legislation and other law of a country	In the United States, there is a federal constitution for national issues. Each state also has a constitution regulating state policies.
Associations and Organizational Services, Systems, and Policies	Relating to groups of people who have joined together in the pursuit of common, noncommercial interests.	This is a broad area, advocacy groups such as the American Association of Retired Persons and the Disability Rights Advocacy Group were discussed earlier in the text. In this chapter, see the discussion on "lobbying."
Media	Oversight of the provision of mass communication through radio, television, newspapers, and Internet.	The Federal Communications Commission regulates interstate and international communications by radio, television, wire, satellite, and cable.
Economic	The overall system of production, distribution, consumption, and use of goods and services.	The Small Business Administration provides small business owners with access to federal, state, and local government resources from a single access point.

Continues

TABLE 21-1   Services, Systems, and Policies   *(continued)*

Category of Services, Systems, and Policies	Descriptor	U.S. Policy Example
Social Security	Providing income support to people who, because of age, poverty, unemployment, health condition, or disability, require public assistance that is funded either by general tax revenues or contributory schemes.	The Social Security Administration manages the U.S. social insurance program consisting of retirement, disability, and survivors' benefits known as Social Security.
Health Services	Services, systems, and policies for preventing and treating health problems, providing medical rehabilitation, and promoting a healthy lifestyle.	The Patient Protection and Affordable Care Act (ACA) is aimed primarily at decreasing the number of uninsured Americans and reducing the overall costs of health care (Pub. L. No. 111-148).
Education and Training	Supports for the acquisition, maintenance, and improvement of knowledge, expertise, and vocational or artistic skills.	The No Child Left Behind Act of 2001 supports standards-based education reform based on the premise that setting high standards and establishing measurable goals can improve individual outcomes in education (20 U.S.C.A. § 6301 et seq.).
Labor and Employment	Services, systems, and policies related to finding suitable work for people who are unemployed or looking for different work, or to support individuals already employed who are seeking promotion.	The Civil Rights Act prohibits unlawful employment discrimination by public and private employers, labor organizations, and training programs (42 U.S.C. § 1971 et seq.).
Political Services	Policies related to voting, elections, and governance of countries, regions, and communities, as well as international political organizations.	Eligibility to vote in the United States is determined by both federal and state law. Only citizens can vote in U.S. elections, and citizenship is governed by federal law. In the absence of a federal law or constitutional amendment, each state is given considerable discretion to establish qualifications for suffrage and candidacy within its own jurisdiction.

SOCIAL JUSTICE

Social justice is a term that relates to the equitable distribution of advantages and disadvantages within a society. Social justice relies on a set of beliefs that every human deserves equal economic, political, and social rights and opportunities. For the most part, the emphasis in social justice is equity within society. In Chapter 1, we showed you the distinction between a medical model of health and a social model of health. This distinction can serve as an analogy to our discussion of social justice.

As health care providers, we often engage in personal relationships with people who may benefit from our support as advocates. On an individual level, each time we write a letter of justification for a piece of equipment or for a needed service, we advocate for our client. This is an important aspect of ethical clinical practice, but it does not reflect a commitment to social justice. To support social justice, health care providers need to focus on the community—not just individuals. An example of working toward social justice would include meeting with local legislators to assure new community development includes accessible sidewalks and

TABLE 21-2	General Principles of the Convention on the Rights of Persons with Disabilities

Respect for inherent dignity, individual autonomy including the freedom to make one's own choices, and independence of persons;

Non-discrimination;

Full and effective participation and inclusion in society;

Respect for difference and acceptance of persons with disabilities as part of human diversity and humanity;

Right to an education;

Right to health care;

Equality of opportunity;

Accessibility;

Equality between men and women;

Respect for the evolving capacities of children with disabilities and respect for the right of children with disabilities to preserve their identities.

playgrounds. If you succeed, your actions will open a door for many people, and society as a whole—beyond your client base. The two areas of social justice that will receive attention in this chapter are initiatives to support population health and initiatives to support social participation.

In 2006, the United Nations promulgated an international treaty titled the **United Nations Convention on the Rights of Persons with Disabilities**. This treaty was a call to action for all UN members to commit to respect and support the rights and dignity of people with disabilities. The guiding principles of this convention are presented in **Table 21-2**. Over 158 representative groups, including the European Union, Canada, and Australia, have endorsed this document. This treaty, commonly referred to as "a convention," is a social justice effort to improve the place of people with disabilities in society on a global scale.

The World Health Organization developed the **World Report on Disability** (WHO/WB, 2011) in response to the convention. In its introduction, it states that "many people with disabilities do not have equal access to health care, education, and employment opportunities; do not receive the disability-related services that they require; and experience exclusion from everyday life activities" (p. xxi). The *World Report on Disability* offers a call to action and identifies barriers to participation faced by people with disabilities. The first of these barriers is inadequate policies and standards. The report expresses concern that policy design does not always take into account the needs of people with disabilities, or existing policies. Further, it found that though standards exist, often no one enforces them. WHO also found problems with service delivery. These problems included poor coordination among services, inadequate staffing, and insufficient training of staff

who were thus unable to provide adequate quality services for people with disabilities.

In support of social justice, rehabilitation professions should get active and vocal on local, regional, and national stages to support both people with disabilities, and the policies needed to increase opportunities for their active participation in community living. You can participate in this advocacy as an individual, as a part of a civic group, or in collaboration with a state and national professional organization such as the American Occupational Therapy Association or the American Physical Therapy Association.

POLICY ON AN INTERNATIONAL SCALE

Laws emerge from the values of the society in which they exist. International law surfaces from compromises and values that multiple countries support. All legal systems incorporate what is sometimes referred to as the **public policy doctrine** in the development, enforcement, and judicial review of its laws and policies. Public policy provides the foundation for the development and review of laws that regulate behavior, either to reinforce existing social expectations, or to encourage constructive change. The public policy doctrine considers the social, moral, and economic values that tie a society together: values that vary in different cultures and change over time. For example, at one time in the United States, it was illegal in some states for people of different races to marry. In reviewing that law, the U.S. Supreme Court found, among other things, that these laws were contrary to public policy and threw them out (*Loving v. Virginia*, 388 U.S. 1 (1967)).

Internationally, leaders often promote a public policy-based response to reflect accepted societal norms and the collective morality of the society. Current events or events that develop over time may trigger public policy-based responses.

In Chapter 1, when we introduced the ICF, we introduced the use of the ICF as a clinical problem-solving tool for rehabilitation practice. A primary purpose of the ICF is to provide a standard language and framework to describe health and health-related conditions as a basis to guide and as a function of the public policy doctrine. The ICF belongs to the WHO family of international classifications, some of which we described in Chapter 1.

The best known of the WHO classification systems is the **ICD-10 (the International Statistical Classification of Diseases and Related Health Problems)**. The ICD-10 is a tool for the classification of diseases, disorders, and other health conditions. The WHO developed the ICD-10 and ICF as complementary tools that, when used together, create a meaningful picture of the experience of health at both the individual and the population level (WHO, 2002). The ICD-10 is the global health information standard for mortality and morbidity statistics. Increasingly, clinicians and researchers use it to define diseases and study disease patterns, as well as manage health care, monitor outcomes, and allocate resources. **Table 21-3** presents early adopters of the ICD-10, who use it in their health care systems to guide reimbursement and resource allocation in their health system. The original ICD-10 document was published in English, and a significant part of the country-specific modifications involve translation and cultural adaptations. The international version of ICD-10 has been translated into 43 languages and is used in about 110 countries as a system to report mortality data, a primary indicator of health status (WHO, 2014).

As you look at this list, you will see that the United States was slow to adopt the ICD-10. The United States did not achieve full implementation of this data system until 2014. This offered a chance for reflection on health policy. All of the countries listed as early adopters of the system have nationalized health care systems administered through their government. The uniformity of their systems' billing and payment systems made rapid change easily attainable. The health care system in the United States provides health care via numerous national programs including, for example, Medicare, Medicaid, Veterans Health, Military Health, and CHIP, and all work differently. Further, some government-provided health care involves private insurance carriers as intermediaries in the billing and payment process, providing many inconsistencies in government-provided health care programs, unlike the early adopters of the ICD-10.

The United States has made attempts to increase uniformity of health information. The **Health Insurance Portability and Accountability Act of 1996 (HIPAA)**, a U.S. law designed to protect the privacy of health care consumers, also included provisions to standardize methods of communicating patient health information while at the same time protecting privacy of protected health information. HIPAA requires the following actions: (1) the continuity of health care coverage for individuals who change jobs without preexisting-condition waiting periods; (2) the management of health information; (3) simplification of the administration of health insurance; and (4) combat of waste, fraud, and abuse in health insurance and health care. Congress has amended this law over time to establish national standards for electronic health care transactions including meaningful use of patients' electronic health records by multiple health care providers. To implement the ICD-10, the process of moving to meaningful use includes extensive changes through the multiple providers and through a series of rulings to

TABLE 21-3 Early Adopters of the ICD-10		
Country	**Name of Variant of the ICD-10**	**Date of Implementation**
Netherlands	ICD-10-nl	1994
Sweden	Clinical modification of ICD-10	1997
Australia	ICD-10-AM (Australian Modification)	1998–1999
Canada	ICD-10-CA	2000
Korea	ICD-10-KM (Korean Modification)	2008
France	Clinical addendum to ICD-10	2005
Germany	ICD-10-GM (German Modification)	2002
Thailand	ICD-10-TM	2007

maintain compliance with HIPAA. These issues, together with the 2010 passage of the Patient Protection and Affordable Care Act (ACA) described later in this chapter, further complicate the preparation for the implementation of the ICD-10 code set.

NATIONAL POLICY

State and federal governments play a primary role in the development of public policy, which they express through laws, regulations, court decisions, and funding mechanisms. For example, in the past decade, in response to strong parent advocacy, states passed laws to require coverage of specific services for people with autism under private health insurance. One treatment favored by some, applied behavior analysis (ABA), an early intensive behavioral support program, is staggeringly expensive. In 2012, it was estimated that some families spend more than $50,000 per year on autism-related therapies (National Conference of State Legislatures, 2012). Private health insurance carriers denied payment of the claims for ABA and other autism-related services, asserting they were not "medically necessary." After much parent and therapist advocacy, as of 2014, 37 states and the District of Columbia enacted legislation to require insurance carriers to provide coverage for autism treatment (Autism Speaks, 2014). Seven more states are pursuing similar legislation.

Not all policy is legislative. The American Psychiatric Association developed the standards to describe and define mental illness and mental health conditions in its *Diagnostic and Statistical Manual (DSM)*. Following a lengthy review process, an updated and revised *DSM-5* changed the standards for the diagnosis of autism, among other conditions. The intent of the change is to clarify the diagnosis and make it consistent with research and scholarly findings. Several advocacy groups and others challenged the changes made because some feared the changed criteria would exclude as many as 40 percent of children considered to have autism under the DSM IV-R. Parents of mildly affected children and advocates worried the new criteria would leave their children out and cause them to lose access to academic, behavioral, and other services (Tanner, 2012). In this case, the American Psychiatric Association is the policy-making body that governs how clinicians of all backgrounds diagnose someone within the psychiatric world.

These two different types of policies relating to autism affect individuals with autism in opposite ways. The autism insurance legislation potentially *increases* the availability of services for people with autism spectrum disorder (ASD); however, the DSM-5 potentially *limits* the number of individuals eligible for those services, because the changes in diagnostic criteria will designate fewer individuals eligible for the new insurance benefits.

Another path toward public policy is through the judicial branch of government—that is, the courts. The U.S. Supreme Court makes policy when it issues decisions on cases it hears, or decides not to hear. For example, in *Olmstead v. LC* (1999), the Court ruled that states could not require individuals with disabilities to live in segregated state institutions to receive services. According to the Court, states must provide a range of services in the community so society does not prevent individuals with disabilities from participating in community life—an opportunity afforded to individuals without disabilities.

Policies do not change by themselves. Occupational and physical therapy practitioners can play key roles in advocacy for public policies that help those they serve. As professionals, readers must endeavor to familiarize themselves with the key public policy initiatives that will affect their practice and the people they serve, and stay current with these issues on an ongoing basis. This chapter examines some of those public policies with which rehabilitation professionals regularly work: the Fair Housing Act, the Individuals with Disabilities Education Act (IDEA), the Americans with Disabilities Act (ADA), Medicare, and the Patient Protection and Affordable Care Act (PPACA). Although this chapter provides readers with background information, readers must keep in mind that, as the previous examples showed, these policies often change based upon the passage of new laws and regulations and appellate court decisions.

ANTIDISCRIMINATION LEGISLATION

Many forms of antidiscrimination legislation serve to identify potential grounds for discrimination and offer areas of protection. Several of these laws are presented in **Table 21-4**. The **Rehabilitation Act of 1973** (also called the *Rehab Act*) was one of the first significant pieces of civil rights legislation for individuals with disabilities (Albrecht, Seelman, & Bury, 2001). Section 504 of the Rehabilitation Act is often cited because it contains language indicating that individuals with disabilities cannot be discriminated against in any program (including public education) that receives federal sources of funding.

In 1990, the U.S. Congress passed the **Americans with Disabilities Act (ADA)**, extending the reach of antidiscrimination law. The ADA prohibits discrimination on the basis of disability in employment, state and local government services, places of public accommodations, transportation, and telecommunication (Americans with Disabilities Act, 1990). By enacting the ADA, Congress expanded the public policy goals of the Rehab Act, broadening its reach to nongovernmental, private entities. **Table 21-5** lists the five titles of the ADA.

TABLE 21-4   Examples of Antidiscrimination Legislation

Title of Legislation	Intent of the Law
The Rehabilitation Act	Prohibits discrimination on the basis of disability in programs conducted by federal agencies, in programs that receive or benefit from federal financial assistance, in federal employment, and in the employment practices of federal contractors. Since the Americans with Disabilities Act (ADA) became law, both the Rehab Act and the ADA use the same standards to determine employment discrimination.
Americans with Disabilities Act (ADA)	The ADA prohibits discrimination on the basis of disability in employment, state and local government services, public accommodations, commercial facilities, transportation, and telecommunications.
Fair Housing Act	This prohibits housing discrimination on the basis of race, color, religion, sex, *disability*, familial status, and national origin. Its coverage includes private housing, housing that receives federal financial assistance, and state and local government housing. It is unlawful to discriminate in any aspect of selling or renting housing or to deny a dwelling to a buyer or renter because of the disability of that individual. It is unlawful to fail to make modifications to policies to allow access to the full enjoyment of the premises.
Air Carrier Access Act	This prohibits discrimination in air transportation by domestic and foreign air carriers against qualified individuals with physical or mental impairments. It applies only to air carriers that provide regularly scheduled services for hire to the public.
Civil Rights of Institutionalized Persons Act (CRIPA)	This law authorizes the U.S. Attorney General to investigate conditions of confinement at state and local government institutions such as prisons, jails, pretrial detention centers, juvenile correctional facilities, publicly operated nursing homes, and institutions for people with psychiatric or developmental disabilities. Its purpose is to allow the attorney general to uncover and correct widespread deficiencies that seriously jeopardize the health and safety of residents of institutions.
The Individuals with Disabilities Education Act (IDEA)	This requires public schools to make available to all eligible children with disabilities a free appropriate public education in the least restrictive environment appropriate to their individual needs. IDEA requires public school systems to develop appropriate individualized education programs (IEPs) for each child. The specific special education and related services outlined in each IEP reflect the individualized needs of each student.
Telecommunications Act	This requires manufacturers of telecommunications equipment and providers of telecommunications services to ensure that such equipment and services are accessible to and usable by people with disabilities.
Architectural Barriers Act (ABA)	This requires that buildings and facilities that are designed, constructed, or altered with federal funds, or leased by a federal agency, comply with federal standards for physical accessibility. ABA requirements are limited to architectural standards in new and altered buildings and in newly leased facilities.
Voting Accessibility for the Elderly and Handicapped Act	This act requires polling places across the United States to be physically accessible to people with disabilities for federal elections. Where no accessible location is available to serve as a polling place, a political subdivision must provide an alternate means of casting a ballot on the day of the election.
The National Voter Registration Act (also known as the "Motor Voter Act")	This act requires all offices of state-funded programs that are primarily engaged in providing services to people with disabilities to provide all program applicants with voter registration forms, to assist them in completing the forms, and to transmit completed forms to the appropriate state official.

Adapted from U.S. Department of Justice, Civil Rights Division, Disability Rights Section (2009)

Title I of the ADA prohibits discrimination against individuals with disabilities in employment by a private, nongovernment employer (*University of Alabama v. Garrett,* 2001). Included in the definition of *discrimination* is the failure to make reasonable accommodations for qualified individuals with a disability. Rehabilitation professionals often become involved in employment cases where their skills can promote better function in the workplace and help determine needed reasonable accommodations.

Some worry that the ADA interferes with business operations and forces employers to do things they do not want to do. However, the ADA does not require that

TABLE 21-5	Americans with Disabilities Act—Five Titles
Title I	Employment
Title II	State and Local Government Services and Transportation
Title III	Public Accommodations
Title IV	Telecommunications
Title V	Miscellaneous Provisions

employers hire everyone with a disability who fills out an employment application. Rather, the ADA aims to level the playing field so individuals with disabilities have an opportunity for employment in positions for which they can perform the essential functions and for which they are qualified. Thus, an employer need not hire an individual with a disability who could not do the job, or was not qualified for the position. Not every employee is entitled to an accommodation in the workplace. There is a formal three-step inquiry process to determine whether an employee needs or is entitled to an accommodation, shown in **Table 21-6**.

The first question is whether the worker is an individual with a disability. There are three definitions of *disability*, and the worker must meet one of them. Workers must show that they have a physical or mental impairment that substantially limits one or more major life activities, a history of such an impairment, or are currently regarded as having such an impairment. If workers meet the definition, the next inquiry is whether they are qualified for the job. Finally, if individuals are qualified individuals with a disability, the final question is whether the requested accommodation is reasonable.

Title II of the ADA applies to services provided by state and local governments. State and local governments must make the programs and services they provide accessible to individuals with disabilities. This could include, for example, access to classes provided at public universities, to voting, and to parks and recreational programs. In the United States, under the ADA, public places such as restaurants and shopping malls must provide wheelchair-accessible bathrooms. These ADA requirements cover all public venues, such as fairs and sports venues. Temporary portable toilets, such as those shown in **Figure 21-1**, are common at outdoor events. Note that even at these temporary events, wheelchair accessibility is required. This helps ensure wheelchair users can participate in all types of public gatherings in the mainstream of community life.

TABLE 21-6	Reasonable Accommodations Decision Progression

Step 1: Is the worker an individual with a disability?

1. A physical or mental impairment that substantially limits one or more major life activities;

2. A history of having had such an impairment; or

3. Regarded as having such an impairment.

***If the worker is not an individual with a disability, the employer does not have to accommodate.

Step 2: Is the worker a qualified individual with a disability?

1. Individual satisfies the requisite skills, experience, education, and other job-related requirements of the job; and

2. Individual can perform the essential functions of such position with or without reasonable accommodations.

***If the worker is not a qualified individual with a disability, the employer does not have to accommodate.

Step 3: Is the accommodation reasonable?

1. How much does the accommodation cost in relationship to the size and budget of the business?

2. Are there tax credits or deductions or outside funding sources to pay for the accommodation?

3. Does the accommodation interfere with the operation of the business or the ability of other employees to perform their duties?

***If it is not reasonable, the employer does not have to accommodate.

Used with permission of ADA Consultants, Inc.

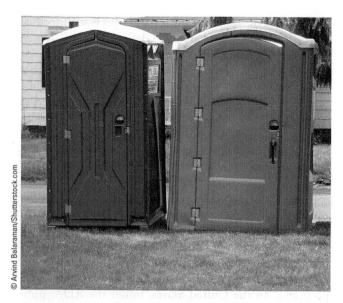

© Arvind Balaraman/Shutterstock.com

Figure 21-1 The portable toilet unit on the right is wider, is flush with the ground, and has support rails inside to accommodate people in wheelchairs.

Title III of the ADA provides that privately owned places of public accommodations must allow access for their customers with disabilities to the goods, services, facilities, and advantages they offer to the public. These places include, for example, theaters, doctors' offices, golf courses, hotels, retail establishments, day care centers, gas stations, and hospitals. This section of the ADA helps those we serve participate in community life. Places of public accommodations are required to make reasonable accommodations for individuals with disabilities so they may enjoy what these accommodations offer to the public. These privately owned places of public accommodation cannot refuse to serve individuals with disabilities, and cannot segregate individuals with disabilities.

Title IV of the ADA sets up a system of telecommunications for individuals with hearing impairments. A relay service is in place to allow communication through telecommunication devices for the deaf (TDD) with those who do not have hearing impairments. These *text telephones* can allow individuals with hearing impairments access to telephone services. New communication, called the CART (Communication Access Realtime Translation) system, allows deaf and hard of hearing individuals to read on their computer screen or other device information presented in an auditory modality. Closed captioning is an example of an application of CART technology. Title IV requires closed-captioning for federally funded public service announcements.

Other countries around the world have similar types of antidiscrimination legislation. Some examples of these include the Disability Discrimination Act (Australia), Human Rights Act (New Zealand), Persons with Disabilities Act (India), and the Human Rights Act (Canada). Each of these laws includes its own definition of discrimination, and its own provisions to address or not address reasonable accommodations.

These and other disability discrimination laws have one significant flaw. They are complaint driven. There are no ADA police checking for compliance. This means the burden is on individuals to understand their rights and figure out how to enforce those rights. This could mean filing an administrative complaint with a government agency or finding a lawyer to file a lawsuit, or both. Although an administrative process is available, many perceive it as adversarial, and agencies may not have the time to properly investigate complaints. Individuals must challenge and defend themselves in a legal arena. This may be both daunting and beyond the fiscal, temporal, and emotional resources available to the individuals (Albrecht, Seelman, & Bury, 2001).

ENTITLEMENT PROGRAMS

An entitlement program is a government program that guarantees benefits (that is, fiscal benefits, housing, or health coverage) to a specified segment of the population. Some examples of entitlement programs at the federal level in the United States include Social Security, unemployment compensation, food stamps, Medicaid, and Supplemental Security Income. The Patient Protection and Affordable Care Act (ACA), Medicare, and Medicaid are health-specific entitlement programs that will be discussed later in this chapter.

Supplemental Security Income (or SSI) is a program that provides financial support to low-income people who are blind, disabled, or aged (65 or older). In this program, "[d]isability means inability to engage in any SGA [substantial gainful activity] by reason of any medically determinable physical or mental impairment which can be expected to result in death, or has lasted or can be expected to last for a continuous period of not less than 12 months" (Social Security Administration, 2005).

Another entitlement program, **Social Security Disability Insurance (SSDI)**, is a federal insurance program managed by the Social Security Administration. This program provides financial support in the form of insurance payments to people who meet the same disability criteria as for SSI. However, unlike SSI, SSDI is not an income-based program. It is an insurance program. In addition to qualifying under Social Security's definition of disability, one must have worked for 40 quarters (of a year) or 10 years (Social Security Administration, 2005). Both of these entitlement programs have limitations. First, although entitlement programs offer support, they do not address the source of problems or create a culture of accommodation and inclusion (Albrecht, Seelman, & Bury, 2001).

Additionally, people who receive SSI disability may face social stigma as others view them as living off welfare, and not as contributing members of society. Conversely, as mentioned in Chapter 19, some people malinger or falsify impairments to receive disability support. This is rare, however. Most claims are denied upon initial application, and most requests for reconsideration of that initial application also are usually denied. Most claimants must go to a hearing to obtain benefits. It is very difficult for individuals to obtain SSI benefits without an attorney. Television stories have implied there are unscrupulous lawyers involved in the SSI benefits system aggravating the belief that malingering is common.

Of intense concern is the fraud involved in claims for services provided under Medicare and Medicaid to recipients of these programs. Providers, including occupational and physical therapists, have billed for services not provided, more expensive services than those actually provided, or services provided by unqualified people. As a result, Congress has funneled money into oversight programs to catch the perpetrators of fraud against these entitlement programs.

HEALTH CARE POLICY

The Patient Protection and Affordable Care Act (referred to as the Affordable Care Act or ACA), passed by Congress in 2010, requires insurance companies to cover all applicants and offer the same rates regardless of preexisting conditions or gender. State governments, corporations, and others have challenged this law in court, and challenges will likely continue.

Prior to ACA, most Americans obtained their health insurance through their employers who purchased group plans through private insurance companies. If one's employer did not provide employer-based health insurance, most people were unable to obtain affordable individual coverage. Over 30 million Americans lacked health insurance coverage. At the same time, health care costs continued to increase.

This created a national problem, because the law required hospitals to treat critically ill people even if they were uninsured. Hospitals incurred debt from caring for the uninsured. They built this debt into the fees they charged paying patients, and this aggravated the rising cost of health care and the cost of health insurance coverage. Congress passed ACA to increase the number of Americans with insurance coverage and, in doing this, reduce the overall costs of health care (Elmendorf, 2011). **Table 21-7** provides an overview of the provisions of ACA. This table does not include changes specific to the Medicare and Medicaid programs that were enacted in response to the ACA.

TABLE 21-7 Requirements of ACA
This act prevents health insurance carriers from discrimination in new plans, by requiring that they issue policies at the same cost or premium amount, for applicants of the same age and in the same geographic location, regardless of any preexisting medical condition. ACA allows carriers to charge higher premiums based on age, and for individuals who smoke (ACA §1201 (1)).
ACA mandates all individuals not covered by an employer health plan, Medicaid, Medicare, or other public insurance program, purchase private insurance coverage or pay a penalty (unless the applicable individual is a member of a recognized religious sect exempted by the Internal Revenue Service, or is deemed to experience financial hardship). This is called the "individual mandate" (Kaiser Family Foundation, 2014a).
States and the federal government established health insurance exchanges or marketplaces in each state, in 2013, to offer individuals and small businesses a vehicle to compare policy benefits and premiums, and buy insurance (with government subsidies or tax credits if eligible). The marketplaces will continue for future coverage purchases (Centers for Medicare and Medicaid Services, 2014).
All nonelderly adults with income up to 138 percent of the federal poverty level (FPL) are eligible for Medicaid if they live in one of the 27 states that expanded Medicaid. Individuals with incomes up to 400 percent of the FPL will be eligible for tax credits, payable in advance, to purchase insurance in the marketplaces. Individuals with incomes between 100 and 250 percent of the FPL are eligible for additional subsidies to help with co-pays and deductibles for the plans they buy through the marketplaces (Angeles, 2013; Kaiser Family Foundation, 2014b).
The Department of Health and Human Services established minimum standards for health insurance policies. These included 10 essential benefits that specifically include rehabilitation, habilitation, and durable medical equipment. ACA also eliminated annual and lifetime caps on insurance coverage (ACA § 2711; Jost, 2013).
The act mandates businesses that employ 50 or more people offer health insurance to employees, or face a penalty, should the government need to provide a subsidy to its employees to purchase insurance. ACA provides small businesses with subsidies to offset the cost of purchasing insurance for their employees through the exchanges or marketplaces (Internal Revenue Service, 2014; Kaiser Family Foundation, 2013).
ACA eliminated co-payments, co-insurance, and deductibles for many preventative health benefits provided under Medicare and new private plans (ACA § 4103; Kaiser Family Foundation, 2011).

Medicare was created in 1965 as Title 18 of the Social Security Act. It is a health insurance program run by the federal government for individuals over age 65 and individuals under 65 with permanent disabilities. Medicare has four parts: *Part A* is hospital insurance. *Part B* is medical insurance. Medicare *Part D* covers prescription drugs. Medicare Advantage Plans, also known as *Medicare Part C*, allows enrollees to receive their Medicare health benefits through a private health insurance plan. ACA winds down the amount of subsidies paid to the private insurance companies that provide coverage under these Medicare Advantage Plans (ACA § 3201). ACA also provides for a Medicare demonstration project to evaluate "bundled payments" to provide integrated care for Medicare beneficiaries (ACA §2704(a)(1)). This differs from Medicare's current "fee-for-service" reimbursement. This concept of "bundled payments" concerns many health care professionals and will be discussed in more detail later in this chapter.

Enacted into law in 1965 as Title 19 of the Social Security Act, Medicaid is a joint federal/state program that provides basic medical care to approximately 36 million medically indigent individuals. These individuals qualify for Medicaid because their income is a certain percentage below the poverty level, they are children or parents (in some states), they are disabled, or they qualify for public assistance programs, such as *Supplemental Security Income (SSI)*. Unlike Medicare, Medicaid recipients do not pay premiums for the health care benefits they receive, because the Medicaid program provides services to the poor and is not an insurance program like Medicare. Section 1331 of ACA gives states the option to create a Basic Health Program (BHP). The BHP is a health benefits coverage program for people with incomes between 138 percent and 200 percent of the federal poverty level (who do not qualify for Medicaid), and are otherwise eligible to purchase coverage through the exchanges/marketplaces. The BHP gives states the flexibility to provide more affordable coverage for low-income residents and improve their continuity of care. Both Medicaid benefits and the BHP benefits must include the 10 essential health benefits specified in the ACA and described later in this chapter (Cassidy, 2014).

ADVOCACY AND POLITICAL ACTION

People with disabilities constitute a discrete minority group within the population. In addition, because of their various limitations and limited resources, people with disabilities often function on the margins of society. As noted earlier in the text, a large proportion of the chronically homeless in the United States are people with mental health conditions. People with I/DD may lack the skills needed to reason or plan strategically to advance themselves or to become leaders

in society. In our society today, the term *disability* implies a medical model mind-set that reflects a lack of capacity one must overcome (medical interventions), compensate for (rehabilitation), or receive charity for (entitlement programs) (Albrecht, Seelman, & Bury, 2001). Areheart (2008) clearly articulates the medical viewpoint when he states that "the medical model views the physiological condition itself as the problem. In other words, the individual is the locus of disability" (p. 186). In this conception, a disability is "a personal, medical problem, requiring an individualized medical solution; that people who have disabilities face no 'group' problem caused by society, or that social policy should be used to ameliorate" (Johnson, 2003 as cited in Areheart, 2008 p. 186).

This medical view of disabilities is seen by many as serving to fragment the disability community by focusing on individual physiological traits, traits that differentiate disabled people. The social model of disabilities rejects this approach and focuses on common societal obstacles that people with disabilities share. In the social model, being "disabled" depends upon deviation from society's construction of normality. People with a disability in society are isolated because of the ways of society, how buildings are built, what is expected in community gatherings. People with a disability face discrimination because society makes no effort to include them. The universal design movement described in Chapter 7 is the result of a social response to disability advocacy. This movement advocates a code of accessibility for use in all new societal infrastructures, both virtual and physical. This movement has broadly influenced many industries and manufacturers. For example, **Figure 21-2** shows a commercially available kitchen cabinet unit (brand name KraftMaid) called a "Pull-Out Table" designed for easy wheelchair access and stowaway storage when not needed. The disability rights

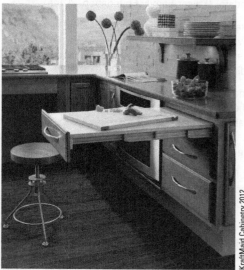

Figure 21-2 The universal design movement has encouraged manufacturers to design products that make everyday environments more usable.

movement arose from the social model of disability described in Chapter 19, and grew to where people with disabilities constitute a political advocacy group.

The rights model complements the social model. The United Nations puts forth the rights model in the *United Nations in the Convention on the Rights of Persons with Disabilities*. The rights model asserts that all humans are entitled to their rights without discrimination. People with disabilities are "rights holders" entitled to determine the course of their own lives like any other members of society. This includes, for example, the right to determine where to live, where to work, and what to eat. Limitations placed on people with disabilities by society, such as architectural barriers, amount to violations of their basic human rights (Landmine Survivors Network, 2007).

POLITICAL ADVOCACY

Political advocacy is a process designed to create positive change. Advocacy by individuals or interest groups organize and plan actions to influence public policy and resource allocation decisions. Advocacy of this type can influence political, economic, and social systems. Common political advocacy activities include media or social media campaigns, public speaking, commissioning and publishing research, and developing voter petitions.

Lobbying is a form of advocacy where advocates directly approach legislators to address an issue or concern.

Individuals or organized groups can lobby. We call people who lobby as a profession, professional lobbyists. Professional lobbyists try to influence legislation on behalf of groups or individuals who hire them. Professional lobbyists play a very influential role in U.S. politics, and because of their role, the national organizations representing each health care profession hire professional lobbyists to identify legislative issues that will have an impact on their profession.

To organize and finance political advocacy initiatives, including funding professional lobbyists, health care organizations in the United States often form a legally separate entity called a political action committee. A political action committee (PAC) is an organization whose main function is to financially support or campaign for (or against) political candidates, ballot initiatives, or legislation. A PAC must comply with federal law. In Chapter 19, we presented you with some political advocacy groups that support people with developmental, mental health, and intellectual disabilities. These groups may sponsor PACs to support the political interests of their constituency.

In addition to advocacy groups for people with disabilities, professional groups also must remain politically active to support both their clients and areas of practice. Some important PACs for rehabilitation professionals are presented in **Table 21-8**. Because elections and the political process have a profound impact on the direction of health care policy in the United States, professional and other advocacy groups view contributions to PACs as crucial.

TABLE 21-8 Examples of Professional Political Action Committees

Professional Organization	PAC Description	Donations in 2012 Election Cycle
American Occupational Therapy Association (2013) *AOTPAC Fact Sheet*	The purpose of AOTPAC is to further the legislative aims of the Association by influencing or attempting to influence the selection, nomination, election, or appointment of any individual to any federal public office, and of any occupational therapist, occupational therapy assistant, or occupational therapy student member of AOTA seeking election to public office at any level. The committee is not affiliated with any political party.	$205,950
American Physical Therapy Association (n.d.) *About PT-PAC*	PT-PAC is the sole fund-raising organization that provides access to and influence of legislators to champion PT legislative interests at the federal level.	$772,850
American Speech-Language-Hearing Association (2012)	ASHA-PAC is the political action committee for the American Speech-Language-Hearing Association.	$88,000
National Association of Rehabilitation Providers and Agencies (2012)	The National Association of Rehabilitation Providers and Agencies Political Action Committee (NARA-PAC) is a voluntary and nonprofit committee consisting of members of NARA and other interested individuals who are concerned about the rehabilitation agency industry and its patients. The PAC is consistent with NARA's motto, "Committed to the Success of PT, OT and SLP Businesses."	N/A

POLICY ISSUES FOR REHABILITATION PROFESSIONALS

No one knows how the changes in health policy brought on by ACA will affect the practice of occupational or physical therapy in the long run. For this reason, the professional organizations (AOTA and APTA) work hard to identify areas of concern to address as the Department of Human and Human Services (HHS) promulgates regulations and various provisions take effect. We present some of the issues that raise professionals' concerns.

ESSENTIAL HEALTH BENEFITS

ACA established health insurance "exchanges" or "marketplaces" to help improve insurance access, choice, cost, and coverage. An exchange or marketplace is typically a web portal that identifies insurance plans that meet federal standards established by the ACA for eligibility for participation within a given state. A qualified insurance plan is required to cover a standard minimum of services. This minimum level of coverage is called the essential health benefits. ACA mandated 10 essential health benefits. They include the following: ambulatory patient services, emergency services, hospitalization, maternity and newborn care, mental health and substance use disorder services (including behavioral health treatment), prescription drugs, rehabilitative and habilitative services (and devices), laboratory services, preventive and wellness services (including chronic disease management), and pediatric services, including oral and vision care (CMS, 2013).

There is some federal guidance on the scope of essential health services, but ultimately each state will independently determine the scope of essential health benefits they will provide. Rehabilitative and habilitative services are one of the designated categories of essential health service. ACA provided that the Institute of Medicine (IOM) study the essential benefits and make recommendations to the secretary of HHS as to how to proceed to implement the 10 essential benefits (IOM, 2012a). APTA and AOTA had input into the IOM's process to develop these recommendations. The IOM defined these terms as follows:

- **Rehabilitation services**: Health care services designed to help a person restore a function. These services may include physical and occupational therapy, speech-language pathology, and psychiatric rehabilitation services in a variety of inpatient or outpatient settings.

- **Habilitation services**: Health care services distinct from rehabilitation, because they help people first attain a particular function rather than restore a function. Examples include therapy for a child who does not yet walk or talk at an expected age of those milestones. Habilitation services may include physical and occupational therapy, speech-language pathology, and other services for people with disabilities in a variety of inpatient or outpatient settings (IOM, 2012a).

Following the IOM's report on implementation of the essential health benefits, HHS issued a rule. The rule required states to choose existing benchmarked insurance plans in their states from which to model the plan offerings on the exchanges/marketplaces. Although HHS required rehabilitative and habilitative services in qualified health plans, because the benefits were determined by the states, the benefits vary from state to state. The result is different benefits definitions from among the 50 states plus the District of Columbia. State plans may include annual visit limits, caps on the amount of therapy costs, or other restrictions for therapy services, as current employer-sponsored plans do. Therefore, state professional associations need to pursue advocacy efforts to ensure its state provides therapy coverage.

POST-ACUTE CARE BUNDLING

The ACA authorizes a voluntary national pilot program on "bundled payments" as well as a demonstration project on "bundled payments." This will involve post-acute services of habilitation and rehabilitation if the facility that offers the services chooses to participate in the program. A *bundled payment* means Medicare provides payment for services delivered across an episode of care, such as a stroke or hip replacement, rather than paying for each service (that is, PT, OT, X-ray) separately. ACA included the bundled payment provisions "to improve care coordination and to control the cost of an episode of care by changing providers' financial incentives" (Dummit, 2011). Under a bundled payment, Medicare pays a lump sum, either prospectively or retrospectively, for all services patients receive during an episode of care. For example, instead of the treatment of a hip fracture generating multiple claims from multiple providers (the surgeon, the anesthesiologist, the radiologists, the hospital, the physical therapist, the occupational therapist, and so on), Medicare compensates the entire team with one bundled payment.

Similarly, in **post-acute care bundling**, Medicare would make one payment to cover the scope of care for the entire recovery period related to the episode. The designated service provider determines how the payments are divided, what services are included, and how long a particular service is provided. This initiative means Medicare would pay a lump sum to a designated entity to cover services provided in a skilled nursing facility, an inpatient rehabilitation facility, and a home health agency for a particular patient. The hospital-based services provider and all of the patient's community-based services providers would need to cooperate and coordinate care. This initiative, although potentially quite beneficial for clients, may result in very limited access, especially to community-based care. No one is really sure how this will work. For this reason, both physical and occupational therapy professional organizations are closely monitoring developments in the regulation and implementation of the bundling payment programs.

TELEHEALTH

Telehealth is the use of electronic information and telecommunications technologies to support long-distance clinical health care (IOM, 2012b). ACA encourages the development of telehealth service delivery models as a strategy to provide cost-effective care. Telehealth programs involve "the application of evaluative, consultative, preventative, and therapeutic services delivered through communication and information technologies" (Cason, 2012, p. CE1). Communication technologies potentially used in telehealth involve many forms of virtual communication including videoconferencing, text messaging, blogging, streaming media, Skype and Google Hangouts communication, and smart phone–based communications.

Clinicians can incorporate telehealth in clinical services such as videoconferencing (real-time telehealth) to assist with service delivery between professionals, or between professional and families. Some federal agencies promote the use of telehealth to address health disparities (HRSA, 2012). For example, in rural West Virginia, access to specialists is limited. Through telehealth videoconferencing, an occupational therapist with expertise in the treatment of children with autism can observe a child in real time while also consulting with the family. In a similar application, not in real time, the family could videotape an event, for example, mealtime participation. Once complete, the family could send the video to the therapist and a telephone conference could follow.

Telehealth also includes the transmission of medical data for disease management (remote monitoring). **Figure 21-3** shows a man using a glucometer. The glucometer is one of many technologies used to help assess and maintain health. Data from this type of device is easily assimilated into telehealth practices.

Telehealth as a growing area of rehabilitation, and habilitation practice offers unparalleled new avenues to aid clients in overcoming access barriers to services. Telehealth as a service delivery model is especially well suited to promote prevention and wellness initiatives (Cason, 2012). There is consistent and strong evidence that telehealth is as (or more) effective when compared to conventional

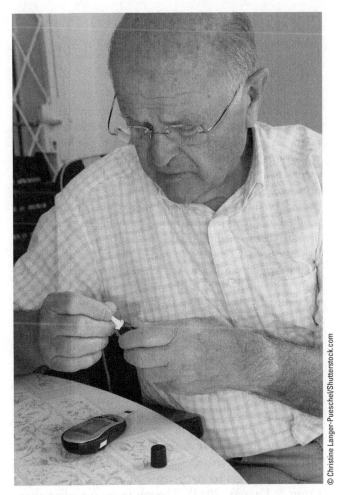

Figure 21-3 This man monitors his glucose level using a glucometer. Through transmission of glucometer readings, alterations in activities or exercise may be made in a timelier manner.

interventions (WHO/WB, 2011). The American Occupational Therapy Association identifies telehealth as an emerging practice niche. This is a growth area for all health care providers that has emerged as a result of global (WHO) and national policy initiatives. A specific application of telehealth for management of individuals with congenital or acquired disability is called "telerehabilitation." Telerehabilitation has emerged as a potential tool for management of many conditions, including stroke. A Cochrane review (Laver et al., 2013) of research into telerehabilitation post-stroke suggests such interventions have promise with respect to delivery of therapy services, especially in underserved areas. At this point, available literature does not support that telerehabilitation is superior to "usual care" across many dimensions of function, such as independence with ADLs. The review points out that it is not necessary to show telerehabilitation is superior to usual care, only that outcomes are comparable. However, the review calls for more stringent study of telerehabilitation, especially with respect to cost comparisons with traditional means of service delivery.

INDIVIDUALS WITH DISABILITIES EDUCATION ACT (IDEA)

The Individuals with Disabilities Education Act (IDEA) was introduced in Chapter 15. Since Congress created this policy, many students have benefited from the provision of educationally relevant services within the school environment. In addition, this legislation allowed numerous therapists a role in the public education sector as related service providers. This increased number of job opportunities resulted in a new awareness of what therapists can contribute outside the medical model.

In 1990, Congress amended the Education for All Handicapped Children Act, changing the name to the **Individuals with Disabilities Education Act**, commonly referred to by the acronym **IDEA**. **Table 21-9** presents the legislative history of this important law. It is important to note that although the scope of this legislation expanded greatly in the decades since its inception, the federal government actually funds less than what the law promises to provide (Aron & Loprest, 2012). With the current political focus on reducing spending, this legislation is likely to continue to face challenges.

Some criticize IDEA in two areas of particular interest to occupational and physical therapists. First, the data over the past 40 years fails to show that students from special education programs participate more in the workforce (Aron & Loprest, 2012). Though many speculate about why, clearly even the most severely disabled children qualify for educational services under IDEA. This means that even children in a permanent vegetative state participate in the school setting, with specialist teachers and therapists.

Because their anticipated educational progress is very limited, some legislators and taxpayers may argue these children can receive adequate care in a less expensive setting. Certainly, these children probably will not actively participate in either school or community settings.

A second area of interest is that IDEA mandates the provision of needed related services to allow students to access and participate in the educational environment. The definition of related services in IDEA includes, but is not limited to, physical therapy, occupational therapy, speech-language pathology, and psychological services. The related services are among the most expensive of the services mandated through IDEA. This breeds contention because the distinction between what is medically necessary and what is educationally relevant is subject to interpretation. For example, a child with tight heel cords may need physical therapy for the medical management of the condition and to improve gait and mobility. Tight heel cords do not limit the child's ability to access the curriculum, educational materials, or interact in the school environment. In this view, the school is not responsible to provide physical therapy services for the child. However, if the child is unable to manage the mobility demands within the school, or if tight heel cords interfere with the child's participation in an adaptive physical education program, one may argue physical therapy *is* educationally relevant.

Many of the lawsuits initiated by parents against local school districts relate to their child's access to services (Wright & Wright, 2012). The determination of "educationally relevant" varies from school district to school district, and has made school districts cautious about recommending related services.

Similarly, IDEA requires that schools provide assistive technology, as needed, to help students access and

TABLE 21-9	Legislative History of IDEA
1975	The Education for All Handicapped Children Act became law.
1990	The law was renamed "Individuals with Disabilities Education Act." (Pub. L. No. 101-476, 104 Stat. 1142). IDEA received minor amendments in October 1991 (Pub. L. No. 102-119, 105 Stat. 587).
1997	The act was expanded to include children between 3 and 21 years of age. It established a process for parents to attempt to resolve disputes with schools and local educational agencies through mediation, prior to initiating a lawsuit. This revision also authorized additional grants for technology, disabled infants and toddlers, parent training, and professional development (Pub. L. No. 105-17, 111 Stat. 37).
2004	IDEA was amended by the Individuals with Disabilities Education Improvement Act of 2004, now known as IDEIA. Several provisions aligned IDEA with the No Child Left Behind Act of 2001, and authorized 15 states to implement three-year IEPs. Congress added provisions related to discipline of special education students, acceptance of a "response-to-intervention" model for students not in special education, and specific requirements about using present levels of functional performance to develop functional goals in the IEPs (Pub. L. No. 108-446, 118 Stat. 2647).
2009	The American Recovery and Reinvestment Act of 2009 (ARRA) allocated $12.2 billion in additional funds for IDEA.

participate in the school environment. IDEA defines an **assistive technology device** as "any item, piece of equipment, or product system, whether acquired commercially off the shelf, modified, or customized, that is used to increase, maintain, or improve functional capabilities of a child with a disability" (20 U.S.C. 1401(1)). Assistive technology varies from simple, inexpensive devices to complicated expensive devices. An example of an expensive piece of assistive technology is a customized power wheelchair, such as the one pictured in **Figure 21-4**. Should the public school purchase this expensive device? Some school districts will purchase this and other expensive assistive technology devices, whereas others may not. However, the purchase may come with strings attached. If the school buys the device, it may

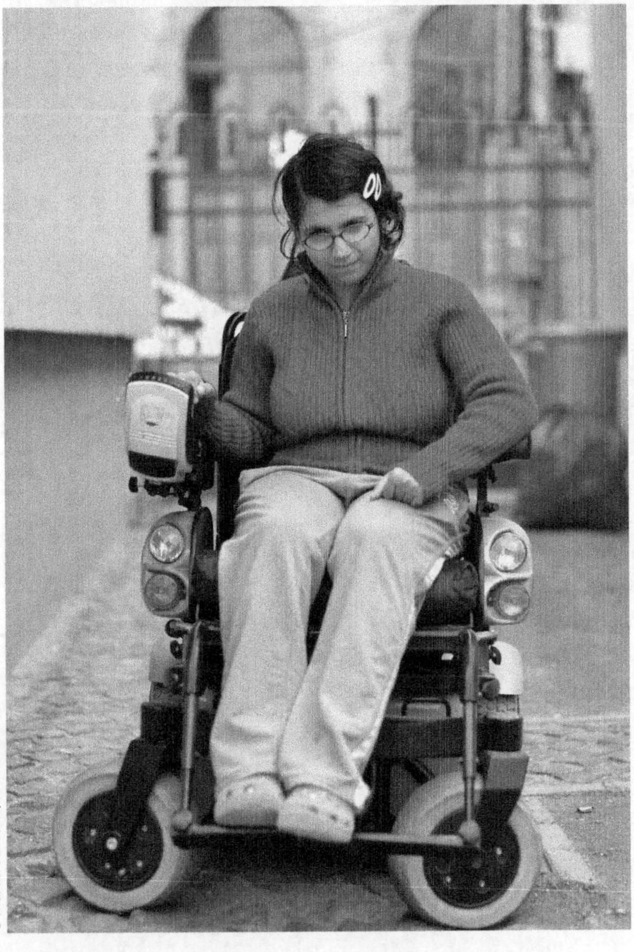

© Marcel Jancovic/Shutterstock.com

Figure 21-4 This adolescent needs her power wheelchair system to access the public school setting.

limit the device's use to the school premises or school activities. This young woman will want to use this device in other settings outside of school. Different school districts around the country will handle this dilemma differently and may develop different policies for different devices.

One of the primary methods for ensuring and financing related services and assistive technology devices, strengthened through IDEA 1997, is the use of *interagency agreements* between the public agency responsible for the child's education and other noneducational public agencies in the state. In this context, an **interagency agreement** is a sharing of resources between different governmental agencies. This includes agencies within the state's health care infrastructure, such as Medicaid. An amendment to the law states that a "noneducational public agency, as described above, may not disqualify an eligible service for Medicaid reimbursement because that service is provided in a school context" (34 C.F.R. § 300.142(b)(1)(ii)). Similarly, a school may defer the purchase of a customized power wheelchair system as "medically necessary," and have the device purchased through the state's health insurance program. This has the advantage of assuring the student owns the device and can use it in any setting.

Wright and Wright (2012) identify limits to the use of public insurance in the school setting. For example, schools may not require parents to sign up or enroll in public insurance programs in order for their child to receive free appropriate public education. Schools may not require parents to incur out-of-pocket expenses, such as deductibles or co-payments to file a claim for services. Finally, schools may not use a child's benefits under a public insurance program if it would cause the family to have to pay for services otherwise covered by the program and required for the child outside of school, or cause them to lose eligibility for home- and community-based services (34 C.F.R. § 300.142(e)).

This seems very clear, but as many states have restricted the number of therapy visits people may receive as part of their Medicaid benefits, the benefits may be exhausted during the school year, leaving the family with no options for coverage of therapy services during the summer break from school. Families must be encouraged to learn what benefits they are entitled to both under IDEA and under Medicaid, and consider what is best for their child and their family. Changes to health care financing and funding also threaten funding for medical equipment and assistive technology devices. Occupational and physical therapists will likely continue to concern themselves with these issues and will need to closely follow them during the process of ACA implementation over time.

SUMMARY

Occupational and physical therapists do not practice in isolation from the politics of policies and laws in the United States. Certain laws protect the rights of those we serve. As professionals, therapists have a professional responsibility to familiarize themselves with laws and policies that affect therapy practice and the lives of those we serve. Advocating for these laws promotes independence for our clients and patients and is part of our professional responsibility.

CASE 1

Mrs. Meena Johnson

While recovering from a fractured hip, Mrs. Johnson is diagnosed with multiple sclerosis. An occupational therapist recommends that her family install grab bars in the bathroom of her apartment and a raised toilet seat. The physical therapist also recommends a parking space close to her apartment due to her limited endurance. A home program is set up for Mrs. Johnson to perform her exercises in her apartment complex's swimming pool. Because she requires assistance in the pool, a member of her church has volunteered to help her in the pool, and the therapists have trained this person to assist her. Shortly before her discharge, the family reports to the therapists that the landlord refused to allow them to put in a grab bar. He also will not give Mrs. Johnson a parking space close to the building, because no one has "reserved" parking in the complex. The family further reports that the complex's pool rules do not allow guests in the pool after 3:00 in the afternoon on weekdays and not at all on weekends. These are the only times her church member can help Mrs. Johnson with her water exercise program. Everyone is frustrated and angry over all of the plans that were made and are now thwarted.

Not all is lost, however. The Fair Housing Amendments Act of 1988 considers Mrs. Johnson's landlord's behavior discrimination—discrimination against individuals with disabilities for housing opportunities. Occupational and physical therapy practitioners can help their clients advocate for their rights in situations like this. This advocacy makes a significant difference in people's lives, and in some situations can make the difference between living independently and living in a nursing home or other institution.

In this case study, it would be a reasonable accommodation to modify the pool rules for Mrs. Johnson so she could enjoy the pool with the assistance of her fellow church member during normally "nonguest" hours. This could be done by adding grab bars to help Mrs. Johnson get in and out of the pool at her cost. It would also be reasonable to assign Mrs. Johnson a parking space close to the building even though no one else has an assigned space. Failure to modify its policies to allow these accommodations would be discrimination. Should Mrs. Johnson face this restriction, she can file a complaint for discrimination to the U.S. Department of Housing and Urban Development at http://www .hud.gov/complaints/housediscrim.cfm.

Guiding Questions

Some questions to consider:

1. How does the situation in which Mrs. Johnson finds herself relate to goals of therapeutic intervention?
2. Compare and contrast "reasonable" versus potentially "unreasonable" accommodations in this situation.
3. Why is advocacy an important mandate for therapists and other health professionals?

CASE 2

Nancy

Nancy, a nurse with post-polio syndrome and arthritic changes, finds herself tiring easily at work. She requests accommodations from her employer to decrease the amount of energy she expends on the job. She suggests that she use a scooter at work to cut down the number of steps she must take during her workday. Nursing management makes it very clear that it cannot possibly imagine "a nurse in a wheelchair." With her employer unwilling to make this accommodation, Nancy files a complaint for employment discrimination with the Equal Employment Opportunity Commission. The Human Resources Department, alerted to the complaint, calls in an occupational therapist for advice on how to make reasonable accommodations in the workplace. The occupational therapist performs a job analysis and determines that the scooter is a safe accommodation that meets Nancy's needs and does not interfere with her job performance except during emergencies. After some hand holding with the nurse managers, the hospital administration allows Nancy to perform her nursing job using a scooter during nonemergency job functions. The occupational therapist recommends relocating the charts to a more convenient location. The final recommendation gives Nancy her own key to the supply closet so she need not go back and forth from the patient rooms to the nurse's station repeatedly to get the key. Staff readily accepts the final recommendations, Nancy's complaint is settled, and Nancy continues in her staff nursing position.

Guiding Questions

Some questions to consider:

1. How did the passage of the Americans with Disabilities Act affect the situation in which Nancy finds herself?
2. The ADA is considered an important piece of civil rights legislation. Discus what this means, and compare it with other civil rights legislation that you know.
3. In Nancy's case, how did the ADA complaint and attitudes of staff and supervisors act as barriers or facilitators?

Speaking of

Oh! The Politics of Health Care!

HUGH MURRAY, PT, DMDT, PRESIDENT,
HUNTINGTON PHYSICAL THERAPY

When I graduated from PT school back in the dark ages, I was excited about my future. I possessed a solid base of knowledge. This solid base was a little information on just about everything. The chance to learn more was on the horizon, and coming toward me hourly. I was excited about life, about gaining more knowledge, and about the

Continues

Speaking of Continued

success I was having with patients in their recovery. I was now flying along, not to be stopped or to even be slowed in my pace toward the goal of learning more and successfully treating *my* patients. I was working in an acute care hospital. The Physical Therapy Department was located between the emergency room and radiology. This was a great location to observe more and enhance my education.

All was going along well until certain events in my life radically changed my rose-colored-glasses perception of health care. I was of the opinion that I could evaluate and treat patients as if I were an island. An island of health care! Evaluating and treating patients with the best education I could achieve, some minimal experience, and the most recent research I read the night before was my life's work. That was my professional track.

This happy little freight train quickly derailed from that track. Here are just a few examples:

- A disgruntled patient confronted me early one morning, stating that workers' compensation had stopped his benefits because of the "noncompliant" letter I sent to his doctor.

- A doctor was upset with me because I told the patient he had a disc problem. What does a diagnosis mean, anyway? Do I have the right to do this—or is it limited to the doctor? The director of the department met with me to provide an "in-service" because Medicare was changing the regulations and now there were certain treatments for which there was no reimbursement. Now I could not provide this service because there was no payment. But I thought I was supposed to provide the best and most appropriate treatment dictated by my professional judgment, not by what would be reimbursed.

- The hospital was unionized, and my fellow employees voted to strike. They walked out and did not return for 28 days. Some employees did not return for 9 months due to scheduling. (I worked 12-hour days for 28 days in Central Supply because the patient census had dwindled.) Administration wants the PT staff to join the union. What does that mean to me personally? Is this professionally ethical?

- In 2009, the state legislature in its great wisdom decided chiropractors can provide physical therapy—but did not conversely decide that physical therapists could provide chiropractic care. In the meantime, the political action committee (PAC) for PT raised $3,000—while the chiropractic PAC raised $40,000. I wonder if this has anything to do with the legislative initiative.

- Our state practice act was up for "review" in 2009; we could all have been unlicensed then. Medicare had a $1,500 cap on physical therapy and speech therapy as one health care provider, but a $1,500 cap on OT as a separate provider. How did that happen???

I did not receive any education regarding these politics in PT school. I still love the profession of physical therapy after gaining more experience over all of these years. But what I know now is, there never was an island for my practice. It was a myth! I am part of a huge political system that impacts my ability to deliver care as well as the scope of care I can legally provide. For that reason, I have worked over the years to become politically informed *and* politically active. I think this is a responsibility we all must accept. I remain in the trenches because I am still excited regarding life, my continuing acquisition of knowledge, and the success I am having with my patients.

But, oh! The politics of health care!

REFERENCES

Albrecht, G., Seelman, K., & Bury, M. (2001). *Handbook of disability studies*. Thousand Oaks, CA: Sage Publications.

Americans with Disabilities Act. (2008). Pub. L. No. 101-336 (1990), as amended by Pub. L. No. 110-325 (ADAAA).

American Occupational Therapy Association. (2013). *AOTPAC fact sheet*. Retrieved from http://www.aota.org/en/Advocacy-Policy /AOTPAC/Fact.aspx

American Physical Therapy Association. (n.d.). *About PT-PAC, mission.* Retrieved from http://www.ptpac.org/about_ptpac/mission

American Speech and Hearing Association. (2012). *ASHA-PAC: Your voice on Capitol Hill.* Retrieved from http://www.asha.org/advocacy/federal/pac/

Angeles, January. (2013). Making health care more affordable: The new premium and cost-sharing assistance. Center on Budge and Policy Priorities. Retrieved from http://www.cbpp.org/cms/?fa=view &id=3190

Architectural Barriers Act, Pub. L. No. 90-480, codified at 42 U.S.C. §4151 et seq. (1968)

Areheart, B. (2008). When disability isn't "just right": The entrenchment of the medical model of disability and the Goldilocks dilemma. *Indiana Law Journal, 83,* 181–232.

Aron, L., & Loprest, P. (2012). Disability and the education system. *Future of Children, 22*(1), 97–122.

Autism Speaks. (2014). Autism Speaks 2014 State Initiative Map! Retrieved from http://www.autismspeaks.org/sites/default/files/docs/gr/states_may.2014_md.pdf

Cassidy, A. (2014). Health policy brief: Basic health program. *Health Affairs,* updated April 17, 2014. Retrieved from http://www.healthaffairs.org/healthpolicybriefs/brief.php?brief_id=113

Cason, J. (2012). Continuing education article: An introduction to telehealth as a service delivery model within occupational therapy. *OT Practice* (April 23). 17(7), CE1–CE7.

Centers for Medicare and Medicaid Services (CMS). (2013) Essential health benefits. Retrieved from http://www.cms.gov/CCIIO/Resources/Fact-Sheets-and-FAQs/ehb-2-20-2013.html

Centers for Medicare and Medicaid Services. (2014). Health insurance marketplaces. Retrieved from http://www.cms.gov/CCIIO/Programs-and-Initiatives/Health-Insurance-Marketplaces/

Civil Rights Act of 1964, 42 U.S.C. §1971 et seq. (1964).

Dummit, L.A. (2011). Medicare's bundling pilot: Including post-acute care services. *National Health Policy Forum Issues Brief, 841.* Retrieved from http://www.nhpf.org/library/issue-briefs/ib841_bundlingpostacutecare_03-28-11.pdf

Education for All Handicapped Children Act of 1975, 20 U.S.C. 33 §1401 et seq. (1975).

Elmendorf, D. (2011). *CBO's 2011 long-term budget outlook.* Congressional Budget Office, p. 44. Retrieved from http://cbo.gov/sites/default/files/cbofiles/attachments/06-21-Long-Term_Budget_Outlook.pdf

Fair Housing Act Amendments Act of 1988, 42 U.S.C. § 3601 et seq. (1988).

Federal Food, Drug, and Cosmetic Act, 21 U.S.C. Chapter 9 (2013).

Health Insurance Portability and Accountability Act of 1996 (HIPAA), Pub. L. No. 104-191, 110 Stat. 1936 (1996)

Health Resources and Services Administration (HRSA). (2012). *The role of telehealth in an evolving health care environment.* Retrieved from http://www.hrsa.gov/ruralhealth/about/telehealth/

Individuals with Disabilities Education Act. 20 U.S.C. 33 §1401 et seq. (1990).

Individuals with Disabilities Education Act Amendments of 1997, codified at 20 USC 33 § 1401 et seq. (1997).

Individuals with Disabilities Education Act (IDEA), 20 U.S.C. § 1400 (2004).

Institute of Medicine (IOM). (2012a). *Essential health benefits: Balancing coverage and cost.* Washington, DC: The National Academies Press.

Institute of Medicine (IOM). (2012b). *The role of telehealth in an evolving health care environment: Workshop summary.* Washington, DC: The National Academies Press.

Internal Revenue Service. (2014). Affordable Care Act tax provisions. Retrieved from http://www.irs.gov/uac/Affordable-Care-Act-Tax-Provisions

Johnson, M. (2003). *Make them go away: Clint Eastwood, Christopher Reeve and the case against disability rights.* Louisville, KY: The Avocado Press, Inc.

Jost, Timothy. (2013). Implementing health reform: The essential health benefits final rule. *Health Affairs* (blog). Retrieved from http://healthaffairs.org/blog/2013/02/20/implementing-health-reform-the-essential-health-benefits-final-rule/

Kaiser Family Foundation. (2014a). The requirement to buy coverage under the Affordable Care Act. Retrieved from http://kff.org/infographic/the-requirement-to-buy-coverage-under-the-affordable-care-act/

Kaiser Family Foundation. (2014b). How will the uninsured fare under the Affordable Care Act? Retrieved from http://kff.org/health-reform/fact-sheet/how-will-the-uninsured-fare-under-the-affordable-care-act/

Kaiser Family Foundation. (2013). Employer responsibility under the Affordable Care Act. Retrieved from http://kff.org/infographic/employer-responsibility-under-the-affordable-care-act/

Kaiser Family Foundation. (2011). Preventive services covered by private health plans under the Affordable Care Act. Retrieved from http://kff.org/health-reform/fact-sheet/preventive-services-covered-by-private-health-plans/

Landmine Survivors Network. (2007). *Disability rights advocacy workbook* (2nd ed.). Retrieved from http://www.handicap-international.fr/kit-pedagogique/documents/ressourcesdocumentaires/apadoption/DisabilityRightsAdvocacyWorkbook2007.pdf

Laver, K. E., Schoene, D., Crotty, M., George, S., Lannin, N. A., & Sherrington C. (2013). Telerehabilitation services for stroke. *Cochrane Database of Systematic Reviews* 12, CD010255. doi:10.1002/14651858.CD010255.pub2

Loving v. Virginia, 388 U.S. 1 (1967).

National Association of Rehabilitation Providers and Agencies. (2012). *The NARA political action committee (NARA-PAC).* Retrieved from http://naranet.org/the-nara-political-action-committee-nara-pac/

National Conference of State Legislatures. (2012). *Insurance coverage for autism.* Retrieved from http://www.ncsl.org/research/health/autism-and-insurance-coverage-state-laws.aspx

No Child Left Behind (NCLB) Act of 2001, 20 U.S.C.A. § 6301 et seq. (2002).

Olmstead v. L.C., 527 U.S. 581 (1999).

Patient Protection and Affordable Care Act (ACA), Pub. L. No. 111-148, 124 Stat. 119 (2010).

Section 504 of the Rehabilitation Act, 29 U.S.C. 701. (1973).

Social Security Administration. (2005). *Supplemental Security Income (SSI)*. Publication No. 05-11000.

Tanner, L. (2012). Doctors want to redefine autism; parents worried. *USA Today*. Retrieved from http://www.usatoday.com /news/health/story/2012-04-05/doctors-change-autism-definition /54047994/1

Telecommunications Act of 1996, Pub. L. No. 104-104, 110 Stat. 56 (1996).

United Nations. (2006). *International convention on the rights of persons with disabilities*. Retrieved from http://www.un.org/disabilities /convention/conventionfull.shtml

University of Alabama v. Garrett, 531 U.S. 356 (2001).

Water Quality Act of 1987, Pub. L. No. 100-4, 101 Stat. 7 (1987).

World Health Organization. (2001). *ICF: International classification of functioning and disability*. Geneva, Switzerland: World Health Organization.

World Health Organization (WHO). (2002). Towards a common language for functioning, disability and health ICF: The International Classification of Functioning, Disability and Health. Retrieved from http://www.who.int/classifications/icf /training/icfbeginnersguide.pdf

World Health Organization. (2014). *International classification of diseases data sheet*. Retrieved from http://www.who.int/classifications /icd/factsheet/en/

World Health Organization/World Bank (WHO/WB). (2011). *World report on disability*. Geneva, Switzerland: World Health Organization. Retrieved from http://whqlibdoc.who.int /hq/2011/WHO_NMH_VIP_11.01_eng.pdf

Wright, P., & Wright, P. (2012). FAQs: Related services. Wrightslaw. Retrieved from http://www.wrightslaw.com/info/relsvcs .faqs.htm

CHAPTER 22

Assessment of Human Performance across the Life Span

Mary Beth Mandich, PT, PhD
Professor and Chairperson, Division of Physical Therapy, West Virginia University, Morgantown, West Virginia and

Anne Cronin, PhD, OTR/L, FAOTA,
Associate Professor, Division of Occupational Therapy, West Virginia University, Morgantown, West Virginia and

Toby Long, PhD, PT,
Associate Professor, Department of Pediatrics, Associate Director for Training, Center for Child and Human Development Director, Division of Physical Therapy, Center for Child and Human Development Georgetown University, Washington, DC

Objectives

Upon completion of this chapter, readers should be able to:

- Describe the strengths and weaknesses of both the top-down and bottom-up models used to assess individuals;

- Differentiate between qualitative and quantitative assessment, including the clinical reasoning process used in the determination of appropriate assessment tools in clinical contexts;

- Discuss the qualities needed in an effective screening assessment;

- Compare and contrast norm-referenced and criterion-referenced assessments;

- Explain how clinical reasoning is used in the assessment process;

- Differentiate between the following three qualitative assessment strategies: structured observation, naturalistic observation and movement analysis; and

- Discuss the reason for the focus on participation as a clinical outcome, and name the challenges to development of objective measurement tools at this level.

Key Terms

assessment

bottom-up assessment

Canadian Occupational Performance
   Measure (COPM)

client

clinical reasoning

criterion-referenced test

developmental assessment

enablement theory

Functional Independence
   Measure (FIM)

movement analysis

naturalistic observation

norm-referenced test

outcome measures

qualitative assessment

quantitative assessment

reliability

screening process

sensitivity

specificity

standardized test

structured observation

top-down assessment

validity

treatment theory

INTRODUCTION

The World Health Organization provides health coding and classification systems that are incorporated into health care documentation standards adopted by most countries so uniform data is available for descriptive and comparative analysis. The ICD-10 (the International Statistical Classification of Diseases and Related Health Problems), which was described in Chapter 21, is the most widely known of these classification and coding systems. The ICD-10 is a code for the medical diagnosis or health condition. Throughout this text, the frame of reference used has been that of another major WHO classification system, that is, the ICF (International Classification of Functioning, Disability and Health). The ICF describes the structure/function and activity/participation dimensions of health outcomes, which are not inherent in the medical diagnosis. The use of these two tools is intended to improve analysis and research into health and health care interventions on a global scale. The ICD-10 is a medical model–based consideration of health conditions, and the ICF offers an integrated biopsychosocial model. **Figure 22-1** is a duplication of a figure presented in Chapter 1 of this text. The discussion of medical and social models is especially important as we consider clinical applications of human performance across the lifespan.

Within the U.S. health care system, documentation of outcomes is a product of a process of accumulation and interpretation of clinical data. The *Guide to PT Practice* 3 (American Physical Therapy Association, 2014) uses the following terminology to characterize this process. *Examination* refers to obtaining data from the patient or client, utilizing both subjective (interview, history) and objective (tests and measures) tools. *Tests and measures* are tools for objective documentation of the client's condition, which should be reliable and valid. Examples of tests and

measures include a variety of familiar clinical tools, such as goniometry, muscle strength testing, balance scales (American Physical Therapy Association, 2001). *Evaluation* is a

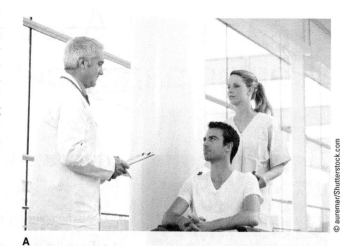

A

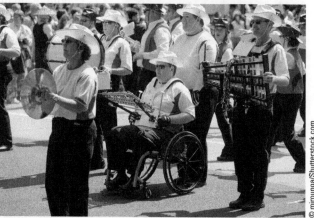

B

Figure 22-1   A. The ICD-10 offers a tool to classify disease (medical model) **B.** The ICF offers a tool to classify function and participation (social model).

TABLE 22-1	What is a Client?
Type of Client	**Description**
People	Includes families, caregivers, teachers, employers, and relevant others.
Groups	Includes community support groups, businesses, industries, or agencies.
Populations	Includes subgroups within a community, such as refugees, veterans who are homeless, and people with chronic health disabling conditions.

American Occupational Therapy Association. (2014). Occupational Therapy Practice Framework: Domain and process (3rd ed.) Bethesda, MD: AOTA Press.

synthesis of the examination results and clinical reasoning to determine if the nature of the problem is within the scope of PT practice and subsequently to establish diagnosis, prognosis and a plan of care. For example, if a woman is referred to therapy for walking on her toes, the examination results will determine if she has limited range of motion, spasticity, and so on. The evaluation will take these findings into account based on clinical knowledge and arrive at a clinical hypothesis, such as idiopathic toe walking or mild cerebral palsy. The *Occupational Therapy Practice Framework: Domain and Process (OTPF)* (AOTA, 2014) describes evaluation as a process that occurs during the initial and all subsequent visits with a client that has the focus of determining what the client wants and needs to do. Assessment is an umbrella term that may encompass the entire process or its component parts. Assessment provides a foundation for clinical reasoning. The nature of assessment is dependent on numerous factors, including the specific assessment environment, purpose, client condition, and available resources. The assessment process is characterized by the use of comprehensive strategies and tools to delineate strengths and needs, to develop appropriate intervention plans and strategies, and to determine change in individuals. A client is the focus of interest in the health care service interaction. Although we typically think of a client as an individual, a client may also be a group or a population. **Table 22-1** presents the definition of client presented in the *OTPF* (AOTA, 2014). This broad view of a client is important, especially for clinicians working in the areas of wellness and public health.

MODELS OF ASSESSMENT

Assessment is a broad term used to characterize important activities for rehabilitation professionals. Assessment strategies may vary in purpose, frame of reference, and scope. However, the outcome of assessment uniformly should be an intervention plan that promotes the clients' ability to perform age-appropriate life roles within an environmental context.

SCREENING VERSUS FOCUSED ASSESSMENT

Models of assessment may be described with respect to their purpose as either *screening* or *focused*. The screening process is a brief general assessment used to identify impairments and to determine if further assessment is needed. Typically, the screening process should be brief, and the test used should be easy to administer by a variety of people (physicians, therapists, nurses, teachers, and, in some cases, parents). Because the purpose of screening is to determine the need for referral and further assessment, screening tools should be characterized by sensitivity and specificity. Sensitivity is the ability of a screening tool to identify individuals who have a condition, such as developmental delay, and differentiate them from the population at large. A sensitive screening tool avoids false negatives, that is, overlooking someone who has a condition. Specificity is the ability of a screening tool to differentiate individuals with a condition at a high level of accuracy, thereby avoiding false positives. A test that lacks specificity would identify many children as having developmental delays, causing undue concerns and costs, when in fact, most of the children identified did not have a problem upon further assessment. As you can see, for many reasons, it is important that screening assessments have high sensitivity and specificity.

Focused assessment may be construed as part of the evaluation process, which is a more complex process, typically following an initial screening. If a formalized screening was not completed, as is sometimes the case in hospital-based referrals, informal medical chart review and client interview can serve as a starting point for the evaluation. The evaluation process includes historical information, current test findings, and clinical judgment about actual or potential health problems/life process occurring with the individual, family, group, or community. The evaluation process is a cyclical and ongoing process that can end at any stage if the problem is solved. *Clinical reasoning* plays an essential role in the evaluation process as the specific approaches to assessment are determined based on the data the expert clinician deems necessary and on the environments in which participation is limited. **Clinical reasoning** is "a situated, practice-based form of reasoning that requires a background of scientific and technological research-based knowledge about general cases, more so than any particular instance. It also requires practical ability to discern the relevance of the evidence behind general scientific and technical knowledge and how it applies to a particular patient. In doing so, the clinician considers the patient's particular clinical trajectory, their concerns and preferences, and their particular vulnerabilities (e.g., having multiple comorbidities) and sensitivities to care interventions (e.g., known drug allergies, other conflicting comorbid conditions, incompatible therapies, and past responses to therapies) when forming clinical decisions or conclusions" (Benner, Hughes, & Sutphen, 2008, p. 4).

BOTTOM-UP VERSUS TOP-DOWN

Assessment strategies are often described as either *bottom-up* or *top-down*. **Bottom-up assessment** is the synthesis of signs and symptoms with chief complaint and past history to determine underlying pathology that may contribute to performance impairments. In a bottom-up approach, individual deficits are first specified in great detail. These elements are then linked together to form larger diagnostic categories. For example, if a person is referred to therapy for a medical condition such as arthritis, a bottom-up assessment would first compile information about strength, range of motion, and cardiovascular status, and then derive how these goals influence activity and participation. A bottom-up evaluation strategy gathers information regarding body-level structure and function and is *diagnostic-prescriptive,* meaning deficits or impairments are delineated in specific areas, leading to a program designed to remediate those deficits. This strategy is most appropriate for (1) assessing the underlying cause of performance problems, and (2) designing intervention that targets impairments such as decreased joint range of motion or muscle weakness. This model, illustrated in **Figure 22-2**, is less helpful when designing functionally orientated intervention plans needed to improve outcomes within the daily lives of individuals.

Conversely, **top-down assessment** is an approach from the social model that considers participation within the context of everyday life. Top-down assessment starts with the big picture first, before considering underlying problems. For example, in top-down assessment, therapists will ask clients what activity/participation dimensions are sources of difficulty. If a client says he has difficulty in self-care, assessment will focus on determining *why*. For example, assessment may determine he lacks strength, sufficient range of motion, or cardiovascular endurance. In a top-down evaluation strategy, a therapist

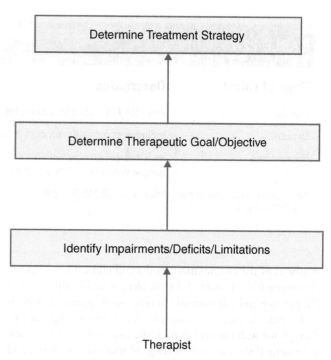

Figure 22-2   Trajectory of a Bottom-Up Assessment Strategy

collects information on areas of activity and participation in the client's natural environment. Therapeutic programs are functionally orientated and are geared to the accomplishment of client-identified outcomes. In the top-down model, illustrated in **Figure 22-3**, *desired outcomes* guide the assessment process. These are statements that describe what the team (clients, parents, caregivers, and professionals) would like to see happen in individuals. Outcomes can be general ("I'd like to see Anna move around") or specific ("Mr. O'Mara needs to walk from his bed to the bathroom"). In either example, the purpose of the assessment is to determine why the person is unable to achieve the desired activities and participation.

Table 22-2 presents these two assessment approaches as they relate to the ICF and ICD-10. The assessment process is informed by both the medical and social models. As health care practitioners, we will need to be fluent in both models and understand the strengths and weaknesses of each in assessment.

Because physical therapy practice emerged from a medical model, the great bulk of assessment procedures historically used in physical therapy reflect this model. A study by O'Neil and colleagues (2006) discovered that, although many assessments targeted activity and body structure/function for individuals with cerebral palsy, only a handful of assessments were geared toward participation. Occupational therapy has historically had a strong participation perspective; however, medical reimbursement for services and specific medically based referral processes have led to the use of similar medical model–based bottom-up assessment tools in occupational therapy practice.

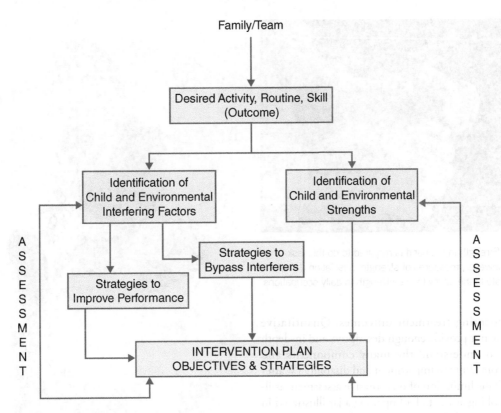

Figure 22-3   Trajectory of a Top-Down Assessment Strategy

Currently, both occupational and physical therapy assessments, for different historical reasons, are weighted toward the bottom-up assessment approach, which represents a medical model.

Several research groups have noted a disproportionate reliance on bottom-up assessments of structure and function in both physical and occupational therapy. Watter and colleagues (2008) noted that, in a review of multidisciplinary assessments for children with developmental coordination disorder, common assessment measures were "bottom heavy" leading to the potential overrepresentation of body structure and function impairments in the assessment process.

QUANTITATIVE VERSUS QUALITATIVE

Assessment tools may be either quantitative or qualitative. **Quantitative assessment** is an assessment approach that uses measurable properties such as range of motion, distance, reaction time, or performance measures to give insight into the integrity and function of the human body. Quantitative assessments are highly valued because they are objective, repeatable, and people can be specifically trained to give the measure in a reliable manner. Quantitative assessment is useful in making a diagnosis, in identifying deviation in development, in determining eligibility for therapy services,

TABLE 22-2	Approaches to Assessment Consistent with the ICF			
	Activity Limitation		**Participation Restriction**	
	Bottom-Up Assessment		*Top-Down Assessment*	
Focus Area	Pathology	Behavioral	Participation	
Conditions	Anatomical, physiological, mental	Performance skill deficits	Performance pattern deficits	Role performance deficits
Interventions	Medical and habilitative/rehabilitative therapies		Adaptations and environmental modifications	Supportive services and social policies

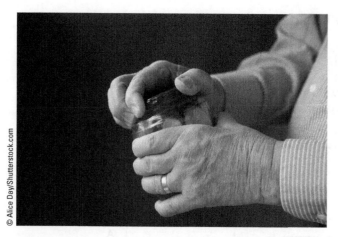

© Alice Day/Shutterstock.com

Figure 22-4   Strength in the hand is required to do this task of opening a jar; however, measures of strength in isolation do not perfectly correlate to the ability to use strength in daily occupations.

and in documenting treatment outcomes. Quantitative assessment may not provide enough descriptive and in-depth information to understand the many components and contexts that contribute to impairment and disability (Watter et al., 2008). This limitation of quantitative assessment is illustrated by looking at the task of opening a jar illustrated in **Figure 22-4**. Although it is easy to get data on grip strength using a quantitative measurement tool such as a dynamometer, grip strength measures are not descriptive of what the individual can or cannot do in everyday life. Absence of grip strength will certainly limit this woman's competence in opening a jar lid; however, good grip strength will not assure that she can perform these tasks. Tests and measures, such as dynamometry, commonly used by therapists are examples of quantitative assessment that will be discussed in greater depth later in this chapter.

Qualitative assessment is an assessment approach that uses observation, knowledge, and clinical reasoning in conjunction with nonstandard assessment tools such as chart review, intervention, visual assessment of movement patterns, and ecological assessments. Qualitative assessments tend to be naturalistic, embedded in the individuals' usual environmental setting, and accommodating of variations in instruction and demonstration to help optimize performance.

Qualitative assessment differs from quantitative assessment in that the test results are not uniform and the validity of the test varies with the skill of the individuals giving and interpreting the test. Qualitative assessment relies on clinical reasoning rather than psychometric properties to make a testing procedure valid. Qualitative assessment is useful in determining function and participation above the body structures and functions level.

The extensive education in anatomy, physiology, kinesiology, human development, and motor control common to the education of occupational and physical therapists provides the foundation for clinical reasoning that supports qualitative assessment, whereas quantitative assessments can

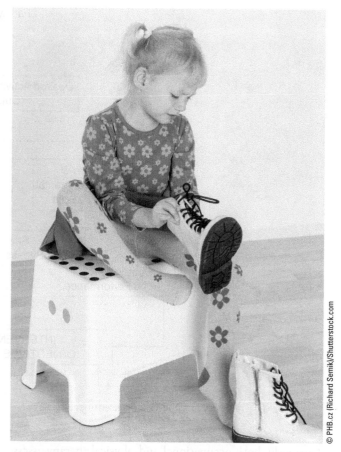

© PHB.cz (Richard Semik)/Shutterstock.com

Figure 22-5   This little girl is putting on her boots. Qualitative assessment of the pattern she uses provides insight into parameters such as postural control, strength, calibration, and flow.

be given by any individual trained in the administration of the test. In **Figure 22-5**, the little girl is putting on her boots. Qualitative assessment, such as the movement analysis presented in **Table 22-3**, would describe the strategy she uses to accomplish this task.

Observation is an important qualitative assessment tool for occupational and physical therapists. **Structured observation** is an assessment strategy that involves the staging of a movement pattern or behavior that the therapist needs to analyze, to observe it carefully and repeat as needed until enough information has been gathered. The balance assessment shown in **Figure 22-8** is an example of a structured observation. Structured observation is an aspect of many assessment procedures. **Naturalistic observation** is a strategy of observing a behavior as it occurs in its natural setting with no attempts at intervention on the part of the clinician. Naturalistic observation is distinct from structured observation in that it occurs in the clients' familiar environment, using the clients' own tools or materials. Asking a client to walk in the clinical setting would be a structured observation, whereas watching the person walk in the park, as shown in **Figure 22-6**, would be a naturalistic observation.

motor task, is presented in **Table 22-3**. The movement analysis in **Table 22-3** was intended to reflect age-related changes in motor performance in healthy, typically developing individuals. When normal movement patterns are well understood, they can provide the basis for clinical reasoning, and the movement analysis can be an effective qualitative assessment strategy for people with impairments or disabilities. Note that a movement analysis may be a naturalistic observation, as is the example presented in **Table 22-3**, or it can be used in a clinical setting as a structured observation.

ICF FRAME OF REFERENCE

Emerging focus on outcomes is increasingly at the level of participation; however, the assessment process, as discussed previously, has deep roots in a model that emphasizes body structure/function and even activity, but not participation. An **outcome measure**, in the context of health care, is a measure of the quality of medical care, the standard against which the end result of the intervention is assessed. The need for better outcome measures that reflect community participation has been widely endorsed by the rehabilitation community. Some assessment tools have been developed to look at specific aspects of community function, and an increasing number of studies seek to document the link between improvements in body structures and function and activity/participation. This entire subject is further complicated by the fact that therapists practicing in institutional settings, that is, hospitals and outpatient clinics, historically have determined participation from report, as they are unable to directly assess participation in natural environments.

Although there is a widespread clinical belief that improvement in body structures and functions reduces activity limitations and participation restrictions, this has not been convincingly demonstrated in the literature. Sullivan and Cen (2011) reported that the direct effect of impairment on participation was not statistically significant; however, the indirect effect through activity was significant. Darrah and colleagues (2008) discussed how goals generated from evaluation directed intervention for children with cerebral palsy. These authors reported 78 percent of therapists identified goals at the level of enhancing function or participation. However, they reported that therapists working with children under the age of 3 were more likely to establish goals at the body function/structure level. An interesting finding from the study by Darrah and colleagues is therapists reported an assumption of translation of outcome, that is, that increases in strength or range of motion (body function) would translate to activity-level goals, such as improved ambulation. These assumptions, were multidirectional, that is, therapists sometimes established goals at the activity level to maintain strength and range of motion. This may not

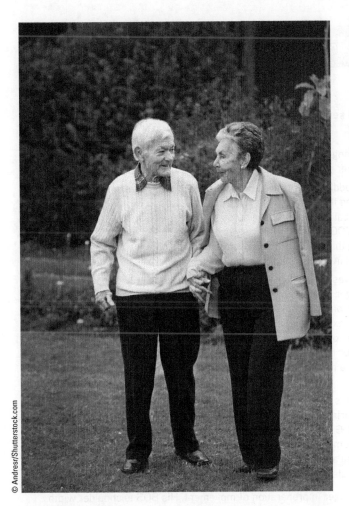

Figure 22-6   Watching this couple walk in the park is an example of a naturalistic observation of gait.

© Andresr/Shutterstock.com

A specific type of qualitative assessment, usually taught early in the educational process for physical and occupational therapists is the movement analysis. **Movement analysis** is an in-depth method of describing, interpreting, and documenting a specific movement pattern. A movement analysis includes a brief description of the movement to be observed. Typically, observers describe at least four aspects of the movement, and describe the movement in stages as it occurs. The first aspect of the movement that is considered is the *postural set,* including the impact of gravity, challenges to balance, and alignment. The second aspect is movement *calibration,* including where the movement strength is needed, how the strength demands change and the grading or controlling of effort to suit the task. The third aspect is *flow.* Flow includes the timing, speed, direction, and quality of movement. Flow is reflected in the coordination of the movement. The final aspect is the *sensory/perceptual* aspect. For the sensory/perceptual aspect of movement analysis the focus is on changes in, or use of sensory information, rather than on a background awareness of posture in a resting position. An example of a completed movement analysis, comparing four individuals performing the same

TABLE 22-3   Example Movement Analysis Comparing Performance across Four Age Groups

TASK OBSERVED: Hanging Up a Hanger

Age of client	Please write a description in a few sentences of the qualitative aspects of the movement pattern used by your subject.
4 years	The child stands statically holding the hanger in preparation of movement. Her base of support (BOS) is about shoulder width apart and her center of gravity (COG) remains along her midline. The *preparatory phase* begins with the toddler performing a weight shift forward as she stumbles to take a step closer to the hanger rod. She grips the hanger while her elbow appears to be in flexion and her shoulder remains in the neutral anatomical position. As she steps forward, her BOS is narrowed slightly and throws her a little off balance. Her COG is also shifted forward as she steps closer to the hanger rod. Little muscle activity is used during this phase of the movement to hold onto the hanger; however, body and vestibular control are essential in moving closer to the hanger rod. The *middle phase* of the movement involves the toddler lifting her arm to place the hanger on the rod. Because she cannot see where the hanger needs to be placed, she makes some placement errors and relies on proprioception to fit the hanger on accurately onto the hanger rod. This movement is accomplished by the muscle strength through flexion of the shoulder and flexion and extension of the elbow, wrist, and hand. The action that occurs is open-chain and transpires proximal to distal. As the arm extends to place the hanger on the hanger rod, the COG is shifted even farther forward and the BOS appears to be fairly narrow, allowing for a more unstable position that intern allows for more dynamic movement. The *final phase* of the movement concludes with retraction of the arm back to its original starting position. Little muscle activity is recruited during this phase as the resistance of the hanger is no longer being placed on the toddlers arm. Her COG returns with a downward force being placed in the center of her body and her BOS remains stable. Somatosensory activity involved touching the hanger and feeling it being placed onto the closet rod as well as feeling her BOS on the ground. The flow of her movement was very rapid and showed poorly calibrated control.
10 years	The child stands statically holding the hanger in preparation of movement. His BOS is shoulder width apart, and little muscle activity is being recruited during this initial phase of the movement. The *preparatory phase* is characterized by a weight shift forward and by gripping the hanger with finger flexion paired with extension of the elbow. The wrist and the shoulder remain in a neutral position. As the weight shift occurs, the COG is shifted forward. The BOS remains stationary but the movement requires more vestibular control. Little strength is required during this phase of the movement. The *middle phase* of the movement is characterized by flexion of the shoulder and slight elbow flexion in order to place the hanger on the rod. This movement is visually guided and the action is an open-chain movement with motion occurring proximal to distal. This stage requires the greatest amount of strength. The *final phase* of the movement is concluded with retraction of the shoulder through extension back to its neutral position. As the arm is returned to neutral, the postural control was reestablished with the COG returning back to its initial position over the BOS. Little muscle activity is being recruited during this phase of the movement. The flow of the movement is well calibrated but occurs rapidly. The resistive force that acts throughout the movement is that of the child's arm and the weight of the hanger. Movement occurred in a cardinal plane occurring in the sagittal plane. Somatosensory activity involved touching the hanger and feeling it being placed onto the closet rod as well as feeling his BOS on the ground.
23 years	The person stands statically in preparation of the movement. Her BOS is stable on the ground and her COG is at her body midline. She holds the hanger in her right hand with her elbow in 90 degrees of flexion, her wrist and shoulder at neutral, and flexion in her hand. Little muscle action is needed. The *preparatory phase* of the movement occurs with a forward weight shift of the body as the student leans forward and takes a step toward the hanger rod. There is no change in her right arm position. As the weight shift occurs, the COG also shifts forward and the BOS is altered as she takes a step forward. Vestibular control is necessary to maintain balance throughout the movement.

Continues

TABLE 22-3 Example Movement Analysis Comparing Performance across Four Age Groups *(continued)*

Age of client	Please write a description in a few sentences of the qualitative aspects of the movement pattern used by your subject.
	The *middle phase* of the movement is characterized by the student engaging in extension of the elbow and flexion of the shoulder to place the hanger onto the rod. The intrinsic and extrinsic muscles of the hand and wrist are also active in holding and releasing the hanger, using visual guidance. This is an open-chain action, and movement occurs proximal to distal. This phase of the movement requires the greatest amount of strength as she lifts the hanger overcoming the resistive forces of both the hanger and the student's arm. Proprioception is also important during this phase to accurately place the hanger on the closet rod. She did look briefly at the target, but did not sustain her gaze, allowing proprioception to guide the bulk of the movement.
	The *final phase* of the movement involves the student retracting her arm after placing the hanger on the rod. The elbow moves through slight flexion and then returns to an extended position. The shoulder extends to return to a neutral position. The BOS remains stationary, and the COG is returned to its original position. This phase requires little muscle activation. The flow of the movement is quick but very well calibrated. Somatosensory activity involved touching the hanger and feeling it being paced onto the closet rod as well as feeling her BOS on the ground.
71 years	The person begins standing statically with her COG at midline. She holds the hanger using the intrinsic and extrinsic muscles of the hand, slight wrist flexion with her elbow flexed at almost 90 degrees.
	The *preparatory phase* of the movement begins with a weight shift forward as she takes two steps to lean into the closet. Her BOS is altered allowing for more dynamic movement to occur. Her COG is also shifted forward. Vestibular control is necessary to maintain balance, and some postural muscle activity is being recruited.
	The *middle phase* of the movement involves extension of the elbow and flexion of the shoulder to place the hanger on the closet rod. The intrinsic and extrinsic muscles of the hand and wrist are also active in holding and releasing the hanger, using visual guidance. Although she is using visual guidance and proprioception, her placement is a little off as she initially lifts the hanger about an inch too high. She then lowers it to accurately place the hanger in the appropriate position. This phase requires the most muscle activation to overcome the resistive forces of the hanger and her arm. This is an open-chain movement, and action occurs proximal to distal.
	The *final phase* of the movement is characterized by retracting the shoulder using the posterior deltoid back to its neutral starting position and flexing the elbow back to 90 degrees using the biceps brachii. The COG is returned to its starting position over top of the BOS. She returns to a static position. Little muscle activity is used during this phase. The flow of the movement was uneven, with slight pauses during the action. As compared to a younger person, her movements were also somewhat slower. Somatosensory activity involved touching the hanger and feeling it being placed onto the closet rod as well as feeling the ground under her feet. There was much more visual attention to the task than was seen in other age groups.

Summary

All age groups provided similar results in their movement patterns; however, the preparatory phase of the toddler was much less stable and occurred with less control than the other three age groups. All age groups engaged in a weight shift forward during the preparatory phase, whether or not they stepped into the closet. The COG was shifted with their weight, and the BOS became less stable, allowing for the dynamic movement to occur. The child and the adult had no trouble placing the hanger on the closet rod, whereas the toddler and the senior struggled a little bit. The toddler could not effectively use visual guidance because of the height of the rod, and may have been more effective with a closet rod closer to eye level. The flow of the movement occurred rapidly and unevenly for the toddler, whereas the child and the adult showed more control and consistency in their movements. The flow of the movement for the senior occurred slowly but was controlled. Vestibular control was established and maintained in each subject; however, the toddler required a little more compensation through taking more steps or using her arm that placed the hanger on the closet rod for stability.

be the case, and the activity-participation dimension of the ICF infers that changes in activity do NOT automatically result in change in participation.

Both Watter et al. (2008) and Ptyushkin et al. (2012) mention the extensive use of discipline-specific assessments used in settings providing rehabilitation services. Watter and colleagues reviewed these discipline-specific tests and commented that there was little overlap between tests and that "the implication for clinical practice is that multiple assessments—across disciplines and across ICF domains—provide optimal description of performance in children with DCD, which is essential for optimal intervention planning" (Watter et al., 2008, p. 347). Although the need for a multidisciplinary viewpoint is acknowledged, Ptyushkin et al. (2012) noted that the multitude of differing measures and differing profession-specific descriptors made outcome measurement difficult. These authors were optimistic about the potential for uniform ICF terminology to allow for the standardization of outcome measures. Simeonsson et al. (2003) stated the ICF could assist in developing proper measurement tools for assessing childhood disabilities by providing a framework that accurately portrays patients' lifestyle and functioning levels. The authors also felt the ICF framework could ultimately allow for culmination of the rights of children with disabilities.

TESTS AND MEASURES

To provide evidence of effectiveness of interventions, both at the individual and group levels, measurement is essential. To that end, measurements must be characterized by **reliability** and **validity**. Reliability may be thought of as equivalent to the stability of the measurement across different examiners and at different times. The former type of reliability is referred to as *inter-rater reliability*, which means how close the measurements would be if taken by two different people. *Test-retest reliability* refers to how stable the measurement is if taken hours or days apart. This type of reliability is important because it differentiates between normal fluctuations in measurement versus true clinical change. Reliability is usually expressed as a correlation between two measures, taken by different individuals or at different times. Validity generally refers to whether an instrument measures what it is supposed to measure. There are several types of validity. One example of validity is *construct validity*. Assessment of pain is an example of a challenge in obtaining construct validity, because it is such a multidimensional concept. However, one way to determine whether a pain scale is valid is to compare it to physical indicators of pain, such as sweating or muscle tension.

Many kinds of tests and measures are used in habilitative and rehabilitative settings, ranging from simple to complex. For example, consider the measurement of a common

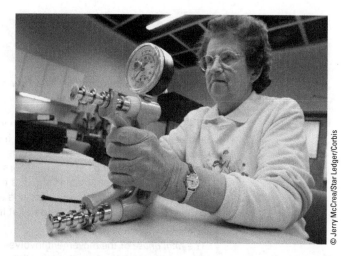

© Jerry McCrea/Star Ledger/Corbis

Figure 22-7   This woman has had a stroke and has been working in occupational therapy to regain the strength in her left hand. By using a dynamometer, the therapist has a quantitative measure of her grip strength.

function such as muscle strength. Muscle strength can be measured by a manual muscle test, which assigns a prescriptive value to the person's ability to move against gravity and resistance. Basic measurement tools, like dynamometers, can be used to measure muscle strength. The range of possibilities in the measurement of muscle strength extends to elaborate technological tests of muscle strength including isokinetic machines, such as the KinCom or BioDex. **Figure 22-7** shows a woman using a dynamometer to test her grip strength. This is a reliable tool, which can be used to diagnose weakness and can be used to measure progress in therapy. Very little instruction is needed for student therapists to learn to use and to interpret the readings on a dynamometer. The dynamometer provides an example of a bottom-up assessment. It measures muscle strength in a standard grasp pattern. This information may be used to identify whether strength is a reason why a woman with rheumatoid arthritis cannot open a jar, as in Figure 22-4. There is no doubt that dynamometers and similar tools will always be a mainstay for both occupational and physical therapists.

Balance is another example of having a range of measurement instruments. At the most basic level, balance may be assessed as simply as using a watch to time how long a person can stand on one leg. **Figure 22-8** shows a therapist displacing a woman's balance to assess her response. The therapist may count or time the number of seconds the woman can hold this pose. The therapist is guarding the woman to assure her safety as her balance is challenged by being asked to hold this position.

Assessment of balance may also be as sophisticated as the virtual reality system shown in **Figure 22-9**. Virtual reality systems are popular because they measure basic parameters of body structure and function, but also simulate activities that represent real-life participation. Another advantage of virtual reality systems is that safety risks are

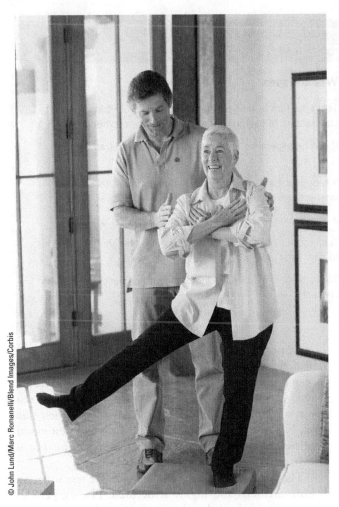

Figure 22-8   A physical therapist is assessing this woman's balance using both qualitative assessment and simple quantitative measures, such as timing the task.

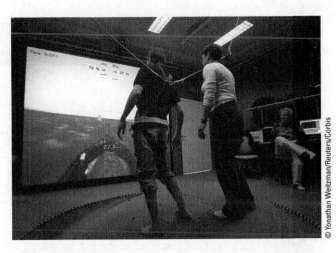

Figure 22-9   This young man had a brain injury and has difficulty with balance. He works here with a virtual reality system that gives the therapist detailed information about his performance at a higher level and with more contextual specificity than is often available.

minimized in the virtual environment, as opposed to the natural environment. However, virtual reality systems remain very expensive, and it is questionable if they give significantly more information than simpler assessments. Such systems may become more common in the future as costs for the virtual technology are reduced.

It is worth considering the level of client engagement and motivation in the types of measurements discussed previously. Although dynamometry and simple balance assessments such as standing on one leg provide insight into strength and balance respectively, the more practice individuals have in the natural context for the task, the greater the likelihood the task will be transferred into the natural environment. Most would agree that practice in the virtual reality environment is likely to be highly engaging and motivating, therefore making the virtual reality assessment tool effective as part of the intervention process.

Although measurements such as dynamometry and balance tests measure isolated parameters, a standardized test is a measurement tool designed to compile numerous measurements. A **standardized test** is a test that is administered and scored in a consistent, or "standard," manner. A standardized test is any test in which the same test is given in a uniform manner to all test takers (Richardson, 2001). A **norm-referenced test** is a type of standardized test that has been given to a large number of individuals that serve as a normative sample (Richardson, 2001). Therapists using a norm-referenced test can compare the performance of individuals tested to those of other "normative" individuals with similar qualities. The underlying construct for a norm-referenced test is the bell curve of score distribution of individuals comprising the normative sample. It is important that the normative sample is representative of the population. For example, a normal distribution of scores for dynamometry should be broken into age and gender classifications, as comparison of scores achieved by a 70-year-old female would not be appropriate based on norms developed on younger male adults. Peters and colleagues (2011) published normative values for adults, differentiated by age and gender, on the standard dynamometer. In this way, the therapist working with the woman in **Figure 22-7** is able to compare her performance to the average performance of women her age.

Standardized tests are often used in the screening process, because they offer objective information to determine whether or not further, more in-depth assessment is required. Standardized tests are also often used as outcome measures, because uniform information can be obtained that is useful for the analysis of not only individuals, but also therapy approaches and rehabilitation programs. Some commonly used standardized tests are **criterion-referenced tests**. Criterion-referenced tests develop a list of items, or criteria, typically performed by a standard sample of the population and evaluate individuals against these criteria. Criterion-referenced tests are very useful in documenting

TABLE 22-4   Strengths and Weaknesses of Standardized Testing

Strengths	Weaknesses
Data analysis is easy because of the quantitative nature of data.	Test situation is artificial and highly structured; it may not be comparable to performance in natural environments.
It allows comparability of common measures across populations.	It can be expensive in terms of materials and training.
It has strong psychometric properties (high measurement validity).	It requires that the person being tested understand the instructions for test performance.
It provides availability of reference group data.	It may not be applicable to people with clinical conditions.
Tests are recognized and respected across disciplines.	Test scores are objective, but may not be meaningful without further interpretation.
It provides data that is comparable across individuals and can be useful in research.	These tests are limited in their ability to capture the unique characteristics of individuals.

progress of individuals toward goals in therapy. An example of a widely used criterion-referenced test is the **Functional Independence Measure (FIM)** (Keith, Granger, Hamilton, & Sherwin, 1987; Granger, 1990). The FIM is a brief 18-item test that provides a uniform system of measurement for disability that is consistent with the ICF. The FIM measures the level of a person's disability and indicates how much assistance is required for the individual to carry out activities of daily living. **Table 22-4** presents the strengths and weaknesses of standardized testing.

Many standardized tests come as a "kit" with a set of standardized test materials and forms. Standardized test kits include an administration manual that describes in detail the purpose(s) of the test and the population for which it was designed. A test manual should include the results of research studies examining the reliability and validity of the tool. In addition, administration and scoring procedures are described in detail. An example of a test with a kit that is widely used by both occupational and physical therapists is the Bruininks-Oseretsky Test of Motor Proficiency, Second Edition (BOT-2) (Bruininks & Bruininks, 2005). The BOT-2 is a test of motor proficiency intended for children and youth. It is based on normative data on individuals between the ages of 4 and 21. This test comes with specific test materials, including a balance beam and tape measures. This is to assure that differences in performance are not due to differences in the materials with which the test is administered.

The BOT-2 is a good tool with which to illustrate the strengths and weaknesses of standardized testing. The BOT-2 has strong psychometric properties (high measurement validity). The first edition of the test was used for more than 25 years before the development of the second edition. This test has been widely used and reported on in both normal and clinical population groups. One of the significant upgrades to the second edition is the use of a normative reference group sample that mirrors the 2000 U.S. census, assuring that it reflects the typical performance of American youths. Motor skills are tested through the use of game-like tasks that are appealing and that are novel. The level of appeal is important because you want the test subjects to be motivated to demonstrate their highest skill level. Novelty is important, because you want to test motor proficiency, not prelearned motor patterns. This test is widely used in diagnosis and in research.

The weaknesses of this test are that the test situation is both artificial and highly structured. Placing pennies on a mat with both hands simultaneously can give the test administrator a lot of information about bimanual motor control, but it is not able to predict performance on important bimanual skills such as handwriting or dressing. The BOT-2 is expensive. The complete test kit, with scoring software, costs around $1,000 dollars. This cost does not include the cost of training therapists in test administration or the time cost for 45 to 60 minutes it takes to administer the test. Because the test items are novel, the person being tested must understand the instructions for test performance, rather than rely on prior knowledge. Although the instructions given during the test are not verbally complex, they do require basic receptive language skills, attention, working memory, and the ability to imitate. In some clinical populations, such as people with autism, the language, attention, and imitation demands may be too extreme. In this case, the children are likely to score very poorly on the test, even though they may have adequate motor proficiency.

Finally, test scores on the BOT-2 are objective. Even in the consideration of children with autism described previously, the children's scores are valid measures of their ability to perform in a standardized manner. The test does not offer an explanation for why the children's performance is poor. A child with hemiplegic cerebral palsy may have a similarly low score to a child with autism. This child may have good language, attention and imitation skills, but will be unable to perform any bimanual tasks. In both cases, the standardized test scores will not be meaningful without further interpretation and will not reflect the unique capabilities and limitations of individual children.

OVERVIEW OF COMMON ASSESSMENTS BY ICF DIMENSION

Literally hundreds of tools are available to occupational and physical therapists to assist in collecting information about an individual's body structures and functions, daily activities, and community participation. Some examples of common assessments will be presented for each of the three categories of function described in the ICF.

BODY STRUCTURES AND FUNCTIONS

The previous examples of grip strength test using a dynamometer and balance testing using both the virtual reality–based movement analysis system and testing using structured observation are all measurement strategies of body function. Many commonly used measures address this ICF dimension, including goniometry or range of motion (ROM), pain scales, girth measurements, and other measurements of strength.

ACTIVITIES OF DAILY LIVING/ INSTRUMENTAL ACTIVITIES OF DAILY LIVING ASSESSMENTS

The Functional Independence Measure (FIM) (Granger, 1990) was introduced earlier in this chapter. The FIM and its pediatric counterpart (WeeFIM) (Granger et al., 1991) assess a person's degree of independence in a variety of ADLs. Items include self-help skills, mobility, communication, social adjustment, and problem solving. The FIM is widely used in rehabilitation settings and is part of a comprehensive outcome database management system. A large literature base describes the FIM's utility. Studies include prediction of the burden of care (Granger, Hamilton, & Gresham, 1988), measure of change in performance following rehabilitation (Heinemann, Linacre, Wright, Hamilton, & Granger, 1994), and prediction of outcome following stroke (Oczkowski & Barreca, 1993). There is less information available on the WeeFIM.

A self-care assessment widely used for children is the Pediatric Evaluation of Disability Inventory (PEDI) (Haley, Coster, Ludlow, Haltiwanger, & Andrellas, 1992). The PEDI determines functional capabilities and performance, monitors progress in functional skill performance, and evaluates therapeutic or rehabilitative program outcomes in children with disabilities. It can also be used for children without disabilities from 6 months to 7 years and 6 months of age. The PEDI is a norm-referenced test with strong psychometric characteristics. The test is divided into three subtests, focusing on functional skills: self-care, mobility, and social function. In addition, environmental modifications and amount of caregiver assistance are systematically recorded. Information can be obtained through parental report, structured interview, or professional observation of a child's functional behavior. The PEDI is a reliable and valid assessment of functional performance in children with significant cognitive and physical disabilities.

A self-care assessment package designed for the population of adults seen in sub-acute rehabilitation settings and nursing homes is the Melville-Nelson Self-Identified Goals Assessment (SIGA) and the Melville-Nelson Self-Care Assessment (SCA). The SIGA is designed to help patients identify meaningful goals for therapy and make judgments as to progress toward those goals. The SCA is designed for the objective analysis of self-care within the scope of Medicare guidelines for assessment. The SIGA and SCA can be used in conjunction with each other, or separately.

DEVELOPMENTAL ASSESSMENT

Another important category of assessments are comprehensive developmental assessments. A **developmental assessment** is a comprehensive standardized evaluation to ascertain the status of a child across all domains of development. This differs from the tests described earlier that had a specific focus, such as motor control or self-care skills. The main goal of a developmental assessment is to determine a child's specific pattern of abilities and needs. Developmental assessments focus on developmental norms across different domains that play important roles in the early identification of developmental problems. Most developmental assessments recommend an interdisciplinary approach to assessment. Typically, developmental assessments are criterion-referenced tests. **Table 22-5** compares the norm-referenced and criterion-referenced types of standardized measurement instruments.

The IDEA legislation requires comprehensive developmental assessment to qualify children for early childhood intervention services. For this reason, many excellent developmental assessments are available for use. The Developmental Profile 3 (DP-3) (Alpern, 2007) is presented here because it is designed to evaluate children from birth through age 12 years, 11 months, presenting one of the widest effective age ranges of the common

TABLE 22-5 Standardized Measurement Instruments

Norm-Referenced	Criterion-Referenced
Standard point score	Cutoff scores
Evaluates individual performance against group	Performance against standard
May or may not be related to therapeutic or instructional content	Content-specific
Normal distribution of scores	Variability of scores not desired
Maximizes differences among individuals	Discriminates
Requires diagnostic skills	Provides information to plan intervention
Not sensitive to effects of therapy	Sensitive to effects of therapy
Not concerned with task analysis	Depends on task analysis
Summative	Formative

developmental tests. Many developmental assessments only evaluate children up to age 5, so the additional scope of this test is an advantage. The DP-3 includes 180 items, each describing a particular skill. The respondents, usually parents, simply indicate whether or not the child has mastered the skill in question. Like many developmental tests, DP-3 yields an overall General Development score as well as scores in each of its five independent scales. The Physical Scale on the DP-3 scores large- and small-muscle coordination, strength, stamina, flexibility, and sequential motor skills. The Adaptive Behavior scale scores the child's ability to cope independently with the environment, including activities of daily living. The Social-Emotional scale measures interpersonal abilities, social and emotional understanding, and functional performance in social situations, including the manner in which the child relates to friends, relatives, and adults. The Cognitive Scale measures intellectual abilities and pre-academic skills. Finally, the Communication Scale measures expressive and receptive communication skills. Within each scale, basal and ceiling scores are used, so you don't have to administer all 180 items. Each scale of the DP-3 has its own norms, allowing the scales to be administered separately, or all at once.

The Alberta Infant Motor Scale (AIMS) (Piper & Darrah, 1993) is an example of a standardized test that is focused on developmental acquisition, which includes some elements of qualitative as well as quantitative performance. The AIMS tests for delays in infants up to 18 months of age and can be used as a screening tool or as part of an assessment to measure gross motor skill maturation over time. The authors of the AIMS clearly indicate that the test is not to be used for older children with known disabilities who are functioning below the 18-month level or to monitor progress of therapy in children with known disabilities.

Developmental assessments include most of the ICF taxonomy, and can give a broad view of a child's overall function. There are few such tests for adults. Assessments like the Canadian Occupational Performance Measure (discussed later in this chapter), although qualitative in format, come the closest to covering the scope of function that a pediatric developmental assessment offers. Since the adoption of the ICF, there has been an increasing interest in a similar broadly conceived comprehensive assessment for adults with disabilities. Even well designed, psychometrically rigorous tests like the FIM do not have adequate research to demonstrate their efficacy as predictors of client outcomes after hospital discharge (Armstrong, Glenny, Stolee, & Berg, 2010; Chumney et al., 2010).

ASSESSMENTS OF PARTICIPATION

One of the earliest assessments of health outcomes that arose from dissatisfaction with typical medical reporting is the Short Form (36) Health Survey (SF-36). Developed and refined throughout the 1980s as a product of the RAND Corporation health insurance experiment in the United States, the SF-36 was designed to obtain patient reported measures of health. The categories of the SF-36 include: Physical Functioning, Social Functioning, Mental Health, Role Limitations (Physical and Emotional), Energy and Vitality, Pain and General Health Perception (Jenkinson, Coulter, & Wright, 1993). As one of the earliest tools of its kind, the SF-36 has been used in numerous studies, including those of effectiveness of rehabilitative therapies for many conditions. There is a web site (www.sf-36.org) where interested parties can review psychometric properties of the instrument, examine related instruments, and obtain permission for use of the SF-36.

The School Function Assessment (SFA) (Coster, Deeney, Haltiwanger, & Haley, 1998) is an assessment of participation within the educational environment that can be used to guide program planning for students with disabilities in kindergarten through sixth grade. Nonacademic tasks divided among those areas assessing level of participation, amount of task assistance or modification, and level of performance in cognitive or physical tasks are judged by teachers and other providers of services in the educational environment. The SFA is a criterion-referenced test, using a judgment-based format to gather information on the typical performance of children from a variety of individuals involved in their education. It yields detailed information across domains and environments that requires collaboration from those that know the students well. The SFA is targeted specifically to an educational environment. Information gathered is directed specifically to the nonacademic components of school functioning and specifically links assessment results to individualized education program (IEP) development.

The **Canadian Occupational Performance Measure (COPM)** (Law, Baptiste, et al., 1994) is designed to obtain the clients' perception of self-care status, as well as productivity, leisure, and social participation. Using a semi-structured interview, the COPM helps clients and family members articulate their difficulties, needs, and goals within naturally occurring activities and routines. The tool has been shown to be responsive to changes noted in performance and personal satisfaction of performance over time in clients receiving therapeutic services (Law, Polatajko, et al., 1994).

Resnik and Plow (2009) did an extensive review of the literature and content analysis to determine participation-related items included in self-report assessments for adults with disabilities. These authors identified five assessment tools that had items linked to all nine of the chapters of the ICF, including the whole scope of the classification system. All five of these assessments will be presented here. These tests are the Community Living Skills Scale, the Assessment of Life Habits, Mayo-Portland Adaptability Scale, the Participation Measure for Post-Acute Care (PM-PAC), and the Psychosocial Adjustment to Illness Scale.

The Community Living Skills Scale (CLSS) (Smith & Ford, 1990) was developed by consumers of a psychosocial rehabilitation (PSR) program as a means of evaluating the impact that the program services had on their functioning. The CLSS is a self-report instrument that measures functioning in the domains of personal care, socialization and relationships, activities and leisure skills, and vocational skills. This scale asks about the frequency of participation (or frequency of problems with participation) in the specified domains of function.

As compared with some of the tests presented earlier in this chapter, the psychometric properties of this test are adequate, but are not a strength. The CLSS was tested with 50 individuals of a mental health consumer group. Although this test was developed in a mental health setting, it may be a useful tool in the assessment of adults with developmental disabilities and people with impairments in cognition, such as people with brain injury or dementia.

The Assessment of Life Habits Scale (LIFE-H) was developed to assess life habits and social participation, and is focused on these skills in people with disabilities (Noreau, Fougeyrollas, & Vincent, 2002). The LIFE-H includes 12 categories: nutrition, fitness, personal care, communication, housing, mobility, responsibilities, interpersonal relationships, community life, education, employment, and recreation. This test was designed for use with people with spinal cord injuries, and psychometric testing of this measure has been used with this population. Like the CLSS, the LIFE-H is a self-report scale. The level of difficulty of tasks and the types of assistance needed are weighted to derive an accomplishment score.

The Mayo-Portland Adaptability Inventory was designed to not only assess the scope of cognitive, physical, and behavioral barriers to community reintegration for individuals with acquired brain injury, but also to assess the effectiveness of rehabilitation programs in accomplishing the outcome of community reintegration. It has three index subscales, including ability, adjustment, and participation. The eight-item Participation Index is a measure of societal participation. The Mayo-Portland Adaptability Inventory is in its fourth edition (Malec, 2005). The Participation Measure for Post-Acute Care (PM-PAC) is a recently developed measure designed specifically with the ICF framework in mind. The PM-PAC is a self-report questionnaire that assesses participation across nine domains. Preliminary psychometric testing has been done on this instrument, with the ultimate goal of creating an adaptive, computerized instrument to assess participation (Gandek, Jette, Sinclair, & Ware, 2006). The Psychosocial Adjustment to Illness Scale was developed by Derogatis (1986) to assess psychological and social adjustment of patients and their families to medical illness. The scale has been used in a number of studies of health-related quality of life in populations with serious illness, such as cancer.

ASSESSMENT AS A GUIDE TO TREATMENT

The assessments described in this chapter are good clinical measures. They assist in the process of diagnosing impairments and functional limitations. They also assist in the treatment planning process. These assessments help specify the mechanism by which a proposed treatment changes its immediate treatment targets, the clients. This approach to assessment is based in treatment theory. **Treatment theory** is described by Whyte and Barrett (2012) as follows: "Treatment theory specifies the mechanism by which a proposed treatment changes its immediate treatment target—referred to here as the treatment object"(p. S103). Whyte and Barrett further explain this model with the example that exercise, in the form of repetitive muscle contraction against a load (the treatment in this example) leads to increased muscle strength in the client (the treatment object). What these authors note is that treatment theory does not address or consider the impact of increased muscle strength on a specific aspect of function. Extending the example of therapeutic exercise for strengthening, Whyte and Barrett (2012) comment that treatment theory does not address the impact of improved muscle strength "on more distal aspects of function such as ambulation. Indeed, the impact of strengthening leg muscles on ambulation depends on a wide range of other coexisting abilities and impairments (e.g., balance, visual perception), as well as environmental factors (e.g., ground surface, lighting), and even social factors (safe home environment)—on which strengthening exercises have no impact" (S103). **Table 22-6** offers specific examples of treatment theory application.

The limitation to treatment theory is that it addresses clinical outcomes, not participation level outcomes. Increasingly, health care consumers and health care payers are looking for evidence that therapy impacts participation in a meaningful (and measureable) manner. An alternative approach, **enablement theory**, emphasizes the individuals and proposes to provide those individuals with adequate power, means, opportunity, or authority to manage their own health and rehabilitation. Enablement theory focuses on the causal interrelationships among variables at different levels. This theory, as proposed by Whyte (2011), is well suited to considering the variable at different levels in the ICF. Through the enablement theory approach, we can respond to the query "If we improve strength, what effects do we expect elsewhere in the ICF classification system?" In this model, the target of treatment (the clinically relevant outcome) is often distal to the object of the treatment. Although this relationship has been simplified for this test, **Figure 22-10** illustrates a possible explanation, applying enablement theory, for why leg

strengthening is causally interrelated with community ambulation. Enablement theory is primarily concerned with linking different entities in the ICF framework, and with what the weightings of those causal links may be.

As rehabilitation practitioners, we may intuitively see these linkages, but our intuitive clinical reasoning may be faulty. As you remember, clinical reasoning improves with the experience and training of the person doing the reasoning. It is not a standard product and is not supported by scientific evidence.

We must be able to understand and apply both treatment theory and enablement theory if we are to be responsible clinicians using an evidence-based approach to practice. Treatment theory supports and guides our efforts to make changes to something within the ICF framework, but it does not predict the distal impact of that change. Enablement theory predicts what will happen elsewhere in the ICF framework if we do change something, but it does not provide the tools for change. This distinction applies equally to assessment and to treatment.

The assessments presented earlier in this chapter have been historically based in treatment theory. As illustrated in **Table 22-7**, treatment theory is an adequate guide for assessment of outcomes at the level of body structure. However, if the level of assessment is focused on body structure and the expected outcome is in the area of activity or participation, then the assessment will not effectively measure the desired outcomes. As mentioned previously, Darrah and colleagues (2008) found pediatric therapists assumed goals written at the structure/function level would automatically promote participation. Enablement theory suggests this is erroneous and the causal relationships illustrated in **Figure 22-10** need to be developed in the plan of care to justify that treatment will enable the desired result at the participation level. **Table 22.7** shows assessments at the level of outcome reflect treatment theory, but enablement theory requires the development of causal links between the assessment and

---

TABLE 22-6 Treatment Theory Examples

Treatment	Object	Essential Ingredients
Progressive resistive exercise	Muscle strength	Repetitive contraction against increasing resistance
Dressing training	Independent dressing in a reasonable length of time	Repeated performance with error feedback about physical strategies
Brandt-Daroff vestibular repositioning exercise	Improved balance	Repetitive movement within the movement planes of the semicircular canals
Computer-based cognitive training	Improved working and short-term memory, attention, and mental processing speed	Individualized game-like computer activities

Adapted from Whyte, J. (2011). Distinguishing treatment and enablement theory, Program book: Accelerating Clinical Trials and Outcomes Research Conference. American Occupational Therapy Association and American Occupational Therapy Foundation.

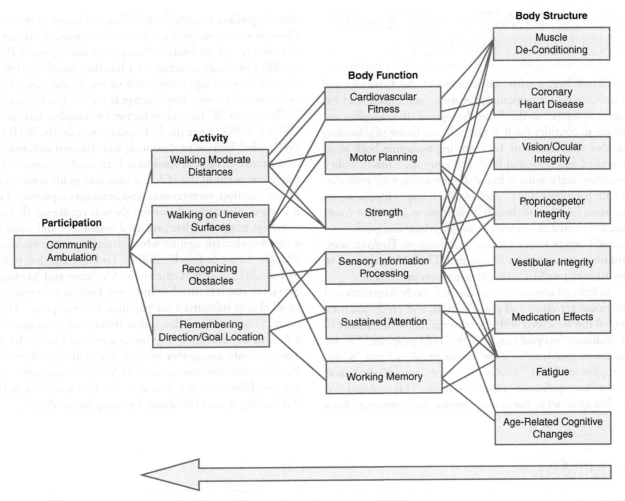

Figure 22-10 This diagram includes a partial presentation of causal relationships within the enablement model. Note that the target of treatment (muscle deconditioning in this example) is distal to the object of treatment (community ambulation).

outcome if the desired outcome is at a different level than the target of the assessment. Increasingly, occupational and physical therapists have been looking beyond this approach, especially in tools that measure the outcomes of therapeutic

intervention. Several assessments of participation have been developed, especially for pediatric population. Assessments of participation such as the SF-36 and the COPM discussed previously embody the concepts of enablement theory.

TABLE 22-7 Levels of Assessment

		Level of Outcome			
		Body Structure	**Body Function**	**Activity**	**Participation**
Level of Assessment	Body structure	*	↓	↓	↓
	Body function		*	↓	↓
	Activity			*	↓
	Participation				*

*Treatment theory suffices.
↓Treatment theory and enablement required.

THE ICF, HEALTH OUTCOMES, AND HEALTH POLICY

This book began with a discussion of the International Classification of Functioning, Disability and Health and has employed the ICF as the theme throughout. It is therefore important to consider the ICF not only as a frame of reference, but also as a framework for reporting outcomes both at an individual and a societal level. For example, a health policy researcher might want to know about outcomes for individuals with paraplegia due to a spinal cord injury. This researcher may want to compare these ICF dimensions across two countries, the United States, with its mix of private and public payers, and Canada, with a national health system. To do so, standard measurements must be recorded. The ICF, when used in this manner, provides such a measurement instrument.

Briefly, all components of the ICF (body structures and functions, activities and participation, and environmental factors) can be scored with the same ordinal scale. A score of "0" indicates "no problem," "1" for "mild problem," "2" for "moderate problem," "3" for "severe problem," and "4" for "complete problem." Scores of "8" for "not specified" and "9" for "not applicable" are also available. This is considered the first qualifier in the coding system. Body structure has a second qualifier ranging from "0" as no change in structure through scores assigned for absence of a part, deviation or deformity, and qualitative change in a body part. A third qualifier for body structure is a location qualifier, that is, right, left, arm, leg, trunk, and so on. In the case of environmental factors, scores range from "0" (no barrier, no facilitator) to "4" (complete barrier or complete facilitator) (WHO, 2001). Since the ICF's acceptance by the WHO in 2001, rehabilitation professionals and affiliated stakeholders in the rehabilitation process have been working towards the implementation of the ICF as a means to guide assessment, documentation, intervention, and outcomes reporting. This is a work in progress; however, there is consensus that the adoption of the ICF has impacted assessment and provides a new benchmark against which assessments are evaluated (Rauch, Sieza, & Stucki, 2008). To illustrate that point, in July 2013, CMS (Centers for Medicare and Medicaid Services) implemented mandatory functional reporting in all claims submitted for payment by therapists. These codes, known as G-Codes, reflect functional status at evaluation, in 10 treatment day increments, and at discharge. The G-Code categories include familiar ICF Activity/Participation dimensions such as Mobility and Self-Care. The modifiers are very similar to the first qualifiers in the ICF coding system (Medicare Learning Network, 2013).

SUMMARY

The last 20 years have seen significant changes in providing therapeutic intervention to individuals with motor dysfunction. These changes have primarily occurred in methods of gathering information about a client's functional status and delivering appropriate functionally oriented services. Therapists are revising traditional service delivery models to reflect the growing emphasis on providing integrated therapeutic services within inclusive settings. The physical and occupational therapists' expertise in motor development, the effects of sensory motor skills on function and other developmental areas, and their ability to analyze tasks is being applied more broadly to the benefit of clients of all ages.

This chapter outlines models of information gathering therapists use to evaluate and assess infants, young children, adolescents, and adults. It also reviewed several measurement tools used by physical and occupational therapists. Instruments are used as a component of the measurement process to (1) screen individuals for potential concerns, (2) evaluate individuals to determine diagnosis or eligibility for services, or (3) assess clients to plan therapeutic intervention or to determine effects of intervention. Therapists should be aware of the purpose of each tool and the information they would like to gain before selecting an instrument. They may need to use a variety of tools and strategies to meet their screening, evaluation, or assessment objectives.

Therapists need to appreciate that the assessment or evaluation of neuromotor, sensorimotor, and functional status can be influenced by the interaction of clients with significant others, the environment, and the individuals' own neurobehavioral state. This is especially critical with very young infants and when establishing intervention priorities, outcomes, and goals and strategies. Collaborating with family members, other professionals, and caregivers will increase the likelihood that the therapists' findings will reflect the individuals' capabilities across environments and current capacities and strengths, as well as identify barriers to optimal development. Individualized assessment of clients' skills should capture movement patterns, components of movement, and the use of movement within a functional activity in addition to sensory processing and developmental skill acquisition.

In creating an information-collection procedure, it is important to determine if your strategies are meeting the guidelines of contemporary service delivery. The checklist for assessment standards in **Table 22-8** is a series of questions used to create systems of assessment that are relevant to clients, the families, and other team members, and can be used to create meaningful therapeutic programs.

TABLE 22-8 Checklist for Assessment Standards

Area of Validity	Questions
Treatment	1. Does the assessment identify feasible goals and objectives?
	2. Does assessment information assist in the selection or use of therapeutic methods or approaches?
	3. Does assessment contribute to evaluating intervention effects?
Social	1. Does assessment identify goals and objectives that are judged as worthwhile and appropriate?
	2. Are assessment methods and materials acceptable to participants?
	3. Does the assessment detect significance of change?
Convergent	1. Are several types of assessment materials and approaches used?
	2. Is information collected from several settings and sources, especially family members and other caregivers?
	3. Are assessments done on more than one occasion?
Consensual	1. Is information pooled and perspectives shared?
	2. Do team dynamics favor collaboration and negotiation?
	3. Are decisions truly consensual?

CASE 1

Andrew

Andrew was born with a congenital heart defect, which was repaired when he was an infant. He has been healthy and has not had any cardiac-related problems since infancy. He has, however, been diagnosed with severe spastic diplegia and language-processing deficits. He uses a walker and wears ankle-foot orthoses (AFOs). His parents, Ms. King, a dentist, and Mr. Hammer, an architect, are very proud of Andrew's school performance thus far. During preschool and early elementary school, he attended a self-contained special education classroom in an elementary school. He did extremely well there and subsequently moved to a third-grade class with typically developing peers. Andrew is now on the playground with children in other grades; he goes on field trips, goes outside the classroom for art, gym, and music, and is handling more homework. He has been followed by the same therapist since preschool. While he was in the special education program, the therapists saw him twice weekly in the therapy room for 30-minute sessions. He is now receiving therapy using a collaborative-consultation model. A three-month review of Andrew's individualized education program (IEP) is coming up. The therapists are part of the review team.

Andrew's condition has been diagnosed, and it has already been determined that he is eligible for special education and related services. Documenting his degree of delay in the acquisition of motor skills and his neuromotor status is unnecessary to review his IEP. At this point, it is important to gather information about Andrew's performance in the classroom and within the school environment. This type of information will allow the team to determine if any additional services and supports are needed to help him meet the expectations of his present environment. The School Function Assessment (SFA) is designed to assess this

Continues

Case 1 *Continued*

type of information and would provide excellent information to the team to determine his needs. This test will be completed by all members of the team who see Andrew throughout the day. They will indicate from their perspective how well Andrew is meeting expectations placed on him. The team members will indicate what types of supports and modifications he needs to accomplish tasks and whether or not he is participating in all activities within the school. The information gained from SFA will help the team delineate areas of strengths and needs and further refine his IEP.

Guiding Questions

Some questions to consider:

1. In this case, the goal of the assessment process is to develop an intervention plan and *not* to qualify Andrew for services. Discuss how the purpose of the assessment may determine the choice of assessment strategy.
2. If the therapist needed to contact Andrew's physician regarding a change in his status regarding his AFOs, or a potential need for Botox, the SFA would not mean anything to the physician. Give an example of some tests and measures that might be useful in communicating Andrew's needs to the physician.
3. The SFA is a criterion-referenced test. Define what is meant by a criterion-referenced test, and describe how such tests are used to guide intervention.

CASE 2

Bill

Bill is a 72-year-old father of three children and grandfather to a 2-year old girl. He practices law about 10 hours a week for the firm he has been a partner in for the last 25 years. He lives in the suburbs of a metropolitan area with his wife, who is a high school principal. The couple has a very active lifestyle. They golf, play tennis (Bill competes nationally in his age group), bike ride, and socialize with friends and family. When Bill was in his mid-40s, he underwent cardiac bypass surgery. Until recently, he has had no residual problems. Recently, he has been diagnosed with congestive heart failure. As an in-patient, he was seen by a physical and an occupational therapist. The PT did a thorough full-system examination and identified several impairments, including limited endurance and generalized weakness. The OT assessed his ADL status, and found limitations in dressing and bathing due to fatigue. He also no longer could participate in daily household management tasks or leisure activities. Bill was continuing to do his law consultation, but feared that he may not be able to continue with this for much longer.

   The World Health Organization's quality of life measure, WHOQOL-BREF (2004) was used to allow Bill to rate his physical capacity, his psychological well-being, his level of independence and environmental support. Bill rated the overall quality of his life as poor, noting that he needed much medical intervention to be able to

Continues

Case 2   *Continued*

participate in his daily life. He also reported that he had some difficulty concentrating and that he did not always feel safe when he was performing daily tasks. He only scored himself at a 36/100 level in physical capacity, reflecting this area as his greatest area of impairment. He scored a 56/100 in both psychological well-being and level of independence, suggesting significant limitations in these areas as well. This assessment gave the OT and PT the information that Bill's environment was very supportive, but that his participation in physical activity was highly valued by him, and his impairment had a powerful negative impact on his quality of life.

Although his impairments in the areas of self-care and leisure were less distressing to him, they had a negative impact on his overall quality of life. The OT and PT working with Bill may have reasoned out this pattern of limitations and its impact on his quality of life, but by using the WHOQOL-BREF, they have an objective measure that will assist not only in therapy planning but also in justifying additional therapy support to help him return to his active lifestyle.

Guiding Questions

Some questions to consider:

1. Discuss how the WHOQOL-BREF assessment provided different information than other tests and measures mentioned in the case, such as endurance or independence with ADLs.
2. Assessment should provide a means to determine treatment effectiveness. How could therapists use the assessments mentioned to establish goals and determine treatment effectiveness.
3. The WHOQOL-BREF assesses participation. Discuss the importance of assessment at the participation level, including how assessment at this level may differ from assessments of activity or function.

Speaking of
Measuring the Unmeasureable

ANNE CRONIN, PhD, OTR/L,
PEDIATRIC OCCUPATIONAL THERAPIST

I hear so often that there is a disconnect between education and clinical practice, that what is taught in the classroom does not always fully prepare students for their clinical experience, and that the demands of the clinical settings do not always support extended assessment periods. The big focus is on functional outcomes, and many tests, even ADL checklists, do not truly reflect functional outcomes. So the choices seem to be to give up assessment altogether, or to figure out ways to assess that support treatment planning and measureable functional outcomes.

Unfortunately, the things I care the most about as a pediatric occupational therapist are somewhat subjective and hard to measure. Questions—such as, Has his social engagement during group interactions improved in the classroom setting?—will not be answered by any test that I do in a one-to-one therapy session. Do I have to schedule time to observe him in the classroom? Can I ask the teacher to do it? Will my observation

Continues

Speaking of *Continued*

count as therapy time? Is this a good use of the 40 minutes a week I spend with this child? The questions go on and on. . .

Then I read this article by Mailloux and colleagues (2007) that introduced an assessment strategy called Goal Attainment Scaling (GAS). GAS is a technique for evaluating individual progress toward goals. GAS is a great approach for those hard-to-measure outcomes. It is both client-centered and functional. GAS is a systematic analysis of functional behavior that involves a standard series of steps. The steps are:

1. Identify areas where an undesirable set of behaviors should be minimized or where a favorable set of behaviors should be increased. These will be the basis for your goals.

2. Narrow your focus to three to five priority goals and determine current or initial performance on outcome goals;

3. Specify a continuum of possible outcomes (for example, worst expected outcome = -2, less than expected outcome = -1, expected outcome = 0, more than expected outcome = $+1$, and best expected outcome = $+2$);

4. Intervene for a specified period;

5. Determine performance attained on each objective; and

6. Evaluate extent of attainment.

In GAS, the outcomes should be not be vague; they should be measurable and specific. Therapists need to be careful not to set up goals that are too easily accomplished or too difficult. The following is an example of a GAS goal for social engagement in group activities within a classroom setting:

$+3$ = Interacts with peers cooperatively, imitates activities

$+2$ = Interacts through adult structuring play with other children 80 percent of occasions

$+1$ = Interactive play in group; interacts with one child or adult less than 50 percent of occasions

0 = Isolated play, will separate from parent within a few minutes, with support from teacher or aide; happily enters playground and classroom; needs intermittent support and encouragement from adult

-1 = Isolated play; will separate from parent after considerable time; will enter playground and classroom following structured support from teacher or aide and bonding time with teacher or aide; totally dependent on adult for support and encouragement

-2 = Isolated play; will not separate from parent; will not enter playground or classroom willingly; totally dependent on parent

-3 = Isolates self from all social and play contact and interactions

GAS has been successfully used in all areas of practice and is increasingly used as a measurement tool in outcomes research (Mailloux et al., 2007). In a clinical setting, clients (or clients' parents) are involved in both the goal setting and analysis of goal attainment. This approach gives a clear agenda for professional conversations and provides a structure for problem definition, evaluation, planning, and reporting.

It is important to always look for better ways to meet your clients' clinical needs. A good, objective, measureable functional outcome may be the thing that makes the therapy approach recognized and reimbursed. It may allow people to continue to receive therapy, when more traditional skill-based goals are not sufficient to support continued treatment. Remember that continuing competence as a clinician means not only keeping up with the latest therapy techniques, but also with the latest assessment techniques.

REFERENCES

Alpern, G. (2007). *Developmental Profile 3 (DP-3)*. Los Angeles, CA: Western Psychological Services.

American Occupational Therapy Association. (2014). *Occupational Therapy Practice Framework: Domain and process* (3rd ed.) Bethesda, MD: AOTA Press.

American Physical Therapy Association. (2014). Guide to physical therapist practice 3.0 (3rd ed.). Alexandria, VA: American Physical Therapy Association. Retrieved from: http://guidetoptpractice.apta.org. Accessed October 30, 2014.

Armstrong, J., Glenny, C., Stolee, P., & Berg, K. (2010). A comparison of two assessment systems in predicting functional outcomes of older rehabilitation patients. *Age & Ageing, 39*(3), 394–399.

Benner, P., Hughes, R. & Sutphen, M. (2008). Clinical reasoning, decision making, and action: Thinking clinically and critically. In R. G. Hughes (ed.), *Patient safety and quality: An evidence-based handbook for nurses* (pp. 1–23). Rockville, MD: Agency for Healthcare Research and Quality.

Bruininks, R., & Bruininks, B. (2005). *Bruininks-Oseretsky test of motor proficiency* (2nd ed.). San Antonio, TX: Pearson Education.

Chumney, D., Nollinger, K., Shesko, K., Skop, K., Spencer, M., & Newton, R. A. (2010). Ability of Functional Independence Measure to accurately predict functional outcome of stroke-specific population: Systematic review. *Journal of Rehabilitation Research & Development, 47*(1), 17–29.

Coster, W., Deeney, T., Haltiwanger, J., & Haley, S. (1998). *School function assessment*. San Antonio: Therapy Skill Builders.

Darrah, J., Wiart L., & Magill-Evans, J. (2008). Do therapists' goals and interventions for children with cerebral palsy reflect principles in contemporary literature? *Pediatric Physical Therapy, 20*(4), 334–339.

Derogatis, L. (1986) The psychosocial adjustment to illness scale (PAIS). *Journal of Psychosomatic Research, 30*(1), 77–91.

Gandek, B., Sinclair, S., Jette, A., & Ware, J. (2006). Development and initial psychometric evaluation of the Participation Measure for Post-Acute Care (PM-PAC). *American Journal of Physical Medicine and Rehabilitation, 86*, 57–71.

Granger, C. (1990). *Functional independence measure*. Buffalo, NY: Uniform Data System for Medical Rehabilitation, State University of New York.

Granger, C., Braun, S., Griswood, K., Heyer, N., McCabe, M., Msau, M., & Hamilton, B. (1991). *Functional independence measure for children*. Buffalo, NY: Uniform Data System for Medical Rehabilitation, State University of New York.

Granger, C. V., Hamilton, B. B., & Gresham, G. E. (1988). The stroke rehabilitation outcome study—Part 1: General description. *Archives of Physical Medicine and Rehabilitation, 69*, 505–509.

Haley, S., Coster, W. J., Ludlow, I. H., Haltiwanger, J. T., & Andrellas, P. (1992). *Pediatric evaluation of disability inventory*. Boston: PEDI Research Group, Department of Rehabilitation Medicine, New England Medical Center Hospital.

Heinemann, A. W., Linacre, J. M., Wright, B. D., Hamilton, B. B., & Granger, C. V. (1994). Prediction of rehabilitation outcomes with disability measures. *Archives of Physical Medicine and Rehabilitation, 75*, 133–143.

Individuals with Disabilities Education Act (IDEA). (2004). 20 U.S.C. § 1400.

Jenkinson, C., Coulter, A., & Wright, L. (1993). Short form (SF-36) health survey questionnaire: Normative data for adults of working age. *British Medical Journal, 306*, 1437–1440.

Keith, R., Granger, C., Hamilton, B., & Sherwin, F. (1987). The functional independence measure: A new tool for rehabilitation. *Advances in Clinical Rehabilitation, 1*, 6–18.

Law, M., Baptiste, S., Carswell, A., McColl, M. A., Polatajko, H., & Pollack, N. (1994). *Canadian occupational performance measure*. Toronto, Canada: CAOT Publications.

Law, M., Polatajko, H., Pollack, N., McColl, M. A., Carswell, A., & Baptiste, S. (1994). Pilot testing of the Canadian Occupational Performance Measure: Clinical and measurement issues. *Canadian Journal of Occupational Therapy, 55*, 63–68.

Malec, J. (2005). The Mayo-Portland Adaptability Inventory. *The Center for Outcome Measurement in Brain Injury*. Retrieved October 3, 2012 from http://www.tbims.org/combi/mpai

Mailloux, Z., May-Benson, T. A., Summers, C. A., Miller, L. J., Brett-Green, B., Burke, J. P., et al. (2007). The issue is—Goal attainment scaling as a measure of meaningful outcomes for children with sensory integration disorders. *American Journal of Occupational Therapy, 61*, 254–259.

Medicare Learning Network (MLN) (2013). MLN Matters: Outpatient therapy functional reporting requirements. Retrieved from www.cms.gov/outreach-and-education/medicare-learning-network-mln/mlnmattersarticles/downloads/se1307.pdf. Accessed 10/30/2014

Noreau, L., Fougeyrollas, P., & Vincent, C. (2002). The LIFE-H: Assessment of the quality of social participation. *Technology & Disability, 14*(3), 113–118.

Oczkowski, W. J., & Barreca, S. (1993). The functional independence measure: Its use to identify rehabilitation needs in stroke survivors. *Archives of Physical Medicine and Rehabilitation, 74*, 1291–1294.

O'Neill, M., Fragala-Pinkham, M., Westcott, S. L., Martin, K. Chiarell, L., Valvano, J., & Rose, R. (2006). Physical therapy clinical management recommendations for children with cerebral palsy-spastic diplegia: Achieving functional mobility outcomes. *Pediatric Physical Therapy, 18*, 49–72.

Peters, M. H., van Nes, S. I., Vanhoutte, E. K., Bakkers, M., van Doorn, P. A., Merkies, I. J., & Faber, C. G. (2011). Revised normative values for grip strength with the Jamar dynamometer. *Journal of the Peripheral Nervous System, 16*(1), 47–50.

Piper, M., & Darrah, J. (1993). *Motor assessment of the developing infant*. Philadelphia: W. B. Saunders.

Ptyushkin, P., Vidmar, G., Burger, H., & Marincek, C. (2012). Use of the International Classification of Functioning, Disability, and Health in traumatic brain injury rehabilitation: Linking issues and general perspectives. *American Journal of Physical Medicine and Rehabilitation, 91*(13), 548–554.

Rauch, A., Cieza, A., & Stucki, G. (2008). How to apply the International Classification of Functioning, Disability and Health (ICF) for rehabilitation management in clinical practice. *European Journal of Physical and Rehabilitative Medicine, 44*(3), 329–342.

Resnik, L., & Plow, M. A. (2009). Measuring participation as defined by the International Classification of Functioning, Disability and Health: An evaluation of existing measures. *Archives of Physical Medicine and Rehabilitation, 90*, 856–866.

Richardson, P. (2001). Use of standardized tests in pediatric practice. In J. Case-Smith (Ed.), *Occupational therapy for children* (pp. 217–245). St. Louis: Mosby.

Simeonsson, R.J., Leonardi, M., Lollar, D., Bjorck-Akesson, E., Hollenweger, J., & Martinuzzi, A. (2003). Applying the international classification of functioning, disability and health (ICF) to measure childhood disability. *Disability and Rehabilitation, 25*(11-12), 602–610.

Smith, M. K., & Ford, J. J. (1990). A client-developed functional level scale: The Community Living Skills Scale (CLSS). *Journal of Social Service Research, 13*(3), 61–84.

Sullivan, K. J. & Cen, S. Y. (2011) Model of disablement and recovery: Knowledge translation in rehabilitation research and practice. *Physical Therapy, 91*(12), 1892–1904.

Watter, P., Rodger, S., Marinac, J., Woodyatt, G., Ziviani, J., Ozanne, A. (2008). Multidisciplinary assessment of children with developmental coordination disorder: Using the ICF framework to inform assessment. *Physical & Occupational Therapy in Pediatrics, 28*, 331–352.

Whyte, J. (2011). Distinguishing treatment and enablement theory, *Program book: Accelerating Clinical Trials and Outcomes Research Conference* Bethesda, Maryland:AOTA. American Occupational Therapy Association and American Occupational Therapy Foundation.

Whyte, J., & Barrett, M. (2012). Advancing the evidence base of rehabilitation treatments: A developmental approach. *Archives of Physical Medicine and Rehabilitation, 93*, S101–S110.

World Health Organization (2004) The World Health Organization Quality of Life (WHOQOL-BREF). Retrieved from http://www .who.int/substance_abuse/research_tools/en/english_whoqol.pdf

World Health Organization (WHO). (2001). *ICF: International classification of functioning, disability and health*. Geneva, Switzerland: World Health Organization.

Glossary

abnormal development A pattern or sequence of behavior acquisition that differs from typical patterns in quality and form.

absolute threshold A term used in neuroscience to indicate the smallest detectable level of a stimulus.

abstract symbols Pictograms and alphabets used in communication to indicate a concept, quality, or abstract idea in a way that is not physically similar to what they represent.

accessibility The quality of being at hand when needed; also the attribute of being easily approached or entered. Providing *accessibility* in an environment means removing barriers that prevent people with activity limitations from the use of services, products, and information available in that environment.

accommodation From Jean Piaget's theory of cognitive development, a change of function in accordance with the environment or modification of the schema.

acculturation The process of an outsider getting used to the way people are, while retaining core cultural values from his or her ethnic cultural upbringing.

achieving stage This is Schaie's stage of early adult thought where previously acquired knowledge is used to establish oneself in the world.

activity The execution of a task by an individual, and an associated construct is the notion of capacity.

activity limitation In the ICF, this phrase is used to replace disability; it refers to restrictions in activities and participation, due to limitations in structure, function, or contextual factors.

activities of daily living (ADL) The daily self-care activities within any of an individual's routine environments (home, leisure, work, and so on). Special equipment such as wheelchairs and adapted vehicles are additional examples of compensations to support ADL.

acquisitive stage The first stage of cognitive development described by Schaie, the stage focuses on task of acquiring information and spans all of childhood and adolescence.

activities and participation (ICF) Aspects of human behavior that deal with the range of tasks and behavior associated with a person's life situation.

acute poverty Poverty that is caused by a particular incident, such as the loss of a job or a major illness when the individuals involved expect to be able to improve their circumstances as the problems are resolved.

adaptive coping An approach to problem solving that aims to master a situation, or expand resources to deal with the situation. It is primarily used as a coping mechanism when individuals feel that they have a realistic chance to effect change.

aerobic capacity Maximum energy the body can generate through aerobic processes; represents the functional capacity of the cardiovascular system.

affective domain Involves feelings, including happiness, sadness, anger, etc., which are all part of the human experience.

521

affordance A perceived or actual property of a thing, primarily those fundamental properties that determine just how the thing could possibly be used.

ageism A type of discrimination that involves prejudice against people based upon their age. Similar to racism and sexism, ageism involves holding negative stereotypes about people of different ages.

age-associated memory impairment (AAMI) Modest loss of memory function in healthy people over age 50; involves complaints of memory impairment with everyday activities.

age-normative influences These are the aspects of development that are chronological. Many age-normative changes are physiological and reflect the maturation of the organism.

aging-associated disease These are true diseases, not a part of healthy aging, that occur with increasing frequency with age.

aging in place The ability to live in one's own home and community safely, independently, and comfortably, regardless of age, income, or ability level.

agonist Muscle considered to be the prime mover of a motion.

Ainsworth, Mary A developmental psychologist known for her work in early emotional attachment with "the strange situation," as well as her work in the development of attachment theory. With Bowlby she studied the effect of early social experience on personality, developed the *strange situation* experimental paradigm, and classified modes of attachment behavior.

allele One member of a pair or series of genes that occupy a specific position on a specific chromosome.

Alzheimer's disease (AD) The most prevalent form of progressive dementia among people aged 65 and older. In Alzheimer's disease, brain cells degenerate and die, causing a steady decline in memory and mental function.

American Sign Language (ASL) A complete, complex language that employs signs made with the hands and other movements, including facial expressions and postures of the body. It is the first language of many deaf North Americans, and one of several communication options available to deaf people.

Americans with Disabilities Act (ADA) Law passed in 1991 that addresses societal limitations through affirmative action and removal of physical barriers.

animal-assisted therapy (AAT) A type of therapy that involves animals as a form of intervention or support for people with social, emotional, or cognitive impairments.

anorexia nervosa A serious mental health disorder primarily affecting adolescent girls and young woman defined in the *Diagnostic and Statistical Manual* 5 (DSM-5) as characterized by a pathologic fear of becoming fat manifesting as excessive restriction of food intake.

antagonist Muscle that acts against the given motion of an agonist muscle.

anticipatory control Alteration or adjustment of the motor program even before any interaction with the environment occurs.

anticipatory grief Characteristics of the grieving process, such as sorrow and disengagement, manifested prospectively, that is, before the loss has actually occurred.

anxiety disorders A group of mental disturbances characterized by anxiety as a central or core symptom.

Applied behavior analysis (ABA) A psychological approach that uses the theory of behaviorism to modify human behaviors as part of a learning or treatment process. By functionally assessing the relationship between a targeted behavior and the environment, the methods of ABA can be used to change that behavior.

articulation The ability to produce individual speech sounds clearly and combine sounds correctly for words.

arthritis A disease condition involving the inflammation of one or more joints. There are over 100 different types of arthritis.

assessment Use of comprehensive strategies and tools to delineate strengths and needs, develop appropriate intervention plans and strategies, and determine change in individuals.

assets Products or objects of economic exchange such as money, goods, property, and other valuables that individuals own and have rights to use.

assimilation Process of changing elements of the environment so they will fit into the current cognitive structure, or schema.

assistive technology (AT) Assistive technology includes any product, instrument, equipment, or technology adapted or specially designed for improving the functioning of a person with disabilities.

assistive technology device Any item, piece of equipment, or product system, whether acquired commercially off the shelf, modified, or customized, that is used to increase, maintain, or improve functional capabilities of individuals with a disability.

associations In the context of birth defects, if two or more defects tend to appear together but do not share the same cause, they are called associations.

associative learning Learning in which individuals learn to predict relationships and draw on long-term memory to make associations; includes classical conditioning, operant conditioning, declarative learning, and procedural learning.

associative play Behavior common in 2-year-old children, in which they enjoy the company of other children but do not organize their play.

astasia An inability in an infant to bear body weight on the legs in the period of integration of primitive postural muscle tone patterns and the emergence of voluntary limb control.

asymmetrical tonic neck reflex (ATNR) Mediates a typical postural set, beginning at birth and peaking over the first 2 months of life; stimulated by turning the head to one side, causing the upper and lower limbs on the side toward which the infant is looking (that is, the face side) to extend while the upper and lower limbs facing the back of the head (the skull side), flex; creates a postural set symbolic of the en guarde position in fencing, so the pattern is sometimes referred to as the *fencing position.*

asynchronous development Describes a situation in which the normal developmental progression is highly uneven.

atherosclerosis A disease condition that develops when a substance called plaque builds up in the walls of the arteries (American Heart Association, 2014). Atherosclerosis narrows the arteries, making it harder for blood to flow through, potentially leading to heart attack or stroke.

attention Mental function that begins prenatally and allows people to focus on something while simultaneously excluding less important information; the key that opens the door to the information-processing system; the process of detecting and orienting to important or desired environmental stimuli.

attention deficit/hyperactivity disorder (ADHD) A neurobehavioral disorder that is characterized by either significant difficulties of inattention or hyperactivity and impulsiveness or a combination of the two with the symptoms occurring before seven years of age.

attitudinal environment The influence of observable beliefs based upon customs, practices, ideologies, values, norms, facts, and religious beliefs.

attitudinal racism Actions based on a set of stereotypical assumptions, feelings, beliefs, and attitudes about or toward a group of people.

attractor well In systems theory of motor control, a preferred pattern; the deeper the attractor well, the more obligatory the pattern.

attunement play A playful social exchange that establishes a connection, such as between newborn and mother.

augmentative/alternative communication (AAC) An area of clinical, research, and educational practice that attempts to compensate and facilitate, temporarily or permanently, for the impairment and disability patterns of individuals with severe expressive, and/or language comprehension disorders.

autism spectrum disorder (ASD) A neurodevelopmental condition diagnosed when the child has moderate to severe problems with socialization and communication, and restricted patterns of behaviors or interests.

autonomic nervous system (ANS) The part of the peripheral nervous system that acts as a control system functioning largely below the level of consciousness, and controls visceral functions.

avoiding reaction A reflexive behavior involving finger extension as infants withdraw and abduct the fingers in response to touch on the hand. This reflexive pattern serves as an automatic mechanism to facilitate finger extension, often resulting in an involuntary, or automatic, release.

Ayres Sensory Integration A theory of brain-behavior relationships that allow us to interact and respond in purposeful ways that depends on adequate organization of sensory information. Intervention based on this theory usually takes place within a specially designed therapeutic environment that allows a therapist to present specific sensory and movement challenges to the child, which gradually increase in complexity over time.

balance The ability to maintain a postural alignment in relation to gravitational forces and physical displacement.

Bandura, Albert Social learning theorist of the twentieth century best known for the concept of modeling.

barrier A factor, such as low socioeconomic status, which limits the individual's access to factors that support health.

behavioral genetics Behavioral genetics is the field of study that examines the role of genetics of behavior in all animals, including humans. Behavioral geneticists study the inheritance of behavioral traits. In humans this is most often seen in twin studies or studies of people who have been adopted.

behavioral state A period of coordinated activity, that in the fetus is punctuated by periods of rest. These are one of the most important aspects of behavior in newborn infants; may be defined as the infants' level of arousal mediating the responsivity to environmental inputs.

behaviorism Theoretical perspective that ascribes to the notion that all behavior can be described by the principles of conditioning.

benign senescent forgetfulness (BSF) Brief transitory episodes of cognitive decline attributable to inattentiveness and distractions.

bimanual coordination The process of using one hand as a lead hand and the other as an assist hand simultaneously to manipulate objects.

biological age An approach to aging that is determined by physiology rather than the chronological passage of time. Biological age refers to the condition of an individual's organ and body systems as well as changes in the performance of motor skills and sensory awareness. A person who has been active and exercised regularly is likely to have a "younger" cardiovascular system than a chronologically younger person with a more sedentary lifestyle.

biologic risk Related to factors in an infant or the mother that are known to have potentially adverse consequences on the infant; may include genetic problems, disease or disability in the mother or infant, maternal age, maternal smoking or drug use during pregnancy, *intrauterine growth retardation* (IUGR), and prematurity.

birth defect Physical abnormalities that are present at birth.

blastocyst Multicellular product of conception during the first week; embryonic tissue (inner cell mass) is first differentiated from extra-embryonic tissue (fetal membranes and placenta).

body functions Physiological aspects of the human organized by functional system, such as mental functions, cardiovascular functions, or movement-related functions.

body image A person's sense of his or her own physical appearance and physical abilities, usually in relation to others within the person's social environment.

body mass index (BMI) A calculation that uses height and weight to estimate how much body fat someone has.

body-on-body righting reaction (BOB) A transitional movement pattern that persists through life and aids in the control of posture. In this pattern, when one leg is flexed and rotated across the midline of the body, a segmental rotation of the trunk, shoulder, and then head follows the initial movement.

body-on-head righting reaction (BOH) A transitional movement pattern that persists through life and aids in the control of posture. When an individual's postural orientation is not vertical, such as in prone, the individual moves the head out of alignment with the body into a vertical position.

body schema An internalized sense of the space that the body occupies.

body structures Body parts and anatomy, such as the nervous system or structures related to movement.

bone remodeling The dynamic balance between the absorption of bone tissue (osteoclastic functions) and simultaneous deposition of new bone (osteoblastic functions).

boomerang generation A term applied to young adults who often choose to cohabitate with their parents after a brief period of living on their own, "boomeranging" back to their place of origin.

bottom-up assessment Perspective in which deficits or impairments are delineated in specific areas, leading to a program model designed to remediate those deficits.

Bowlby, John Psychiatrist who studied social development and attachment in children, including ethologic work. He examined the effects of mother-child separation.

bridge employment Any paid work after an individual retires or starts receiving a pension.

bronchopulmonary dysplasia (BPD) Progressive scarring of the lungs, creating a emphysematous-like function that is caused by many factors but is probably most closely related to prolonged ventilation of immature lungs.

bulimia Also called bulimia nervosa, bulimia is a mental health disorder defined in DSM-5 as abnormal binge eating followed by induced vomiting or purging, occurring at least on a weekly basic (American Psychiatric Association, 2013). Many (but not all) people with bulimia also have anorexia nervosa.

bullying A form of aggressive behavior perpetuated by either an individual or a group that involves the use of force or coercion directed repeatedly toward particular victims.

calculation functions An ICF category including determination, approximation, and manipulation of mathematical symbols and processes.

calibration Judgment of force, speed, and directional control necessary to accomplish a task.

Canadian Occupational Performance Measure (COPM) A qualitative assessment tool using a semistructured interview. It has been shown to be responsive to changes noted in performance and personal satisfaction of performance over time in clients receiving therapeutic services.

cancer A term used for diseases in which abnormal cells divide and result in the uncontrolled growth of abnormal cells in the body. Cancer is not just one disease but many diseases. There are more than 100 different types of cancer, a major health problem facing people of all ages.

capacity A construct related to the individual's ability to perform a task in a controlled environment, such as a rehabilitation setting. Capacity represents, as the term implies, what the individual could do in an optimum setting with extrinsic factors controlled.

cardiopulmonary system A key physiologic system in mediating behavior, particularly motor behavior; supports characteristics of motor performance such as endurance.

cardiovascular fitness The combined efficiency of the heart, lungs, and vascular system in delivering oxygen to the working muscle tissue so that prolonged physical work can be maintained. When you exercise regularly, you can increase your cardiovascular fitness as your heart becomes more efficient at pumping blood and oxygen to the body, and the body becomes more efficient at using that oxygen.

career An organized path of work pursued over some length of time.

Case, Robbie Developmental psychologist who elaborated upon Piaget's theory of cognitive development, emphasizing innate abilities with social and cultural influences.

causal attributions The explanatory attributions people make to help them understand the world around them and to seek reasons for a particular event. Attributions can be explanatory, that is, "I did well on the test because I studied hard," or they can be interpersonal, that is, "I did poorly on the test because my neighbors made so much noise I could not sleep."

central nervous system (CNS) The brain and spinal cord; the parts of the nervous system that do not leave the protective covering of the skull and vertebral column.

cephalocaudal Relating to a head-to-tail direction along the long axis of the body.

cerebral palsy (CP) An umbrella term encompassing a group of nonprogressive, noncontagious motor conditions that result in musculoskeletal impairments in infancy. In neurological terms, cerebral palsy is not a single condition, but the manifested symptoms that are secondary to many kinds of cerebral damage.

Chess, Stella Theorist who, with Alexander Thomas, developed a classic system for describing and categorizing temperament.

children with special health care needs A legal definition for the purposes of policy and health care access that indicates children who have or are at increased risk for a chronic physical, development, behavioral, or emotional condition and who also require health and related services of a type or amount beyond that required by children generally.

chondroskeleton The well-formed cartilaginous skeleton identified at the lowest portion of the skull, the spine, rib cage, scapulas, and extremities by the 10th to 11th week postconceptual age.

chronic disease/health problem A disease or serious health condition that persists for a long time. A chronic disease is one lasting three months or more, by the definition of the U.S. National Center for Health Statistics.

chronic obstructive pulmonary disease (COPD) The occurrence of chronic bronchitis or emphysema, a pair of commonly coexisting diseases of the lungs in which the airways become narrowed.

chronic poverty The expectation of poverty as a way of life that occurs when individuals hold little hope for improvement in their circumstances.

chronic sorrow Recurrent sorrow that occurs when parents encounter repetitively the limitations from their child's enduring impairments.

chronic stressor Chronic stress is a long-term or continuous state of nervous arousal where individuals perceive that the demands on them are greater than their ability to meet those demands. Chronic stressors include enduring problems, conflicts, and threats that people face in their everyday lives that persist over time.

civic engagement The commitment to working to make a difference in the civic life of our communities and developing the combination of knowledge, skills, values, and motivation to make that difference. It means promoting the quality of life in a community, through both political and nonpolitical processes.

classical conditioning Process that enables learning to occur from repeatedly pairing some neutral stimulus with a stimulus that evokes a response.

client The focus of interest in the health care service interaction. Although we typically think of clients as individuals, clients may also be a group, an organization, or a population.

client-centered care A dynamic strategy in which both professionals and clients work together in a collaborative manner to meet the needs of the client.

clinical reasoning A situated, practice-based form of reasoning that requires a background of scientific and technological research-based knowledge about general cases, more so than any particular instance. It also requires practical ability to discern the relevance of the evidence behind general scientific and technical knowledge and how it applies to a particular patient. In doing so, the clinician considers the patient's particular clinical trajectory, their concerns and preferences, and their particular vulnerabilities (for example, having multiple comorbidities) and sensitivities to care interventions (for example, known drug allergies, other conflicting comorbid conditions, incompatible therapies, and past responses to therapies) when forming clinical decisions or conclusions.

closed-loop theory Proposed by Jack A. Adams to describe motor skill development based on a sensory feedback loop.

cognitive appraisal A process of trusting individuals' personal interpretation of an event or illness in determining their emotional reaction.

cognitive domain Involves thought, and includes the ability to express one's self through written and spoken language, the ability to read, think, and perform tasks from planning through completion.

cognitive flexibility The ability to consider alternatives and change strategies or approaches to a problem. This is associated with working memory.

cognitive map Mental manipulations of remembered sensory experiences superimposed on a desired task.

cognitive monitoring A form of metacognition that involves self-examination of what you are currently doing, what you will do next, and how effectively the activity is serving to meet your intended purpose.

cohabitation A living arrangement in which two adults who are not legally married are in a sexual relationship and share domestic tasks and responsibilities.

coincidence-anticipation timing The ability to initiate and complete a motor pattern with the arrival of a moving object at a previously set interception point.

collectivistic cultural characteristics The principles or system of ownership and control of the means of production and distribution by the people collectively, usually under the supervision of a government.

communication Term that encompasses the ability of humans to interact in ways that enable them to share such functions as basic needs, wants, desires, and ideas.

communication bill of rights Document developed by the National Joint Committee for the Communicative Needs of Persons with Severe Disabilities that emphasizes the importance of communication to quality of life.

comparator In motor control theories, used to refer to a neural body, such as the cerebellum, that has access to both expected or programmed and actual or received sensory input about the motor program.

competence promotion Competence promotion involves education and public health initiatives designed to increase resilience.

conceptional age Common terminology associated with dating the age of the preterm infant. Also called *postconceptual age.*

concrete operations In Piaget's theory of cognitive development, the third stage, typically roughly equivalent to that displayed by school-age children. In this stage, children perform manipulations on the environment using organized cognitive structures. Key characteristics displayed by children in this phase are reversibility of actions and mastery of conservation tasks.

concrete symbols The use of actual objects, gestures (such as raising arms to say "pick me up"), and sounds (such as barking to mean dog) as an aid to communication.

congenital infections Newborn infant infections contracted before or at birth from the mother.

congestive heart failure A condition in which the heart works inefficiently and fails to pump enough blood through all the organs within the body.

consciousness A global mental function; involves a level of arousal that permits responsiveness to the environment.

consolidation stage The fifth of Super's (1985) eight stages of career exploration and development. Here individuals respond to actual work experiences; a vocational path is selected that offers the best chance to obtain satisfaction.

constructive play Play that involves making or building things; develops at age 3 to 4 years and closely parallels the development of manipulation and fine motor skills and executive functions like planning, sequencing, and error detection.

constructivist theories Theories of learning and an approach to education that lays emphasis on the ways that people create meaning of the world through a series of individual constructs.

contextual factors In the ICF, those factors that influence how a person is able to respond to a given condition; these factors are intrinsic (personal) or extrinsic (environmental).

continuing care retirement community A planned residential arrangement, usually including apartments and townhouses, that include social, recreational, meal, and housekeeping services for a monthly fee. These communities include a range of housing levels from independent housing through nursing care, so that as more skilled care is needed, individuals can remain within their social community for as long as possible.

continuous career path model Models of career development such as those of Ginzberg and Super that consider a career path as continuous from completion of formal education to retirement.

control parameters The conditions in existence at the time the task is executed. A control parameter could be a function of change in any one of the subsystems considered in dynamical systems theory.

Convention on the Rights of Persons with Disabilities A document developed through the United Nations (UN) that was a call to action for all UN members to commit to the protection of the rights and dignity of persons with disabilities.

co-occupation Co-occupations are characterized by an ongoing interaction between the occupations of one individual and another that sequentially shapes the occupations of both people. Many adult occupations, including the occupation of parenting, are co-occupations, involving two or more people who are active in building a shared meaning and have shared goal in the performance of either necessary or chosen occupations.

cooperative play Behavior typical of middle childhood, as in team games where there is social interaction in a group setting, with a sense of group identity.

coping Expending conscious effort to solve personal and interpersonal problems in a manner that overcomes or minimizes stress or conflict.

co-regulation When one person, (e.g., the child) takes an action (buying a nutritious lunch) in response to another person's action (parent's request). In this example, both the parent and the child shares control of everyday behaviors.

coronary heart disease A prevalent cardiovascular disease associated with age, caused by a narrowing of the coronary arteries, which results in a decreased supply of blood and oxygen to the heart. CHD includes myocardial infarction, commonly referred to as a heart attack, and angina pectoris, or chest pain.

criterion-referenced test Type of formative assessment that examines the number of items or criteria individuals can successfully complete as compared with a standard completed by a normative group; is sensitive to intervention and can help guide therapy.

critical period A highly sensitive period during which a developing infant is at greatest risk for congenital anomalies or developmental disabilities should the developmental process be interrupted or altered; also refers to limited time in which a developmental event can occur, the time when an organism is most receptive to learning a certain kind of behavior.

cruising An infant mobility pattern that involves moving the hands along furniture or other environmental features while taking steps sideways to move in a desired direction.

crystallized intelligence Intelligence that reflects the acquired and accumulated education, knowledge, and skills of individuals.

crystallization (stage of career choice) In Super's theory, the stage characteristic of early adolescence where only general ideas regarding a career are formulated.

cultural awareness The recognition that there are other ways of viewing the same scenario.

cultural broker A communicator who works to bridge or mediate between groups or people of differing cultural backgrounds to reduce conflict or produce change.

cultural competence A set of congruent behaviors, attitudes, and policies that come together in a system, agency, or among professionals and enable that system, agency, or those professions to work effectively in cross-cultural situations. Often replaced by the more accurate term *cultural effectiveness* in contemporary works.

cultural fluidity An understanding of cultural differences and how they manifest in everyday occupations that allow individuals to consider their own primary culture as a reference point from which new values and beliefs are considered and understood.

culture A complex construct that includes the sum of experiences, values, beliefs, ideals, judgments, and attitudes that shape meaning to human occupations. Culture is learned as people experience the complexity of social life, and although much of culture is conscious, over time culture becomes deeply embedded in personality and becomes largely unconscious.

cumulative impact The impact resulting from increasing or frequent influences during the developmental period being considered.

deafness A degree of poor hearing such that a person is unable to understand speech through hearing even in the presence of amplification.

deceleration stage The fourth of Super's adult stages of career development. This includes the preretirement phase, during which individuals' attention is on continuing to meet the minimum requirements of the job rather than on enhancing their position. It culminates in leaving the workforce.

declarative learning Learning that individuals are conscious of and make a conscious effort to support; this predominates as individuals attempt to learn a new skill at any age and requires both awareness of and attention to the task.

degrees of freedom In any system, the number of factors that are free to vary. In the context of this book, the flexibility in the motor program is referred to as its degree of freedom.

dementia A disease state that results in the deterioration of intellectual faculties such as judgment, concentration, and especially memory.

depression A mental health disorder that involves the body, mood, and thoughts that often results in a lack of energy and difficulty in maintaining concentration or interest in life. This condition, also called a mood disorder, interferes with daily life, normal functioning, and causes pain for both the person with the disorder and those who care about him or her.

determinants Factors that influence overall health and well-being, including biologic factors, behaviors, social and physical environments, and public policies and interventions.

development The changes in performance that are heavily influenced by maturational processes.

developmental assessment A comprehensive standardized evaluation to ascertain the developmental status of children across all domains of development.

developmental delay Describes failure of child to acquire normative age-related behaviors; implies the ability to "catch up." Developmental delay may be global or focal. In some cases, delays in all areas of development or the delay may be restricted to only some areas, such as motor or language development.

developmental disability Pervasive and chronic developmental delay, often with scatter in the acquisition patterns of developmental milestones.

developmental milestones Skills typical within a culture to a specific age group; useful for screening children, but do not give adequate information to determine whether a delay is based on neuromotor or environmental causes.

developmental niche The developmental niche is seen as the interaction of the individual's physical and social cultural milieu, including customs, child rearing practices, and beliefs of parents about caretaking that dynamically impacts the developmental trajectory of the individual through the lifespan. Each of the aspects of the developmental niche is dynamic and adapts based on the age, gender, temperament, developmental level, and talents of the individual.

developmentally appropriate care An approach to newborn infant care that seeks to minimize the iatrogenic effects of prematurity by increasing sensitivity of caregivers to infant cues.

developmental systems theory A collection of models of biological development and evolution that argue that the emphasis the modern evolutionary considerations places on genes and natural selection as explanation of living structures and processes is inadequate.

developmental theory A theory that addresses changes that are attributed proportionately more to maturation than to environmental experience.

developmental theory of vocational choice Proposed by Ginzberg and associates (1951), a theory that describes a continuous process of occupational choice following a developmental progression that begins in childhood and spans into the early adult years.

Dewey, John A theorist who believed in the biologic and social bases to learning, and emphasized the school as an instrument of social progress; a major influence on American education systems.

diabetes mellitus A group of metabolic diseases in which a person has high blood sugar, either because the body does not produce enough insulin or because cells do not respond to the insulin that is produced.

difference threshold A term used in neuroscience to describe the smallest change in stimulation that a person can detect.

disability Inability to pursue life tasks and roles because of physical or mental impairment.

disability fraud The receipt of payment(s) intended for the people with disabilities by one who should not be receiving them.

disability paradox The difference noted between self-reported health and assessment of health by others. Individuals with severe impairments may not self-identify as "disabled" and may report high levels of quality of life based in supportive contextual factors and personal perceptions of well-being and life satisfaction.

disability rights movement An organized political and social action movement to raise public awareness and secure equal opportunities and rights for people with disabilities.

disablement Sociologic concept commonly used to describe the impact of a disease or disability on human function, recognizing that functional states associated with health conditions are not identical to the conditions themselves.

discontinuous career paths Career paths interrupted or deferred by child rearing, need for additional education, disability, and other family needs are increasingly the norm.

discriminative touch Aspects of touch that we think consciously about, like how hard, smooth, or curved an object is.

domestic violence A pattern of abusive behaviors by one partner against another in an intimate relationship such as marriage, dating, family, or cohabitation.

Down syndrome Fairly common genetically based developmental disorder caused by an extra 21st chromosome; physical characteristics and mental retardation are commonly associated with this syndrome.

ductus arteriosus Passageway between the pulmonary trunk and the aorta that normally closes within the first few hours after birth.

dynamic postural stability Type of active, adaptive control that allows an individual to change movements without stopping or losing balance; begins around 5 years of age.

dynamic visual acuity The ability to accurately identify a moving target. This can be the ability to perceive objects accurately while actively moving the head. Alternatively, the person's head can be stable and the object can be moving!

dynamical systems theory Has its roots in a theory of human physics, which refers to self-organization of complex particles; states that behavior at any given point in time is the result of variable interactions of a number of complex systems and that behavior is emergent.

early intervention In the context of Part C of IDEA, this is the process of providing services, education, and support to young children who are deemed to have an established condition, those who are evaluated and deemed to have a diagnosed physical or mental condition (with a high probability of resulting in a developmental delay), an existing delay, or a child who is identified as at risk of developing a problem that may impede their development.

early programming A conceptual focus of life course theory. The literature in human development shows that early experiences can "program" an individual's future health and development (USHHS, 2010a). This early programming can have either a positive or a negative effect on the health of an individual.

eating disorder Any of a range of psychological disorders characterized by abnormal or disturbed eating habits including anorexia nervosa and bulimia.

ectoderm Among the three primary embryonic cell layers, the one that results in the surface layer of cells forming the skin.

effector system of motor control Musculoskeletal system; key in executing motor behavior.

efficacy The personal sense that you are competent and effective in your life roles.

egalitarianism A preference for affirmation of the individual allowing for negotiation in authority relationships.

elder abuse A single, or repeated act, or lack of appropriate action, occurring within any relationship where there is an expectation of trust that causes harm or distress to an older person. Elder abuse can take various forms such as physical, psychological or emotional, sexual, and financial abuse.

elder cottage housing opportunities (ECHO) Temporary, movable, self-contained houses designed to enable older people to live near family and/or caregivers to prevent them from having to be institutionalized.

embodied cognition The construct that active movement and physical "doing" influences our cognition, just as the mind influences bodily actions.

embryonic period Period extending to the end of the 8th week after conception, at which point all major body structures have been formed.

emergent control In motor control theories, the ability to alter how a task is performed in accordance with current environmental circumstances.

emerging adulthood period A phase of the life span between adolescence and full-fledged adulthood that primarily applies to individuals who do not have children and who do not have sufficient income to become fully financially independent.

emotional functions Functions that include specific mental functions related to the feeling and affective reactions of individuals, as well as mental regulation of the appropriateness and degree of emotion within an individual's social and environmental context.

empiricist school Based on belief that the formation of associations between various sensations is the foundation of perception.

enablement theory An approach to health policy and assessment that emphasizes individuals and proposes to provide that individuals with adequate power, means, opportunity, or authority to manage their own health and rehabilitation. Enablement theory focuses on the causal interrelationships among variables at different levels.

endoderm Germ layer from which are formed the digestive system, many glands, and part of the respiratory system.

energy and drive functions ICF functions that include the physiologic and psychological mechanisms that result in the individual's energy level, motivation, appetite, craving (including craving for substances that can be abused), and impulse control.

engrossment The sense of absorption, preoccupation, and interest that fathers have in their newborn child.

entrainment Rudimentary variation of a linked behavioral and social exchange present at birth.

environmental constraints Prevailing environmental conditions that help shape the movement to be executed.

environmental factors Features that make up the physical, social, and attitudinal environment in which people live and conduct their lives.

environmental modifications Internal and external physical adaptations to the home, which are supportive in ensuring the health, welfare, and safety.

environmental risk Related to factors in an infant's environment that may have a potentially adverse effect on the infant, such as low socioeconomic status (SES), inadequate parental caregiving, neglect or abuse, poor nutrition, etc.

epiblast Outer layer of a blastula that gives rise to the ectoderm.

epigenesis Epigenesis describes the development of an organism as it moves from a relatively unstructured state to a more ordered and differentiated state over the course of developmental time.

epigenetics The study of heritable changes in gene expression or cellular phenotype caused by mechanisms other than changes in the underlying DNA sequence.

epiphysis The end portion of a long bone, initially separated from the shaft (diaphysis) by a section of cartilage.

Erikson, Erik One of the few true life span theorists; his psychosocial theory-related developmental stages to a series of life tasks, or crises that need to be resolved.

essential health benefits The Affordable Care Act of 2010 requires that health insurance plans sold to individuals and small businesses provide a minimum package of services in 10 categories called "essential health benefits." But rather than establishing a national standard for these benefits, the Department of Health and Human Services (HHS) has decided to allow each state to choose from a set of plans to serve as the benchmark plan in their state.

essential tremor Involuntary shaking (tremors) often in the hands. Essential tremors worsen with movement and are aggravated by emotional stress, fatigue, and extremes of temperature.

equilibrium reactions Complex patterns involving rotational movements along the body axis in order to maintain balance that are considered neurologically mature because their presence indicates the integration of earlier primitive and transitional motor patterns.

establishment stage The third of Super's stages of career development. In this stage, individuals are in actual work situations, and a suitable field is selected. Efforts are made to secure a long-term place in the chosen career.

ethnicity Generally refers to the influence of both race and culture on behavior and may also refer to shared traits, customs, language, religion, and ancestry.

ethnocentric Characterized by or based on the attitude that one's own group is superior.

evaluation process A cyclical and ongoing process that includes historical information, current test findings, and clinical judgment about actual or potential health problems/life process occurring with individuals, families, groups, or communities.

evolutionary psychology Evolutionary psychology is defined as the application of evolutionary biology to psychology, including the notion that the human brain, as the source of behavior, has specialized mechanisms which evolved to solve recurrent problems encountered by the organism in the environment.

executive attention The individual's ability to regulate his or her responses, particularly in conflict situations where several responses are possible.

executive functions Control or oversight functions of thought; the mental processes that organize our thoughts for action, including the processes of initiating, abstraction, problem solving, cognitive flexibility, and judgment.

executive stage The fourth of Schaie's stages in which the task is of broadening focus from the personal domain to the community or societal level, typically occurring later than the responsible stage in middle adulthood but not necessarily exhibited by all adults.

experience of self and time functions ICF-based specific mental functions related to the awareness of one's identity, body, position in the reality of one's environment, and of time.

exploration stage The first adult stage in Super's career development model during which people begin to specify and implement a career choice. Different roles are tried and various employment options are explored.

expressive communication The use of language to communicate thoughts, ideas, or feelings. Expressive communication may be spoken, signed, or written language.

expressive/overt communication Communication with others that may be gestural, vocal, signed, written, or produced through an augmentative communication device. Expressive communication most typically involves the use of language.

eye-hand coordination Skillful use of the hand under visual guidance; precedes the development of fine hand and eye control.

facilitator A factor that supports healthy participation.

failure to thrive (FTT) A diagnostic term that indicates insufficient weight gain or inappropriate weight loss.

family-centered care An approach to the health care of infants and children that assures the health and well-being of children and their families through a respectful family-professional partnership. It honors the strengths, cultures, traditions, and expertise that everyone brings to this relationship. Family-centered care is the standard of practice that results in high-quality services.

family development theory Family development theory emphasizes the evolution of families over time. A central defining attribute of family development theory is that its focus is on families rather than individuals.

fast twitch (type II) muscle fibers Muscle fibers that use anaerobic metabolism to create fuel, making them much better at generating short bursts of strength or speed than slow fibers. However, they fatigue more quickly.

fear of falling (FOF) Multifactorial problem with high incidence in older adults; associated with poorer health status and functional decline.

fetal alcohol syndrome (FAS) Syndrome caused by excessive maternal consumption of alcohol during pregnancy; typically includes microcephaly, developmental delay, and dysmorphism in the child.

fetal period The longest period of prenatal development, extending from approximately the 9th week after conception until the moment of birth. This period involves extensive growth as well as complex structural and physiologic refinement of the tissues, organs, and systems that were formed during the embryonic period.

fetal viability Exists when a fetus is sufficiently developed to live outside the uterus.

figure-ground perception Ability to separate an object of regard from its surroundings.

fine motor control Includes the volitional, coordinated use of the eyes, hands, and muscles of the mouth.

finger dexterity The ability to make precisely coordinated movements of the fingers of one or both hands to use or manipulate very small objects.

flexibility In musculoskeletal terms, this is the range of motion available to joints during functional activity.

flow Term used to describe the smoothness and fluidity of movement.

fluid intelligence Capacity to use unique kinds of thinking to solve unfamiliar problems by utilizing short-term memory, creating concepts, perceiving complex relationships, and engaging in abstract reasoning.

foramen ovale Opening between the two atrial chambers of the heart that normally closes within the first two weeks after birth.

formal relationships An association based on employment or social interactions between two parties, who are linked because of a mutual affiliation or goal. Often these relationships are with people in positions of authority, but they may also be with subordinates and equals.

frame of reference Theoretical perspective or viewpoint that organizes the approach to client management.

Freud, Sigmund Father of psychoanalysis; developed familiar concepts such as id, ego, and superego; one of the originators of psychological interventions.

function Action or ability for which a person or thing is specially fitted, used, or responsible for.

Functional Independence Measure (FIM) A brief 18-item test that provides a uniform system of measurement for disability that is consistent with the ICF. The FIM measures the level of a person's disability and indicates how much assistance is required for the individual to carry out activities of daily living.

gag reflex Elicited by touch of the posterior half to third of the tongue or the soft palate/uvula region; plays an important role in feeding development in preterm infants.

games with rules Play activities that have explicit rules that are agreed upon by all parties and involve the cooperative play of at least two people.

gastroesophageal reflux (GER) A heartburn-like condition created by stomach content refluxing into the esophagus that is extremely common in premature infants; can produce behaviors such as incoordination in swallowing, feeding aversion, and arching.

gender identity The sense of identification with either the male or female sex, as manifested in appearance, behavior, and other aspects of a person's life.

Generation Y The generation born in the 1980s and 1990s, typically regarded as increasingly familiar with digital and electronic technology.

genomics Genomics is the study of the genetic code in the context of the genome.

genotype The genotype is the genetic makeup of a cell, an organism, or an individual (that is, the specific allele makeup of the individual).

germinal (pre-embryonic) period Period that lasts approximately two weeks from conception and ends when the unicellular zygote has implanted in the uterus and has become an embryo, a complex multicellular organism capable of producing all of the organs and tissues of the body.

Gesell, Arnold Pioneer in the study of child development who published extensively from his work with developmental norms, and was a strong supporter of the maturationist or "nature" school.

Gestalt school Characterized by belief that perception is not a perfect, photographic representation of the world, nor is it a sum of sensations, but that it has a psychological form that represents the world without being identical to it.

gestational age (same as menstrual age) Direct estimate of the duration of the pregnancy, dated from the mother's last menstrual period.

Gibson, Eleanor Perceptual theorist who studied perceptual development and believed that perception is a function of learning to attend to salient features of a stimulus.

global mental functions Functions that underlie the other mental activities, including consciousness, energy, and drive, and are crucial to all human activity; they also are important predictive factors in rehabilitation outcomes.

global psychosocial functions Essential mental abilities that allow individuals to integrate aspects of social experience, personality, and emotions to provide a foundation for the formation of the interpersonal skills.

graphomotor skills The collections of conceptual and perceptual motor skills involved in drawing and writing.

gray power A phrase coined in the 1980s to describe the organized influence exerted by elderly people as a group, especially for social or political purposes or ends.

group homes Small, residential facilities located within a community and designed to serve people with chronic disabilities. These homes usually have six or fewer occupants and are staffed 24 hours a day by trained caregivers.

habilitation services Health care services that help people keep, learn, or improve skills and functioning for daily living.

habits Ingrained behaviors that can be performed without conscious thought.

hand dominance The consistent and more proficient use of the preferred hand in functional and skilled tasks.

hand preference Consistent choice of the same hand for complex skilled tasks; usually developed by the age of 4.

haptic perception Active memory of touch, texture, shape, temperature, and weight that allows an individual to tell you that she has, for example, a penny in her hand even in the absence of sight.

Hayflick limit The ability of cells to divide and replicate is limited to some genetically predetermined amount referred to as the Hayflick limit. The ability of cells to reproduce is decreased as one begins to age.

health A state of complete physical, mental, and social well-being, not merely the absence of disease and infirmity (WHO, 1948). It includes the motivation to become engaged in life, a sense of control over one's actions, and a desire to interact and connect with others, and perhaps most importantly, engages the individual's self-esteem.

health behavior An action taken by individuals that results in supporting health or preventing illness. Some common health behaviors are exercising regularly, eating a balanced diet, and maintaining regular sleep habits.

health belief model This model was developed to study utilization of preventive health services. The model suggests people will change their behavior if they feel they are at risk for an illness or injury that is sufficiently dangerous to warrant action.

health disparity Health disparity refers to the differences in the quality of health and health care across different populations that includes differences in the incidence of disease, health outcomes, or access to health care across racial, ethnic, and socioeconomic groups.

health equity The study of differences in the quality of health and health care across different populations.

Health Insurance Portability and Accountability Act of 1996 (HIPAA) A U.S. law designed to protect the privacy of health care consumers. HIPAA requires the following actions: (1) the continuity of health care coverage for individuals who change jobs; (2) the management of health information; (3) simplification of the administration of health insurance; and (4) combat of waste, fraud, and abuse in health insurance and health care. An aspect of this law was to establish national standards for electronic health care transactions.

health literacy The degree to which individuals have the capacity to obtain, process, and understand basic health information needed to make appropriate health decisions and services needed to prevent or treat illness.

health promotion The provision of information that makes positive contributions to the health of consumers, whether they are individuals, families, employers, or community groups. Health promotion is also the promotion of healthy ideas and concepts to motivate individuals to adopt healthy behaviors.

Health Traditions Model An approach to understanding the diverse health beliefs and social expectations of families.

health trajectory A health trajectory is a predicted pattern of health or disablement that is likely given the internal and external influences on individuals as they develop and mature. Health trajectories may be started and change over an individual's life course. The LCT considers health trajectories not just for individuals, but also trajectories for groups such as populations and communities.

health-related quality of life (HRQOL) A multidimensional concept that includes domains related to physical, mental, emotional, and social functioning. It goes beyond direct measures of population health, life expectancy, and causes of death, and focuses on the impact health status has on quality of life.

Healthy People 2020 An initiative of the U.S. Surgeon General to focus efforts to improve the health of the nation. Healthy People 2020, includes almost 600 objectives encompassing 42 different topic areas with five major goals. These are: (1) to identify nationwide health improvement priorities; (2) to increase public awareness and understanding of the determinants of health, disease, and disability and the opportunities for progress; (3) to provide measurable objectives and goals that are applicable at the national, state, and local levels; (4) to engage multiple societal sectors to take actions to strengthen policies and improve practices that are driven by the best available evidence and knowledge; and finally (5) to identify critical research, evaluation, and data collection needs (U.S. Department of Health and Human Services, 2012).

hearing impairment A broad term covering individuals with hearing loss ranging from mild to profound (deaf). A hearing impairment has a significant effect on the other components of language.

hemispheric specialization (also called *brain lateralization*) The end result of the brain maturation that allows the hemispheres to work separately and more efficiently.

heritability The term used to describe the amount of variability in the phenotype that is attributable to the genotype.

hierarchical models Theory tying the acquisition of developmental milestones to the level of brain maturation; the models explain human motor behavior, with the cerebral cortex ultimately determining the form and function of human movement.

high-risk infant Infants with medical challenges, including those born prematurely, are likely to spend some time in a NICU and then be discharged to family care; infants preparing to be discharged from the NICU that continue to have significant health problems or health conditions that leave them vulnerable to the development of additional health or developmental problems.

hippotherapy Use of horseback riding to accomplish therapeutic goals such as improved strength, balance, and posture.

history-normative influences These are the social/environmental influences on development that affect a cohort in time.

home establishment and management The scope of activities and occupations involved in obtaining and maintaining personal and household possessions and environment (e.g., home, yard, garden, appliances, vehicles), including maintaining and repairing personal possessions (clothing and household items) and knowing how to seek help or whom to contact.

homebound Going out of the house once a week or less.

HomeFit A collaborative initiative between the American Association of Retired Persons and the American Occupational Therapy Association is designed to educate people 50+ and their family members on how to make their homes more "livable" by incorporating a universal design concept.

hospice A specialized type of care for people who are expected to have less than six months to live and who are not seeking a cure for their condition.

hypertension Sometimes called arterial hypertension, is a chronic medical condition in which the blood pressure in the arteries is elevated.

hypotonia Hypotonia involves decreased resting tension in the muscles (muscle tone). Hypotonia may suggest the presence of central nervous system dysfunction, genetic disorders, or muscle disorders.

hypoxic ischemic encephalopathy (HIE) Lack of oxygen due to asphyxia that can cause injury to the nervous system of preterm infants.

iatrogenic health problems Medical or psychological problems that result from medical treatment.

identity formation The establishment of a distinct personality of an individual that helps him or her identify their newly forming place in society and life.

incidence The measure of the number of new cases of a health condition occurring in a population during a certain period of time.

inclusion Philosophy that all students in school, regardless of strengths/weaknesses, are part of the school community.

inclusive design Developing systems, products, or websites flexible enough to serve the broadest possible range of users. It provides access to users with disabilities and provides better usability for everyone.

individualistic cultural characteristics Typical of a culture that values assertiveness in reaching goals, with emphasis on individual over collective welfare.

Individuals with Disabilities Education Act (IDEA) The Individuals with Disabilities Education Act (IDEA) is a United States federal law that governs how states and public agencies provide early intervention, special education, and related services to children with disabilities. It addresses the educational needs of children with disabilities from birth to age 21.

infant mortality rate An estimate of the number of infant deaths for every 1,000 live births. This is an important and often reported number because this statistic is often used as an indicator to measure the health and well-being of a nation.

inferior pincer grasp Developmental grasp pattern using the distal pads of the thumb and forefinger, with the ulnar fingers inhibited and the thumb in opposition.

in-hand manipulation The process of using one hand to adjust an object for more effective placement or for release; the object remains in that hand and usually does not come in contact with a surface during in-hand manipulation.

instrumental activities of daily living (IADL) Activities of daily living that typically involve cognitive sequencing of chains of behavior; examples include complex tasks, often involving some tool or instrument, such as setting the table, picking up toys, washing vegetables, and folding washcloths.

integrated employment Paid work in the general labor market for people with disabilities, where the proportion of workers with disabilities does not exceed the natural proportions in the community (unlike sheltered workshops).

intellectual disability (ID) The current terminology suggested to replace the term *mental retardation* in the United States. There are three areas in which criteria must be met for this diagnosis: The person must have an IQ below 70, have the onset of these problems before age 18, and demonstrate difficulty with adaptive functioning.

intellectual functions Skills required for individuals to understand and constructively integrate information from all types of mental function, functions that develop and change over the life span and are influenced by experience, environmental contexts, and learning.

intelligibility The proportion of a speaker's output that a listener can readily understand. In typical development, as children learn to talk, they not only gain speech sounds, but those sounds also become more understandable to those around them.

intentional behavior Communication strategy used by typically developing children between 3 and 8 months of age. This state is still considered unintentional communication because, although the children intentionally engage in a behavior, what that behavior communicates must be determined through interpretation of a caregiver.

interactive behaviors All active behaviors that are directed at gaining the attention of others.

interagency agreement A sharing of resources within governmental agencies. This includes the state health care infrastructure that includes Medicaid and IDEA.

interdependence A cultural value supporting the belief that closeness is the key to all relationships.

International Classification of Functioning, Disability and Health (ICF) Classification system published by the World Health Organization to provide a scientific basis for understanding and studying functional states associated with health conditions with a focus on emphasizing health and de-emphasizing the concept of disability.

International Statistical Classification of Diseases and Related Health Problems (ICD-10) The ICD-10 is a tool for the classification of diseases, disorders, and other health conditions. The ICD-10 and ICF are planned to be complementary tools that, when used together, create a meaningful picture of the experience of health at both the individual and the population level.

interprofessional education (IPE) A curriculum-based initiative in health care in which two or more professions learn with, from, and about each other to improve collaboration and quality of care through planned and structured encounters.

interuterine growth retardation (IUGR) A term applied to infants who failed to reach obstetrical growth norms while in utero.

intraventricular hemorrhage (IVH) Fragile blood vessels near the ventricles of the brain that can rupture, causing injury to the nervous system of preterm infants.

jaundice An increase in bilirubin that causes an infant's skin to have a yellowish cast.

kangaroo care In care of premature infants, the concept of providing warmth from the temperature of the parents' skin, by placing the baby inside the parents' clothing and against the skin; replaces the warming incubator or isolette.

keeper of the meaning One of Vaillant's six adult life tasks. This task involves passing on the traditions of the past to the next generation. Becoming a "keeper of the meaning" allows one to link the past to the future.

kernicterus Caused by excessive bilirubin levels that may lead to damage to certain parts of the brain.

kinkeeper Family members who work at keeping in touch with family members or at keeping family members in touch with one another. Individuals who fulfill the role of keeping others informed about what is happening in the family, organizing get-togethers, and encouraging direct interactions. Kinkeeping serves to facilitate access of members of the kin network to one another.

kinesthetic perception Interpretation of information regarding relative position of body parts, body in space, and awareness of position and movement.

Knowledge of Performance (KP) In motor learning/ control theory, the knowledge of qualities of the movement.

Knowledge of Results (KR) In motor learning/ control theory, the knowledge of the outcome of the movement; essential for motor learning.

Kohlberg, Lawrence Student of Piaget, who is known for his theory of moral development.

kyphosis A curving of the spine that causes a bowing of the back, which leads to a forward-bending or slouching posture.

labyrinthine righting reactions Mediate antigravity behaviors that include a number of upper brainstem–mediated responses that either align the body with respect to gravity or the support surface or rotate the body parts into alignment with each other, thereby permitting the individual to change positions, as in rolling.

language A learned code, or system, of rules that make it possible for us to communicate ideas and express wants and needs.

language decoding The ability to recognize written representations of words. Through decoding, learners develop an understanding of letter-sound relationships, including knowledge of letter patterns to represent words. It is only through the development of language decoding that individuals learn that alphabetic symbols can be combined in endless variety to express language.

language disorder Problem with the comprehension or production of the language components morphology, syntax, semantics, and pragmatics that interferes with functional communication to a significant degree.

language impairment Any difference or limitation in the comprehension (understanding) or production (speaking) of the language code that results in a difference in communication but does not interfere with it.

lateral grasp (also called a *scissors grasp*) Prehension pattern holding a small object between the lateral side of the radial fingers and the thumb.

learned helplessness Disabling type of social learning in which a person learns that there is no way to succeed after repeatedly experiencing failure, resulting in a passive failure to attempt unfamiliar tasks.

learning Acquisition of new behavior, heavily influenced by environmental exposure as well as feedback and practice.

learning disability (LD) A neurologically based impairment that affects the brain's ability to process and respond to information. Although this diagnostic label is used more broadly in some parts of the world, in the United States, this term is used when children's level of achievement is substantially below what is expected by their intelligence level.

leisure Time that is not relegated to specific work or purpose but is used for enjoyment; leisure time has varying characteristics at different ages across the life span.

leisure competence The understanding of what leisure activities are meaningful and rewarding for you as an individual.

life course health development model A model proposed by Halfon and Hochstein (2002) that considers health as more than the absence of disease and as something that is affected by multiple determinants over the life course.

life course theory (LCT) is a multidisciplinary paradigm for the study of people's lives, structural contexts, and social change.

life expectancy An estimate of how long a person is expected to live at a certain point in time.

Lifestyle Redesign A copyrighted approach to improving health and wellness by preventing and managing chronic conditions through building healthier lifestyles with community-based small groups led by a trained facilitator that was developed through research in Well Elderly studies (Clark & Azen, 1997; Clark et al. 2001). This approach has been extended to many other populations than the elderly.

limbic system Part of the brain that controls needs, drives, and innate behaviors; very old and buried deep within the cerebral cortex.

linguistic competence The capacity of an organization and its personnel to communicate effectively, and convey information in a manner that is easily understood by diverse audiences including people of limited English proficiency, those who have low literacy skills or are not literate, and individuals with disabilities.

literacy Ability to read written language.

lobbying A form of advocacy where a direct approach is made to legislators on an issue or concern. Lobbying may be done by individuals and by organized groups.

locomotor pattern Type of mobility pattern in which the body as a whole is moved, or translated, through space.

long-term memory Memory for an indefinite period of time; storage is widely distributed in the brain.

lordosis The inward curvature of a portion of the lumbar and cervical vertebral column.

low back pain A common musculoskeletal symptom that may be either acute or chronic.

low vision A level of vision that is 20/70 or worse and cannot be fully corrected with conventional glasses.

maintenance stage The third of Super's adult stages of career development. This stage is characterized by constancy: (1) *holding on* (stagnating or plateauing), or (2) *keeping up* (updating or enriching). Continuity, stress, safety, and stability tend to be the standard.

malingering The act of intentionally feigning or exaggerating physical or psychological symptoms for personal gain.

marriage A social union or legal contract between people called spouses that legally identifies kinship and in which committed interpersonal relationships, usually intimate and sexual, are acknowledged.

Maslow, Abraham Theorist who developed a theory of hierarchy of needs, from the most basic physiologic needs to self-actualization.

maturation The process of an individual growing biologically, socially, and emotionally over time changing gradually from a simple to a more complex level of function.

mature rotary neck righting A transitional movement pattern that persists through life and aids in the control of posture. In this pattern, when the head and neck are rotated across the midline of the body, a segmental rotation of the shoulder, trunk, and then pelvis follows the initial movement.

McGraw, Myrtle Theorist known for her study of motor development, including the Johnny and Jimmy twin studies, designed to assess the relative impact of nature versus nurture.

meconium Thick, tarry substance that is usually voided in utero as well as for the first few days postnatally.

Medicaid Enacted into law in 1965 as Title 19 of the Social Security Act, a joint federal/state program that provided basic medical care for medically indigent individuals. The Patient Protection and Affordable Care Act of 2010 has absorbed the older Medicaid program into its scope.

medical model Emphasizes the person, and that person's impairments, as a cause of disability; it is the traditional approach presented in rehabilitation literature.

Medicare A federal health insurance program for individuals over the age of 65, created in 1965 as Title 18 of the Social Security Act. The Patient Protection and Affordable Care Act of 2010 has led to a restructuring of Medicare reimbursement from "fee-for-service" to "bundled payments."

medication reconciliation The process of comparing a patient's medication orders to all of the medications that the patient has been taking.

medication toxicity A state of illness that occurs when people have accumulated too much of a drug in their bloodstream, leading to adverse effects within the body.

meme An element of a culture or system of behavior that may be considered to be passed from one individual to another through communication. A meme can be transmitted from one person to another through writing, speech, gestures, videos, or other forms of communication.

mental functions of language Described in the ICF as recognizing and using signs, and recognizing and using symbols as they relate to a language.

mental function of sequencing complex movements Defined in the ICF as the mental aspect of sequencing and coordinating complex, purposeful movements.

mental health disorder Any condition characterized by impairment of an individual's normal cognitive, emotional, or behavioral functioning, and caused by social, psychological, biochemical, genetic, or other factors, such as infection or head trauma.

mesenchymal cells Cells of mesodermal origin that are capable of developing into connective tissues, blood, and lymphatic and blood vessels.

mesoderm Germ layer that forms many muscles, the circulatory and excretory systems, and the dermis, skeleton, and other supportive and connective tissue. It also gives rise to the notochord.

metabolic equivalent unit (MET) A measure of aerobic capacity. One MET is equal approximately to the body's utilization of 3.5 ml O_2 per kilogram of body weight per minute (ml O_2/kg/min).

metacognition Refers to the use of cognitive skills that provide the basis for transfer and generalization of learned skills to daily functioning; includes monitoring functions and executive functions that help us plan, organize, execute, and evaluate our day-to-day activities.

metacognitive knowledge What individuals know about themselves and others in terms of self, task, and problem solving.

metacognitive process The regulation of thought and control of thoughts.

metalinguistic awareness Ability to engage in introspective tasks that reflect one's use of language.

metamemory A type of metacognition that involves a conscious awareness of one's memory capabilities and the intentional use strategies to aid memory.

minimal-stimulation protocols Caregivers attempt to cluster caregiving procedures such that premature or sick infants have the ability to settle into quiet behavioral states and rest between disturbances.

mixed-use development A community development strategy that combines two or more different types of land uses, such as residential, commercial, employment, and entertainment uses, in close proximity.

modeling Part of Bandura's social learning theory that proposes that children do not need to be directly reinforced to learn certain social skills; rather, they can learn by watching and receiving vicarious reinforcement.

morbidity Rate of incidence of a disease or disability within a population.

Moro reflex Key pattern used in all neonatal assessment to determine neurologic integrity; an infant's head is dropped backward, stimulating the vestibular system of the inner ear and causing abduction of the arms, followed by adduction of the arms across the chest.

morphology Study of word structure, including alterations in word structure to change word meaning.

mortality Death rate in a given population.

motor behavior Any performance of movement that can be observed or documented.

motor control Study of the neurobiologic processes underlying human movement.

motor learning Both a specific type of learning and an approach to therapeutic intervention following injury that is directed toward searching for a motor solution that emerges from an interaction of an individual with the task and the environment.

movement analysis An in-depth method of describing, interpreting, and documenting a specific movement pattern.

multitrauma A medical term describing the condition of a person who has been subjected to multiple traumatic injuries, such as a serious head injury in addition to a serious burn.

mutation A change of the DNA sequence within a gene or chromosome of an organism resulting in the creation of a new character or trait not found in the parental type.

myelination Developmental process of building a myelin sheath on the nerves to insulate the fibers and ensure that messages sent by nerve fibers are not lost en route.

National Prevention Strategy An initiative of the U.S. Surgeon General's office that aims to guide the nation in the most effective and achievable means for improving health and well-being. This strategy envisions a prevention-oriented society where all sectors recognize the value of health for individuals, families, and society, and work together to achieve better health for all Americans.

nativist school Perspective that genetic predisposition and innate ability largely explain the development of perception.

naturalistic observation A strategy of observing a behavior as it occurs in its natural setting with no attempts at intervention on the part of the clinician.

naturally occurring retirement community (NORC) A community that was not originally designed for older adults, but that through natural evolution, now contains a large proportion of residents who are 60 or more years old.

neglect This may include the failure to provide sufficient supervision, nourishment, or medical care, or the failure to fulfill other needs for which victims are helpless to provide for themselves. This term may apply to a child, a person with I/DD, or to a frail older person.

negotiability Ability to access a feature of the environment and use it for its intended purpose in a manner acceptable to the person.

neonatal abstinence syndrome (NAS) This is a condition reflecting postpartum behavioral and physiologic effects on the neonate of exposure to drugs in utero. Infants born with NAS are subjected to higher levels of mortality and morbidity.

neonatal intensive care unit (NICU) A specialized nursery prepared to take care of infants who require resuscitation and mechanical ventilation.

neonatal neck-righting reaction First of the rotary righting reactions to develop that allow infants to transfer from one postural set to another, that is, prone to supine.

neonatal period Period of the first four weeks after birth.

neural connectivity Physical links between areas of the brain that share common developmental trajectories. Brain studies show that areas with high neural connectivity activate together during a task.

neural plate Region of embryonic ectodermal cells that lie directly above the notochord.

neural tube defect A major birth defect caused by abnormal development of the neural tube, the structure that is present during embryonic life that gives rise to the central nervous system; among the most common of birth defects resulting in infant death and serious disability.

neurogenesis Process by which new nerve cells are generated.

neuromotor behavior The most prescriptive of the neonatal characteristics; includes the behavior of the newborn that is a direct reflection of the parts of the central nervous system.

neuroplasticity The ability of the human brain to change as a result of one's experience, that the brain is "plastic" and "malleable," and structural and functional changes in the brain are driven by environmental experience.

nonassociative learning Learning in which individuals do not rely on memory or prior experiences to associate with the sensory experience; this is important in learning physical and motor skills, resulting in both transient and long-term modulation at the synaptic level, as well as in rehabilitation of movement disorders.

nonnormative Developmental tasks or challenges are considered nonnormative when they are achieved in a manner that is not consistent with general patterns and experiences seen within the population, such as adapting to a disease or disability.

nonnormative influences Influences on human development and aging that are not necessarily associated with chronological age or historical time, yet play an important role in development, such as poverty, illness, physical abuse, or injury.

normalization Normalization reflects an internalization of the specialized habits and routines associated with activity limitations to such a degree that they are integrated as ordinary personal and family occupations. The normalization process represents the successful integration of activity limitations into daily occupations in a manner that enhances function.

normative Developmental tasks or challenges are considered normative when they are achieved in a manner that is consistent with general patterns and experiences seen within the population, such as the usual timing and sequence associated with learning to walk or to read.

norm-referenced test Summative assessment in which individual performance is evaluated against the standard deviation of scores obtained from a normative group or population; scores are typically presented as standard scores, z scores, or stanines, referenced to the bell-shaped curve; useful for diagnosis but not sensitive to intervention effects.

notochord Hollow chord at the embryo's midline formed when mesenchymal cells migrate upward between the ectodermal and endodermal layers. The vertebral column will form around this rodlike structure. The notochord provides some stability to the embryo and also serves as "the primary inductor" of early embryonic development.

nursing home A blanket term for a wide variety of institution-based living arrangement facilities that provide 24-hour supervised care.

obesity The term used for ranges of weight that are greater than what is generally considered healthy for a given height. Body mass index (BMI) is the standard used to judge weight. An adult who has a BMI of 30 or higher is considered obese.

object play (also play with objects) Manipulation of objects in an intrinsically motivated activity that is not focused on some externally imposed goal.

occupation An occupation is a meaningful action in the context of a person's life.

occupational balance The extent to which an individual's pattern of occupation is perceived by that person to be satisfactory, fulfilling, and compatible with that individual's values and goals.

occupational deprivation The condition when something external to an individual results in limiting his or her opportunity to participate in valued occupations.

occupational engagement The process of individuals doing occupations in a manner that fully involves their effort, drive, and attention.

occupational identity The subjective sense of capacity and effectiveness for participation in a chosen task. Occupational identity encompasses those things that people find interesting and satisfying to do, the roles and relationships that are sustained through participation, and a sense of comfort and familiarity with the routines associated with a chosen life path.

occupational model Theoretical model that focuses on competence in performance of desired human occupations.

occupational roles Patterns of behavior that are often culturally defined and that an individual actively identifies with. Occupational roles offer guidance about expected behaviors and responsibilities in specific defined situations and influence the individuals' aspirations and choice of vocational paths.

Occupational Therapy Practice Framework A classification scheme by the American Occupational Therapy Association that organizes client factors, performance skills, areas of occupation, performance patterns, and context.

occupational transition A major change in the occupational repertoire of a person. This transition may be gradual, as in healthy aging, or more abrupt as would follow a disabling injury or illness. In all cases, an occupational transition is a period of lifestyle change in which one or several occupations change, disappear, or are replaced with others.

ocular cataract A clouding that develops in the lens of the eye or in its envelope (lens capsule), varying in degree from slight to complete opacity.

oligohydramnios Insufficient amount of amniotic fluid, sometimes associated with kidney problems in the fetus.

onlooker play Behavior that occurs when children watch other children play without engaging in the play activity themselves.

open-loop theory A motor learning theory proposed by Richard Schmidt that argues that a motor response *schema* exists, consisting of a set of rules for directing movement. The actual sensory consequences, obtained through feedback, are compared to the expected sensory consequences, generated as part of the schema and response specifications.

operant conditioning Type of behavioral conditioning in which the behavioral response is strengthened in the presence of reinforcers.

optical righting reaction A vision-dependent transitional movement pattern that persists throughout life. When the visual field appears tilted, an individual uses visual information to seek a vertical orientation for the body. This response can conflict with the vestibular/gravity-mediated righting responses in some environments, causing disorientation.

orientation functions Defined in the ICF as the general mental functions of knowing and ascertaining one's relation to self, to others, to time and to one's surroundings. Orientation functions include functions of orientation to time, place, and person; orientation to self and others; disorientation to time, place, and person.

orofacial clefts Common birth defect pattern including cleft lip or cleft palate. Cleft lip and cleft palate are birth defects that occur when a baby's lip or mouth do not form properly.

oral motor reflexes Reflexes specific to the muscle actions of the mouth and oral area.

organogenesis The development of major organs and organ systems, such as the heart and lungs; occurs during the embryonic period.

orientation functions An awareness of who you are, where you are, and what time it is.

orthostatic hypotension An abnormal decrease in blood pressure when a person stands up. This may lead to fainting.

ossification Formation of bone.

osteoarthritis A disease condition caused by the degeneration of joint cartilage and the underlying bone, most common from middle age onward. It causes pain and stiffness, especially in the hip, knee, and thumb joints.

osteoporosis A disease condition when the body fails to form enough new bone, when too much old bone is reabsorbed by the body, or both. This disease has a high incidence and prevalence, especially in women, in which imbalance between bone resorption and bone formation leads to susceptibility to fracture.

outcome measure A measure of the quality of medical care, the standard against which the end result of the intervention is assessed.

palliative care An approach to health care that concentrates on reducing the severity of disease symptoms, and supports a positive quality of life in the presence of illness. This is ideally a multidisciplinary approach that supports both the patient and the family through addressing the physical, emotional, spiritual, and social concerns that arise with serious illness.

palliative coping An emotion-focused form of coping in which the main objective is to feel better through the management of the emotional response to a stressful situation in order to relinquish oneself of the psychological or physical impact.

palmar grasp Earliest voluntary grasp characterized by a pronated hand and flexion of all fingers to hold an object against the palm without use of the thumb.

palmar grasp reflex Involuntary pattern that occurs in response to pressure in the palm, causing an infant's fingers to curl around the examiner's finger, appearing to be a grasp.

paralanguage Nonverbal elements of communication that are used to modify meaning and convey emotion within a cultural context.

paralinguistic communication The use of manner of speaking to communicate particular meanings.

parallel play Developmentally typical play pattern at 2 to 4 years, when children are not mature enough to sustain interaction with others. Children bring toys or establish play space near others, yet play independently.

parenting The conscious decision to promote and support the physical, emotional, social, and intellectual development of children from infancy to adulthood.

parenting stress A particular type of psychological stress related to caring for children that is appraised by the parent as taxing or exceeding his or her resources. Parenting stress can be associated with both normative (adolescent risk-taking behaviors) and nonnormative (child illness or disability) factors influencing the parent. Parenting stress is often associated with the accumulation of demands with which the parents must cope.

Parkinson's disease (PD) A progressive disorder primarily impacting older adults that affects movement and cognition. PD is characterized by slowed movements (bradykinesia), resting tremor, and postural reflex impairment leading to balance problems.

Part B of the Individuals with Disabilities Education Act Through Part B, assistance for education of all children with disabilities in their educational pursuits through special education services from the age of 3 to 21.

Part C of the Individuals with Disabilities Education Act Through Part C, evaluation and special services are to be provided to infants and toddlers at no cost to the parents. When the infant is medically stable and residing in the family home, supportive health services including occupational and physical therapy, come to the child's home to provide family education, support, and therapy for the infant.

participation Participation within the context of the ICF is involvement in a life situation, most typically life tasks or actions.

participation restriction An ICF qualifier; the negative qualifier for participation, which indicates the person is functioning toward the disability part of the continuum of function.

patent ductus arteriosus Failure of the ductus arteriosus to close; often seen in premature infants.

Patient Protection and Affordable Care Act (ACA) Legislation aimed at decreasing the number of uninsured Americans and reducing the overall costs of health care. Additional reforms are aimed at improving health care outcomes and streamlining the delivery of health care. PPACA requires insurance companies to cover all applicants and offer the same rates regardless of preexisting conditions or gender.

Pavlov, Ivan Russian psychologist responsible for description of the classical conditioning paradigm (Pavlov's dogs).

perceptual functions Functions that include the mental processes of matching sensations with meaning by using information from an individual's sensory environment.

perceptual motor skills Controlled, volitional motor acts that respond in a dynamic way to sensory perceptions.

performance skills Skills that involve the ability to physically perform within the environment and that can be measured by attributes such as goal achievement, accuracy, and speed.

peripheral nervous system (PNS) Consists primarily of nerves and nerve roots that connect the control centers of the CNS to external sites, such as muscles, glands, or skin.

periventricular leukomalacia (PVL) Characterized by necrosis and cavitation of the white matter of the brain and may develop following a vascular insult, such as intraventricular hemorrhage, or in isolation, presumably due to some insult to the neural tissue.

persistent fetal circulation Occurs when the shunting of blood persists beyond the perinatal period and is treated by aggressive oxygenation through special ventilators or through *extracorporeal membrane oxygenation (ECMO)*.

persistent pulmonary hypertension High vasomotor tone in the pulmonary vasculature, which helps to keep the fetal circulation away from the lungs and moving through the ductus and foramen ovale. In a normal term birth, these vascular beds should open postpartum, allowing blood flow into the lungs for oxygenation. Failure to do so is considered persistent pulmonary hypertension.

personal factors Contextual influences on function and activity limitation that are intrinsic, such as gender, age, temperament, and personality.

phasic bite reflex Elicited by pressure on the gums, with a normative response being an up-and-down motion of the jaw, that often accompanies feeding behavior.

phenotype The composite of an organism's observable characteristics or traits, behavior, and products of behavior. Phenotypes result from the expression of an organism's genes as well as the influence of environmental factors and the interactions between the two.

phonology Rules governing combinations of phonemes to produce words that have meaning.

physical environment The natural and man-made features of the space a person occupies.

physical play Physical (body) play includes active rough-and-tumble activity and fine motor practice. Exercise activities related to children's developing whole-body and hand-eye-coordination also fall into this category.

physiologic immaturity Present in preterm infants; adversely affects the development of the lungs, because their development in the last postnatal trimester in utero is in large part what enables the successful transition to extrauterine life at term birth.

Piaget, Jean Twentieth-century psychologist who presented one of the most comprehensive and accepted theories of cognitive development for its time; his theories have influenced numerous subsequent psychological and educational systems.

placing reaction Reaction present in both hands and feet that is facilitated by stroking the back of the hand or top of the foot against a tabletop, causing an infant to lift the limb in flexion, then extend the limb as if to place it on the table.

plagiocephaly A term used to describe flattening of one side of the skull with contralateral skull bulging in the frontal area.

plantar grasp reflex Pattern representing primitive attempt at balance that occurs in response to pressure across the metatarsal heads, just under the toes, causing grasping by the toes.

plasticity (also neuroplasticity) The ability to modify behavioral or neural systems in response to changes in the internal or external environment.

play Activity that is intrinsically motivated and engaged in for pleasure. Play reflects individual differences and preferences and becomes more complex as one matures.

play with objects Manipulation of objects in an intrinsically motivated activity that is not focused on some externally imposed goal.

pluripotent stem cells Primordial cells that may still differentiate into various specialized types of tissue elements.

political action committee (PAC) Any organization whose main function is to financially support or campaign for (or against) political candidates, ballot initiatives, or legislation.

political advocacy A process by which individuals or an interest group organize and plan actions to influence public policy and resource allocation decisions. Advocacy of this type can influence political, economic, and social systems.

polyhydramnios An excess of amniotic fluid; may be associated with leakage of fluid from the fetus into the amniotic sac.

population health The health outcomes of a group of individuals, including the distribution of such outcomes within a group.

positive stress The sense of pressure that results from challenging experiences that are short-lived. Positive stress is stress that results in learning and positive growth.

positive support reactions One of the key patterns seen in standing, where extension through the lower limbs is mediated when infants are held in vertical suspension and the feet are placed on the surface; occurs without true weight bearing and must be integrated to permit true weight bearing and walking to occur.

post-acute care bundling Reimbursement strategy proposed by the Patient Protection and Affordable Care Act in which one payment would be made that is intended to cover the scope of care for the entire recovery period related to an episode.

postconceptional age Common terminology associated with dating the age of a preterm infant.

poster child A child who has a disease and is pictured in posters to solicit funds for combating the disease.

post-traumatic stress disorder (PTSD) A severe anxiety disorder that can develop after exposure to any event that results in psychological trauma.

postural control Ability to control your body's position in space, to remain erect in spite of changes in the surface you are walking on.

postural equilibrium Process of maintaining, through postural adjustments, the center of mass over the base of support.

postural set Alignment of body parts at any given point in time.

postural stability Ability to keep the body balanced and aligned.

postural support reaction A normal developmental reaction that occurs when an infant is held in vertical suspension and the feet are placed on the surface. The positive support reaction mediates extension through the lower limbs.

posture Alignment of the body at any given point in time, including both biomechanical and neuromotor elements.

poverty The state of not having sufficient basic resources.

power grasp Used for managing large or heavy objects; includes cylindrical grip, spherical grip, hook grip, and lateral prehension.

pragmatics The social rules for talking, or the rules governing what we say and how we say it.

praxis Ability of the brain to conceive, organize, and carry out a sequence of unfamiliar actions. Also known as motor planning.

pre-academic skills The skills that a child must learn (such as matching shapes or colors, one-to-one correspondence, and other concepts) before learning more complex academic skills (such as reading, math, and spelling).

precision grasp Grip patterns involving an unsupported hand and active wrist extension. Some examples of precision grasp are "chuck," or *tripod grips*, *pincer grasp* (the fingertips press against each other), and *lateral prehension* (pad-to-side; key grip).

prefrontal cortex The anterior part of the frontal lobes of the brain. The prefrontal area of the brain is an area of high neural connectivity, including strong connections with the limbic system and the striatal system.

prehension Using the hands for grasping, holding, and manipulation of objects.

pre-intentional behavior A normal form of communication in typically developing children between 0 and 3 months of age who communicate even though the behavior is not under the individuals' own control, but rather reflects their general state (hungry), and caregivers interpret the meaning from their body movements, facial expressions, and sounds.

prelinguistic period Period from birth to 12 months in which developmental changes in cognitive motor and social domains occur; when the period ends, the child can use words to refer to things.

presbyastasis Balance and dizziness resulting in disequilibrium in the absence of overt pathology.

presbycusis Age-related inner-ear dysfunction that diminishes auditory acuity and is the most common cause of hearing loss in adults.

presbyopia Most common visual problem in older adults; loss of accommodation or ability to focus on near objects.

presymbolic communication Communication that does not use symbols such as words or signs. This kind of communication therefore does not have a shared meaning for others.

pretense/sociodramatic play Pretense/ sociodramatic play, also called social play, includes all forms of pretend play including dressing up and role-playing. Pretense play typically emerges during solitary play in the second year as children's language skills grow to support their imagination. Through the preschool years, children's pretense play expands and becomes more social, involving others into their pretend world.

preterm infant An infant born at less than 37 weeks gestation.

prevention The management of factors that could lead to impairment, disease, or disability so as to maintain and support optimal levels of function and participation.

prevention programs Targeted programs are delivered to large groups without any prior screening for the risk status of the individual program recipients. A targeted determinant of health is typically the focus of the program, which is designed to address a known population at risk.

prevention science An interdisciplinary field with roots in disciplines such as developmental, community, and clinical psychology, as well as psychiatry, public health, epidemiology, and psychopathology.

primary prevention Efforts designed to protect people from acquiring an illness or injury. Immunization from infectious diseases is a classic example of primary prevention that addresses biologic health risks.

primitive stepping Spontaneous and reciprocal flexion of one leg and extension of the other in alternating patterns in response to an infant being tipped slightly forward; occurs without true weight bearing and must be integrated to permit true weight bearing and walking to occur.

procedural learning Learning of tasks that are performed automatically, such as the development of skill in areas like sports and playing musical instruments; occurs after declarative learning is complete.

process skills Skills that allow the transfer and adaptation of previously learned tasks to novel or altered situations.

products and technology Natural or human-made products, equipment, and technology in an individual's immediate environment that are gathered, created, produced, or manufactured. It is recognized that any product or technology can be used to improve the function of an individual with an activity limitation and thus be considered "assistive technology."

programmed aging theories Theories of aging that state that life expectancy is predetermined with cells programmed to divide a certain number of times.

proprioceptors Sensory receptors located in muscles, tendons, joints, and ligaments that provide information about position and movement of the body in space.

protective factor Opposite of risk factor. Protective factors are personal or environmental factors that insulate or counteract the potential negative impact of risk factors.

protective reactions Protective reactions, in postural control, are localized reactions to displacement or unexpected postural change. These reactions vary in degree from limb-specific to whole-body reactions based on the degree of displacement. Protective reactions involve a pattern of abduction and extension.

proxemics The study of the nature, degree, and effect of the spatial separation individuals naturally maintain and of how this separation relates to environmental and cultural factors is the study of such interaction distances and other culturally defined uses of space.

proximodistal From the center, or midline, moving outward.

psychological age An approach to aging that is determined by an individual's ability to adapt, solve problems, and cope with life events rather than the chronological passage of time.

psychomotor abilities (also psychomotor functions) Mental functions of control over physical and motor skills; they include the ability to originate (plan) and initiate (begin) movements, monitor and adjust motions in progress, perform learned tasks automatically without conscious direction, and pace, limit, or end movement based on activity demands.

psychomotor domain Involves movement and includes all the activities that give an individual mastery over the environment; encompasses both cognitive and affective behavioral domains through cognitive ability, motivation, and affect.

public policy doctrine The body of principles that underpin the operation of legal systems in each state or nation. This addresses the social, moral, and economic values that tie a society together—values that vary in different cultures and change over time. Public policy doctrine leads to the development and review of laws that are used to regulate behavior either to reinforce existing social expectations or to encourage constructive change. Public policy doctrine may be initiated in response to a current event or it may be developmental over time reflecting accepted societal norms and the collective morality of the society.

pulmonary hypertension A disease condition involving high blood pressure in the arteries of the lungs (the pulmonary arteries). Over time, the pulmonary arteries narrow, making the right side of the heart work harder as it takes higher pressure to force blood through the narrowed arteries.

purposeful sensory experience Any intentional use of the senses to gain information or experience.

qualitative assessment An assessment approach that uses observation, knowledge, and clinical reasoning in conjunction with nonstandard assessment tools such as chart review, intervention, visual assessment of movement patterns, and ecological assessments.

quality of life The phrase *quality of life* refers to a perception of fulfillment both of basic and of complex needs in daily life, leading to life satisfaction.

quantitative assessment An assessment approach that uses measurable properties such as range of motion, distance, reaction time, or performance measures to give insight into the integrity and function of the human body.

racism A belief that race is the primary determinant of human traits and capacities and that racial differences produce an inherent superiority of a particular race. As an action, racism is the act of discriminating against people of difference races or ethnic origins.

radial digital grasp An early grasp pattern in which an object is held distally (in the fingers rather than the palm) and the child grasps an object with the thumb, index and middle fingers.

raking A developmental grasp pattern that involves using all of the fingers in a raking motion to slide small objects into the palm to pick them up. This grasp does not persist in typically developing children beyond one year.

random error theories This group of theories (also called the *stochastic theories*) consists of theories based on random events occurring over time, and includes free radical generation, gradual wear and tear, mutation over time, and differences in metabolic rate.

reaction time Time delay between presentation of a stimulus and motor response to that stimulus.

Rebuilding Together This is the name of a nonprofit organization providing critical home repairs, modifications, and improvements for America's low-income homeowners.

receptive communication An individual's ability to receive and interpret verbal and/or nonverbal messages.

reference group Any group that individuals use as a standard for evaluating themselves and their own behavior.

reflex Stereotypic obligatory response to a given stimulus.

Rehabilitation Act of 1973 One of the first significant pieces of civil rights legislation for individuals with disabilities; Section 504 is often mentioned because it said that any program that received federal funding, such as public education and transportation, could not discriminate against people with disabilities. This act has been revised and amended several times since its 1973 passage.

rehabilitation services Health care services that help people keep, get back, or improve skills and functioning for daily living that have been lost or impaired because they were sick, hurt, or disabled. These services may include physical and occupational therapy, speech-language pathology, and psychiatric rehabilitation services in a variety of inpatient or outpatient settings.

reinforcement Consequence to an action that modifies the likelihood of the action being repeated.

religion The commitment or devotion to religious faith or observance.

reliability Stability of a test instrument or assessment tool. A reliable instrument is one that will yield similar scores when testing is repeated in a short time frame (test-retest) or is done by different examiners (inter-rater).

religiosity Attitudes and behaviors that connect individuals to specific organized faith practices.

resilience A concept that describes the emergence of a desired outcome despite periods of stress and change. The ability to weather each period of disruption and reintegration leaves the person better able to deal with the next change.

respiratory distress syndrome Condition caused by immaturity of the lungs, which results from an infant being born too soon; present in nearly all preterm infants; attributable to a lack of surfactant.

responsible stage Stage 3 described by Schaie, in which adults are mainly concerned with protecting and supporting, raising families, and building careers most typically experienced in early and middle adulthood.

restrained formal communication Form of communication characterized by governing one's emotions or passions and adhering to traditional standards of correctness without emotion content.

retinopathy of prematurity (ROP) Condition caused by abnormal vascularization of the eye and related to levels of oxygenation; can range from mild to severe, and in the most severe cases, infants with ROP are blind.

retirement community A residential development designed for older adults who are generally able to care for themselves. Typically these communities are age-restricted or age-qualified and the community offers shared services or amenities, such as meal preparation and maid services.

rheumatoid arthritis (RA) A chronic and systemic inflammatory disorder that may affect many tissues and organs, in addition to the joints. RA can be a disabling and painful condition, leading to loss of functioning and mobility.

righting reaction A category of transitional movement patterns that help individuals maintain a vertical alignment with respect to gravity during movement and position change.

risk factor Personal or environmental factor, as defined in the ICF (World Health Organization, 2002), that leaves the individual at risk or susceptible to injury, disease, impairment, or death.

risk reduction A concept in prevention science that involves reducing risk factors.

role strain The feeling of anxiety and tensions that arises when there is a conflict in the demands of roles, when individuals do not agree with the assessment of others concerning their performance in their role, or from accepting roles that are beyond their capacity.

romantic relationship A relationship between partners that is both emotionally and sexually oriented.

rooting reflex Elicited by perioral touch; is the vestige of early patterns allowing newborns of other species born with their eyes closed to seek out the maternal teat.

routine A prescribed, detailed sequence of actions to be followed regularly, that is customary to the individual.

rule of thirds Approach to aging proposed by Sloan in 1992; in this conception, aging is considered a combination of three things: (1) normal age-related changes plus, (2) the effects of disuse, and (3) the effects of age-related diseases. With this *rule of thirds*, an increased focus on fitness emerged that continues to be central to contemporary views on successful aging.

sandwich generation Term used to describe the role of middle-aged adults who are "sandwiched" between older and younger cohorts in the population. Additionally, this term serves to describe a middle-aged adult who is concurrently serving in a role of both parent to her own children and adult child of a parent.

sarcopenia An age-related decline in muscle mass and thereby muscle strength.

school readiness Mastering of prerequisite developmental criteria for success in the school environment; there are no agreed-upon criteria, but in general a child must be healthy both physically and emotionally.

screening process A brief general assessment used to identify impairments and to determine if further assessment is needed.

Sears, Robert Social learning theorist who combined a number of perspectives, including psychoanalytic and behavioral; he theorized that a child imitates the mother because this is reinforcing.

secondary prevention Efforts to reduce the duration, severity, and sequelae of an illness or a disability.

self-actualization Highest level in Maslow's hierarchy, defined as the need to become all one can be.

self-advocacy As presented by the disability rights movement, the term indicates that people with disabilities should be able and allowed to speak for themselves, rather than have experts or authority figures determine their fate.

self-assessed health Individuals' perception of their general well-being and quality of life.

self-concept The composite of ideas, feelings, and attitudes that the individual has about his or her own identity, worth, capabilities, and limitations.

self-determination A concept reflecting the belief that all individuals have the right to direct their own lives. Used in relation to the transition from high school to adult lifestyles, people who have self-determination skills have a stronger chance of being successful in employment, household management, and interpersonal relationships.

self-disclosure The act of revealing private information, such as the personal feelings of one person toward another.

self-efficacy Belief in one's personal power to change things, to organize and implement effective strategies to deal with potential situations that may be novel, unpredictable, or stressful.

self-management skills Methods, skills, and strategies by which individuals can effectively direct their own activities toward the achievement of objectives, and includes goal setting, decision making, focusing, planning, scheduling, task tracking, self-evaluation, and self-intervention.

self-regulation Individuals' capacity to alter their behaviors in accordance to some standards, ideals, or goals either stemming from internal or societal expectations.

self-representation A group's overall evaluation or appraisal of the worth of individuals within the group.

semantic memory The memory of concept and word meanings.

semantics A parameter of language that refers to meaning in context.

senescence The term used to describe the process of biological aging.

sensitive period An extended period of time during development when an individual is especially receptive to specific types of environmental stimuli, and therefore the individual more predisposed to learning.

sensitivity In assessment, such as screening, the ability to pick an individual with the target condition, such as developmental delay, out of the population, thereby avoiding false negatives. A highly sensitive instrument means individuals are not missed in identification.

sensorimotor praxis (motor planning) The ability of the brain to conceive, organize, and carry out a sequence of unfamiliar actions.

sensorineural hearing loss Hearing loss due to problems with the inner ear or end organ of hearing.

sensory modulation disorder (SMD) A subtype of sensory processing disorder in which individuals react in atypical ways to sensory input, often resulting in the perception of typically innocuous sensations as irritating, unpleasant, or painful.

sensory perceptual memory The first step in the process of memory that allows for the perceptual analysis that filters information deemed unimportant and moves forward information deemed as important.

sensory processing A complex set of neurobiologic functions that enable the brain to understand what is going on both inside the body and in all of the environmental contexts in which an individual engages.

service animals Working dogs trained to perform specific tasks relating to their owners' disability.

sexual interest A psychological experience that pertains to a person's desire to engage in sexual behavior. Sexual interest is distinct from sexual activity, the act of actually engaging in sexual behaviors.

sexual orientation An enduring pattern of attraction that may be emotional, romantic, sexual, or some combination of these to another person.

sexuality The state of being sexual, including not only the physical act but also the more complicated elements of emotion, physiologic drive, pregnancy, birth control, and sexually transmitted disease.

sheltered workshop A facility-based workplace that provides a supportive environment where physically or mentally challenged people can acquire job skills and vocational experience.

sick role A social role described by Talcott Parsons in 1959 in which a sick individual is exempt from normal social role responsibilities, such as going to work.

situated learning Learning that occurs through purposeful sensory experiences in the context that the learned behavior is needed.

skill Behavior acquired through learning.

Skinner, B. F. The best-known of the behaviorists; developed principles of reinforcement as ways to study and control behavior.

sleep functions Periods of reversible mental disengagement from one's immediate environment accompanied by characteristic physiologic changes.

sleep hygiene The habits, environmental factors, and practices that may influence the length and quality of one's sleep.

slow twitch (type I) muscles fibers Muscle fibers that are more efficient at using oxygen to generate more fuel for continuous, extended muscle contractions over a long time.

small for gestational age (SGA) Used to describe infants born at less than the 10th percentile for weight based on gestational age.

social age An approach to aging that is determined by habits, beliefs, and attitudes rather than the chronological passage of time. For example, a young adult may have had to take on the role of supporting a family while still in her teens, and may have struggled socially and economically, so that she has taken on the cautious, conservative behavior of a much older person.

social capital The presence (or absence) of some tangible resource that is valued within a social network, something that will afford the owner of the resource preferential treatment.

social cognitive theory Theory that people acquire skills and perform new behaviors by enacting them, being reinforced for performance, and observing others. This theory suggests that behavior influences, and is influenced by, personal and environmental factors.

social competence Smooth sequence of social skills applied in a dynamic way across various social contexts.

social knowledge The understanding of appropriate social behavior, including decoding and interpreting social cues, searching and selecting an optimal response, and undertaking the correct action.

social learning Acquisition of behaviors within a social context.

social model Model that sees society rather than the individual as the problem, viewing disability as a society-created problem.

social referencing Comparison of self to peers; often begins in the school-age child.

Social Security Disability Insurance (SSDI) A federal insurance program managed by the Social Security Administration. This program provides income supplements to people who are physically restricted in their ability to be employed because of a notable disability.

societal-level risk factors Risk factors such as teenage pregnancy and maternal drug and alcohol abuse.

solitary play Play behavior that typically emerges around 2 years of age when children are focused on an activity that they enjoy without including others in the play activity.

somatic awareness Information about the state of the body (touch, pressure, temperature, pain, etc.).

somatosensory General sensory input to the central nervous system from the body, typically touch and pressure.

somesthesia The faculty of bodily perception including information from all of the sensory systems associated with the body.

spatial awareness Understanding of both near and far space around an individual; assessed by the accuracy of locating items in that space.

Special Olympics International program dedicated to empowering children and adults with disabilities to become more physically fit, respected, and productive through sports training and competition.

special senses Those senses that are unique and supplied by cranial nerves, such as vision, hearing, and taste.

specific mental functions Functions of memory, language, and calculation; more easily quantified than the global functions and more often a focus of intervention following brain injury.

specificity In screening assessments, it is the ability to accurately separate the individual with the condition, such as developmental delay, from the population at large, avoiding false positive identification. A highly specific instrument means individuals are not told they have a problem when they actually do not.

speech Oral form of language.

speech disorders Speech sound disorders (phonology), voice disorders (voice generation), and fluency disorders (stuttering).

spirituality Belief in an inner path that gives meaning, purpose, and direction to life and life choices.

stability limit The farthest that an individual can shift his mass off center without altering his base of support.

standardized tests Measurement instruments in which the procedures used to collect the information and score performance are the same across examiners.

static postural stability Ability to maintain the preferred posture when the body is still; includes the ability to remain upright while sitting in a chair or to stand quietly when waiting in line without leaning against support or sitting.

static visual acuity Refers to the ability to discern details when both the person and the target are static; useful for reaching and grasping objects and the basic hand skills required in infancy and early in the preschool years; permits the development of eye-hand coordination.

statutory blindness (also called *legal blindness*) The person's best corrected visual acuity is 20/200 or less in the better eye, or a visual field limitation such that the widest diameter of the visual field, in the better eye, subtends an angle no greater than 20 degrees.

stereotypy Intrinsic nonpurposeful movement pattern that repeats itself.

stigma A social mark of disgrace associated with a particular circumstance, quality, or person.

stranger anxiety An innate mistrust or wariness of new or unfamiliar people.

stress Emotional state, generally considered to be unpleasant, that occurs when people are facing a demanding situation that is appraised by them as taxing or exceeding their resources and endangering their well-being.

stress hardiness A mindset exhibited by individuals that makes them resistant to the negative impacts of stressful circumstances and events.

striatal system Influences the planning and modulation of movement pathways, supports the executive function processes, and is activated by stimuli associated with reward and novel or intense stimuli (also known as the neostriatum or striate nucleus).

structured observation An assessment strategy that involves the staging of a movement pattern or behavior that the therapist needs to analyze, so that it can be observed carefully and repeated as needed until enough information has been gathered.

subculture A cultural subgroup differentiated in some way from the dominant cultural group.

substance abuse Overindulgence in and dependence on an addictive substance, especially alcohol or a narcotic drug; in pregnancy, the use of drugs and alcohol that can result in negative long-term effects for the infant.

subsyndromal depression A pattern of depressive symptoms that are not severe enough to meet the full diagnostic criteria for a depressive disorder.

successful aging models Emphasize the importance of adaptation and emotional well-being in successful aging. For most senior citizens, subjective quality of life is more important than the absence of disease and other objective measures relating to physical and mental health.

suck-swallow reflex The most basic of the neonatal motor behaviors that is associated with the intake of nourishment.

suckling Process of pressing the nipple or teat to the hard palate and using a process of positive pressure, or expression, to obtain milk.

superior pincer grasp Developmental grasp pattern using the distal tips of the thumb and forefinger for precision, with the ulnar fingers inhibited and the thumb in opposition.

Supplemental Security Income (SSI) A program that provides stipends to low-income people who are either aged (65 or older), blind, or disabled.

supported employment An approach to helping people with disabilities participate in the competitive labor market, helping them find meaningful jobs and providing ongoing support from a team of professionals.

sustainability The creation and maintenance of conditions under which humans and nature can exist in productive harmony.

symbolic communication Communication that involves a shared message between a sender and receiver.

symbolic play Symbolic (imaginative) play emerges late in the preschool period, as children gain language skills. Symbolic play is the ability of children to use objects, actions, or ideas to represent other objects, actions, or ideas as play. This type of play supports the development of children's abilities to express ideas, feelings, and experiences. This expression can be in any media including language, painting, drawing, music, and craft activities.

symmetrical tonic neck reflex (STNR) The STNR is a tonic reflex initiated by an infant's head position. When the head and neck are in extension, extensor tone increases in the upper trunk and limbs, with an increase in flexion in the lower limbs. Conversely, when the head and neck are in flexion, flexor tone increases in the upper trunk and limbs, with an increase in extension in the lower limbs.

synaptic pruning The process of preserving the most-used neurons, synapses, and dendrites while gradually eliminating synaptic connections that are not used.

synaptogenesis The building of specialized junctions at which a nerve cell communicates with a target cell.

syndromes In the context of birth defects, a pattern of multiple birth defects that occur together and have a similar cause.

syntax Rules governing word order in a language.

systemic family development model (SFD) A process-oriented model grounded in systems theory, this model recognizes that all families share a common process of development; however, within individual families there is variation in how this process manifests.

technology-dependent children Children who cannot survive without a medical technology such as mechanical ventilation or parenteral nutrition. These technology-dependent children are more medically unstable and in their follow-up care will require more frequent medical visits, hospital admissions, and they will place greater care demands on parents and other family members.

telehealth The use of electronic information and telecommunications technologies to support long-distance clinical health care.

temperament Collection of inborn differences among individuals that is closely associated with personality; the constitutional disposition of an individual to react in a particular way to situations.

temporal awareness Perception of time as it relates to the planning, sequencing, and altering of movement.

temporal discounting When people discount the potential long-range impacts of decisions, focusing instead on immediate rewards.

teratogen Agent that causes the production of physical defects in the developing embryo.

term infant The name used for a newborn infant that is born at 37 weeks or more in gestational age.

tertiary prevention Efforts including the rehabilitation, adaption, and accommodation that occur after an illness or injury to maintain and support optimal levels of function and participation.

Thomas, Alexander Theorist who, with Stella Chess, developed a classic system for describing and categorizing temperament.

thought functions Specific functions related to the presence and development of ideas that emphasize the control of thought in terms of pace, content, and form.

toddling Immature walking pattern characterized by rapidity, wide base of support, and limited rotary movement between shoulder and pelvis.

tolerable stress Difficulty coping caused by adverse life experiences that are more intense than those causing positive stress, but that are still relatively short-lived. Examples of tolerable stress would include death of a parent, a natural disaster, or a frightening accident.

tonic labyrinthine reflex Reflex that plays a role in mediating the gravity dependency of human newborns based on the position of the head (body) in space; when infants are prone, systemic flexion is facilitated, and when they are supine, systemic extension is facilitated, pulling them into gravity.

top-down assessment Assessment in which desired outcomes guide strategy.

torticollis Congenital damage to the sternocleidomastoid muscle in the neck that results in a shortening or excessive contraction of the muscle, resulting in both limited range of motion in both rotation and lateral neck bending.

toxic stress Stress that results from intense adverse experiences that may be sustained over a long period of time. This is the type of stress associated with child abuse or chronic neglect. In these situations, children are unable to effectively manage the stress, and the stress response system gets activated for a prolonged amount of time. Toxic stress can lead to permanent changes in the development of the brain.

transfer pattern Type of mobility pattern that allows individuals to transfer from one postural set to another, as from lying down to sitting.

transient developmental delay This type of delay is often seen in infants who had a difficult perinatal course, and it seems that the brain as well as other body systems take some time to recover.

transtheoretical model This model developed by Prochaska is widely used for a variety of health behaviors (Prochaska et al., 1994). It is an integrative, biopsychosocial model to conceptualize the process of intentional behavioral change.

Trauma-Informed Pediatric Care A strategy in pediatric and infant care that involves incorporating an understanding of the impact of traumatic stress on ill or injured children and families while treating the medical aspects of trauma.

traumatic brain injury (TBI) A nondegenerative, noncongenital injury to the brain from an external mechanical force, possibly leading to permanent or temporary impairment of cognitive, physical, and psychosocial functions, with an associated diminished or altered state of consciousness.

treatment theory A medical approach to health and illness that specifies the mechanism by which a proposed treatment changes its immediate treatment target—referred to here as the treatment object.

trimester system System in which the human gestational period is divided into periods of three months, each being one-third of the length of a pregnancy.

trophoblast In the first week of pregnancy, the outer layer of the blastocyst that will give rise to the placenta and other tissues.

type 2 diabetes A disease that results from insulin resistance, a condition in which cells fail to use insulin properly, sometimes combined with an absolute insulin deficiency. This form was previously referred to as non-insulin-dependent diabetes mellitus (NIDDM) or "adult-onset diabetes."

uncertainty in illness theory (UIT) Developed by Merle Mishel in 1988, the UIT explains how uncertainty develops in patients with an acute illness and how patients deal with this uncertainty.

United Nations Convention on the Rights of Persons with Disabilities In 2006, the United Nations promulgated this international treaty as a call to action for all UN members to commit to respect and support of the rights and dignity of people with disabilities.

universal design Designing the physical environment, as in the personal home, in such a manner as to be accessible to people of all ages and various levels of physical abilities.

unoccupied play The earliest, least mature class of play in which children are not actively playing; they may be observing, or even standing in one spot or performing random movements.

use-dependent brain plasticity The capacity of the brain to remodel itself based on the activity patterns and environmental demands on individuals. Use-dependent brain plasticity plays a major role in the recovery of function after injury to the brain and helps explain patterns of cognitive changes associated with aging.

useful field of view (UFOV) The visual area over which information can be extracted at a brief glance without eye or head movements. In most people, the size of the UFOV decreases with age, reflecting reduced attentional resources, and less ability to ignore distracting information.

Vaillant, George A physician and scientist interested in successful aging and in human happiness. He wrote the book *Aging Well,* which has been very influential in the study of healthy aging.

validity In test instruments or assessment tools, it means that an instrument measures what it is supposed to measure, therefore accurately representing the performance of an individual being tested.

values Broad preferences concerning appropriate courses of action or outcomes.

vascular dementia A general term describing cognitive problems that are caused by brain damage from impaired blood flow to the brain.

vascularization Growth of blood vessels into a tissue or organ, with the result that the oxygen and nutrient supply is improved.

ventricular septal defect An abnormal opening between the left and right ventricles.

very low birth weight infants Infants weighing 1500 g or less.

Vygotsky, Lev Russian theorist who studied cognitive development with an emphasis on sociocultural influence.

virtual (digital) play Intrinsically motivated activity using an electronic device such as television, video game, or computer for the purpose of enjoyment.

virtual environment Computer or other technology-driven social network of real and virtual human interaction at a communal or larger group level that operates for reasons of tradition, culture, business, pleasure, information exchange, institutional organization, legal procedure, governance, human betterment, social progress, spiritual enlightenment, among other reasons.

visitability A movement to change construction practices so that virtually all new buildings, whether or not designated for residents who currently have mobility impairments, offer at least one zero-step entrance on an accessible route leading from a driveway or public sidewalk, interior doors providing at least $31\frac{3}{4}$ inches (81 cm) of unobstructed passage space, and toilet facilities on the main floor.

visual accommodation The process during which the eye adjusts its focus, whether to near or far objects, in order to gain visual clarity.

visual discrimination Ability to discriminate visual details, the perception of depth, spatial relations, and directional orientation.

visual disorder Abnormality of the eye, the optic nerve, the optic tracts, or the brain that may cause a loss of visual acuity or visual fields.

visual scanning Short, rapid changes of fixation from one point in the visual field to another, also known as saccadic eye movement.

vocation A "calling," or "life's work"; the term is typically used in describing the affective attachment one has to a career.

voice Voice is the sound made as air from our lungs is pushed through our larynx which is a product of anatomy, respiratory pattern and learning. In the context of alternative and augmentative forms of communication, it is the audible output of electronic communication devices reflecting and individuals efforts at communication.

Watson, John First American behaviorist; he viewed the stimulus-response relationship as the essential one between organism and environment.

welfare A term used to describe those government programs that provide benefits and economic assistance to no- or low-income Americans.

wellness Triangulated concept including physical, psychosocial, and spiritual health and well-being.

white coat syndrome A fear or increased level of stress when dealing with doctors and others (wearing white coats) in health care settings.

work Meaningful activity that helps us define our position in society, is an outlet for creativity, is a source of social stimulation, and provides fulfillment.

work-life balance How you spend your time working and relaxing, recognizing that what you do in one fuels your energy for the other.

working memory The type of human memory in which past events are associated with present events.

World Report on Disability A report developed in response to the UN *Convention on the Rights of Persons with Disabilities* and offers a call to action identifying barriers to participation for people with disabilities.

zone of proximal development (ZPD) From Vygotsky's theory, refers to the child's preparedness to learn such that minimal support from the environment will result in learning.

Index

Note: figures are indicated by "*f*" and tables by "*t*".

M

T